Yves Pommier
Editor

DNA Topoisomerases and Cancer

Humana Press

Editor
Yves Pommier
Laboratory of Molecular Pharmacology
Center for Cancer Research
National Cancer Institute, National Institutes of Health
Bethesda, MD, USA
pommier@nih.gov

ISBN 978-1-4614-0322-7 e-ISBN 978-1-4614-0323-4
DOI 10.1007/978-1-4614-0323-4
Springer New York Dordrecht Heidelberg London

Library of Congress Control Number: 2011937449

Printed on acid-free paper

Humana Press is part of Springer Science+Business Media (www.springer.com)

Preface

This book brings together a unique collection of chapters that provide detailed information on human topoisomerases. It covers current knowledge on human DNA topoisomerases, their targeting by anticancer drugs and carcinogenic lesions, the clinical use of topoisomerase inhibitors and the various pathways and cellular responses involved in the repair of topoisomerase-mediated DNA damage.

Contributors to this book are world class scientists who have made key discoveries in the field. I wish to thank them for their time, enthusiasm and for making this book a collection of complementary articles covering the topoisomerase field both from basic biology and therapeutic viewpoints.

I dedicate this book to Dr. Kurt W. Kohn who in 1979 suggested that a topoisomerase should be the target of anticancer drugs. Kurt Kohn inspired me to work on DNA topoisomerases starting in 1981 and has remained a precious collaborator ever since.

Bethesda, MD   Yves Pommier

Contents

Contributors

Mounira Amor-Guéret Institut Curie, Centre de Recherche, Centre Universitaire Orsay, France

Céline Auzanneau INSERM U916 VINCO, Institut Bergonié & University of Bordeaux, Bordeaux cedex, France

Karim Bahmed Molecular Pharmacology Department, St. Jude Children's Research Hospital, Memphis, TN, USA

Laura Baranello "G. Moruzzi" Department of Biochemistry, University of Bologna, Bologna, Italy

Piero Benedetti Department of Biology, University of Padova, Padua, Italy

James M. Berger Department of Molecular and Cell Biology, QB3 Institute, University of California at Berkeley, Berkeley, CA, USA

Jeffrey Berk Molecular Pharmacology Department, St. Jude Children's Research Hospital, Memphis, TN, USA

Davide Bertozzi "G. Moruzzi" Department of Biochemistry, University of Bologna, Bologna, Italy

Mary-Ann Bjornsti Department of Pharmacology and Toxicology, University of Alabama at Birmingham, Birmingham, AL, USA

Giovanni Capranico "G. Moruzzi" Department of Biochemistry, University of Bologna, Bologna, Italy

James J. Champoux Department of Microbiology, School of Medicine, University of Washington, Seattle, WA, USA

Stefanie Hartman Chen Department of Biochemistry, Duke University Medical Center, Durham, NC, USA

William Dahut Center for Cancer Research, National Cancer Institute, National Institutes of Health, Bethesda, MD, USA

Benu Brata Das Laboratory of Molecular Pharmacology, Center for Cancer Research, National Cancer Institute, National Institutes of Health, Bethesda, MD, USA

Shyamal D. Desai Department of Biochemistry and Molecular Biology, LSU Health Sciences Center-School of Medicine, New Orleans, LA, USA

Thomas S. Dexheimer National Chemical Genomic Center, National Institutes of Health, Rockville, MD, USA

Patrick Forterre Institut de Génétique et Microbiologie, Univ Paris-Sud, 91405, Orsay Cedex, France

CNRS UMR 8621, and Institut Pasteur, 25 rue du Docteur Roux, 75015, Paris, France

Takahisa Furuta Center for Clinical Research, Hamamatsu University School of Medicine, Hamamatsu, Japan

Stefan Gajewski Institut für Molekulare Biowissenschaften, Karl Franzens Universität, Humboldtstrasse, Graz, Austria

Department of Structural Biology, St Jude Children's Research Hospital, 262 Danny Thomas Place, Memphis, Tennessee, USA

Giuseppe Giaccone Medical Oncology Branch, National Cancer Institute, Bethesda, MD, USA

François Goldwasser Department of Clinical Oncology, Hopital Cochin, Paris, France

Christopher Heery Center for Cancer Research, National Cancer Institute, National Institutes of Health, Bethesda, MD, USA

Tao-shih Hsieh Department of Biochemistry, Duke University Medical Center, Durham, NC, USA

Shar-yin N. Huang Laboratory of Molecular Pharmacology, Center for Cancer Research, National Cancer Institute, National Institutes of Health, Bethesda, MD, USA

Yan Makeyev New York University Langone Medical Center, New York, NY, USA

Christophe Marchand Laboratory of Molecular Pharmacology, Center for Cancer Research, National Cancer Institute, National Institutes of Health, Bethesda, MD, USA

Jessica Marinello "G. Moruzzi" Department of Biochemistry, University of Bologna, Bologna, Italy

Olivier Mir Department of Clinical Oncology, Hopital Cochin, Paris, France

Margarita Mishina Molecular Pharmacology Department, St. Jude Children's Research Hospital, Memphis, TN, USA

Franco Muggia New York University Langone Medical Center, New York University, NY, USA

John L. Nitiss Department of Biopharmaceutical Sciences, University of Illinois College of Pharmacy, IL, Chicago

Karin C. Nitiss Molecular Pharmacology Department, St. Jude Children's Research Hospital, Memphis, TN, USA

Neil Osheroff Departments of Biochemistry and Medicine (Hematology/Oncology), School of Medicine, Vanderbilt University, Nashville, TN, USA

Yves Pommier Laboratory of Molecular Pharmacology, Center for Cancer Research, National Cancer Institute, National Institutes of Health, Bethesda, MD, USA

Philippe Pourquier INSERM U916 VINCO, Institut Bergonié & University of Bordeaux, Bordeaux cedex, France

Arun Rajan Medical Oncology Branch, National Cancer Institute, Bethesda, MD, USA

Jean-François Riou Régulation et Dynamique des Génomes, INSERM U565, Muséum National d'Histoire Naturelle, Paris, Cedex, France

Anna Rogojina Molecular Pharmacology Department, St. Jude Children's Research Hospital, Memphis, TN, USA

Philippe Rougier University of Versailles, Ambroise Paré Hospital, Paris, France

Ilaria Dalla Rosa Laboratory of Molecular Pharmacology, Center for Cancer Research, National Cancer Institute, National Institutes of Health, Bethesda, MD, USA

Aman Seth Molecular Pharmacology Department, St. Jude Children's Research Hospital, Memphis, TN, USA

Eroica Soans Molecular Pharmacology Department, St. Jude Children's Research Hospital, Memphis, TN, USA

Stéphanie Solier Laboratory of Molecular Pharmacology, Center for Cancer Research, National Cancer Institute, National Institutes of Health, Bethesda, MD, USA

Olivier Sordet Cancer Research Center of Toulouse, INSERM-Université de Toulouse, Institut Claudius Regaud, Toulouse Cedex, France

Beverly A. Teicher Developmental Therapeutics Program, National Cancer Institute, Rockville, MD, USA

Jianhong Wu Department of Biochemistry, Duke University Medical Center, Durham, NC, USA

Hongliang Zhang Laboratory of Molecular Pharmacology, Center for Cancer Research, National Cancer Institute, National Institutes of Health, Bethesda, MD, USA

Chapter 1
Introduction and Historical Perspective

Patrick Forterre

1.1 Introduction

The discoveries of DNA supercoiling and DNA topoisomerases by Jerome Vinograd and James Wang, respectively, have been two of the most important breakthrough in biology during the second part of the last century (Vinograd et al. 1965; Wang 1971). Unfortunately, these discoveries have not received the credit they merit outside of the community of scientists interested in the DNA structure and DNA biological roles. The fact that James Wang has not (yet) been rewarded by the Nobel Prize is astonishing, considering the importance of DNA topoisomerases in both fundamental chemistry and medicine (as testified by this book). More generally, the study of DNA topology and DNA topoisomerases is not given appropriate credit in life science and these topics are still missing from too many biological degree courses at universities. To play down the importance of DNA topology is highly damaging for someone whose aim is to understand how modern living organisms thrive on our planet. DNA topoisomerases are major elements in cellular life and the plethora of natural antibiotics and antitumor drugs that target DNA topoisomerases testify for their importance. By chance for DNA topologists, DNA topoisomerases are not only fascinating examples of the creative power of natural selection, but also extremely important tools for clinical therapy. The study of DNA topoisomerases and DNA topology is therefore one of these blessed fields in which it's possible to follow your fatal attraction for academic science while working with the prospect of gaining useful insights in societal issues.

P. Forterre (✉)
Institut de Génétique et Microbiologie, Univ Paris-Sud, 91405 Orsay Cedex, France

CNRS UMR 8621, and Institut Pasteur,
25 rue du Docteur Roux, 75015, Paris, France
e-mail: forterre@pasteur.fr

Y. Pommier (ed.), *DNA Topoisomerases and Cancer*, Cancer Drug Discovery and Development, DOI 10.1007/978-1-4614-0323-4_1,

The field of DNA topology and DNA topoisomerases has been recently extremely well covered (including the historical dimension) in the James Wang book "*untangling the double helix*" (Wang 2009a, see also Wang 2009b). In this chapter, I will also follow an historical presentation of the discovery of DNA topoisomerases to help the readers become familiar with the diversity of these enzymes and their various personalities. As in many other fields of biology, the studies of DNA topology and topoisomerases has been entangled for a long time with prejudices born from the focus of most biologists on a few number of model organisms. We are still misled by the division of the living world between "prokaryotes" and "eukaryotes" (Pace 2006). Early molecular biologists thought that the molecular world was relatively simple and that "*Anything that is true of E. coli must be true for elephants*" (an answer to a question to Monod that followed a lecture he gave in 1954). This turned out to be wrong, except for the big picture (the genetic code and the basic principles of information processing). As a rule, Eukarya and Bacteria are equipped with quite different sets of enzymes (sometimes not even homologous) to perform similar functions. This rule is especially valid for enzymes involved in various DNA transactions. The first DNA polymerase discovered by Arthur Kornberg in *E. coli* in 1956 is unrelated to major eukaryotic DNA polymerases discovered years later. Similarly, the first DNA topoisomerase discovered by James Wang, the *E. coli* ω proteins, is specific for bacteria.

Enzymes involved in DNA manipulation are surprisingly diverse, and the world of DNA topoisomerases is not an exception. This is well illustrated by the odd nomenclatures of these enzymes that combine historical numerology (Topo I, II, III, IV, V, VI), mechanistic distinction (type I, type II, type IA, type IB) and evolutionary classification (Topo IA, Topo IB, Topo IC, Topo IIA, Topo IIB) (Forterre and Gadelle 2009). It is difficult for the newcomers in front of this conundrum to enter the fields of DNA topoisomerases without some hesitations. We hope that the historical presentation in that chapter will help the reader to understand the logic of the various topoisomerases names and to become progressively familiar with their connections.

Testifying for the surprise of biochemists confronted with the unexpected high number of new DNA topoisomerases discovered between 1980 and 1990, James Wang wrote in 1991 a review untitled, "*DNA topoisomerases, why so many?*" (Wang 1991). The diversity of DNA topoisomerases reflects in fact both their various functions and the diversity of the living world itself. Not only *E. coli* and elephants are quite divergent from each other in term of molecular biology, but they are not even the only two types of organisms present on our planet. This was revealed by the revolution in our vision of the living world brought at the end of the seventies by the work of Carl Woese and his colleagues. These authors demonstrated in 1977 that the modern living world is fundamentally divided into three distinct evolutionary cell lineages: Archaea (formerly archaebacteria), Bacteria (formerly eubacteria), and Eukarya (formerly eukaryotes) (Woese and Fox 1977; Woese et al. 1990), making the eukaryote/prokaryote dichotomy obsolete (Pace 2006).

Table 1.1 Historical discoveries of the major families and superfamilies of DNA topoisomerases

1970	Protein ω	*Escherichia coli* (b)	Wang (1971)
1971	Swivelase	*Mus musculus* (e)	Champoux and Dulbecco (1971)
1976	DNA gyrase	*Escherichia coli* (b)	Gellert et al. (1976)
1979	T4 Topo II	*Escherichia coli* (bT4)	Liu et al. (1979)
1980	Topo II (e)	*Xaenopus levis* (e)	Baldi et al. (1980)
1984	Reverse gyrase	*Sulfolobus acidocaldarius* (a)	Kikuchi and Asai (1984)
1984	Topo III (b)	*Escherichia coli* (b)	Srivenugopal et al. (1984)
1989	Topo III (e)	*Saccharomyces cerevisiae* (e)	Wallis et al. (1989)
1990	Topo IV	*Escherichia coli* (b)	Kato et al. (1990)
1993	Topo V	*Methanopyrus kandleri* (a)	Slesarev et al. (1993)
1997	Topo VI	*Sulfolobus shibatae* (a)	Bergerat et al. (1997)

Archaea have been "*hidden before our eyes*" for a long time, because they look like bacteria under the microscope. However, molecular studies demonstrated without doubt that they are clearly distinct from the two other domains (for a brief presentation of Archaea to unfamiliar molecular biologists, see Forterre and Gadelle 2009). Archaea turned out to be a goldmine for DNA topologists. As soon as they were scrutinized for their DNA topoisomerases, molecular biologists discovered in these fascinating microbes a specific set of DNA topoisomerases with unique properties. Hence, whereas DNA topoisomerases I, II, III, and IV, were isolated from *E. coli* (numbered by the order of the proteins discoveries in this model organism), DNA topoisomerases V and VI were isolated from two distinct archaea, *Methanopyrus kandleri* and *Sulfolobus shibatae*, respectively (Slesarev et al. 1993; Bergerat et al. 1997) (Table 1.1). The discovery that intracellular DNA is not supercoiled in archaea that lack DNA gyrase (Charbonnier and Forterre 1994) also has great significance. It teaches us that global negative supercoiling is not the "normal" state of cellular DNA, but a unique characteristic of organisms harboring a DNA gyrase. The ubiquity of this fascinating enzyme in the domain Bacteria reminds us that bacteria are not primitive organisms, but rather sophisticated bugs with unique molecular devices that allowed them to be the most abundant organisms in the biosphere.

The comparative study of DNA topoisomerases in the three domains of life has raised unexpected evolutionary problems. Indeed, whereas most proteins involved in information processes can be nicely segregated in three distinct versions, each of them corresponding to one of the three domains, this is not the case for DNA topoisomerases (Forterre and Gadelle 2009). It's a challenge now to make sense of the diversity of these enzymes and to propose new hypotheses on their origin and evolution based on phylogenomic analyses. I will not shy to go in that direction at the end of this chapter, with the hope to attract more scientists into current discussions on these exciting evolutionary issues.

1.2 The Topological Problem and the Discovery of DNA Supercoiling

1.2.1 The Double Helix: Beautiful but Challenging

The DNA structure model proposed by Watson and Crick in 1953 was immediately endorsed by many biologists since it solves elegantly, at once, the problem of the nature of genetic information and the mechanism for the transmission of this information from one generation to the other (Watson and Crick 1953a). The beauty of the double helical structure has always fascinated human minds and the double helix is now one of the icons of modern science. However, the helical nature of the molecule was by no means related to the nature of DNA as genetic material, but a consequence of the stereochemistry of the chemical bonds that link the various atoms of the molecule. The double helical structure was gorgeous, but Watson and Crick immediately realized that it also raised a critical problem for the biological function of DNA. They wrote in their 1953 Cold Spring Harbor paper, "*As in our model the two chains are wrapped around each others, it is essential that they could be unwound to be separated...although it is difficult at the moment to see how these processes occur without everything getting tangle, we do not feel that this objection will be insuperable*" (Watson and Crick 1953b). Others were less optimistic and Max Delbrück wrote in a letter to Watson the same year, "*I am willing to bet that the plectonemic coiling of the chains in your structure is radically wrong.*" These scientists thus immediately realized that the double helical DNA structure has introduced a new problem in modern biology: How to separate, thus unwound, the two strands of the helix in the course of processes such as DNA replication. This seemed a daunting task, especially considering the incredible length of the molecule and its extreme packaging inside cells.

The problem became even worse when John Cairns demonstrated 10 years later the circular nature of the bacterial chromosome (Cairns 1963a). In a circular molecule, the two DNA strands form continuous curves that are entangled by topological links. Such links cannot be removed unless the continuity of at least one of the two strands is broken somewhere to let the other strand pass across. This is exemplified by what occurs when a covalently closed circular DNA is denatured by alkaline treatment (Vinograd and Lebowitz 1966). The two strands remain wrapped around each other into a random coiled structure (Fig. 1.1). In that structure, the previous turns of the double helix have been transformed into pure topological links. The geometry of the system has been dramatically changed, but the number of topological links (dubbed the Linking number, Lk) remains the same before and after denaturation. For that reason, the Lk is called a topological invariant. The Watson and Crick model thus introduced a mathematician problem at the heart of the cellular information processing mechanism. To understand the magnitude of this problem, let us consider what's happens when a bacterial chromosome of 4 Mb is replicated. Since one turn of the double helix corresponds roughly to 10.5 bp, it means that about 390,000 topological links should be eliminated in the process of replication (which means

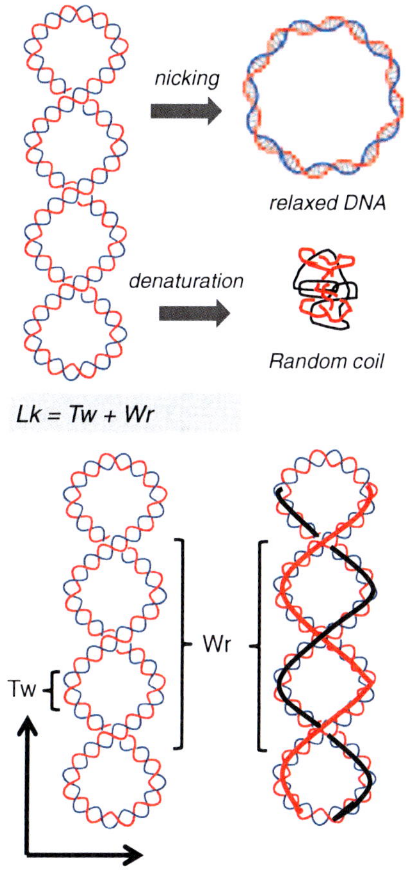

Fig. 1.1 Basic topological tenets (see the text for explanation)

about 30 links per second if the chromosome is replicated in 20 min, as in the case of some bacteria). What is the mechanism responsible for this Herculean task? This formidable and challenging question became "THE" topological problem associated to DNA replication. To solve this problem on paper, Cairns predicted the existence of a specific chromosomal structure, a swivel, allowing the free rotation of one DNA strand around the other (Cairns 1963b), but the chemical and/or physical nature of this swivel was a big question mark.

1.2.2 Small Circles and the Magic Equation

Whereas the first discussions on DNA topology in the fifties and early sixties were purely theoretical, DNA topology became an experimental science in the late sixties through the work of molecular biologists who were studying viral DNA structure.

These workers did not solve the topological problem but, unexpectedly, brought to light another one, the role and origin of intracellular DNA supercoiling. This story is worth to be reminded (Lebowitz 1990). In early sixties, several research teams have started to investigate small DNA viruses known to induce tumor in model mammals, such as polyoma viruses or SV40. They soon discovered that the genomes of these viruses were circular double-stranded DNA, like bacterial ones (Weil and Vinograd 1963). In 1965, Vinograd and his collaborators, while analyzing polyoma virus DNA by ultracentrifugation on sucrose gradients, noticed the existence of two forms with different sedimentation coefficients, a major form (form I) that migrated rapidly, and a minor form (form II) that migrated slowly (Vinograd et al. 1965). They thought first that one of these forms was circular and the other linear (broken DNA). However, upon examination by electron microscopy, it turned out that both forms were circular. Careful examination of the images led the authors to notice that form I DNA was characterized by multiple crossovers. From this observation, Vinograd and his colleagues hypothesized that this DNA was supercoiled, i.e., that the double helix winds around itself to produce a super-helix.

This was a great time when, in a few years, the DNA supercoiling theory was elaborated, first by biologists alone, and later on in collaboration with mathematicians. Amazingly, the famous equation relating the Linking number (Lk) of two closed curves to the twist (Tw) and writhe (Wr) of their axis (Lk = Tw + Wr) was first empirically proposed by biologists (Vinograd and Lebowitz 1966) before being demonstrated by mathematicians a few years later (Fuller 1971). In this equation, whereas the Linking number is a topological invariant, Tw and Wr are geometrical parameters that depend on the physical environment of the DNA molecule (temperature, ionic strength, ligands). The twist and writhe formally described the path of two interlinked closed circular curves in the three dimensional space. For most biologists, it is more intuitive to think in term of turns and superturns, as Vinograd and Lebowitz did when they proposed the equation $\alpha = \beta + \tau$, in which α (the linking number) was called the topological winding number, β the turn number, and τ the superturn number. However, the twist and writhe are only equivalent to the number of turns (β) and superturns (τ), if the DNA molecule is constraint in two dimensions (Fig. 1.1). Nevertheless, once assumed, the Vinograd and Lebowitz version of the topological equation is still useful for biologists, because the number of turns and superturns can be easily determined experimentally. The turn number corresponds to the DNA length (in base pairs) divided by the length of the helical path (roughly 10.4 bp in physiological conditions), whereas the superturn number can be obtained from agarose gel electrophoresis (see below). Figure 1.2 depicts a small exercise that could help to understand why the formation of a superturn introduces a link in a circular DNA duplex.

1.2.3 Negative Supercoiling; The Natural Form of DNA?

The equation Lk = Tw + Wr predicts the existence of either positive or negative superturns (Fig. 1.3). In a relaxed DNA, Lk = Tw. If the superhelix winds in the same direction as the double-helix itself, the superturns are positive (Wr > 0) because the

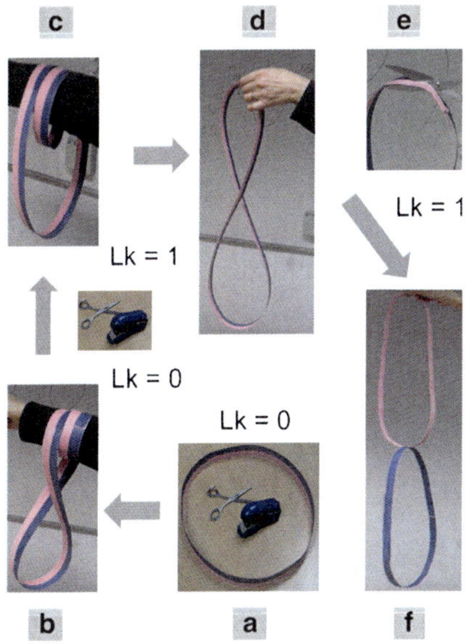

Fig. 1.2 Home-made exercise to illustrate several concepts in DNA topology. (**a**) The material you need a nuclease (scissor), a ligase (stapler) and a relaxed circular DNA (semi-rigid ribbon paper). For simplicity, the two DNA stands (*pink and blue*) are not intertwisted but lye side by side (Lk = 0 since Tw = 0); (**b**) wrapping the DNA circle around your arm introduces a toroidal superturn around your arm (either positive or negative, depending of the sense of your wrapping) and a compensatory plectonemic superturn in the free part of the circle to maintain the Lk constant; (**c**) a topoisomerase activity (scissor plus stapler) has relaxed the free DNA, introducing a modification of Lk by one unit; (**d**) removing DNA from your arm transforms the toroidal superturn into a plectonemic superturn; (**e**) use a helicase (a scissor again) to separate the two DNA strands; (**f**) once completely separated the two strands are still physically linked, showing that the plectonemic supercoiling in D indeed corresponds to a topological link between the two edges of the ribbon (or the two DNA strands for the demonstration)

double-helix turns are themselves positive per definition, the DNA then exhibit an excess of topological link compared to a relaxed DNA of the same size (Lk > Tw). On the contrary, if the super-helix winds in the opposite direction, the superturns are negative (Wr < 0) and the DNA exhibits a linking deficit (Lk < Tw). In both cases, the supercoiling of the DNA molecule is explained by the impossibility to adjust the twist to the value of the Lk. Indeed, the twist can only fluctuate in a narrow range because of the rigidity of the double helical structure. The stress induced either by Lk excess or deficit is actually compensated by modification in both the twist and the writhing of the molecule. This topological stress, ΔLk, corresponds to the difference between the Lk of the DNA molecule and the (theoretical) Lk (Lko) that would allow the same molecule to be relaxed. The topological stress is thus distributed between the twist and writhing of the molecule (ΔLk = Lk − Lko = ΔTw + ΔWr).

By playing with the equation Lk = Tw + Wr, it is very easy to understand the effect of drugs or physical parameters (temperature, ionic strength) on DNA topology. For instance, addition of ethidium bromide (EtBr) or increasing temperature, that both unwind the double-helix, reduce the number of turns in a DNA molecule of finite

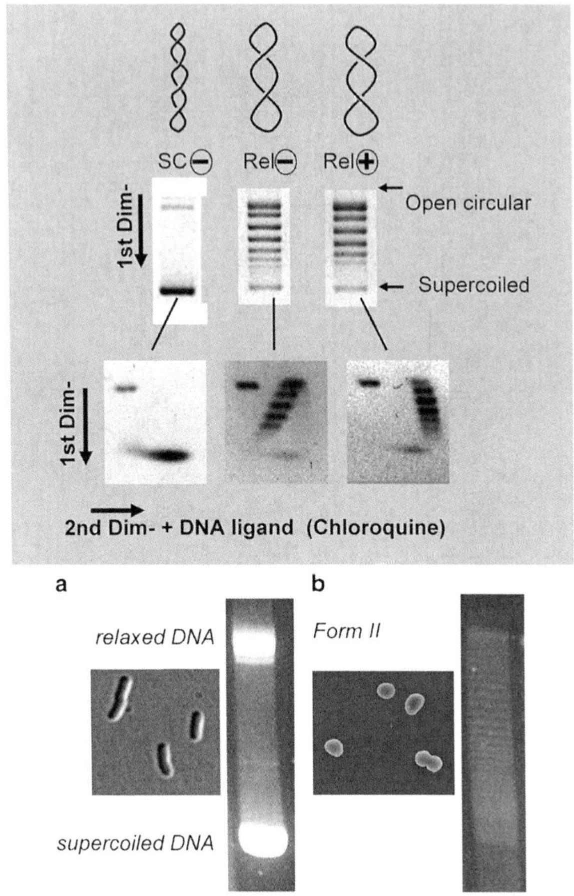

Fig. 1.3 Positively and negatively supercoiled DNA. *Upper panel*: Topoisomers with Lk varying by one unit can be separated in a one dimensional agarose gel, whereas positively and negatively supercoiled topoisomers with the same number of superturns can be discriminated by two dimensional gel electrophoresis. The migration in the second dimension in presence of a DNA intercalator decreases the number of turns, introducing positive superturns to maintain the Lk constant (Lk = Tw + Wr). This reduces the number of absolute superturns in a negatively supercoiled DNA that migrates more slowly (*left arch*) and increases the number of absolute superturns in a positively supercoiled DNA that migrates more rapidly (*right arch*). *Lower panel*: The archaeal/bacterial shuttle plasmid pCL70 is negatively supercoiled when isolated from the bacterium *E. coli* (**a**), whereas its exhibit a broad distribution of partially relaxed topoisomers (**b**) when isolated from the archaeon *Thermococcus kodakaraensis* (M. Gaudin and P. Forterre, unpublished data)

length, and thus increase the number of superturns, such that Lk remains constant. In both cases, this induces positive supercoiling. Conversely, decreasing the number of turns by increasing the ionic strength (screening the repulsive negative charges of the DNA backbone) or by adding drugs, such as netropsin, that binds the DNA minor groove and overwound the double helix, induce negative supercoiling.

The possibility to manipulate DNA topology using EtBr allowed Vinograd and his colleagues to discover that small circular double-stranded DNA isolated from either eukaryotes (viral genomes) or bacteria (plasmids) are negatively supercoiled (Radloff et al. 1967; Roth and Helinski 1967; Vinograd et al. 1968). The same turned out to be true for the bacterial chromosome when Karl Drlica succeeded to isolate the intact bacterial "nucleoids" (a *tour de force* realized in the seventies and rarely repeated from that time) (Drlica and Worcel 1975). Interestingly, the level of supercoiling turned out to be similar in "eukaryotic" and "prokaryotic" covalently closed circular DNA, about one superturn for about 180 base pair (or else 17 helical turns). This corresponds to a supercoiling density (originally defined as the number of superturns divided by the linking number, $\sigma = \tau/\alpha$) of about – 0.06. The supercoiling density (a measure of the stress induced in the DNA molecule by the supercoiling) is now defined as the "*specific linking difference*" $\alpha = \Delta Lk/Lk_{o.}$

Some scientists originally believed that DNA supercoiling observed in vitro was an "artefact" of the DNA isolation procedure, i.e., that negative supercoiling was induced by the differences between the physical environment of DNA in cells and test tubes (differences in ionic strength and/or in association with other molecules). However, other soon realized that negative supercoiling could have biological relevance, since it favors unwinding of the double helix. Indeed, a negatively supercoiled DNA corresponding to a Lk deficit, local melting of such DNA reduces this deficit (lowering the turn number) producing a slight relaxation of the molecule. This process is energetically favorable, supercoiling being correlated to an energetic stress ($\sigma = \Delta Lk/Lk_O$). Negative supercoiling of DNA thus would a priori facilitate all processes that require transient DNA unwinding such as activation of replication origins, opening of some promoters, or else initiation of various recombination or repair mechanisms.

Amazingly, despite the potential interest of negative DNA supercoiling as an "active form" of DNA, the supercoiling observed in vitro turned out to be indeed an artefact of isolation procedure in the case of eukaryotic DNA. This DNA is indeed mostly relaxed in the cell, when it is organized into nucleosome-like structure. It only became negatively supercoiled after the removal of histones. The wrapping of DNA around histones in the nucleosome corresponds to a "toroidal" supercoiling (Fig. 1.2c). When histones are removed, toroidal supercoiling is transformed into "plectonemic" supercoiling (Fig. 1.2d), the type of supercoiling first observed by Vinograd and colleagues in naked DNA. Once biochemists realized that negative supercoiling in eukaryotes originate from the nucleosome structure (Germond et al. 1975), a main question became: What is the source of negative supercoiling in "prokaryotes" that lack histone? Could it be that DNA is also organized in nucleosome-like structures in bacteria, but more labile and difficult to characterize, Griffith (1976).

In any case, the discovery of negative supercoiling in natural DNA did not solve the topological problem that was still as mysterious as before at the beginning of the seventies. The two different aspects of DNA topology that remained challenging at that time, the DNA replication topological problem and the origin of negative supercoiling in bacteria, were finally solved together in the seventies when scientists discovered that a same class of enzymes, DNA topoisomerases, were responsible for both the resolution of topological problems and the introduction of negative superturns into bacterial DNA.

1.3 The Discovery of DNA Topoisomerases

1.3.1 The Protein ω and Swivelase

The first DNA topoisomerase was discovered in 1971 in *Escherichia coli* by James Wang who was studying the supercoiling of *E. coli* DNA (Wang 1971). The relaxing activity of this new type of enzyme was discovered serendipitously, in measuring the superhelicity of negatively supercoiled plasmids in crude extract (for an historical account, see Wang 2009b). The protein responsible for the relaxing activity was purified and turned out to be a monomer of around 100 kDa, combining nuclease and ligase activities in a single polypeptide. This bacterial protein was initially named omega, referring the parameter of angular velocity, because its activity was tested using ultracentrifugation (Wang 1971). Although the discovery of the ω protein was a breakthrough, it was at the same time frustrating. Indeed, the ω protein could not be the swivel predicted by John Cairns because it was only able to relax negatively supercoiled DNA, whereas unwinding of the parental strands for DNA replication (reducing the number of turns) produces positive supercoiling (refer to the equation). However, a *bona fide* swivelase, relaxing both negatively and positively supercoiled DNA, was discovered soon after by Champoux in extracts of nuclei from mouse-embryo cells (Champoux and Dulbecco 1972). So for some time, the topological problem seems to be resolved in eukaryotes, but not in prokaryotes.

Studies performed with the *E. coli* ω proteins and the eukaryotic "swivelase" (or untwisting enzyme) laid the foundation for our understanding of the mechanism of action of enzymes later to be called topoisomerase (Kirkegaard and Wang 1978). Fundamentally, these enzymes have the ability to change the Lk of a covalently closed DNA duplex. James Wang thus rightly claimed that DNA topoisomerases are "mathematicians," since they modify neither the chemical composition nor the length or the sequence of the molecule but "only" a topological property. To perform this task, DNA topoisomerases should nevertheless work as chemists, introducing transient break(s) in at least one of the two DNA strands. At the end of the reaction, DNA is again covalently closed. Importantly, although DNA ligase needs energy to create a new bond, the ligase activities performed by the ω proteins and swivelases are ATP independent. Indeed, both proteins introduce transient single-strand breaks in the DNA molecule and store the energy gained during the cleavage reaction in a transient covalent linkage between DNA and a tyrosine of the protein in order to use it later on for their ligase activity. In this covalent intermediate, the ω protein is transiently linked to the 5′ end of the single-stranded break, whereas the swivelase is linked to the 3′ end (Fig. 1.4). This early observation becomes later on the basis to discriminate

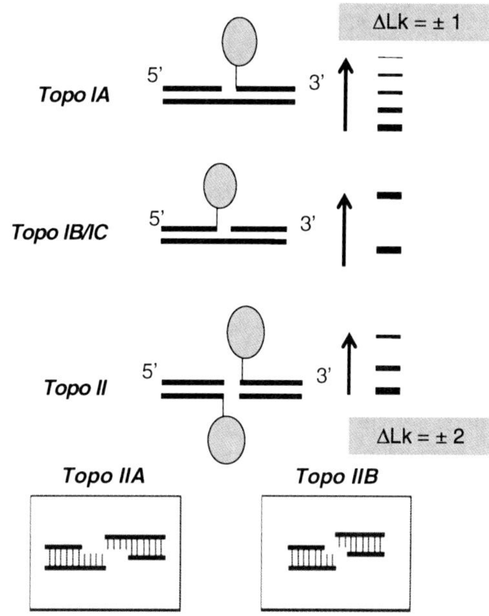

Fig. 1.4 Mechanistic features of the different DNA topoisomerase families

mechanistically between two classes of type I DNA topoisomerases, type IA (omega protein) and type IB (swivelase). The basic reaction mechanism revealed in studying the ω protein and the swivelase (cleavage, formation of a transient covalent protein/DNA intermediate and ligation) turned out later on to be common to all DNA topoisomerases. This mechanism is also partly common to relaxases and rolling-circle replication proteins encoded by some plasmids, as well as to some integrases and transposases encoded by viruses and plasmids. However, these proteins are site-specific, whereas DNA topoisomerases lack strong sequence preference, testifying for their ability to work at the whole genome level.

In the mid-seventies, a technological revolution occurred in the fields of DNA topology; Keller introduced the use of agarose gel electrophoresis as a simple and powerful tool to visualize the different topoisomers present in a population of DNA molecules (Keller 1975). Molecules with various degree of supercoiling indeed exhibit different electrophoretic motilities. This method not only allows to distinguish relaxed from supercoiled DNA much more rapidly than the tedious sucrose ultracentrifugation method previously used; it also allows to count easily the number of superturns and to distinguish populations of topoisomers only differing by a ΔLk of one (Fig. 1.3). Furthermore, by moving the gel by 90° and running plasmid DNA in a second dimension in the presence of an intercalating agent (chloroquine or ethidium bromide), it was even possible to discriminate between negatively and positively supercoiled topoisomerase (2-D gel electrophoresis) (Fig. 1.3). The introduction of agarose gel electrophoresis boosted considerably the number of laboratories involved in the study of DNA topology in the following decades, leading to a great leap in the discovery of new DNA topoisomerases.

1.3.2 The Discovery of DNA Gyrase

A milestone in the history of DNA topoisomerases was the discovery of DNA gyrase by Howard Nash and Martin Gellert (Gellert et al. 1976). The existence in *E. coli* extract of an ATP dependent activity that could introduce negative superturns into a relaxed DNA was deduced from experiments set up to establish an in vitro system for site specific recombination by the bacteriophage lambda integrase (Mizuuchi and Nash 1976). The integration occurred in vitro when a negatively supercoiled plasmid was used as substrate, but not with a relaxed plasmid, except (this was the crucial observation) if ATP was added in the system. This suggested that an ATP-dependent enzyme present in the extract has introduced negative superturns in the relaxed substrate. The postulated enzyme was readily purified by Martin Geller and called DNA gyrase. DNA gyrase turned out to be a heterotetramer, composed of two distinct subunits, GyrA and GyrB (Gellert et al. 1976 ; Sugino et al. 1977, Higgins et al. 1978).

The discovery of DNA gyrase had a lot of biological implications. In a crucial experiment, Gellert and co-workers shown that a plasmid DNA isolated from a coumermycin treated *E. coli* cell was relaxed, indicating that DNA gyrase (and not an unidentified bacterial analogue of histone) is responsible for the negative supercoiling of bacterial DNA (Gellert et al. 1976). Furthermore, since DNA gyrase was able to use as substrate either a relaxed or a positively supercoiled DNA, it was a good candidate for the title of "bacterial swivelase". The discovery of DNA gyrase thus killed two birds at once: solving both the topological problem linked to DNA replication (how to relax positive superturns) and explaining the origin of negative supercoiling. This discovery also revealed very different origins for in vivo negative supercoiling in "prokaryotes" and eukaryotes, passive wrapping of DNA around histone core in eukaryotes, active (ATP-dependent) supercoiling by DNA gyrase in "prokaryotes" (in fact in Bacteria and only in some Archaea, see below). Last but not least, DNA gyrase turned out to be the target of two classes of antibiotics that were already known to inhibit DNA replication but whose target had been previously elusive, coumarins (novobiocin and coumermycin) and quinolone (whose prototype is nalidixic acid). Studies of drug resistant mutants identified the targets of quinolones and coumarins as GyrA and GyrB, respectively (Gellert et al. 1976, 1977; Sugino et al. 1977).

How such a tiny object as an enzyme could introduce superturns into a giant DNA molecule? This was a fascinating question for biologists in the seventies. The first models proposed to explain the supercoiling activity of DNA gyrase were based on the idea that all topoisomerases introduce transient single-stranded breaks in the DNA (Liu and Wang 1978a; Mizuuchi et al. 1980). Two crucial observations helped to delineate the correct model. Firstly, incubation of DNA gyrase with a DNA molecule in the presence of nalidixic acid produces double-stranded breaks (Sugino et al. 1977). This suggested that DNA gyrase produces in fact transient double-stranded breaks (not single-stranded) during the supercoiling reaction. Secondly, a large DNA fragment (around 100 base pairs) of circular DNA could be wrapped around

DNA gyrase in vitro into a positive toroidal superturns, introducing a compensatory negative superturn in the segment of DNA not bound to the enzyme (Liu and Wang 1978b; Morrison and Cozzarelli 1979). From that point, introduction of a negative superturn in the original DNA substrate requires to eliminate the positive supercoiling formed by the DNA segment wrapped around the enzyme, while stabilizing the unconstraint plectonemic negative supercoiling in the rest of the DNA molecule. How this could happen? Brown and Cozzarelli found the right answer to this mechanistic problem in proposing that the DNA segment positively wrapped around the enzyme crosses the double-stranded break, becoming negatively wrapped (Brown and Cozzarelli 1979). In this "sign inversion" model, DNA gyrase introduces two negative superturns at each reaction cycle, modifying the Lk by step of two. This prediction was nicely confirmed by using as substrate for DNA gyrase a population of topoisomers with unique Lk (Brown and Cozzarelli 1979).

1.3.3 Type I and Type II DNA Topoisomerases

Shortly after discovery of DNA gyrase, Bruce Alberts and colleagues discovered that the bacteriophage T4 encodes a DNA topoisomerase that relaxes DNA in the presence of ATP (Liu et al. 1979). This was surprising, relaxation being an energetically favorable reaction. Alberts and colleagues demonstrated that, similar to DNA gyrase, the T4 enzyme makes transient double-stranded breaks and changes the Lk by steps of two. Based on these observations, they proposed the nomenclature type I and type II DNA topoisomerases (Liu et al. 1980). Type I DNA topoisomerase (Topo I) introduces transient single-strand breaks during the reaction of topoisomerization, whereas type II DNA topoisomerase (Topo II) introduces transient double-strand breaks (Fig. 1.4). In the course of their studies, Alberts and colleagues noticed that treatment of double-stranded circular DNA with large amounts of T4 DNA topoisomerase produces knotted DNA circles (Liu et al. 1980). This was a consequence of the ability of this viral Topo II to force a DNA double-helix to pass through the DSB in the same molecule. Kreuzer and Cozzarelli 1980 discovered shortly thereafter that DNA gyrase was also able to knot or unknot a circular DNA duplex but also to catenate or decatenate two DNA rings (Kreuzer and Cozzarelli 1980). Decatenation and unknotting turned out to be general properties of Topo II, explaining why these enzymes are essential in all organisms to segregate the daughter chromosomes at the end of chromosomal replication (DiNardo et al. 1984; Uemura et al. 1987).

In a few years, ATP-dependent decatenation or relaxation activities were readily detected in extracts of various eukaryotic cells, such as *Drosophila melanogaster*, *Xenopus laevis* eggs or else mammalian tissue culture cells, and several laboratories succeeded to purify various eukaryotic Topo II (Miller et al. 1981; Baldi et al. 1980; Benedetti et al. 1983; Halligan et al. 1985). Surprisingly, these enzymes turned out to resemble T4 Topo II, as they all lack gyrase activity. The idea that "*what is true for E. coli should be true for the elephant*" being still prevalent, many scientists believed at that time that a true equivalent of bacterial DNA gyrase remained to be discovered in eukaryotes (Francke and Margolin 1981). However, the quest for an eukaryotic gyrase was in vain.

The eukaryotic Topo II (ubiquitous in this domain) are different from DNA gyrase not only by their lack of gyrase activity but also by their structures and drug sensitivities. Whereas DNA gyrases are heterotetramers, eukaryotic Topo II are homodimers. Eukaryotic Topo II are only slightly sensitive to coumarins and resistant to most quinolones. In turn, DNA gyrases are only slightly sensitive to drugs affecting eukaryotic Topo II. The saga of eukaryotic DNA topoisomerase inhibitors started in 1984 when Leroy Liu and co-workers reported that several antitumor drugs, such as m-AMSA, adriamycin, or epipodophyllotoxin interfere with the breakage-reunion reaction of mammalian Topo II (Nelson et al. 1984; Tewey et al. 1984a, b; Chen et al. 1984; Ross et al. 1984) mimicking the effect of quinolones on DNA gyrase. The next year, it was found that the eukaryotic Topo IB (swivelase) was itself the target of a well-known antitumor drug, camptothecin in 1985 (Hsiang et al. 1985). This opened a Pandora box for the study of DNA topoisomerases and induced many pharmaceutical as well as academic laboratories to focus on DNA topoisomerases and the mechanism of action of their drugs (see the accompanying chapters 9–13). New compounds were subsequently discovered in already known drug families, as well as new families with different modes of action (Pommier et al. 2010).

1.4 DNA Topoisomerases, Why so Many?

The prokaryote/eukaryote paradigm still reigned supreme in the seventies and the first discovered DNA topoisomerases seemed to follow this simple scheme, with one Topo I and one Topo II in each "kingdom" (the ω protein and DNA gyrase in prokaryotes, the swivelase and Topo II in eukaryotes). However, this situation changes rapidly in the eighties. Novel biochemical studies, and isolation of new genes encoding DNA topoisomerases, led to the discovery of additional unexpected DNA topoisomerases. Two new DNA topoisomerases were isolated from *Escherichia coli*, called respectively DNA topoisomerase III (Topo III) and IV (Topo IV) (Srivenugopal et al. 1984; Kato et al. 1990), whereas a gene encoding a new Topo I homologous to *E. coli* Topo III was discovered in *Saccharomyces cerevisiae* (Wallis et al. 1989). Fortunately, the sequencing of the DNA topoisomerase genes in the eighties opened the possibility to classify these enzymes based on sequence similarity (common ancestry), introducing some rationality in the growing topoisomerase zoo (Figs. 1.5 and 1.6). The *E. coli* and *Saccharomyces cerevisiae* Topo III turned out to be evolutionary related to the *E. coli* ω protein (encode by the gene *topA*), being thus new members of the Topo IA family (DiGate and Marians 1989; Wallis et al. 1989). Importantly, sequence comparison revealed that Topo IA (ω protein/ Topo III) and Topo IB (swivelase) were not only mechanistically different, but also

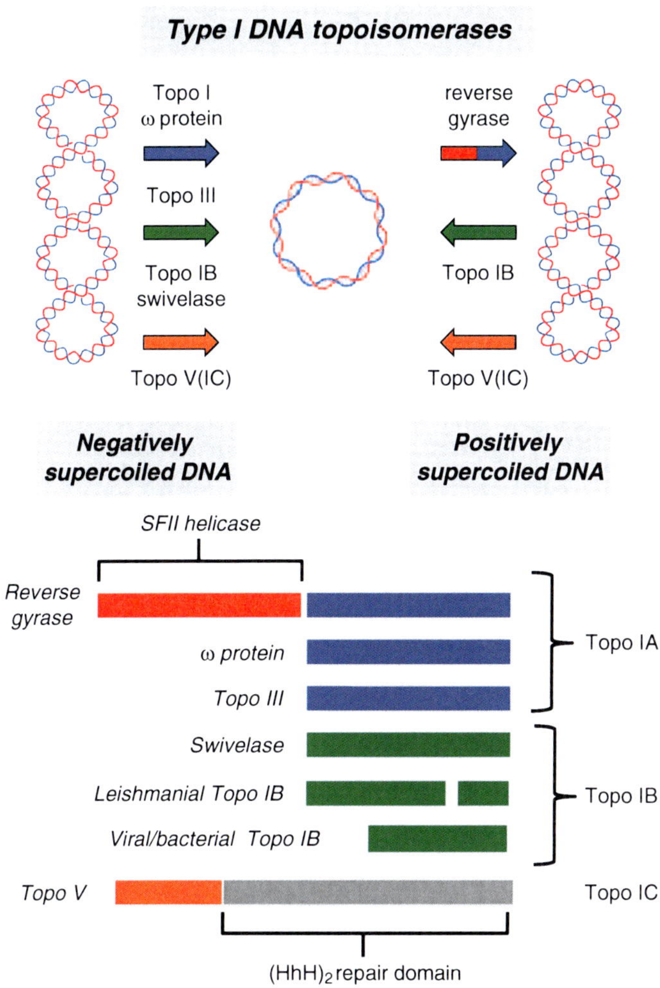

Fig. 1.5 Families and subfamilies of type I DNA topoisomerases; major reactions and homologous relationships. Homologous proteins or protein domains are drawn with same color

non homologous, exhibiting no sequence similarities (it is therefore quite confusing that in *E. coli*, the gene encoding Topo III, a Topo IA has been named unfortunately *topB*) (Fig. 1.5). The independent origin of Topo IA and Topo IB was later on confirmed by structural analyses. Topo IB seems evolutionary related to tyrosine recombinase (Cheng et al. 1998), whereas Topo IA apparently originated by tandem duplication of an ancestral fold (the topofold) that contained some typical folds of nucleic acid binding proteins also present in Topo II, but in different arrangement (Duguet et al. 2006).

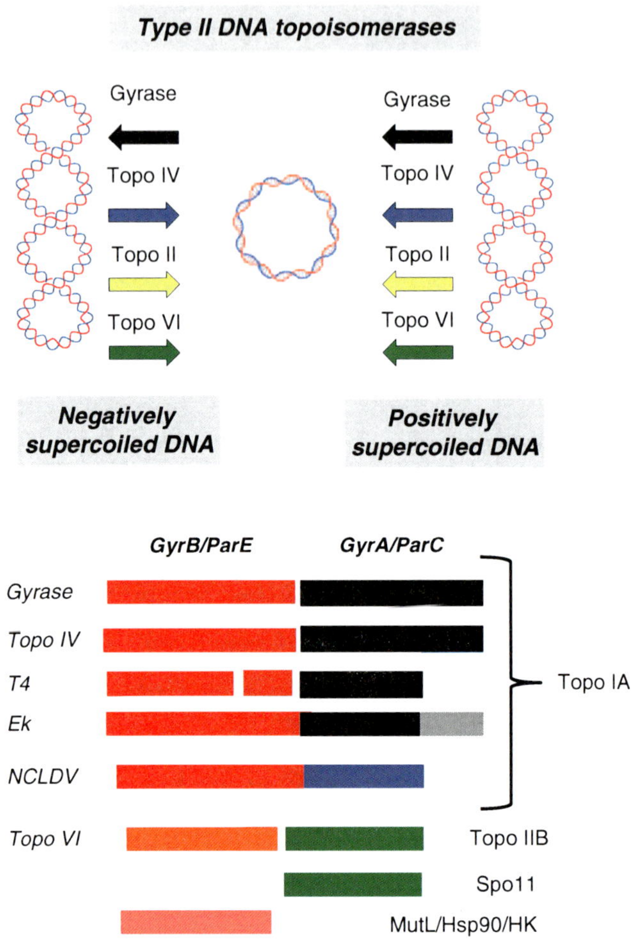

Fig. 1.6 Families and subfamilies of type II DNA topoisomerases; major reactions and homologous relationships. Homologous proteins or protein domains are drawn with same color

1.4.1 Topo IA and IB Are Not Homologous and Have Different Modes of Action

Mechanistic models based on biochemical experiments, structural studies, and later on, single-molecule analyses confirmed that Topo IA and Topo IB use very different reaction mechanisms (Lima et al. 1994; Mondragon and DiGate 1999, for recent review, see Schoeffler and Berger 2008). Topo IA, which has a toroidal shape, binds DNA in such a way that the two strands cannot freely rotate one around the other. They use an active strand passage mechanism to force one strand to cross the other only once per reaction cycle. This mechanism changes the Lk strictly by increments of one ($\Delta Lk = \pm 1$) (Fig. 1.4). In contrast, the mechanism of Topo IB involves the free rotation of one DNA strand around the other until religation occurs (the DNA nevertheless remaining strongly bond to the Topo I during that reaction (Koster et al. 2005)). Although Topo I are often defined as enzymes that change the Lk by step of 1, the controlled rotation mechanism catalyzed by Topo IB can actually changes the Lk by more than one during a single cleavage/religation cycle (Fig. 1.4).

1.4.2 Topo IIA Are Diverse but Homologous

In contrast to Topo I, sequence analyses revealed that all Topo II known in the eighties belong to a same protein family (Fig. 1.6). The Gyr A and Gyr B subunits of DNA gyrase are indeed homologous to the N-terminal and the central domain of eukaryotic Topo II, respectively (although sequence similarities are quite low, except in conserved motives) (Uemura et al. 1986; Giaever et al. 1986; Wyckoff et al. 1989). The *E. coli* DNA Topo IV is functionally similar to eukaryotic Topo II (only relaxing positively and negatively supercoiled DNA) but is more closely related to DNA gyrase in sequence and structure, being a heterotetramer made of two subunits, dubbed ParC and ParE, that are homologous to GyrA and GyrB, respectively (Kato et al. 1992). The three subunits of the T4 Topo II turned out to be also homologous to the bacterial and eukaryotic enzymes (Wyckoff et al. 1989). The protein encoded by gene 52 is homologous to GyrA, whereas the proteins encoded by genes 60 and 39 are homologous to the N and C terminal regions of GyrB, respectively. All these homologous Topo II share a similar mechanism, producing double-stranded breaks with the GyrA subunit (or its homologous subunits/domains) linked in 5′ of the two cleaved stands; the two cleavage sites being separated by four base pairs overhanging.

1.4.3 Topo IIA as Complex Molecular Machines

Biochemical and structural studies of *E. coli* DNA gyrase and *S. cerevisiae* Topo II subdomains suggested in the nineties a "two gates model" to explain the mechanism of action of Topo II (Roca and Wang 1994; Lima and Mondragón 1994; Lindsley et al. 1996; Berger et al. 1996, for a recent review, see Schoeffler and Berger 2008). The crystal structure of a large fragment of yeast Topo II reveals a heart-shaped dimeric protein with a large central hole and two gates at opposite ends. This suggests that a first DNA segment (the G-segment, G for gate) enters into the enzyme cavity through the top gate, at the N-termini (between the two B subunits). Once in the cavity, the G segment is cleaved and covalently linked to both A subunits. A second DNA duplex (the T-segment, T for transported) can then enter via the top gate (dubbed the N gate) into the enzyme cavity. The T-segment is then transported through the cleaved duplex, and expelled through the second gate located at the C-termini (the C-gate). This complex set of reactions involves large conformational changes to move the two DNA duplexes through the gates. Biochemical experiments and resolution of Topo IIA complexed to intact or cleaved revealed that these concerted allosteric movements are triggered by DNA and ATP binding (Roca and Wang 1992; Dong and Berger 2007; Schmidt et al. 2010) *(for more details, see chapter 4)*. In the case of DNA gyrase, the sign inversion model requires the wrapping of the G-segment around the enzyme to form a toroidal positive superturn. Indeed, the C-terminal domains of gyrase exhibit a beta-propeller spherical structure with positively charged residues allowing DNA wrapping at its surface (Corbett et al. 2004; Hsieh et al. 2004, 2010; Ruthenburg et al. 2005; Kramlinger and Hiasa 2006). In Topo IV, the propeller structure is disturbed, probably explaining why the enzyme cannot wrap DNA *(for more details, see chapter 4 and 9)*.

1.5 The In Vivo Role of DNA Topoisomerases

1.5.1 Homeostatic Control of Supercoiling

The discovery of new DNA topoisomerases in the eighties raised the question of their specialization in distinct biological roles (Schmid and Sawitzke 1993). This turned out to be a complicated task, considering the variety of pathways involved and the difficulty to untangle the direct and indirect effect of drugs, especially those inducing the formation of stable protein DNA complex that poison the cell by interfering with replication and transcription. In *E. coli*, the detection of compensatory mutations in DNA gyrase and ω protein mutants established early on that their antagonistic activities (supercoiling and relaxation) cooperate to control the level of chromosomes and plasmids superhelical density (DiNardo et al. 1982; Pruss et al. 1982). This homeostatic control is based on the different responses of gyrase and ω protein gene promoters to supercoiling; whereas the promoters of the *gyrA* and *gyrB* genes are activated by relaxation, the promoter of the *topA* gene (encoding the ω protein) is activated by negative supercoiling (Tse-Dinh 1985). It was shown later on that Topo IV also participates in this homeostatic control (Zechiedrich et al. 2000).

Negative supercoiling is an essential feature of bacterial chromosomes. The initiator protein DNA requires a negatively supercoiled template to open the replication origin at the initiation step of DNA replication (Funnel et al. 1987) and the transcription of a number of genes also requires negatively promoters to be located on negatively supercoiled DNA (Pruss and Drlica 1989). However, the level of negative supercoiling can fluctuate in a narrow range, with fundamental biological consequences. DNA gyrase being an ATP dependent enzyme, the intracellular superhelical density is dependent of the ratio between ATP and ADP intracellular concentrations (Hsieh et al. 1991a, b). The level of intracellular free (unconstraint) negative supercoiling is thus directly coupled to the energetic state of the cell by the enzymatic activity of DNA gyrase. As a consequence, the energetic state of the bacterial cell can directly affect the pattern of gene expression. This is because promoters respond differentially to variations in superhelical density depending on their sequence and organization; some are activated, others are repressed, still others are unaffected by increasing (or decreasing) negative supercoiling (Pruss and Drlica 1989; Peter et al. 2004). The overall transcription pattern in bacteria can be therefore adjusted to fluctuations in the cellular energetic state via modification of DNA gyrase activity (Cheung et al. 2003). Variation in supercoiling density occurs at different stages of growth (stationary versus exponential phase) and can be also triggered by modification of environmental parameters, such as temperature, or osmotic stress (Lopez-Garcia et al. 2000). Accordingly, the enzymatic activity of DNA gyrase allows bacteria to adjust rapidly and efficiently the global gene expression pattern to variation in the environment. A spectacular example is the control by DNA topology of the oscillation in gene expression involved in the cyanobacterial circadian clock mechanism (Vijayan et al. 2009). The possibility to control the pattern of gene expression in such an elegant way could explain the extraordinary evolutionary success of bacteria. Indeed, DNA gyrase is a universal bacterial enzyme (with only one exception, see below), indicating that the Last Bacterial Common Ancestor (LBCA) already benefited from the advantage provided by this fascinating enzyme.

In Eukarya, the linker DNA between nucleosomes is in a relaxed state (Sinden et al. 1980). The nucleosome fiber should be disrupted to transform the toroidal negative superturns around the histone core into plectonemic negative superturns that could facilitate DNA melting. This chromatin remodeling procedure requires a cascade of complex events (such as various histones chemical modifications) and cannot rival for elegance with the simplicity and efficiency of the gyrase-based mechanism operating in bacteria. In traditional evolutionary scenarios, it is therefore difficult to understand, why DNA gyrase has been lost in Eukaryotes, supposed to be "higher" organisms. In fact, DNA gyrase seems to be a real bacterial invention, testifying for the originality of this domain. Some Archaea have borrowed DNA gyrase for bacteria. They probably also used this enzyme to adjust their pattern of gene expression to the environment, but this remains to be demonstrated. However, similar to eukaryotes, most archaea lack DNA gyrase and their plasmids are relaxed or slightly negatively supercoiled, possibly via interaction with eukaryotic-like histones (Charbonnier and Forterre 1994; Musgrave et al. 2000). Thus, negative supercoiling of intracellular DNA should not be considered as a general feature of terrestrial life, but as a characteristic of organisms containing DNA gyrase (see the Fig. 1.3a, b and figure legend). It is important to distinguish negative supercoiling produced by DNA gyrase from transient negative (or positive) supercoiling that are produced by the interaction of DNA with DNA binding proteins and processes such as transcription and replication to fully appreciate the difference in physiology between cells with or without DNA gyrases.

1.5.2 Solving Topological Problems Related to DNA Replication and Chromosome Organization

Theoretically, DNA topoisomerases can be involved in the resolution of the DNA replication topological problem either by relaxing positive superturns in front of the replication forks or by resolving the entanglement of the two daughter chromosomes behind the fork (Champoux and Been 1980). In practice, it seems that topological stress during the elongation stage of DNA replication mainly occurs in the form of positive supercoiling, whereas the formation of catenanes occurs mainly at the termination step, when the topological stress that accumulate cannot be transformed in positive superturns in the vanishing region located between the two converging replication forks. This explains why stress-induced during elongation can be eliminated either by Topo I (providing it can relax positive superturns) or by a Topo II, whereas chromosome segregation cannot properly occur without a Topo II.

Both DNA gyrase and Topo IV can a priori solve the topological problems raised by DNA replication in bacteria by relaxing positive superturns in front of replication forks. Many bacteria, such as Mycobacteria, only contain DNA gyrase (i.e., no Topo IV), indicating that this enzyme can perform these different tasks in addition to supercoil DNA. In Bacteria with two Topo IIA, Topo IV appears to be specialized in chromosome decatenation. The genes encoding its two subunits (*parC* and *parE*) were indeed first identified as genes involved in chromosome partition (Kato et al. 1992) and *E. coli* Topo IV is a better decatenase than DNA gyrase in vitro (Ullsperger and Cozzarelli 1996). In *E. coli*, Topo IV could also play an important role in coordinating the events that occur during chromosome segregation, as suggested by its physical interaction with the segregation motor protein FtsK (Espeli et al. 2003) and the chromosome condensing MukB (Hayama and Marians 2010; Li et al. 2010).

In Eukarya, positive superturns induced in front of replication forks can be removed by either by Topo IIA or Topo IB. Genetic studies in yeast suggested early on that these two enzymes indeed cooperate for this task (Kim and Wang 1989). These studies also show that DNA replication can progress (more slowly) in the absence of either Topo IIA or Topo IB, indicating that elimination of positive superturn (the only reaction possible when Topo IIA is absent) is sufficient to allow progression of the fork. Topo IIA is thus dispensable for the elongation step of DNA replication but, as expected, is essential for chromosome segregation (DiNardo et al. 1984; Uemura et al. 1987; Baxter and Diffley 2008). In Eukarya, DNA topoisomerases are also required during chromatin formation to eliminate the positive superturns produced to compensate the negative wrapping of DNA around nucleosomes. Again, both Topo IIA and Topo IB could perform this task a priori. However, in vitro experiments with reconstituted yeast minichromosome suggest that Topo IIA is much more efficient than Topo IB for this task (Salceda et al. 2006). The authors suggested the cross-inversion mechanism of Topo II allows this enzyme to work at juxtaposition of DNA segments in linker regions free of histones, whereas the strand rotation mechanism of topo IB cannot operate efficiently on DNA covered with nucleosomes. Finally, the formation of higher order structures in the eukaryotic chromosomes also depends on DNA topoisomerases (Uemura et al. 1987; Adachi et al. 1991; Warburton and Earnshaw 1997). Both Topo IB and Topo II seem to be involved in chromosome condensation/decondensation and Topo II, which is a major component of the chromatin, could play a structural role in the organization of the eukaryotic chromosome (Belmont 2006; Nitiss 2009).

1.5.3 Solving Topological Problems Related to Transcription

Whereas the topological problem associated to DNA replication was suspected from theoretical consideration, even before the discovery of DNA topoisomerases, a role for these enzymes in transcription was not anticipated. It's only in 1987 that Liu and Wang realized that progression of RNA polymerases along DNA should induce waves of positive and negative superturns in front and behind the transcription forks, respectively (the twin-domain model Liu and Wang (1987)). Indeed, RNA polymerases being attached to polysomes cannot rotate freely around the transcribed DNA, inducing rotation of the double helix instead. This stress is amplified during transcription of membrane proteins that anchor the whole DNA/RNA complex to the cell envelope. In proposing their model, Liu and Wang were inspired by earlier experiments in which plasmids isolated from *E. coli* cells treated with DNA gyrase inhibitors were positively supercoiled (Lockshon and Morris 1983), whereas plasmids isolated from *E. coli* mutant of the protein ω exhibited an excess of negative superturns (Pruss and Drlica 1986). A particular aspect of the topological problem linked to transcription is the formation of R-loops behind the transcription machinery. The transient excess of negative supercoiling behind the moving RNA polymerase can indeed locally unwind the DNA double helix, stabilizing the RNA/DNA hybrid form between the transcribed strand and the messenger RNA.

In Bacteria, DNA gyrase, Topo IV, and protein ω seem to cooperate to relax the positive and negative superturns that accumulate in front and behind moving RNA polymerases (Khodursky et al. 2000). The protein ω is especially important to prevent R-loop formation by relaxing negative superturns behind the fork (Drolet 2006). In Eukarya, the waves of supercoiling produced by transcription can be relaxed a priori either by Topo IIA or Topo IB. The specific roles of these two DNA topoisomerases seem to differ according to the organisms and (for multicellular organisms) to different tissues. For a given organism, this role can also vary depending of the gene transcribed and/or the level of transcription. DNA topoisomerases appear to be especially important in highly transcribed genes, such as rRNA genes. A recent study, coupling genetic and cytological studies (chromatin spreading) in yeast, has highlighted different roles for Topo IIA and Topo IB in the transcription of rRNA genes (French et al. 2011). In a Topo IIA mutant, transcription is slow down and stops prematurely, suggesting that Topo IIA is mainly involved in relaxation positive torsion in front of the fork. This can be explained by the possibility for topo II to relax nucleosomal fibers using the cross-inversion mechanism. In contrast, in a Topo IB mutant, the rate of transcription is not affected but unwinding regions (bubbles) accumulates. These bubbles originate from the formation of R-loops that are processed by RNAse H as indicated by the study of a Topo IB/RNAse H double mutant. This suggests that, similar to protein ω in bacteria, Topo IB is mainly required to relax negative superturns behind transcription forks.

The stress induced by transcription might have important consequences on transcription itself. The waves of negative supercoiling behind the polymerase can activate a downstream promoter, whereas the wave of positive superturns in front can inactivate upstream promoters. Hence, the transcription patterns of genes determine the superhelicity of their immediate environment (Dröge and Nordheim 1991; Ljungman and Hanawalt 1992). This phenomenon has probably a major role in the dynamic structuration of the chromosome. In Bacteria, the chromosome is divided into many discrete topological domains corresponding to small-supercoiled loops that are randomly distributed without fixed location (Staczek and Higgins 1998; Krasilnikov et al. 1999; Postow et al. 2004). It is likely that transcription, together with the activity of gyrase and Topo IV, determine in most part the structure and superhelicity of these loops. The same situation could occur in eukaryotes, since their chromosomes is divided in topological loops often corresponding to transcription units.

1.5.4 Topo III, a DNA Topoisomerase for Recombination Intermediates

In contrast to other Topo I, Topo III are not required to solve topological problems associated to replication or transcription, neither to control intracellular supercoiling. The biological role(s) of Topo III remain mysterious for a long time. This was quite frustrating, considering the presence of this DNA topoisomerase in all studied organisms. Finally, the biological role of Topo III was determined from genetic studies followed more recently by biochemical characterization of their interactions with various partners. Mutants of Topo III exhibit hyper-recombination phenotypes and both in vivo and in vitro studies suggest that their main role is to prevent excessive recombination by disrupting Holliday junctions and resolving recombination intermediates. They seem to be especially important to remove topological blocks induced by recombination at arrested replication forks (Wu and Hickson 2006; Plank et al. 2006). To perform these tasks, Topo III works hand in hand with helicases. In Bacteria, Topo III interacts with the RecQ helicase, whereas in Eukarya, they interact with RecQ homologues, such as the Sgs1 helicase in yeast or the BLM and WRN helicases in animals (Aggarwal and Brosh 2009). In Eukarya, the Topo III and BLM/Sgs1 helicase associate with a third protein, RmI1, to form the dissolvasome, or RTR (RecQ-Topoisomerase-Rm1) complex (Mankouri and Hickson 2007; Seki et al. 2006; Shimamoto et al. 2000). Inactivation of this complex results in hyper-recombination, gross chromosomal rearrangements, chromosome segregation defects, and human disease. DNA topoisomerase III and the RTR complex also colocalize and interact with telomere binding proteins (Temime-Smaali et al. 2008).

Considering the critical functions of DNA topoisomerases in all processes associated to the expression, structuration, and replication of the genetic information, these enzymes are the major factors of genome stability and maintenance. As a consequence, different DNA topoisomerases are associated to check point controls in Eukarya. (Conti et al. 2007; Nitiss 2009).

The critical roles of DNA topoisomerases in so many essential cellular functions help us to understand why these proteins are the targets of many warfare compounds produced by competitors in life struggle. Molecular marvels of life, DNA topoisomerases are also the Achilles' heel of organisms. To inactivate its DNA, topoisomerase appears to be one of the smartest way to get rid of your rivals – a property that we learn now how to use for our own benefit.

1.6 Archaea: A Goldmine for New DNA Topoisomerases

The diversity of DNA topoisomerases first appeared to be linked to their functionality. This mechanistic view was finally challenged by discoveries made in an apparently unrelated field. In the eighties, the discovery by Carl Woese of a third domain of life on our planet, Archaebacteria (later on renamed Archaea) (Woese and Fox 1977) led to the unexpected discovery of completely new DNA topoisomerases.

1.6.1 Reverse Gyrase: An Environmental Topoisomerase

The first archaeal DNA topoisomerase was discovered by Kikuchi and Asai who reported in 1984 an unusual ATP-dependent positive supercoiling activity in the thermoacidophilic archaeon *Sulfolobus acidocaldarius* (Kikuchi and Asai 1984). They described the enzyme responsible for this activity (christened reverse gyrase) as a four subunits type II DNA topoisomerase. This was probably due to a contamination of their preparation by the archaeal RNA polymerase that indeed co-purify in the first steps of reverse gyrase purification (unpublished result). Indeed, further characterization of the *S. acidocaldarius* positive supercoiling activity revealed that, surprisingly, this reaction was catalyzed by a monomeric type I DNA topoisomerase (Forterre et al. 1985; Nakasu and Kikuchi 1985). This was unexpected for two reasons: Firstly, all type I DNA topoisomerases previously isolated were ATP-independent and secondly, the only enzyme previously known to supercoil DNA (DNA gyrase) was a type II enzyme. This conundrum was solved in 1993 by the isolation and sequencing of the reverse gyrase gene (Confalonieri et al. 1993), followed a few years later by resolution of the enzyme structure (Rodríguez and Stock 2002). It turned out that reverse gyrase is a composite protein formed by the fusion of a Topo IA module with an ATP-dependent SF2 helicase-like module (for reviews, see D'Amaro et al. 2007; Nadal 2007) (Fig. 1.5). The two domains tightly cooperate to produce supercoiling, as shown by reconstituted experiments performed with recombinant domains (Declais et al. 2000; Valenti et al. 2008) or more recently with the reverse gyrase of the archaeon *Nanoarchaeum equitans* in which each domain is encoded by a separate gene (Capp et al. 2010).

Being built on a type I enzyme, reverse gyrase cannot use for supercoiling the sign inversion type mechanism of DNA gyrase. Slesarev and Kozyavkin proposed in 1990 a simple two steps model to explain how reverse gyrase could supercoil DNA. In the first step, reverse gyrase recognizes a single-stranded region in a DNA duplex and binds the two denatured DNA segment in a specific mutual orientation; in a second step, ATP hydrolysis is coupled to a conformational change that triggers the strand transfer in such a way that the Lk is increased by one unit (Slesarev and Kozyavkin 1990). This model was based on the observation that an artificially inserted single-stranded loop in a close DNA duplex stimulates the positive supercoiling activity of reverse gyrase (Slesarev and Kozyavkin 1990). It was also known that binding of reverse gyrase to DNA induces unwinding in the absence of ATP, suggesting that the binding by itself induces local separation of the two DNA strands (Jaxel et al. 1989). Several aspects of this model have been now validated by structural and enzymatic studies performed on reverse gyrases from different organisms (Rodríguez and Stock 2002; Hsieh and Plank 2006; Ganguly et al. 2011). The "helicase" module has no helicase activity but appears to act as a protein motor driving ATP dependent conformational change in the protein/DNA complex. A small inserted region in the helicase domain, dubbed the "latch" seems to play a crucial role in coupling the conformational change induced by ATP in the helicase domain to conformational change in the topoisomerase domain. It remains to determine the relative orientation of the two DNA segments in the course of the reaction. This will probably require solving the structure of several reverse gyrase DNA complexes.

Since positively supercoiled DNA exhibits an excess of topological links compared to a relaxed DNA, it was suggested early on that positive supercoiling by reverse gyrase, an enzyme isolated from hyperthermophilic organisms, is required to prevent DNA denaturation at high temperature. Two observations have now strengthened the connection between reverse gyrase and life in hot environments. Firstly, comparative genomic revealed that all organisms (either archaea or bacteria) with an optimal growth temperature above 80°C (hyperthermophiles by definition) have at least one reverse gyrase, whereas reverse gyrase is systematically absent in mesophilic organisms (Forterre 2002a). Secondly, a null reverse gyrase mutant is thermosensitive and cannot grow above 90°C (Atomi et al. 2004). However, how precisely reverse gyrase protect DNA against the effect of temperature in vivo remains unclear. The finding that the episomal form of viral DNA in *Sulfolobus shibatae* is positively supercoiled initially suggested that chromosomal DNA in hyperthermophiles was positively supercoiled (Nadal et al. 1986). This was put into question later on, when it was discovered that plasmids present in hyperthermophiles harboring reverse gyrase are relaxed or slightly negatively supercoiled at physiological temperature (Charbonnier and Forterre 1994). Even worse, it was found that a few hyperthermophiles harbor a classical gyrase (in addition to reverse gyrase) and that plasmids isolated from these hot-loving species are negatively supercoiled (Guipaud et al. 1997; Lopez-Garcia et al. 2000).

The finding of negative supercoiling in hyperthermophiles might appear surprising at first sight, but this should not be the case. Indeed, because of topological constraints that favor renaturation in a topologically closed DNA, a negatively supercoiled plasmid is as stable as a positively supercoiled one at very high temperature (Marguet and Forterre 1994). Accordingly, the role of reverse gyrase cannot be to introduce positive superturns at the whole chromosome level. However, it might be essential to counteract locally the effect of temperature. This might be even critical in regions that already exhibit a linking deficit, such as topological domains behind replication or transcription forks. Hsieh and Plank, who have shown that reverse gyrase efficiently anneals two complementary single-stranded circles, hence suggested that reverse gyrase acts as a sentinel searching for unwound DNA or bubble regions (Hsieh and Plank 2006). The association of reverse gyrase with RNA polymerase in *Sulfolobus* (personal observation) suggests for instance that this enzyme might be especially important to reduce the waves of negative supercoiling during transcription.

Another problem for DNA in hyperthermophiles is DNA cleavage following temperature-induced depurination, because any break in the double helix removes the topological links that protect against DNA denaturation (Marguet and Forterre 1994). Reverse gyrase could possibly play a role in preventing this phenomenon in vivo, since this enzyme protects DNA against degradation in vitro (Kampmann and Stock 2004). However, this remains to be demonstrated. Finally, several reports by the group of Ciamarella suggest that reverse gyrase is somehow involved in DNA repair in hyperthermophiles. The reverse gyrase of *S. solfataricus* is indeed recruited to the nucleoid structure after UV irradiation and interacts with repair DNA polymerase (Napoli et al. 2004; Valenti et al. 2009).

1.6.2 Topo V, the Lonesome Type I DNA Topoisomerase

Following the discovery of reverse gyrase, a few scientists became interested into archeal DNA topoisomerases. At the end of the eighties, a young Russian biochemist, Alexei Slesarev described the first archaeal Topo III (Slesarev et al. 1991), he reported 2 years later the exciting discovery of an enzyme resembling eukaryotic Topo IB in the hyperthermophilic archaeon *Methanopyrus kandleri*, a methanogen growing up to 110°C. This enzyme can indeed relax both positively and negatively supercoiled DNA and forms 3′-link with DNA. Slesarev christened this new DNA topoisomerase, Topo V (Slesarev et al. 1993). Topo V is unique among all known topoisomerases by combining topoisomerase and DNA repair activities into a single polypeptide. The DNA topoisomerase activity is located in an N-terminal domain of around 40 kDa whereas a large C-terminal domain (around 60 kDa) exhibits an apurinic/apyrimidinic (AP) site-processing activity (Belova et al. 2002). This C-terminal domain is formed by 24 repeats of helix-hairpin-helix (HhH) motives that confer salt resistance and processivity to Topo V (Belova et al. 2002; Pavlov et al. 2002) (Fig. 1.5). Finally, the extreme thermophilic character of Topo V (the enzyme was tested active up to 122°C) allows this enzyme to fully unwind a DNA duplex at high temperature by combining thermal driven unwinding and topoisomerase unlinking (Kozyavkin et al. 1995).The mechanistic similarity between Topo V and Topo IB has been definitely established recently by showing that Topo V relaxes DNA in one step, via a constrained swiveling mechanism, similar to that for type IB (Taneja et al. 2007). However, resolution of the three dimensional structure of the N-terminal Topo V topoisomerase domain revealed a novel protein fold completely unrelated to the Topo IB structure (Taneja et al. 2006). Topo V should therefore be considered as the prototype of a third family of type I DNA topoisomerases, Topo IC (Forterre 2006) (Fig. 1.5). The most intriguing aspect of Topo V is certainly that its gene has still no homologue in organisms other than

M. kandleri. In other word, if not for the work of Slesarev, this protein would be still annotated today as uncharacterized. This led us to wonder how many new DNA topoisomerases hidden in the ORFans jungle are just waiting to be awaked by the curious and lucky biochemists.

1.6.3 DNA Topoisomerase VI, an Archaeal Enzyme with Sexy and Green Homologues

The search for Topo II in the crenarchaeon *Sulfolobus shibatae* led, in the nineties, to the discovery of a new family of Topo II (Bergerat et al. 1994, 1997). The *Sulfolobus* Topo II seemed a first sight similar to bacterial Topo IV: an heterotetramer A2B2 that lacks gyrase activity. However, when the genes encoding its two subunits (A and B) were isolated, this archaeal enzyme turned out to be dramatically different from all Topo II previously discovered (Fig. 1.6). One of its subunit (by chance the B one) exhibited only low sequence similarities with the N-terminal region of the B subunits of previously known Topo II whereas its A subunit exhibited no sequence similarity to A subunits of any Topo II known at that time (Bergerat et al. 1997). The archaeal Topo II, then dubbed DNA topoisomerase VI (Topo VI), is therefore the prototype of a new family of Topo II, Topo IIB (Topo II homologous to DNA gyrase being now called Topo IIA). A significant difference between Topo IIA and Topo IIB is that Topo IIB produce two base pairs overhang after DNA cleavage, instead of four in the case of Topo IIA (Buhler et al. 2001).

Although distinct, Topo IIA and IIB exhibit a similar organization; their B subunits bear the ATP binding site, whereas their A subunits contain the tyrosine responsible for DNA cleavage. Structural analyses allowed defining more clearly their evolutionary relationships. The lack of similarity between the Topo IIA and Topo IB A subunits was confirmed by the resolution of the structure of the A subunit of the *M. jannashii* Topo VI (Nichols et al. 1999). Although all Topo II contain similar folds, such as Toprim domain (also present in Topo IA), and CAP-like domains, these folds are organized in different orders and the overall structure of the two proteins is not similar. The B subunits of Topo IIA and Topo IIB are homologous, as deduced from their structural comparison, although they share only limited sequence similarities (Corbett and Berger 2003). These similarities are concentrated in the N-terminal region, which corresponds to the ATP binding site. The discovery of archaeal Topo VI indeed helps to define a new ATP-binding site that corresponds to a specific protein fold dubbed the Bergerat fold (Bergerat et al. 1997; Dutta and Inouye 2000). Beside Topo II, the Bergerat fold is present in the chaperone Hsp90, the DNA repair protein MutL, and histidine kinases. These proteins have been grouped in the GHKL family (for Gyrase, Hsp90, Kinase, MutL family) a nomenclature that, unfortunately, forgets the archaeal Topo II (Dutta and Inouye 2000). Importantly, some drugs that interact with the Bergerat fold can inhibit several proteins of this family. In particular, radicicol, a well-known inhibitor of Hsp90, inhibits both Topo IIA and Topo IIB (Gadelle et al. 2005, 2006).

Importantly, structural studies of archaeal Topo VI allowed for the first time to solve the complete structure of a Topo II. The group of Berger solved the structure of the closed form of the *Methanosarcina mazei* Topo VI (Corbett et al. 2007), whereas the group of Herman van Tilbeurgh solved the structure of the open form of the *S. shibatae* Topo VI (Graille et al. 2008). Comparison of these two structures allows to nicely visualize the conformational changes that occur during the reaction of topoisomerization by a Topo II at the atomic level (Fig. 1.7). Topo IIB most likely follow the two gates model previously proposed for Topo IIA (although the open form whose structure has been solved only corresponds to the top gate, those used for the entrance of the two DNA segments). It remains to solve the structure of a DNA Topo VI complexes to precise the mechanism of action of Topo VI.

The discovery of archaea Topo VI had a great impact in two unrelated fields of eukaryotic molecular biology: meiotic recombination and plant growth. Sequencing of the Topo VI genes in 1997 revealed that the Topo VI A subunit is homologous to the eukaryotic protein Spo11 (Spo for sporulation). The biological role of Spo11 was unknown, at that time, except for its probable involvement in meiotic recombination. However, it was just discovered that meiotic recombination is initiated by double-strand breaks and that a protein is covalently linked in 5′ ends of these breaks (De Massy et al. 1995; Liu et al. 1995). This immediately suggested that Spo11 was this topoisomerase-like protein and, as a consequence, that Spo11 was responsible of chromosome cleavage during meiosis (Bergerat et al. 1997). This prediction was confirmed by site-directed mutagenesis of the yeast *S. cerevisiae* Spo11, guided by sequence comparison of the archaeal and yeast proteins. Replacement of the only tyrosine conserved between Spo11 and the A subunit of Topo VI by a phenylalanine turned out to inhibit the formation of meiotic-induced double-strand breaks in vivo (Bergerat et al. 1997). Finally, Spo11 was found covalently linked in 5′ ends of the chromosome breaks during meiotic recombination in *S. cerevisiae* (Keeney et al. 1997). The evolutionary link between Topo VI and Spo11 thus testifies for a surprising connection between Archaea and the origin of sex in Eukarya.

A few years after its discovery in archaea, a closely related Topo IIB was detected in plant. The *A. thaliana* genome harbors three SPO11 genes (homologues of the Topo VI A subunit) but also one gene encoding a homologue of the Topo VI B subunit. This suggested that a complete Topo VI was operational in plants. Although this enzyme has not yet been purified, genetic evidences now strongly support this hypothesis (Hartung et al. 2002; Hartung and Puchta 2001; Sugimoto-Shirasu et al. 2002, 2005; Yin et al. 2002). Mutations in any one of the two subunits of Topo VI from *A. thaliana* has a dramatic effect on plant growth and they produce a dwarf phenotype. This results from inhibition of chromosomal polyploidization, a process known as endoreduplication. Indeed, normal plant cells expend their size by multiplying the number of their chromosomes up to 32, and the size of the plant itself is directly linked to the size of the cells. In Topo VI mutants, multiplication stops at eight chromosomes copies, reducing cell size. The dramatic effect induced by the inhibition of endoreduplication is illustrated in Fig. 1.7 by the differences in the leave surfaces of a wild type and a Topo IV mutant of *A. thaliana*. The leaves of

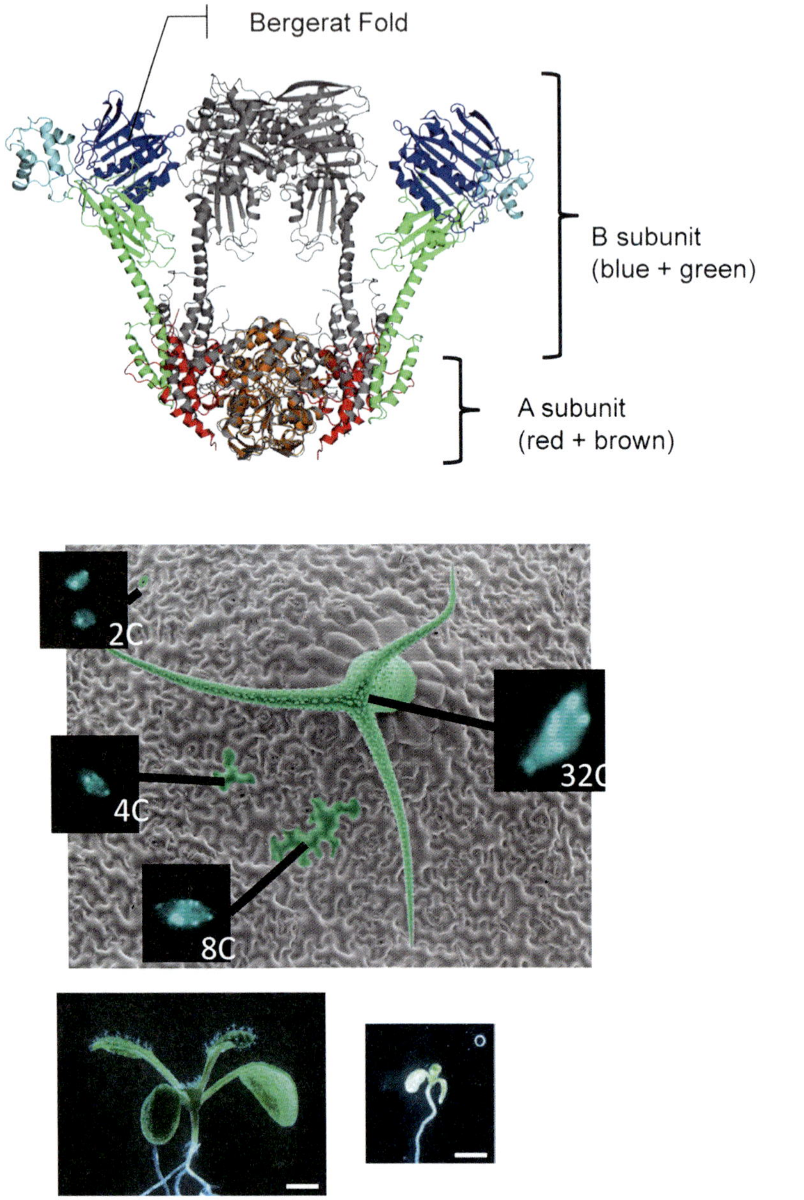

Fig. 1.7 *Upper panel*: structure of *Sulfolobus shibatae* DNA topoisomerase VI (type IIB DNA topoisomerase). The different domains of the open form whose structure has been resolved by X-rays diffraction are in colors. The closed form whose structure has been modeled is in *gray* (adapted from Graille et al. 2008). *Lower panel*: Comparison of wild type and Topo IIB mutant of *Arabidopsis thaliana*. (**a**) The surface of *A. thaliana* leaves is made of cells with different number of homologous chromosomes (from 2N to 32N). This number determines the size of the cells and of the plant. Cells with 32 homologous chromosomes exhibit tricorns that form filaments at the leaves surfaces in the wild type plant. (**b**) In a mutant of the Topo IIB B subunit (HYP6), cells with 16 and 32 homologous chromosomes are absent; as a consequence, plant is small with soft leaves (courtesy of Dr Sugimoto-Shirazu)

A. thaliana are characterized by giant trichomes cells with 32 chromosomes. In Topo VI mutants, these cells are absent and leaves are both small and smooth.

The discovery of Topo IIB has provided us with a second model of type II DNA topoisomerases and raised interesting questions regarding the interaction of drugs and Topo II. Indeed, although the A subunits of Topo IIA and IIB are structurally unrelated, Topo IIB appears to be sensitive to several antibiotics and antitumor drugs that mainly interact with the A subunit of Topo IIA during the cleavage step of the topoisomerization reaction (Bergerat et al. 1994, D. Gadelle, unpublished observation). It will be important to determine precisely the similarities and differences between the mode of action of these drugs on Topo IIA and Topo IIB, with the aim to target specifically one or the other. Indeed, Topo IIB could become important drug targets of their own, since, for instance, genome analysis suggests the existence of a Topo IIB in *Plasmodium* species (Malik et al. 2007).

Finally, the discovery of Topo IIB has dramatically exemplified the importance to take into account the diversity of the living world to mine for new forms of already well-known enzymatic activity. For a long time, such search has been mainly driven by the curiosity of a few scientists and success was dependent on both luck and the choice of the good organism. After the genomic revolution, our search for new enzymes can be guided by *in silico* data and, as a consequence, the search for new model systems could be rationalized. Hence, as new genomes' sequences become available, it become possible to draw an exhaustive landscape of topoisomerases covering more or less the entire living world. We will briefly summarize the state of the art of this landscape below, although we should remain aware that many lineages (kingdoms) in the three domains of life are still only known from their 16S rRNA (phylotype). One could therefore expect some surprises from a project such as the phylogeny-driven "Genomic Encyclopedia of Bacteria and Archaea" (Wu et al. 2009) and similar ones in eukaryotes. This is well illustrated by the recent discovery of eukaryotic-like Topo IB in the sequence of two genomes from Thaumarchaea, a group of Archaea that was for a long time only known by their phylotypes (Brochier-Armanet et al. 2008b).

1.7 Phylogenomics of DNA Topoisomerases

In this chapter, I will illustrate the phylogeny of the various DNA topoisomerase families by schematic trees, adapted (and updated) from phylogenies performed by Simonetta Gribaldo (Forterre et al. 2007).

1.7.1 Topo IA (Fig. 1.8)

Until recently, one or several Topo IA genes were present in all genomes whose sequences were available; Topo IA being the only universal DNA topoisomerases. However, Topo IA genes turned out to be absent from the genomes of two

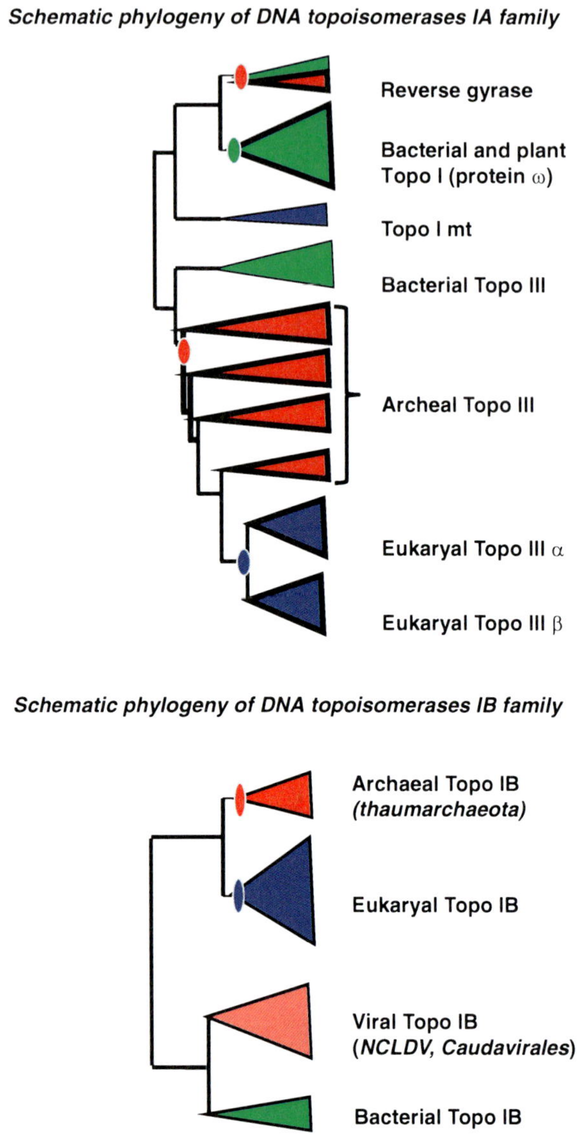

Fig. 1.8 Schematic phylogenetic tree of type IA (*upper panel*) and Type IB (*lower panel*) DNA topoisomerases (adapted from Forterre et al. 2007). Bacterial DNA topoisomerases are in *green*, archaeal DNA topoisomerases in *red* and eukaryal DNA topoisomerases in *blues*. *Circles* indicate that the corresponding DNA topoisomerase subfamily was probably present in the last common ancestor of the domain

Thaumarchaea that harbor a Topo IB gene instead (Brochier-Armanet et al. 2008b). Phylogenetic analysis identifies several monophyletic groups of Topo IA, but cannot resolve with confidence their evolutionary relationships.

A first group of Topo IA is formed by bacterial orthologues of the *E. coli* protein ω, often simply called bacterial Topo I (gene *topA*). The protein ω is universal in Bacteria and was therefore most likely present in the Last Bacterial Common Ancestor (LBCA). The protein ω has been transferred from Bacteria to Plants with

DNA gyrase (see below). Plants are the organisms with the greatest complement of DNA topoisomerases, since they contain the classical eukaryotic DNA topoisomerases (IA, IB, IIA), the bacterial ones (protein ω and DNA gyrase) and a Topo IIB. Topo IA related to bacterial proteins ω were also transferred in the genomes of two giant related viruses of the NCLDV superfamily (NucleoCytoplasmic Large DNA Viruses), the Acanthamoeba polyphaga mimivirus (Raoult et al. 2004), and the Cafeteria roenbergensis *virus (Crov)* (Fischer et al. 2010). These viruses infect protists that prey on bacteria, suggesting that they have acquired their bacterial protein ω from a bacterium living as an endosymbiony in their infected hosts.

The closest relative of bacterial protein ω in the Topo IA family is the topoisomerase domain of reverse gyrase. In agreement with this grouping, reverse gyrase cleaves, preferentially, DNA at sequences that are similar to those cleaved by *E. coli* protein ω (Kovalsky et al. 1990). Several hyperthermophilic archaea of the phylum Crenarchaea and bacteria of the order Aquificales contain two reverse gyrases that originated by gene duplication in these respective lineages (Brochier-Armanet and Forterre 2007). The transcription pattern of the two *Sulfolobus solfataricus* reverse gyrases indicates a functional differentiation of these two proteins, suggesting at least two different functional roles for reverse gyrase in vivo (Garnier and Nadal 2009).

A group of TopoIA more closely related to bacterial protein ω and reverse gyrase than to eukaryotic Topo III (see below) has been recently identified in the mitochondria of Trypanosoma (Socca and Shapiro 2008). These Topo IA, dubbed TopIA(mt) are required to resolve late theta structures in the replication of kinetoplastid DNA (kDNA). Being essential for the survival of the parasite and very divergent from classical eukaryotic Topo IA (Topo III, see below), Topo IA(mt) is a promising new target for drugs against Trypanosomids.

Beside protein ω, several phylums of bacteria, such as Proteobacteria, Firmicutes, Bacteroidetes, or Verrucomicrobiales, contain a homologue of the *E. coli* Topo III (gene *topB*). Topo III homologues are missing from other important bacterial phylums, such as Cyanobacteria, *Thermus/Deinococcus*, Planctomycetes, Chlamydiae, or else Thermotogales. It is thus difficult to decide if Topo III was already present in the LBCA or if it has been introduced in the bacterial domain by plasmids or viruses (Topo III being indeed encoded by a few plasmids). Finally, several related groups of Firmicutes harbor a second quite divergent Topo III, which has been called Topo IIIβ. Unlike classical bacterial Topo III, The Topo IIIβ of *Bacillus cereus*, only exhibits weak relaxation activity and no decatenation activity on replication intermediates (Li et al. 2006).

All archaea, except some thaumarchaea, harbor one or two Topo IA. These archaeal Topo IA branch in between bacterial and eukaryotic Topo III in the Topo IA tree. In agreement with this grouping, the Topo III from the archaeon *Sulfolobus solfataricus* cleaves preferentially DNA at sequences that bear more resemblance with sequences preferred by *E. coli* Topo III than by *E. coli* protein ω (Dai et al. 2003). These data suggest naming these enzymes Topo III as well (Forterre et al. 2007). Four subgroups of archaeal Topo III can be identified by phylogenetic analysis and some archaea harbor two Topo III of different subgroups. The last archaeal common ancestor (LACA) thus contained at least one Topo III, possibly more.

Only a few studies have been reported on archaeal Topo III (Chen and Huang 2006). In particular, it is not known if archaeal Topo III interact with helicase in dissolvasome–like structure and which helicase(s) is (are) involved. It should be interesting to know if some archaeal Topo III could also cooperate with Topo VI to control the level of superhelicity and/or to help in the segregation of chromosomes.

All eukaryotes harbor at least one Topo III. Metazoans, plants, and some protists (but not fungi) contain two Topo III named Top3α and Top3β (the single *S. cerevisiae* Topo III corresponding to Topo IIIα) (Forterre et al. 2007; Scocca and Shapiro 2008). The Last Eukaryotic Common Ancestor (LECA) thus probably contained already two Topo III genes. Phylogenetic analysis indicates that TopIIIα and TopIIIβ originated probably by duplication in the proto-eukaryotic lineage and are more closely related to one of the four archaeal subgroups (Forterre et al. 2007). Archaea and eukaryotic Topo III are thus paraphyletic, another incongruence between the Topo IA tree and the universal tree based on rRNA and universal proteins. Most studies on eukaryotic Topo III apparently have been done on TopIIIα, although the literature is usually not clear on that point. To make things more complicated, Topo IIIα exists in two versions in vertebrates, one present in the nucleus and the other in the mitochondria. The mitochondrial version is created by alternative translation initiation of the same mRNA that encodes the nuclear version (Wang et al. 2002).

1.7.2 Topo IB (Fig. 1.8)

For a long time, Topo IB (swivelase) was only known in eukaryotes (where it is systematically present) and in poxviruses (a subgroup of NCLDV). Later on, Topo IB genes were discovered in the genomes of some bacteria (Krogh and Shuman 2002) of mimivirus (Raoult et al. 2004; Benaroch et al. 2006) and of Thaumarchaea (Brochier-Armanet et al. 2008b). In eukaryotes, Trypanosoma and Leishmania harbor an atypical heterodimeric Topo IB (Bodley et al. 2003). The large subunit contains an additional N-terminal domain fused to part of the core Topo IB domain, whereas the small subunit harbors the C-terminal Topo IB region containing the active tyrosine. This enzyme is the focus of active work to identify new agents against Trypanosomes and Leishmania (Das et al. 2008). In vertebrates, the DNA topo IB gene has been duplicated, and one of the two Topo IB, Top1mt, is now specifically present in mitochondria (Zhang et al. 2001).

The eukaryotic and archaeal Topo IB group together in phylogenetic analysis and are larger than their bacterial and viral counterparts, indicating that Topo IB was probably present in the last common ancestor of Archaea and Eukarya (Brochier-Armanet et al. 2008b). The patchy distribution of Topo IB in Bacteria and its presence in viruses suggest that this enzyme might have been introduced in Bacteria from viruses or plasmids. This hypothesis is supported by the recent discovery of a Topo IB encoded in the genomes of NCLDV other than poxviruses (mimivirus and *CroV)* (Raoult et al. 2004; Fischer et al. 2010) and in the genome of a giant bacteriovirus (Yamada et al. 2010). Whereas original phylogenetic analyses suggested that mimivirus Topo IB had been recruited from bacteria (as in the case of ω protein), new analyses including these sequences group all viral Topo IB, including those of mimivirus, in a monophyletic cluster that itself groups with bacterial Topo IB (C. Brochier-Armanet and PF unpublished result).

1.7.3 Topo IC

As already mentioned, Topo IC illustrates to the extreme the diversity of situation encountered in analyzing the phylogenomic distribution of DNA topoisomerases. Whereas Topo IA is nearly ubiquitous, Topo IC has been detected until now in only one archaeal genome (*Methanopyrus kandleri*). Since this enzyme is complex, corresponding to a large new fold, it is unlikely that it originated suddenly de novo in that lineage. Phylogenetic analyses have shown that *Methanopyrus kandleri* is not an early branching archaeon, as sometimes proposed, but emerged within euryarcheae, at the base of so called group I methanogens (Brochier et al. 2004). The most likely explanation to the loneliness of Topo IC is that this enzyme was recruited by *M. kandleri* from a virus/plasmid whose free form has not yet been isolated.

1.7.4 Topo IIA (Fig. 1.9)

All bacteria and eukaryotes (and some archaea) contain one or several Topo IIA. Phylogenetic analysis shows a clear distinction between eukaryotic and bacterial Topo IIA (Forterre et al. 2007). Bacterial Topo IIA include gyrase and Topo IV. DNA gyrases, which form a monophyletic group of closely related sequences, are present in all bacteria. A DNA gyrase was therefore certainly present in the LBCA. Interestingly, the group of J. Berger isolated and characterized recently a "DNA gyrase" without gyrase activity in *Aquifex aeolicus*, the most hyperthermophilic bacterium known today. This "gyrase" harbors a modified GyrA box in its C-terminal domain (Guipaud and Forterre 2001) and phylogenetic analysis indicates that it has "recently" lost its gyrase activity (Tretter et al. 2010). It is tempting to suggest that this loss corresponds to an adaptation to life at high temperature (*A. aeolicus* contains two reverse gyrase genes). However, one should remind that a few *bona fide* hyperthermophiles, such as *Thermotoga maritima* (a bacterium) and *Archaeoglobus fulgidus* (an archaeon) have an active DNA gyrase (Guipaud et al. 1997; Lopez-Garcia et al. 2000).

Several DNA gyrases are present in Archaea of the phylum euryarchaeota. In contrast, DNA gyrase is absent in other euryarchaea as well as in crenarchaea and thaumarchaea, the two other major archaeal phyla. All archaea harboring gyrase are mesophiles, with the exception of *A. fulgidus*. Some of these archaea (halophiles and methanogens) are sensitive to gyrase coumarins inhibitors, indicating that gyrase is essential in these archaea (Sioud et al. 1988; Sioud and Forterre 1989,

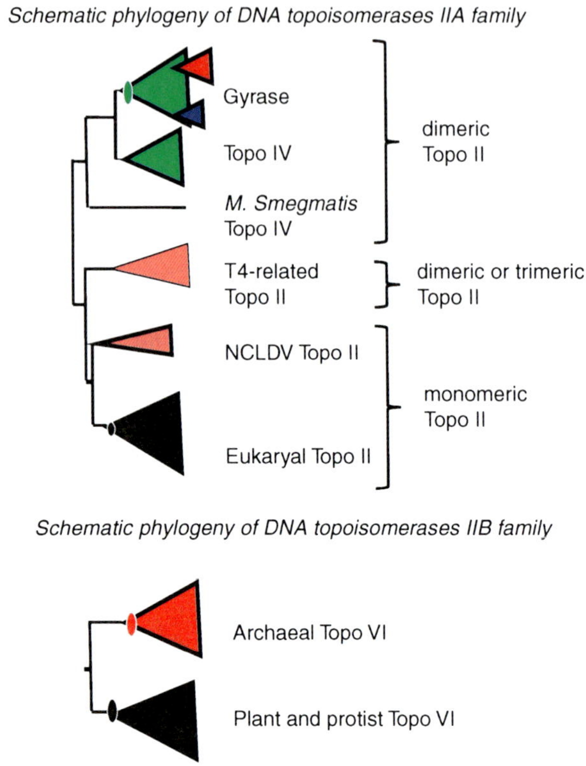

Fig. 1.9 Schematic phylogenetic tree of type IIA DNA topoisomerases (*upper panel*) and type IIB DNA topoisomerases (*lower panel*) (adapted from Forterre et al. 2007). Bacterial DNA topoisomerases are in *green*, archaeal DNA topoisomerases in *red* and eukaryal DNA topoisomerases in *blues*. *Circles* indicate that the corresponding DNA topoisomerase subfamily was probably present in the last common ancestor of the domain

Holmes and Dyall-Smith 1991). An archaeal gyrase was purified and characterized from *Thermoplasma acidophilum* by Yamashiro and Yamagishi (2005) who could confirm its supercoiling activity in vitro. Phylogenetic analysis has clearly shown that archaeal gyrases have been recruited from bacteria by lateral gene transfer (Forterre et al. 2007).

Bacterial gyrase genes have been also transferred to plants, via the chloroplast route. The *A. thaliana* DNA gyrase subunits branch with those of cyanobacteria in phylogenetic analysis and can complement *E. coli* gyrase mutants (Forterre et al. 2007; Cho et al. 2004). Genetic analyses have shown that the DNA gyrase of *A. thaliana* is involved in the segregation of chloroplast DNA (Cho et al. 2004). Interestingly, DNA gyrase of *A. thaliana* is targeted to reach both chloroplasts and mitochondria (Wall et al. 2004). DNA gyrase genes are also present in the human malarial parasite *Plasmodium falciparum* and in other *Plasmodium* species (most likely via the chloroplastic route too, through secondary endosymbiois). The DNA gyrase of *P. falciparum* is indeed targeted exclusively to the apicoplast, an indispensable plasmid-like organelle, and is essential for apicoplast DNA replication (Dar et al. 2007; Raghu Ram et al. 2007). Beside Topo VI, already discussed, the DNA gyrase of *Plasmodium* should become another target for the search of new antimalarial drugs (Garcia-Estrada et al. 2010). *Plasmodium is* indeed sensitive to specific DNA gyrase inhibitors, such as fluoroquinolones (Anquetin et al. 2004). It should be especially interesting to find drugs that would target both gyrase and Topo VI (absent in human), without affecting the human Topo IIA, to prevent the rapid emergence of dug resistance.

Several bacteria contain orthologues of *E. coli* Topo IV, or other Topo IIA without gyrase activity but closely related to Topo IV and DNA gyrases. These enzymes are usually named Topo IV, although they do not form a monophyletic group in phylogenetic analysis (Forterre et al. 2007). It is unclear if a Topo IV was indeed present in the LBCA and if Topo IV derived from DNA gyrase or vice versa. An unusual "Topo IV" has been discovered in *Mycobacterium smegmatis* (Jain and Nagaraja 2005). Although this Topo IIA forms a monophyletic group with DNA gyrases and Topo IV in the Topo IIA tree (Forterre et al. 2007), it is very divergent from both of them. Jain and Nagaraja (2005) reported that this atypical *M. smegmatis* Topo IIA introduce positive supercoiling in vitro. This enzyme thus could be a very interesting target for structural and evolutionary studies of Topo IIA.

The genomes of many bacteriophages related to T4 have been sequenced in recent years. They infect hosts from very divergent bacterial species. Topo II encoded by these viruses form a monophyletic group that branch in-between bacterial and eukaryotic Topo IIA in the Topo IIA tree, very far from the Topo IIA of their hosts (Forterre et al. 2007). We have seen previously that the T4 Topo II is a heterohexamer. However, in most viruses of the T4 superfamily, the Topo IIA is a heterotetramer, with fusion of the homologues of T4 genes 60 and 39.

All eukaryotes encode one or two closely related homodimeric Topo IIA. In particular, mammals contain two nuclear isoforms of Topo IIA, dubbed Topo IIα (Top2α) and Topo IIβ (Top2β), and a mitochondrial Topo IIA derived from nuclear Topo IIβ by proteolysis (Low et al. 2003). These enzymes are very divergent from bacterial Topo IIA in term of sequence (except for conserved motives). In particular, their C-terminal domains are unrelated to those of bacterial Topo IIA. These C-terminal domains are unstructured and themselves poorly conserved between different eukaryotic Topo II. They seem to be targets for the regulation of DNA topoisomerase activities. The great divergence between eukaryotic and bacterial Topo IIA and the fact that eukaryotic Topo IIA have no archaeal orthologue is intriguing. It is unlikely that eukaryotic Topo IIA originated from bacterial ones via the mitochondrial route, considering the extent of their divergence. In agreement with this assumption, topoisomerases that clearly migrated via the mitochondrial or chloroplastic routes, such as DNA gyrase and protein ω, branch within their original clad in phylogenetic trees (Forterre et al. 2007) and some of them can still complement their bacterial homologue in vivo (Cho et al. 2004).

The divergence between eukaryotic and bacterial Topo IIA, together with the position of T4 Topo IIA in-between those two groups has suggested a viral origin for Topo IIA (Gadelle et al. 2003; Forterre and Gadelle 2009). A viral origin for eukaryotic Topo IIA is indeed suggested by the existence of Topo II encoded by NCLDV that branches at the base of the eukaryotic Topo IIA tree (Forterre et al. 2007). These enzymes lack the C-terminal domain present in other Topo IIA and are therefore the smallest known Topo IIA. The Topo IIA from two Chlorella viruses have been purified and biochemically characterized. The DNA of the Chlorella virus PBCV-1 (Paramecium bursaria chlorella virus-A) is highly methylated. Interestingly, PBCV-1 Topo IIA exhibit a high DNA cleavage activity which is reduced on DNA methylated DNA substrates (Dickey et al. 2005), suggesting that these enzyme can discriminate between viral and host DNA.

1.7.5 Topo IIB (Fig. 1.9)

Topo IIB are present in all Archaea, except Thermoplasmatales which contain DNA gyrase. In Archaea that also harbor a DNA gyrase, the genes encoding the two Topo VI subunits co-localize with the two genes encoding DNA gyrase, suggesting a functional linkage between DNA gyrase and Topo VI in these archaea. Several Topo VI present in archaea containing DNA gyrase posses a short additional domain in the A subunit with an immunoglobulin-like fold whose function is unknown (Schoeffler and Berger 2008). It is tempting to speculate that this domain could allow Topo VI to associate with DNA gyrase. Topo IIB have been transferred in a handful of bacteria, where they also coexist with Topo IIA (Forterre et al. 2007).

In Eukarya, Topo IIBs are present in plants and some protists. Phylogenetic analysis suggests that Topo IIB was present in the common ancestor of Archaea and Eukarya (Malik et al. 2007). The single orthologue of the Topo VI A subunit in opisthokonts (Spo11, called Rec12 in *Saccharomyces pombe*) is involved in meiosis and the structural studies of the archaeal enzyme has provided an important tool to dissect the function of eukaryotic Spo11. Plants have three orthologues of the Topo VI A subunit, two being possibly involved in meiosis. Some protists contain several orthologues of the Topo VI A subunit (two for instance in *Plasmodium*). Surprisingly, phylogenetic analysis of Topo VI A subunit homologues in eukaryotes cannot allow to discriminate between the protist proteins corresponding to Spo11 and those corresponding to the Topo VI A subunit, suggesting a complex history of these proteins in the eukaryotic domain (S. Gribaldo, unpublished observation).

1.7.6 DNA Topoisomerases and the Tree of Life

Table 1.2 indicates the families and subfamilies of DNA topoisomerase that were most likely present in the last common ancestors of each domain of life (inferred from phylogenomic analysis, see Forterre and Gadelle 2009). In some cases, a question mark indicates that this question remains open. This table highlights the fact that most DNA topoisomerase families or subfamilies are present in only one or two domains, or even in a subset of a particular domain. Interestingly, very similar patterns of phylogenomic distribution are observed with other proteins involved in various mechanisms dealing with DNA (replication, repair, deoxynucleotide biosynthesis) (for the case of DNA polymerases, see Filée et al. 2002, for ribonucleotide

Table 1.2 DNA topoisomerases present in the ancestors of the three domains of life (LUCA) and in ancestors of each domain. The data are from comparative genomic analyses (see Forterre and Gadelle 2009). Question marks indicate uncertainty on the presence or not of these topoisomerases in the ancestor

Last bacterial common ancestor
DNA gyrase
Protein ω
Topo III?
Topo IV?
Last archaeal common ancestor
Reverse gyrase
Topo III
Topo IB
Topo VI
Last Eukaryal Common Ancestor
Topo IB
Topo II
Topo III α
Topo III β
Topo VI?
Last Universal Common Ancestor
Topo IA?
Gene transfers
Bacterial DNA gyrase to some Archaea
Bacterial DNA gyrase to Viridiplantae
Bacterial protein ω to Viridiplantae
Archaeal Topo VI to few Bacteria
Archaeal reverse gyrase to thermophilic bacteria

reductases, see Lundin et al. 2010). Several hypotheses can explain the puzzling phylogenomic distribution of enzymes involved in DNA synthesis and manipulation (Mushegian and Koonin 1996; Edgell and Doolittle 1997; Leipe et al. 1999; Forterre 1999, 2002b).

One can first imagine that LUCA already harbored one or even several members of all families and subfamilies of these proteins (in our case DNA topoisomerases) and that several of them were lost in the different stem branches leading to the three domains, and/or during the internal diversification of these domains. This hypothesis implies a rather complex LUCA with a DNA genome and, for instance, at least two different DNA replication mechanisms (and both Topo IIA and Topo IIB). LUCA was, for sure, an already rather complex cell, since it contained ribosomes with at least 34 proteins (those present in the universal set), a complete set of tRNA synthetases, and several tRNA modification enzymes (Koonin 2003). Furthermore, recent data suggest that LUCA was more sophisticated than previously thought, with possibly already cellular compartmentation (Forterre and Gribaldo 2010).

The scenario of a complex LUCA thus appears at first sight reasonable. However, such scenario cannot easily explain some data, such as the presence of Topo V in *M. kandleri* only, or else the existence of specific viral versions in several DNA topoisomerases families.

A second hypothesis is that LUCA only harbored a subset of modern proteins involved in DNA metabolism (for instance one Topo IA and one Topo II (A or B) in the case of DNA topoisomerases) and that others were introduced later on, during domain diversification. These new proteins might have been invented in these lineages or recruited from now extinct lineages of cells or viruses that existed at the time of LUCA or shortly after the divergence of the three domains. This scenario also implies that some enzymes were displaced in modern lineage by functional analogues. For instance, if LUCA harbored a Topo IIA, this enzyme was displaced by Topo IIB in the lineage leading to Archaea.

Finally, one can explain the odd phylogenomic distribution of DNA synthesis and replication proteins by assuming that LUCA still had an RNA genome (Mushegian and Koonin 1996; Forterre 2002b). In that case, DNA and DNA replication mechanisms (including DNA topoisomerases) were introduced independently in the different stem branches, and/or during the internal diversification of the three domains of life. The idea of an RNA-based LUCA seems odd to biologists who use to think of the RNA world as a world of RNA molecules thriving in an abiotic soup (the original concept of the RNA world indeed). However, since the transition of RNA to DNA has required complex protein-enzymes, such as ribonucleotide reductases and reverse transcriptases, it is clear that the late RNA world was in fact a word of complex cells with RNA genomes (being able to produce sophisticated enzymes) (Forterre 2005). LUCA might have been such a complex RNA cell, whose RNA genome was faithfully replicated and repaired (Poole and Logan 2005).

The hypothesis of an RNA-based LUCA seems in contradiction with the existence of a few enzymes working at the DNA level in the universal protein set, such as DNA dependent RNA polymerases or Topo IA (Leipe et al. 1999). However, these enzymes might have been introduced independently in the three domains post-LUCA or changed their specificity (from RNA to DNA) after the transition from RNA to DNA genomes. For instance, the incongruence between the Topo IA and the rRNA trees suggests that Topo IA was in fact not present in LUCA but that various subfamilies of Topo IA were introduced independently in the three domains (Forterre et al. 2007). Alternatively, if LUCA harbored a Topo IA, this enzyme might have been involved in RNA metabolism, since both *E. coli* and eukaryotic Topo III exhibit site-specific ribonuclease activity (DiGate and Marians 1992; Sekiguchi and Shuman 1997).

In summary, it is not possible today to determine with present data when DNA genomes (and DNA topoisomerases) originated, i.e., before or after LUCA. This question will be possibly solved in the future when more sequence data will be available from presently poorly studied cellular and viral groups (in particular, those many groups of archaea, bacteria, and eukarya – and their viruses – for which we still have no cultivated representatives), but we cannot bet on this. In any case, in all three hypotheses previously described, one has to explain how DNA topoisomerases originated in the first place?

1.8 Origin of DNA Topoisomerases

Since RNA obviously preceded DNA (a modified RNA form) in the course of evolution (Freeland et al. 1999; Forterre 2002b, 2005), one can safely assume that many enzymes involved in DNA metabolism originated from enzymes initially involved in RNA metabolism (for instance, DNA polymerases from RNA polymerases). However, this assumption cannot be made in the case of DNA topoisomerases, since RNA topoisomerases do not exist (or have not yet been discovered). The genomes of complex RNA cells might have been composed of multiple chromosomes of small linear dsRNA molecules (less than 100 kb). In that case, "DNA" topoisomerases only appeared after the transition from RNA to DNA genomes genomes. It has been suggested that DNA topoisomerases appeared indeed relatively late in the evolution of the DNA replication machinery, i.e., after the origin of DNA primase/polymerase, helicases, and accessory proteins required to produce long DNA duplexes (Forterre and Gadelle 2009). But why DNA and DNA replication mechanisms originated in the first place?

Two hypotheses have been proposed to explain the transition from RNA to DNA, either DNA was selected over RNA because of its greater stability (due to the lack of the reactive oxygen in 2′ of the ribose) or because the first organisms with DNA genomes were immune to mechanisms used by their competitors to inactivate RNA genomes (Lazcano et al. 1988; Forterre 2002b). Both hypotheses can be somehow combined if DNA originated first in a viral lineage since, beside making viral DNA immune to cellular mechanism targeting RNA, DNA genomes could have retained their infectious potential for longer time than RNA genomes when stored in virions without possibility of active repair. If DNA first originated in a virus, with first DNA viruses infecting RNA cells, various mechanisms of DNA replication might have originated independently in different viral lineages before DNA was transferred to cells (Forterre 2002b; Koonin et al. 2006). This scenario could explain why DNA viruses (or plasmids derived from viruses) encode many enzymes involved in DNA replication, recombination, and/or repair, that have presently no homologues in the three cellular domains, such as SFIII helicases and rolling-circle initiation proteins, or which have only distant relatives, such as protein-primed DNA polymerases of the B family or viral specific DNA topoisomerases. In other word, the greater diversity of DNA replication mechanisms in the virosphere would testify for the origin of these mechanisms among viruses, much like the greater diversity of genetic traits in Africans compared to other populations testifies for the origin of *Homo sapiens* in Africa.

The viral origin of DNA (and DNA replication proteins, including DNA topoisomerases) can easily explain why enzymes involved in DNA metabolism exhibit phylogenetic patterns that do not easily fits with the universal tree of life. One can imagine that several non homologous (but analogous) proteins originated independently in different viral lineages to perform the same task (replicate DNA, unwind the double-helix or solve topological problems) and that only a subset of them were transferred later on more or less randomly in cellular lineages. In this scenario, viral specific DNA topoisomerase such as Topo IIA of T4-related viruses, Topo IIA, and Topo IB of NCLDV would correspond to subfamilies of DNA topoisomerases that have never been transferred to cells.

The viral origin of DNA topoisomerases is supported by the existence of structural and/or mechanistic similarities between some DNA topoisomerases and viral (plasmidic) specific proteins. In particular, a viral origin for Topo IB is suggested by structural and mechanistic similarities of these enzymes with viral integrase (tyrosine recombinases) (Cheng et al. 1998) and protelomerases that generate hairpin ends at the extremities of chromosomal viral or plasmidic linear DNA (Huang et al. 2004). This probable evolutionary link is strengthened by the fact that tyrosine recombinases exhibit DNA topoisomerase activity in vitro. In fact, Topo IB appears to be a subfamily of a large family of viral/plasmidic enzymes involved in viral integration and/or replication.

More generally, DNA topoisomerases appears mechanistically related to the large class of enzymes involved in the resolution and/or recombination of viral and plasmid genomes or else in viral/plasmidic replication, such as relaxase, transposases, integrases, or site-specific endonuclease involved in the initiation of rolling circle (RC) replication (Koepsel et al. 1985; Pansegrau et al. 1994; Jo and Topal 1995; Marsin et al. 2000; Yang 2010). For instance, Yang suggested that serine recombinase, mostly encoded by plasmids and viruses, use a strand passage mechanism for DNA recombination, reminiscent of DNA topoisomerization by Topo II (Yang 2010). The Rep proteins involved in RC replication of viruses and plasmids are also mechanistically related to DNA topoisomerases; they exhibit both nuclease and ligase activities and form a phosphotyrosine link in 5′ of the DNA after cleavage, resembling Topo IA. Strikingly, these Rep proteins often exhibit DNA topoisomerase activity in vitro (Koepsel et al. 1985; Marsin et al. 2000). The various families of DNA topoisomerases thus probably originated from endonuclease able to produce transient nicks into DNA for various purposes. Topo I probably evolved from single-stranded endonucleases, whereas Topo II originated later. The catalytic subunits of Topo IIA and IIB might have originated first by the dimerization of a single-stranded endonucleases to produce double-strand endonuclease. The endonuclease activity of Spo11 (a Topo IIB subunit A homologue) in meiotic recombination could be a relic of such activity. Two different dimeric nucleases, associated with evolutionary related Bergerat, fold proteins to produce Topo IIA and IIB, respectively.

As other DNA replication proteins, DNA topoisomerases were built by combining protein domains common to various RNA or DNA manipulating enzymes. These domains were recruited via natural selection during the evolution of DNA replication apparatus from the melting pot of protein folds created during the late RNA/protein world. The same folds were often used for different proteins that cannot be considered as true homologues, even if they share homologous folds in their structure. This is the case for Topo IA, Topo IIA, and Topo IIB that share the Toprim fold (for Topoisomerase primase) (Aravind et al. 1998; Berger et al. 1998). Beside DNA topoisomerase, this fold is present in the catalytic center of DnaG-like primase, nucleases of OLD family, RecR family of DNA repair proteins and serine recombinases (Aravind et al. 1998; Yang 2010). The Toprim domain corresponds to an ancient fold that was probably already present in the RNA world since it has been detected in ribonuclease (Rnase M5) involved in 5S rRNA maturation (Allemand et al. 2005). Recently, resolution of the structure of a eukaryotic Topo IIA covalently linked to a cleaved DNA molecule has suggested a common and atypical mechanism for metal DNA cleavage by Topo IA and Topo II (A and B) (Schmidt et al. 2010). It will be interesting to determine if this mechanism is also shared by RNAse M5. If this is the case, it might be that the origin of the DNA cleavage mechanism of major several DNA topoisomerases can be traced back to the RNA world.

1.9 Perspectives

The discovery of DNA supercoiling and DNA topoisomerases has opened a fascinating field of investigation to biologists. The rich history of this field has been driven by inspired scientists, theoretical considerations, serendipitous discoveries, and technical developments. In recent years, the wealth of data obtained from genome sequencing has progressively opened new lines of investigations. However, although the outcome of comparative genomics and phylogenomic studies has fully exposed now the diversity of DNA topoisomerases, the prejudice toward the first historically characterized ones is still there, and many molecular biologists and biochemists have still to take into account new visions introduced by evolutionists. For instance, very few laboratories are working on plant DNA topoisomerases or on DNA topoisomerases from protists. Eukaryotic Topo IIB have not yet been purified and characterized and generally speaking, our knowledge of Topo IIB lack well behind those of Topo IIA. The studies of drugs acting on DNA topoisomerases have been restricted to a few DNA topoisomerases that are especially important targets for therapeutic action. This make a lot of sense in terms of immediate benefit, but I would bet that more drugs-targets, important for both fundamental and applied research, are hidden in the world of DNA topoisomerases. Mycobacteria resistant to current antibiotics and various eukaryotic parasites (Plasmodium, kinetoplastids, Leishmania) already appear to be promising targets for new therapeutic applications of DNA topoisomerase research. In that context, it is worth noting that the prokaryote/eukaryote division is still operational and potentially misleading for drug development. Indeed, drugs labeled once and for all as antibiotics are then rarely tried against cancer cells, and drugs labeled as once and for all antitumor are then rarely try against bacteria, although they often target proteins with homologues in these two domains. The focus on a few model enzymes also led to underestimate the diversity within protein family, and one often still don't know how this diversity can translate in term of drug sensitivity. Considering how research on DNA topology and topoisomerases unfold (the historical pattern), and how various topoisomerases are actually related to each other (the evolutionary pattern) can help to bypass some artificial barriers that probably still slows down the discovery process.

Finally, one can predict that the Pandora box opened by the genomic era will not dry up soon. New subfamilies and possibly new families of DNA topoisomerases should be hidden within genomes already sequenced or yet to be sequenced. This is especially true if the hypothesis of viral (plasmidic) origin for DNA topoisomerases is correct. We only know a minute fraction of viral and plasmidic (VP) diversity and the enormous amount of VP in the biosphere encode an incredible number of genes encoding ORFans proteins. It is reasonable to assume that some of them encode new DNA topoisomerases that are waiting for adventurous biochemists. The quest for these new DNA topoisomerases should be a must for curious scientists willing to complete the exploration of the molecular biosphere.

Acknowledgment I thank Daniele Gadelle and Marc Nadal for some references and critical comments on some aspect of this manuscript. I am grateful to Anna Bizard for the two-D gels in Fig. 1.3 and Sugimoto-Shirasu for the spectacular pictures of *Arabidopsis* wild type and Topo IIB mutant.

References

Adachi Y, Luke M, Laemmli UK (1991) Chromosome assembly in vitro : Topoisomerase II is required for condensation Cell 64:137–148

Aggarwal M, Brosh RM (2009) WRN helicase defective in the premature aging disorder Werner syndrome genetically interacts with topoisomerase 3 and restores the top3 slow growth phenotype of sgs1 top3. Aging (Albany NY) 1(2):219–233

Allemand F, Mathy N, Brechemier-Baey D, Condon C (2005) The 5S rRNA maturase, ribonuclease M5, is a Toprim domain family member. Nucleic Acids Res 33(13):4368–4376

Anquetin G, Rouquayrol M, Mahmoudi N, Santillana-Hayat M, Gozalbes R, Greiner J, Farhati K, Derouin F (2004) Synthesis of new fluoroquinolones and evaluation of their in vitro activity on Toxoplasma gondii and Plasmodium spp. Guedj R, Vierling P. Bioorg Med Chem Lett 14(11):2773–2776

Aravind L, Leipe DD, Koonin EV (1998) Toprim a conserved catalytic domain in type IA and II topoisomerases, DnaG-type primases, OLD family nucleases and RecR proteins. Nucleic Acids Res 26:4205–4213

Atomi H, Matsumi R, Imanaka T (2004) Reverse gyrase is not a prerequisite for hyperthermophilic life. J Bacteriol 186:4829–4833

Baldi MJ, Benedetti P, Mattoccia E, Tocchini-Valentini GP (1980) In vitro catenation and decatenation of DNA and a novel eucaryotic ATP-dependent topoisomerase. Cell 20:461–467

Baxter J, Diffley JF (2008) Topoisomerase II inactivation prevents the completion of DNA replication in budding yeast. Mol Cell 30(6):790–802

Belmont AS (2006) Mitotic chromosome structure and condensation. Curr Opin Cell Biol 18(6):632–638

Belova GI, Prasad R, Nazimov IV, Wilson SH, Slesarev AI (2002) The domain organization and properties of individual domains of DNA topoisomerase V, a type 1B topoisomerase with DNA repair activities. J Biol Chem 277:4959–4965

Benarroch D, Claverie JM, Raoult D, Shuman S (2006) Characterization of mimivirus DNA topoisomerase IB suggests horizontal gene transfer between eukaryal viruses and bacteria. J Virol 80:314–321

Benedetti P, Baldi MI, Mattoccia E, Tocchini-Valentini GP (1983) Purification and characterization of Xenopus laevis topoisomerase II. EMBO J 2(8):1303–1308

Berger JM, Gamblin SJ, Harrison SC, Wang JC (1996) Structure and mechanism of DNA topoisomerase II. Nature 379(6562):225–232

Berger JM, Fass D, Wang JC, Harrison SC (1998) Structural similarities between topoisomerases that cleave one or both DNA strands. Proc Natl Acad Sci USA 95(14):7876–7881

Bergerat A, Gadelle D, Forterre P (1994) Purification of a DNA topoisomerase II from the hyperthermophilic archaeon Sulfolobus shibatae. A thermostable enzyme with both bacterial and eucaryal features. J Biol Chem 269(44):27663–27669

Bergerat A, de Massy B, Gadelle D, Varoutas PC, Nicolas A, Forterre P (1997) An atypical topoisomerase II from Archaea with implications for meiotic recombination. Nature 386:414–417

Bodley AL, Chakraborty AK, Xie S, Burri C, Shapiro TA (2003) An unusual type IB topoisomerase from African trypanosomes. Proc Natl Acad Sci USA 100(13):7539–7544

Brochier C, Forterre P, Gribaldo S (2004) Archaeal phylogeny based on proteins of the transcription and translation machineries: tackling the *Methanopyrus kandleri* paradox. Genome Biol 5(3):R17

Brochier-Armanet C, Forterre P (2007) Widespread distribution of archaeal reverse gyrase in thermophilic bacteria suggests a complex history of vertical inheritance and lateral gene transfers. Archaea 2:83–93

Brochier-Armanet C, Boussau B, Gribaldo S, Forterre P (2008a) Mesophilic Crenarchaeota: proposal for a third archaeal phylum, the Thaumarchaeota. Nat Rev Microbiol 6:245–252

Brochier-Armanet C, Gribaldo S, Forterre P (2008b) A DNA topoisomerase IB in Thaumarchaeota testifies for the presence of this enzyme in the last common ancestor of Archaea and Eucarya. Biol Direct 3:54

Brown PO, Cozzarelli NR (1979) A sign inversion mechanism for enzymatic supercoiling of DNA. Science 206(4422):1081–1083

Buhler C, Lebbink JH, Bocs C, Ladenstein R, Forterre P (2001) DNA topoisomerase VI generates ATP-dependent double-strand breaks with two-nucleotide overhangs. J Biol Chem 276:37215–37222

Cairns J (1963a) The bacterial chromosome and its manner of replication as seen by autoradiography. J Mol Biol 6:208–213

Cairns J (1963b) The chromosome of *E. coli. Cold Spring Harbour Symp Quant Biol* 28 (1963b) 43–46

Capp C, Qian Y, Sage H, Huber H, Hsieh TS (2010) Separate and combined biochemical activities of the subunits of a naturally split reverse gyrase. J Biol Chem 2010 285(51):39637–39645

Champoux JJ, Bean MD (1980) Topoisomerase and the swivel problem. In: Alberts BM (eds) Mechanistic studies of DNA réplication and genetic recombination. ICN-UCLA Symposia on Molecular and Cellular Biology, Vol 19, pp 809–815 Academic Press, New York

Champoux JJ, Dulbecco R (1972) An activity from mammalian cells that untwists superhelical DNA-a possible swivel for DNA replication (polyoma-ethidium bromide-mouse-embryo cells-dye binding assay). Proc Natl Acad Sci USA 69:143–146

Charbonnier F, Forterre P (1994) Comparison of plasmid DNA topology among mesophilic and thermophilic eubacteria and archaebacteria. J Bacteriol 176:1251–1259

Chen GL, Yang L, Rowe TC, Halligan BD, Tewey KM, Liu LF (1984) Nonintercalative antitumor drugs interfere with the breakage-reunion reaction of mammalian DNA topoisomerase II. J Biol Chem 259(21):13560–13566

Chen L, Huang L (2006) Oligonucleotide cleavage and rejoining by topoisomerase III from the hyperthermophilic archaeon *Sulfolobus solfataricus*: temperature dependence and strand annealing-promoted DNA religation. Mol Microbiol 60:783–794

Cheng C, Kussie P, Pavletich N, Shuman S (1998) Conservation of structure and mechanism between eukaryotic topoisomerase I and site-specific recombinases. Cell 92:841–850

Cheung KJ, Badarinarayana V, Selinger DW, Janse D, Church GM (2003) A microarray-based antibiotic screen identifies a regulatory role for supercoiling in the osmotic stress response of Escherichia coli. Genome Res. 13(2):206–215

Cho HS, Lee SS, Kim KD, Hwang I, Lim JS, Park YI, Pai HS (2004) DNA gyrase is involved in chloroplast nucleoid partitioning. Plant Cell 16(10):2665–2682

Confalonieri F, Elie C, Nadal M, de La Tour C, Forterre P, Duguet M (1993) Reverse gyrase: a helicase-like domain and a type I topoisomerase in the same polypeptide. Proc Natl Acad Sci USA 90:4753–4757

Conti C, Seiler JA, Pommier Y. (2007) The mammalian DNA replication elongation checkpoint: implication of Chk1 and relationship with origin firing as determined by single DNA molecule and single cell analyses. Cell Cycle. 6:2760–2767

Corbett KD, Berger JM (2003) Structure of the topoisomerase VI-B subunit: implications for type II topoisomerase mechanism and evolution. EMBO J 22:151–163

Corbett KD, Shultzaberger RK, Berger JM (2004) The C-terminal domain of DNA gyrase A adopts a DNA-bending beta-pinwheel fold. Proc Natl Acad Sci USA 101(19):7293–7298

Corbett KD, Benedetti P, Berger JM (2007) Holoenzyme assembly and ATP-mediated conformational dynamics of topoisomerase VI. Nat Struct Mol Biol 14:611–619

D'Amaro A, Rossi M, Ciaramella M (2007) Reverse gyrase: an unusual DNA manipulator of hyperthermophilic organisms. J Biochem 56:103–109

Dai P, Wang Y, Ye R, Chen L, Huang L (2003) DNA topoisomerase III from the hyperthermophilic archaeon *Sulfolobus solfataricus* with specific DNA cleavage activity. J Bacteriol 185:5500–5507

Das BB, Ganguly A, Majumder HK (2008) DNA topoisomerases of Leishmania: the potential targets for anti-leishmanial therapy. Adv Exp Med Biol 625:103–115 Review

Dar MA, Sharma A, Mondal N, Dhar SK (2007) Molecular cloning of apicoplast targeted Plasmodium falciparum DNA gyrase genes: unique intrinsic ATPase activity and ATP-independent dimerization of PfGyrB subunit. Eukaryot Cell 6(3):398–412

De Massy B, Rocco V, Nicolas A. The nucleotide mapping of DNA double-strand breaks at the CYS3 initiation site of meiotic recombination in Saccharomyces cerevisiae. EMBO J 1995 Sep 15;14(18):4589–98

Declais AC, Marsault J, Confalonieri F, de La Tour CB, Duguet M (2000) Reverse gyrase, the two domains intimately cooperate to promote positive supercoiling, J Biol Chem 275:19498–19504

Dickey JS, Van Etten JL, Osheroff N (2005) DNA methylation impacts the cleavage activity of Chlorella virus topoisomerase II. Biochemistry 44:15378–15386

DiGate RJ, Marians KJ (1989) Molecular cloning and DNA sequence analysis of *Escherichia coli* topB, the gene encoding topoisomerase III. J Biol Chem 264:17924–17930

DiGate RJ, Marians KJ (1992) *Escherichia coli* topoisomerase III-catalyzed cleavage of RNA. J Biol Chem 267:20532–20535

DiNardo S, Voelkel KA, Sternglanz R, Reynolds AE, Wright A (1982) *Escherichia coli* DNA topoisomerase I mutants have compensatory mutations in DNA gyrase genes. Cell 31:43–51

DiNardo S, Voelkel K, Sternglanz R (1984) DNA topoisomerase II mutant of Saccharomyces cerevisiae: topoisomerase II is required for segregation of daughter molecules at the termination of DNA replication. Proc Natl Acad Sci USA 81(9):2616–2620

Dong KC, Berger JM (2007) Structural basis for gate-DNA recognition and bending by type IIA topoisomerases. Nature 450(7173):1201–1205

Drlica K, Worcel A (1975) Conformational transitions in the Escherichia coli chromosome: analysis by viscometry and sedimentation. J Mol Biol 98(2):393–411

Dröge P, Nordheim A (1991) Transcription-induced conformational change in a topologically closed DNA domain. Nucleic Acids Res 19(11):2941–2946

Drolet M (2006) Growth inhibition mediated by excess negative supercoiling: the interplay between transcription elongation, R-loop formation and DNA topology. Mol Microbiol 59(3):723–730

Duguet M, Serre MC, Bouthier de La Tour C (2006) A universal type IA topoisomerase fold. J Mol Biol 359:805–812

Dutta R, Inouye M (2000) GHKL, an emergent ATPase/kinase superfamily. Trends Biochem Sci 25:24–28

Edgell DR, Doolittle WF (1997) Archaea and the origin(s) of DNA replication proteins. Cell 89:995–998

Espeli O, Lee C, Marians KJ (2003) A physical and functional interaction between Escherichia coli FtsK and topoisomerase IV. J Biol Chem 278(45):44639–44644
Filée J, Forterre P, Sen-Lin T, Laurent J (2002) Evolution of DNA polymerase families: evidences for multiple gene exchange between cellular and viral proteins. J Mol Evol 54:763–773
Fischer MG, Allen MJ, Wilson WH, Suttle CA (2010) Giant virus with a remarkable complement of genes infects marine zooplankton. Proc Natl Acad Sci USA 107(45):19508–11953
Forterre P (1999) Displacement of cellular proteins by functional analogues from plasmids or viruses could explain puzzling phylogenies of many DNA informational proteins. Mol Microbiol 33(3):457–465
Forterre P (2002a) A hot story from comparative genomics: reverse gyrase is the only hyperthermophile-specific protein. Trends Genet 18:236–237
Forterre P (2002b) The origin of DNA genomes and DNA replication proteins. Curr Opin Microbiol 5:525
Forterre P (2005) The two ages of the RNA world, and the transition to the DNA world: a story of viruses and cells. Biochimie 87:793–803
Forterre P (2006) Three RNA cells for ribosomal lineages and three DNA viruses to replicate their genomes: a hypothesis for the origin of cellular domain. Proc Natl Acad Sci USA 103:3669–3674
Forterre P (2006) DNA topoisomerase V: a new fold of mysterious origin. Trends Biotechnol 24:245–247
Forterre P, Gadelle D (2009) Phylogenomics of DNA topoisomerases: their origin and putative roles in the emergence of modern organisms. Nucleic Acids Res 37(3):679–692
Forterre P, Gribaldo S (2010) Bacteria with a eukaryotic touch: a glimpse of ancient evolution? Proc Natl Acad Sci USA 107(29):12739–12740
Forterre P, Gribaldo S, Gadelle D, Serre MC (2007) Origin and evolution of DNA topoisomerases. Biochimie 4:427–446
Forterre P, Mirambeau G, Jaxel C, Nadal M, Duguet M (1985) High positive supercoiling in vitro catalyzed by an ATP and polyethylene glycol-stimulated topoisomerase from *Sulfolobus acidocaldarius*. EMBO J 4:2123–2128
Francke B, Margolin J (1981) Effect of novobiocin and other DNA gyrase inhibitors on virus replication and DNA synthesis in herpes simplex virus type 1-infected BHK cells. J Gen Virol 52(Pt 2):401–404
Freeland SJ, Knight RD, Landweber LF (1999) Do proteins predate DNA? Science 286:690–692
French SL, Sikes ML, Hontz RD, Osheim YN, Lambert TE, El Hage A, Smith MM, Tollervey D, Smith JS, Beyer AL (2011) Distinguishing the Roles of Topoisomerases I and II in Relief of Transcription-Induced Torsional Stress in Yeast rRNA Genes. Mol Cell Biol 31(3):482–494
Fuller FB (1971) The writhing number of a space curve. Proc Natl Acad Sci USA 68:815–819
Funnell BE, Baker TA, Kornberg A. (1987) In vitro assembly of a prepriming complex at the origin of the Escherichia coli chromosome. J Biol Chem. 262:10327–10334
Gadelle, Bocs DC, Graille M, Forterre P (2005) Inhibition of archaeal growth and DNA topoisomerase VI activities by the Hsp90 inhibitor radicicol. Nucleic Acids Res 33:2310–2317
Gadelle D, Graille M, Forterre P (2006) The HSP90 and DNA topoisomerase VI inhibitor radicicol also inhibits human type II DNA topoisomerase. Biochem Pharmacol 72:1207–1216
Gadelle D, Filée J, Buhler C, Forterre P (2003) Phylogenomics of type II DNA topoisomerases. Bioessays 3:232–242
Garnier F, Nadal M (2008) Transcriptional analysis of the two reverse gyrase encoding genes of *Sulfolobus solfataricus* P2 in relation to the growth phases and temperature conditions. Extremophiles 12(6):799–809
García-Estrada C, Prada CF, Fernández-Rubio C, Rojo-Vázquez F, Balaña-Fouce R (2010) DNA topoisomerases in apicomplexan parasites: promising targets for drug discovery. Proc Biol Sci 277(1689):1777–1778
Ganguly A, Del Toro Duany Y, Rudolph MG, Klostermeier D (2011) The latch modulates nucleotide and DNA binding to the helicase-like domain of *Thermotoga maritima* reverse gyrase and is required for positive DNA supercoiling. Nucleic Acids Res 39:1789–1800

Gellert M, Mizuuchi K, O'Dea MH, Itoh T, Tomizawa JI (1977) Nalidixic acid resistance: a second genetic character involved in DNA gyrase activity. Proc Natl Acad Sci USA 74:4772–4776

Gellert M, O'Dea MH, Itoh T, Tomizawa J (1976) Novobiocin and coumermycin inhibit DNA supercoiling catalyzed by DNA gyrase. Proc Natl Acad Sci USA 73(12):4474–4478

Germond JE, Hirt B, Oudet P, Gross-Bellark M, Chambon P (1975) Folding of the DNA double helix in chromatin-like structures from simian virus 40. Proc Natl Acad Sci USA 72(5):1843–1847

Giaever G, Lynn R, Goto T, Wang JC (1986) The complete nucleotide sequence of the structural gene TOP2 of yeast DNA topoisomerase II. J Biol Chem 261(27):12448–12454

Graille M, Cladière L, Durand D, Lecointe F, Gadelle D, Quevillon-Cheruel S, Vachette P, Forterre P, van Tilbeurgh H (2008) Crystal structure of an intact type II DNA topoisomerase: insights into DNA transfer mechanisms. Structure 16:360–370

Griffith JD (1976) Visualization of prokaryotic DNA in a regularly condensed chromatin-like fiber. Proc Natl Acad Sci USA 73(2):563–567

Guipaud O, Forterre P (2001) DNA gyrase from *Thermotoga maritima*. Methods Enzymol 334:162–171

Guipaud O, Marguet E, Noll KM, de la Tour CB, Forterre P (1997) Both DNA gyrase and reverse gyrase are present in the hyperthermophilic bacterium *Thermotoga maritime*. Proc Natl Acad Sci USA 94:10606–10611

Halligan BD, Edwards KA, Liu LF (1985) Purification and characterization of a type II DNA topoisomerase from bovine calf thymus. J Biol Chem 260(4):2475–2482

Hartung F, Puchta H (2001) Molecular characterization of homologues of both subunits A (SPO11) and B of the archaebacterial topoisomerase 6 in plants. Gene 271:81–86

Hartung F, Angelis KJ, Meister A, Schubert I, Melzer M, Puchta H (2002) An archaebacterial topoisomerase homolog not present in other eukaryotes is indispensable for cell proliferation of plants. Curr Biol 12:1787–1791

Hayama R, Marians KJ (2010) Physical and functional interaction between the condensin MukB and the decatenase topoisomerase IV in Escherichia coli. Proc Natl Acad Sci USA 107(44):18826–18831

Higgins NP, Peebles CL, Sugino A, Cozzarelli NR (1978) Purification of subunits of *Escherichia coli* DNA gyrase and reconstitution of enzymatic activity. Proc Natl Acad Sci USA 75:1773–1777

Holmes ML, Dyall-Smith ML (1991) Mutations in DNA gyrase result in novobiocin resistance in halophilic archaebacteria. J Bacteriol 173:642–648

Hsiang YH, Hertzberg R, Hecht S, Liu LF (1985) Camptothecin induces protein-linked DNA breaks via mammalian DNA topoisomerase I. J Biol Chem 260(27):14873–14878

Hsieh LS, Rouviere-Yaniv J, Drlica K (1991) Bacterial DNA supercoiling and [ATP]/[ADP] ratio: changes associated with salt shock. J Bacteriol 173(12):3914–3917

Hsieh LS, Burger RM, Drlica K (1991) Bacterial DNA supercoiling and [ATP]/[ADP]. Changes associated with a transition to anaerobic growth. J Mol Biol 219(3):443–450

Hsieh TJ, Farh L, Huang WM, Chan NL (2004) Structure of the topoisomerase IV C-terminal domain: a broken beta-propeller implies a role as geometry facilitator in catalysis. J Biol Chem 279:55587–55593

Hsieh TS, Plank JL (2006) Reverse gyrase functions as a DNA renaturase: annealing of complementary single-stranded circles and positive supercoiling of a bubble substrate. J Biol Chem 281:5640–5647

Hsieh TJ, Yen TJ, Lin TS, Chang HT, Huang SY, Hsu CH, Farh L, Chan NL (2010) Twisting of the DNA-binding surface by a beta-strand-bearing proline modulates DNA gyrase activity. Nucleic Acids Res 38(12):4173–81

Huang WM, Joss L, Hsieh T, Casjens S. Protelomerase uses a topoisomerase IB/Y-recombinase type mechanism to generate DNA hairpin ends. J Mol Biol 2004 Mar 12;337(1):77–92

Jain P, Nagaraja V (2005) An atypical type II topoisomerase from *Mycobacterium smegmatis* with positive supercoiling activity. Mol Microbiol 58:1392–1405

Jaxel C, Nadal M, Mirambeau G, Forterre P, Takahashi M, Duguet M. (1989) Reverse gyrase binding to DNA alters the double helix structure and produces single-strand cleavage in the absence of ATP. EMBO J. 8:3135–3139

Jo K, Topal MD (1995) DNA topoisomerase and recombinase activities in Nae I restriction endonuclease. Science 267:1817–1820

Kampmann M, Stock D. (2004) Reverse gyrase has heat-protective DNA chaperone activity independent of supercoiling. Nucleic Acids Res. 32:3537–3545

Kato J, Nishimura Y, Imamura R, Niki H, Hiraga S, Suzuki H (1990) New topoisomerase essential for chromosome segregation in E. coli. Cell 63(2):393–404. Erratum in: Cell 1991

Kato J, Suzuki H, Ikeda H (1992) Purification and characterization of DNA topoisomerase IV in *Escherichia coli*. J Biol Chem 267:25676–25684

Keeney S, Giroux CN, Kleckner N (1997) Meiosis-specific DNA double-strand breaks are catalyzed by Spo11, a member of a widely conserved protein family. Cell 88:375–384

Keller W (1975) Determination of the number of superhelical turns in simian virus 40 DNA by gel electrophoresis. Proc Natl Acad Sci USA 72:4876–4880

Kikuchi A, Asai K (1984) Reverse gyrase-a topoisomerase which introduces positive superhelical turns into DNA. Nature 309:677–681

Kim RA, Wang JC (1989) Function of DNA topoisomerases as replication swivels in *Saccharomyces cerevisiae*. J Mol Biol 208:257–267

Kirkegaard K, Wang JC (1978) *Escherichia coli* DNA topoisomerase I catalyzed linking of single-stranded rings of complementary base sequences. Nucleic Acids Res 5:3811–3820

Khodursky AB, Peter BJ, Schmid MB, DeRisi J, Botstein D, Brown PO, Cozzarelli NR (2000) Analysis of topoisomerase function in bacterial replication fork movement: use of DNA microarrays. Proc Natl Acad Sci USA 97(17):9419–9424

Koonin EV. (2003) Comparative genomics, minimal gene-sets and the last universal common ancestor. Nat Rev Microbiol. 1:127–136

Koonin EV, Senkevitch TG, Dolja VV (2006) The ancient Virus World and evolution of cells. Biol Direct 1:19

Koepsel RR, Murray RW, Rosenblum WD, Khan SA (1985) The replication initiator protein of plasmid pT181 has sequence-specific endonuclease and topoisomerase-like activities. Proc Natl Acad Sci USA 82(20):6845–9684

Koster DA, Croquette V, Dekker C, Shuman S, Dekker NH (2005) Friction and torque govern the relaxation of DNA supercoils by eukaryotic topoisomerase IB. Nature 434:671–674

Kovalsky OI, Kozyavkin SA, Slesarev AI. (1990) Archaebacterial reverse gyrase cleavage-site specificity is similar to that of eubacterial DNA topoisomerases I. Nucleic Acids Res. 18:2801–2805

Kozyavkin SA, Pushkin AV, Eiserling FA, Stetter KO, Lake JA, Slesarev AI (1995) DNA enzymology above 100 degrees C Topoisomerase V unlinks circular DNA at 80–122 degrees C. J Biol Chem 270:13593–13595

Kramlinger VM, Hiasa H (2006) The "GyrA-box" is required for the ability of DNA gyrase to wrap DNA and catalyze the supercoiling reaction. J Biol Chem 281:3738–3742

Kreuzer KN, Cozzarelli NR (1980) Formation and resolution of DNA catenanes by DNA gyrase. Cell 20(1):245–254

Krogh BO, Shuman S (2002) A poxvirus-like type IB topoisomerase family in bacteria. Proc Natl Acad Sci USA 99:1853–1858

Lazcano A, Guerrero R, Margulis L, Oró J (1988) The evolutionary transition from RNA to DNA in early cells. J Mol Evol 27:283–290

Lebowitz J (1990) Through the looking glass: the discovery of supercoiled DNA. Trends Biochem Sci 15:202–207

Leipe DD, Aravind L, Koonin EV (1999) Did DNA replication evolve twice independently? Nucleic Acids Res 27:3389–3401

Li Y, Stewart NK, Berger AJ, Vos S, Schoeffler AJ, Berger JM, Chait BT, Oakley MG (2010) Escherichia coli condensin MukB stimulates topoisomerase IV activity by a direct physical interaction. Proc Natl Acad Sci USA 107(44):18832–18837

Li Z, Hiasa H, DiGate R (2006) Characterization of a unique type IA topoisomerase in *Bacillus cereus*. Mol Microbiol 60(1):140–151

Lindsley JE (1996) Intradimerically tethered DNA topoisomerase II is catalytically active in DNA transport. Proc Natl Acad Sci USA 93:2975–2980

Lima CD, Mondragón A. Mechanism of type II DNA topoisomerases: a tale of two gates. Structure 1994 Jun 15;2(6):559–60

Lima CD, Wang JC, Mondragon A (1994) Three-dimensional structure of the 67K N-terminal fragment of *E. coli* DNA topoisomerase I. Nature 367:138–146

Liu J, Wu TC, Lichten M (1995) The location and structure of double-strand DNA breaks induced during yeast meiosis: evidence for a covalently linked DNA-protein intermediate. EMBO J 14(18):4599–4608

Liu LF, Wang JC (1978a) *Micrococcus luteus* DNA gyrase: active components and a model for its supercoiling of DNA. Proc Natl Acad Sci USA 75(5):2098–102

Liu LF, Wang JC (1978b) DNA-DNA gyrase complex: the wrapping of the DNA duplex outside the enzyme. Cell 15(3):979–984

Liu LF, Wang JC (1987) Supercoiling of the DNA template during transcription. Proc Natl Acad Sci USA 84(20):7024–7027

Liu LF, Liu CC, Alberts BM (1979) T4 DNA topoisomerase: a new ATP-dependent enzyme essential for initiation of T4 bacteriophage DNA replication. Nature 28:456–461

Liu LF, Liu CC, Alberts BM (1980) Type II DNA topoisomerases: enzymes that can unknot a topologically knotted DNA molecule via a reversible double-strand break. Cell 19:697–707

Ljungman M, Hanawalt PC. (1992) Localized torsional tension in the DNA of human cells. Proc Natl Acad Sci USA 89:6055–6059

Lopez-Garcia P, Forterre P, Van der Oost J, Erauso G (2000) Plasmid pGS5 from the hyperthermophilic archaeon *Archaeoglobus profundus* is negatively supercoiled. J Bacteriol 182:4998–5000

Lockshon D, Morris DR (1983) Positively supercoiled plasmid DNA is produced by treatment of *Escherichia coli* with DNA gyrase inhibitors. Nucleic Acids Res 11:2999–3017

Low RL, Orton S, Friedman DB. (2003) A truncated form of DNA topoisomerase IIbeta associates with the mtDNA genome in mammalian mitochondria. Eur J Biochem:4173–4186

Lundin D, Gribaldo S, Torrents E, Sjöberg BM, Poole AM. (2010) Ribonucleotide reduction – horizontal transfer of a required function spans all three domains. BMC Evol Biol.10:383–387

Malik SB, Ramesh MA, Hulstrand AM, Logsdon JM (2007) Protist homologs of the meiotic Spo11 gene and topoisomerase VI reveal an evolutionary history of gene duplication and lineage-specific loss. Mol Biol Evol 24:2827–2841

Mankouri HW, Hickson ID (2007) The RecQ helicase-topoisomerase III-Rmi1 complex: a DNA structure-specific "dissolvasome"? Trends Biochem Sci 32:538–546

Marguet E, Forterre P (1994) DNA stability at temperatures typical for hyperthermophiles. Nucleic Acids Res 22(9):1681–1686

Marsin S, Marguet E, Forterre P (2000) Topoisomerase activity of the hyperthermophilic replication initiator protein Rep75. Nucleic Acids Res 28:2251–2255

Miller KG, Liu LF, Englund PT (1981) A homogeneous type II DNA topoisomerase from HeLa cell nuclei. J Biol Chem 256:9334–9339

Mizuuchi K, Fisher LM, O'Dea MH, Gellert M (1980) DNA gyrase action involves the introduction of transient double-strand breaks into DNA. Proc Natl Acad Sci USA 77:1847–1851

Mizuuchi K, Nash HA (1976) Restriction assay for integrative recombination of bacteriophage lambda DNA in vitro: requirement for closed circular DNA substrate. Proc Natl Acad Sci USA 73:3524–3528

Mondragon A, DiGate R (1999) The structure of *Escherichia coli* DNA topoisomerase III. Structure 7:1373–1383

Morrison A, Cozzarelli NR (1979) Site-specific cleavage of DNA by *E. coli* DNA gyrase. Cell 17:175–84

Musgrave D, Forterre P, Slesarev A. (2000) Negative constrained DNA supercoiling in archaeal nucleosomes. Mol Microbiol. 35:341–349

Mushegian AR, Koonin EV (1996) A minimal gene set for cellular life derived by comparison of complete bacterial genomes. Proc Natl Acad Sci USA 93:10268–10273

Nadal M, Mirambeau G, Forterre P, Reiter WD, Duguet M (1986) Positively supercoiled DNA in a virus-like particle of an archaebacterium. Nature 321:256–258

Nadal M (2007) Reverse gyrase: an insight into the role of DNA-topoisomerases. Biochimie 89:447–455

Nakasu S, Kikuchi A (1985) Reverse gyrase dependent type I topoisomerase from Sulfolobus. EMBO J 4:2705–2710

Napoli A, Valenti A, Salerno V, Nadal M, Garnier F, Rossi M, Ciaramella M (2004) Reverse gyrase recruitment to DNA after UV light irradiation in *Sulfolobus solfataricus*. J Biol Chem 279(32):33192–33198

Nelson EM, Tewey KM, Liu LF (1984) Mechanism of antitumor drug action: poisoning of mammalian DNA topoisomerase II on DNA by 4′-(9-acridinylamino)-methanesulfon-m-anisidide. Proc Natl Acad Sci USA 81(5):1361–1365

Nichols MD, DeAngelis K, Keck JL, Berger JM (1999) Structure and function of an archaeal topoisomerase VI subunit with homology to the meiotic recombination factor Spo11. EMBO J 18:6177–6188

Nitiss JL.(2009) DNA topoisomerase II and its growing repertoire of biological functions. Nat Rev Cancer.9:327–37

Pace NR (2006) Time for a change. Nature, 441(7091):289

Pansegrau W, Schröder W, LankaE (1994) Concerted action of three distinct domains in the DNA cleaving-joining reaction catalyzed by relaxase (TraI) of conjugative plasmid RP4. J Biol Chem 269:2782–2789

Pavlov AR, Belova GI, Kozyavkin SA, Slesarev AI (2002) Helix-hairpin-helix motifs confer salt resistance and processivity on chimeric DNA polymerases. Proc Natl Acad Sci USA 99(21):13510–13515

Peter BJ, Arsuaga J, Breier AM, Khodursky AB, Brown PO, Cozzarelli NR (2004) Genomic transcriptional response to loss of chromosomal supercoiling in *Escherichia coli*. Genome Biol 5(11):R87

Plank JL, Wu J, Hsieh TS. (2006) Topoisomerase IIIa and Bloom's helicase can resolve a mobile double Holliday junction substrate through convergent branch migration. Proc Natl Acad Sci USA 103:11118–11123

Pommier Y, Leo E, Zhang H, Marchand C (2010) DNA topoisomerases and their poisoning by anticancer and antibacterial drugs. Chem Biol 17:421–433

Poole AM, Logan DT (2005) Modern mRNA proofreading and repair: clues that the last universal common ancestor possessed an RNA genome? Mol Biol Evol 22:1444–1455

Pruss GJ, Drlica K (1986) Topoisomerase I mutants: the gene on pBR322 that encodes resistance to tetracycline affects plasmid DNA supercoiling. Proc Natl Acad Sci USA 83:8952–8956

Pruss GJ, Drlica K (1989) DNA supercoiling and prokaryotic transcription. Cell 56(4):521–522

Pruss GJ, Manes SH, Drlica K (1982) *Escherichia coli* DNA topoisomerase I mutants: increased supercoiling is corrected by mutations near gyrase genes. Cell 31:35–342

Radloff R, Bauer W, Vinograd J (1967) A dye-buoyant-density method for the detection and isolation of closed circular duplex DNA: the closed circular DNA in HeLa cells. Proc Natl Acad Sci USA 57:1514–1521

Raghu Ram EV, Kumar A, Biswas S, Kumar A, Chaubey S, Siddiqi MI, Habib S (2007) Nuclear gyrB encodes a functional subunit of the Plasmodium falciparum gyrase that is involved in apicoplast DNA replication. Mol Biochem Parasitol 154:30–39

Raoult D, Audic S, Robert C, Abergel C, Renesto P, Ogata H, La Scola B, Suzan M, Claverie JM (2004) The 1.2-megabase genome sequence of Mimivirus. Science 306:1344–1350

Roca J, Wang JC (1992) The capture of a DNA double helix by an ATP-dependent protein clamp: a key step in DNA transport by type II DNA topoisomerases. Cell 71:833–840

Roca J, Wang JC (1994) DNA transport by a type II DNA topoisomerase: evidence in favor of a two-gate mechanism. Cell 77:609–616

Rodríguez AC, Stock D (2002) Crystal structure of reverse gyrase: insights into the positive supercoiling of DNA. EMBO J 21:418–426

Ross W, Rowe T, Glisson B, Yalowich J, Liu L (1984) Role of topoisomerase II in mediating epipodophyllotoxin-induced DNA cleavage. Cancer Res 44:5857–5860

Roth TF, Helinski DR (1967) Evidence for circular DNA forms of a bacterial plasmid. Proc Natl Acad Sci USA 58:650–657

Ruthenburg AJ, Graybosch DM, Huetsch JC, Verdine GL (2005) A superhelical spiral in the *Escherichia coli* DNA gyrase A C-terminal domain imparts unidirectional supercoiling bias. J Biol Chem. 280:26177–84

Salceda J, Fernández X, Roca J (2006) Topoisomerase II, not topoisomerase I, is the proficient relaxase of nucleosomal DNA. EMBO J 25:2575–2583

Schmid MB, Sawitzke JA. (1993) Multiple bacterial topoisomerases: specialization or redundancy? Bioessays 15:445–449

Schoeffler AJ, Berger JM (2008) DNA topoisomerases: harnessing and constraining energy to govern chromosome topology. Q Rev Biophys 41:41–101

Scocca JR, Shapiro TA (2008) A mitochondrial topoisomerase IA essential for late theta structure resolution in African trypanosomes. Mol Microbiol 67:820–829

Seki M, Nakagawa T, Seki T, Kato G, Tada S, Takahashi Y, Yoshimura A, Kobayashi T, Aoki A, Otsuki M, Habermann FA, Tanabe H, Ishii Y and Enomoto T (2006) Bloom helicase and DNA topoisomerase IIIa are involved in the dissolution of sister chromatids. Mol Cell Biol 26:6299–6307

Sekiguchi J, Shuman S (1997) Site-specific ribonuclease activity of eukaryotic DNA topoisomerase I. Mol Cell 1:89–97

Shimamoto A, Nishikawa K, Kitao S, Furuichi Y (2000) Human RecQ5b, a large isomer of RecQ5 DNA helicase, localizes in the nucleoplasm and interacts with topoisomerases 3a and 3b. Nucleic Acids Res 28:1647–1655

Sinden RR, Carlson JO, Pettijohn DE (1980) Torsional tension in the DNA double helix measured with trimethylpsoralen in living *E. coli* cells: analogous measurements in insect and human cells. Cell 21:773–783

Sioud M, Possot O, Elie C, Sibold L, Forterre P (1988) Coumarin and quinolone action in archaebacteria: evidence for the presence of a DNA gyrase-like enzyme. J Bacteriol 170:946–953

Sioud M, Forterre P (1989) Ciprofloxacin and etoposide (VP16) produce a similar pattern of DNA cleavage in a plasmid of an archaebacterium. Biochemistry 28:3638–3641

Slesarev AI, Kozyavkin SA (1990) DNA substrate specificity of reverse gyrase from extremely thermophilic archaebacteria. J Biomol Struct Dyn. 7:935–942

Slesarev AI, Zaitzev DA, Kopylov VM, Stetter KO, Kozyavkin SA (1991) DNA topoisomerase III from extremely thermophilic archaebacteria. ATP-independent type I topoisomerase from *Desulfurococcus amylolyticus* drives extensive unwinding of closed circular DNA at high temperature. J Biol Chem 266:12321–12328

Slesarev AI, Stetter KO, Lake JA, Gellert M, Krah R, Kozyavkin SA (1993) DNA topoisomerase V is a relative of eukaryotic topoisomerase I from a hyperthermophilic prokaryote. Nature 364:735–737

Schmidt BH, Burgin AB, Deweese JE, Osheroff N, Berger JM (2010) A novel and unified two-metal mechanism for DNA cleavage by type II and IA topoisomerases. Nature 465:641–644

Staczek P, Higgins NP (1998) Gyrase and Topo IV modulate chromosome domain size in vivo. Mol Microbiol 29:1435–1448

Sugimoto-Shirasu K, Roberts GR, Stacey NJ, McCann MC, Maxwell A, Roberts K (2005) RHL1 is an essential component of the plant DNA topoisomerase VI complex and is required for ploidy-dependent cell growth. Proc Natl Acad Sci USA 102:18736–18741

Sugimoto-Shirasu K, Stacey NJ, Corsar J, Roberts K, McCann MC (2002) DNA topoisomerase VI is essential for endoreduplication in Arabidopsis. Curr Biol 12:1782–1786

Sugino A, Peebles CL, Kreuzer KN, Cozzarelli NR (1977) Mechanism of action of nalidixic acid: purification of Escherichia coli nalA gene product and its relationship to DNA gyrase and a novel nicking-closing enzyme. Proc Natl Acad Sci USA 74:4767–4771

Srivenugopal KS, Lockshon D, Morris DR (1984) *Escherichia coli* DNA topoisomerase III: purification and characterization of a new type I enzyme. Biochemistry 23(9):1899–1906

Postow L, Hardy CD, Arsuaga J, Cozzarelli NR (2004) Topological domain structure of the Escherichia coli chromosome. Genes Dev 18(14):1766–1779

Krasilnikov AS, Podtelezhnikov A, Vologodskii A, Mirkin SM (1999) Large-scale effects of transcriptional DNA supercoiling in vivo. J Mol Biol 292(5):1149–1156

Taneja B, Patel A, Slesarev A, Mondragon A (2006) Structure of the N-terminal fragment of topoisomerase V reveals a new family of topoisomerases. EMBO J 25:398–408
Taneja B, Schnurr B, Slesarev A, Marko JF, Mondragón A (2007) Topoisomerase V relaxes supercoiled DNA by a constrained swiveling mechanism. Proc Natl Acad Sci USA 104 (37): 14670–14675
Temime-Smaali N, Guittat L, Wenner T, Bayart E, Douarre C, Gomez D, Giraud-Panis MJ, Londono-Vallejo A, Gilson E, Amor-Guéret M, Riou JF (2008) Topoisomerase IIIalpha is required for normal proliferation and telomere stability in alternative lengthening of telomeres. EMBO J 27(10):1513–1524
Tewey KM, Chen GL, Nelson EM, Liu LF (1984) Intercalative antitumor drugs interfere with the breakage-reunion reaction of mammalian DNA topoisomerase II. J Biol Chem 259(14):9182–9187
Tewey KM, Rowe TC, Yang L, Halligan BD, Liu LF (1984) Adriamycin-induced DNA damage mediated by mammalian DNA topoisomerase II. Science 226(4673):466–468
Tretter EM, Lerman JC, Berger JM (2010) A naturally chimeric type IIA topoisomerase in Aquifex aeolicus highlights an evolutionary path for the emergence of functional paralogs. Proc Natl Acad Sci USA 107:22055–22059
Tse-Dinh YC (1985) Regulation of the Escherichia coli DNA topoisomerase I gene by DNA supercoiling. Nucleic Acids Res 13:4751–4763
Uemura T, Morikawa K, Yanagida M (1986) The nucleotide sequence of the fission yeast DNA topoisomerase II gene: structural and functional relationships to other DNA topoisomerases. EMBO J 5:2355–2361
Uemura T, Ohkura H, Adachi Y, Morino K, Shiozaki K, Yanagida M (1987) DNA topoisomerase II is required for condensation and separation of mitotic chromosomes in *S. pombe*. Cell 50:917–925
Ullsperger C, Cozzarelli NR (1996) Contrasting enzymatic activities of topoisomerase IV and DNA gyrase from *Escherichia coli*. J Biol Chem 271:31549–31555
Valenti A, Perugino G, D'Amaro A, Cacace A, Napoli A, Rossi M, Ciaramella M (2008) Dissection of reverse gyrase activities: insight into the evolution of a thermostable molecular machine Nucleic Acids Res 36:4587–4597
Valenti A, Perugino G, Nohmi T, Rossi M, Ciaramella M (2009) Inhibition of translesion DNA polymerase by archaeal reverse gyrase. Nucleic Acids Res 37:4287–4295
Vijayan V, Zuzow R, O'Shea EK (2009) Oscillations in supercoiling drive circadian gene expression in cyanobacteria. Proc Natl Acad Sci USA 106:22564–22568
Vinograd J, Lebowitz J, Radloff R, Watson R, Laipis P (1965) The twisted circular form of polyoma viral DNA. Proc Natl Acad Sci USA 53:1104–1111
Vinograd J, Lebowitz J (1966) Physical and topological properties of circular DNA. J Gen Physiol 49:103–125
Vinograd J, Lebowitz J, Watson R (1968) Early and late helix-coil transitions in closed circular DNA. The number of superhelical turns in polyoma DNA. J Mol Biol 33(1):173–197
Wall MK, Mitchenall LA, Maxwell A (2004) *Arabidopsis thaliana* DNA gyrase is targeted to chloroplasts and mitochondria. Proc Natl Acad Sci USA 101:7821–7826
Wallis JW, Chrebet G, Brodsky G, Rolfe M, Rothstein R (1989) A hyper-recombination mutation in *S. cerevisiae* identifies a novel eukaryotic topoisomerase. Cell 58:409–419
Wang JC (1971) Interaction between DNA and an *Escherichia coli* protein omega. J Mol Biol 55:523–533
Wang JC (1991) DNA topoisomerases: why so many? J Biol Chem 266:6659–6662
Wang JC (2009a) Untangling the double-helix: DNA entanglement and the action of the DNA topoisomerases. Cold Spring Harbor, New York, Cold Spring Harbor Laboratory Press
Wang JC (2009b) A journey in the world of DNA rings and beyond. Annu Rev Biochem 78:31–54
Wang Y, Lyu YL, Wang JC (2002) Dual localization of human DNA topoisomerase IIIalpha to mitochondria and nucleus. Proc Natl Acad Sci USA 99:12114–12119
Warburton PE, Earnshaw WC (1997) Untangling the role of DNA topoisomerase II. In: Mitotic chromosome structure and function. Bioessays 19:97–99. Review

Watson JD, Crick FH (1953a) Genetical implications of the structure of deoxyribonucleic acid. Nature 171:964–967

Watson JD, Crick FH (1953b) The structure of DNA. Cold Spring Harb Symp Quant Biol 18:123–131

Weil R, Vinograd J (1963) The cyclic helix and cyclic coil forms of polyoma viral DNA. Proc Natl Acad Sci USA 50:730–738

Wyckoff E, Natalie D, Nolan JM, Lee M, Hsieh T (1989) Structure of the Drosophila DNA topoisomerase II gene. Nucleotide sequence and homology among topoisomerases II. J Mol Biol. 205:1–13

Woese CR, Fox GE (1977) Phylogenetic structure of the prokaryotic domain: the primary kingdoms. Proc Natl Acad Sci USA 74:5088–5090

Woese CR, Kandler O, Wheelis ML (1990) Towards a natural system of organisms: proposal for the domains Archaea, Bacteria, and Eucarya. Proc Natl Acad Sci USA 87: 4576–4579

Wu D, Hugenholtz P, Mavromatis K, Pukall R, Dalin E, Ivanova NN, Kunin V, Goodwin L, Wu M, Tindall BJ, Hooper SD, Pati A, Lykidis A, Spring S, Anderson IJ, D'haeseleer P, Zemla A, Singer M, Lapidus A, Nolan M, Copeland A, Han C, Chen F, Cheng JF, Lucas S, Kerfeld C, Lang E, Gronow S, Chain P, Bruce D, Rubin EM, Kyrpides NC, Klenk HP, Eisen JA (2009) A phylogeny-driven genomic encyclopaedia of Bacteria and Archaea. Nature 462:1056–1060

Wu L, Hickson ID (2006) DNA helicases required for homologous recombination and repair of damaged replication forks. Annu Rev Genet 40:279–306

Yamada T, Satoh S, Ishikawa H, Fujiwara A, Kawasaki T, Fujie M, Ogata H (2010) A jumbo phage infecting the phytopathogen *Ralstonia solanacearum* defines a new lineage of the Myoviridae family. Virology 398:135–147

Yamashiro K, Yamagishi A (2005) Characterization of the DNA gyrase from the thermoacidophilic archaeon Thermoplasma acidophilum. J Bacteriol 187:8531–8536

Yang W (2010) Topoisomerases and site-specific recombinases: similarities in structure and mechanism. Crit Rev Biochem Mol Biol 45:520–534

Yin Y, Cheong H, Friedrichsen D, Zhao Y, Hu J, Mora-Garcia S, Chory J (2002) A crucial role for the putative Arabidopsis topoisomerase VI in plant growth and development. Proc Natl Acad Sci USA 99:10191–10196

Zechiedrich EL, Khodursky AB, Bachellier S, Schneider R, Chen D, Lilley DM, Cozzarelli NR (2000) Roles of topoisomerases in maintaining steady-state DNA supercoiling in *Escherichia coli*. J Biol Chem 275:8103–8113

Zhang H, Barceló JM, Lee B, Kohlhagen G, Zimonjic DB, Popescu NC, Pommier Y (2001) Human mitochondrial topoisomerase I. Proc Natl Acad Sci USA 98:10608–10613

Chapter 2
Human DNA Topoisomerase I: Structure, Enzymology and Biology

James J. Champoux

2.1 Introduction

DNA topoisomerases that change the linking number of torsionally-strained DNA by introducing a temporary interruption into one strand of DNA belong to the type I family of topoisomerases (for review see (Champoux 2001)). Those enzymes that generate a double-strand break by cleaving both strands of DNA in a staggered fashion are referred to as type II topoisomerases. To conserve the energy required for the religation reaction, DNA cleavage in both cases is accompanied by the covalent attachment of the topoisomerase to a phosphate at the site or sites of breakage. If the attachment of a type I topoisomerase occurs to a 5′ phosphate, the enzyme belongs to the type IA subfamily; if attachment is to a 3′ phosphate, the enzyme belongs to the type IB subfamily. For type I enzymes, during the lifetime of the covalent complex, DNA topology is changed by the passing of one DNA strand through another.

Humans code for two type IB topoisomerases that are paralogues: One is the nuclear enzyme, referred to as Top1 and the other is the topoisomerase found in the mitochondrion, referred to as mt-Top1 (Zhang et al. 2001). The mt-Top1 is encoded in nuclear genes and is described in Chap. 2. The primary focus of this review is the structure of human Top1 as it relates to enzyme catalysis and cellular function. The mechanism of action of the anticancer drugs belonging to the camptothecin (CPT) family is also discussed (Hsiang et al. 1985; Porter and Champoux 1989; Staker et al. 2002). A number of earlier reviews provide a comprehensive background to the subject and summarize the earlier literature (Champoux 2001; Leppard and Champoux 2005; Wang 1996, 2002).

J.J. Champoux (✉)
Department of Microbiology, School of Medicine,
University of Washington, Health Sciences Bldg, 1959 N.E. Pacific Street,
98195, Box 357735 Seattle, WA, USA
e-mail: champoux@u.washington.edu

Y. Pommier (ed.), *DNA Topoisomerases and Cancer*, Cancer Drug Discovery and Development, DOI 10.1007/978-1-4614-0323-4_2,

2.2 Structure of Human Top1

2.2.1 *Crystal Structure and Domain Properties*

A ribbon diagram of the co-crystal structure of the bi-lobed 91 kDa human Top1 protein clamped around a 22 base pair duplex DNA is shown in Fig. 2.1a with the color scheme depicting the domain structure of the enzyme (Redinbo et al. 1998; Stewart et al. 1996). Following the same color scheme, Fig. 2.1b shows the names and arrangement of the domains along a linear representation of the protein. The N-terminal domain comprising the first 214 amino acids is largely disordered, protease sensitive, highly hydrophilic, and poorly conserved among the eukaryotic type

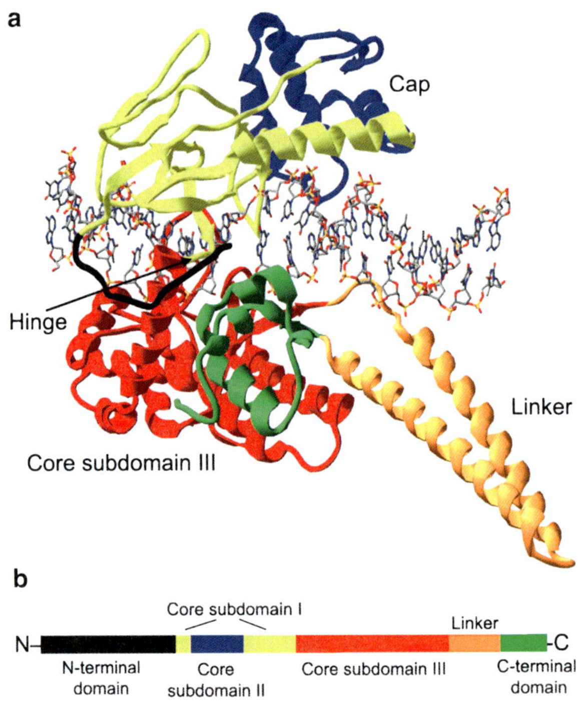

Fig. 2.1 The domain structure of human Top1. The domains of the protein are shown in both parts (**a**) and (**b**) with the following color schemes: *black*, N-terminal domain (residues 1–214); *yellow*, core subdomain I (residues 215–232 and 319–433); *blue*, core subdomain II (residues 233–318); *red*, core subdomain III (residues 434–635; *orange*, linker domain (residues 636–712); and *green*, C-terminal domain (residues 713–765). (**a**) Ribbon diagram of the co-crystal structure of human Top1 containing a 22 base pair duplex oligonucleotide (pdb entry 1K4T) (Staker et al. 2002) was drawn using Swiss-Pdb Viewer software (v3.7) (Glaxo Wellcome Experimental Research) (Guex et al. 2009). The only N-terminal domain residues visible in the crystal structure are those from positions 201–214. The "Cap" region comprising subdomains I and II (*yellow and blue*) is labeled as is the "Hinge" found at the boundary between subdomains I and III. (**b**) The domain structure of human Top1 is depicted on a linear representation of the protein

IB enzymes. Although amino acids from 201 to 214 are present in published crystal structures (shown as a black coil in Fig. 2.1a) (Staker et al. 2002), no structural information is available for the remainder of the N-terminal domain. The highly-conserved core domain extends from amino acid 215 to position 635 and can be subdivided into the three subdomains indicated in Fig. 2.1. Together, core subdomains I and II (shown in yellow and blue) constitute what has been referred to as the "cap" of the enzyme; a pair of α-helices within the cap that assume the shape of a V has been termed the "nose cone." A hinge is likely located at the junction between the cap and core subdomain III (yellow-red boundary, Fig. 2.1a) that enables the protein clamp to close and open as DNA binds and unbinds from the enzyme. On the opposite side of the protein from the hinge, two opposing loops extend from subdomains I and III and interact in the closed clamp form of the enzyme via six amino acids and one salt bridge to form what is referred to as the "lips" region. A poorly-conserved, protease-sensitive region referred to as the linker forms a 77 amino acid long flexible coiled-coiled structure that protrudes conspicuously from the remainder of the protein (Redinbo et al. 1999). The linker connects the core domain of the protein to the conserved C-terminal domain comprising the amino acids from position 713 to the end of the 765 amino acid-protein. The C-terminal domain contains the active site Tyr723 that becomes covalently attached to the DNA end during the formation of the covalent intermediate.

2.2.2 Domain Interactions and Functions

Although the N-terminal domain is dispensable for DNA relaxation activity *in vitro*, the presence of several nuclear localization signals (Alsner et al. 1992; Mo et al. 2000) and sites for the binding of interacting proteins (see Sect. 2.4) make it essential *in vivo*. A region of the N-terminal domain extending from residues 191 to 206 has been shown to reduce the processivity of the enzyme and to be required for efficient blunt-end ligation, implicating these residues in binding DNA downstream of the cleavage site (Frohlich et al. 2004; Lisby et al. 2001). Further evidence that this region of the N-terminal domain contacts the DNA is the finding that a deletion mutant lacking the residues from 191 to 206 or the W205G mutant protein allow faster DNA rotation during the nicked state (Frohlich et al. 2004). In addition, Trp205 is required for the inhibitory effects of CPT on the relaxation of negative, but not positive supercoils, whereas the WT enzyme is inhibited by CPT in both types of reactions (Frohlich et al. 2007). This last observation suggests that Trp205 and perhaps neighboring residues in the N-terminal domain are involved in the hindrance of strand rotation by bound CPT during the relaxation of negative supercoils (see Sect. 2.3.2).

All of the active site residues are contained with the core and C-terminal domains of the protein (Fig. 2.1a) and indeed fragment reconstitution experiments indicate that these two domains represent the minimal requirement for enzymatic activity *in vitro* (Stewart et al. 1997). Although this observation indicates that the linker domain is dispensable for enzyme activity, the rate of religation relative to the WT enzyme is increased in mutants lacking the linker or in the A653P mutant enzyme (Fiorani et al. 2003; Stewart et al. 1997), suggesting some form of communication between the linker and the active site that acts to prolong the cleaved state in the WT enzyme. Although a form of the protein missing the N-terminal domain and the Cap has all of the residues required for catalysis and binds DNA with an affinity similar to that of the full-length enzyme, it nonetheless lacks enzymatic activity (Yang and Champoux 2002). Apparently, the Cap region of the protein is important for proper positioning of the bound DNA and/or activating the enzyme for catalysis. Unlike cleavage, the Cap is not required for the religation step of the reaction (Yang and Champoux 2002).

The function of the linker domain remains a puzzle. Besides prolonging the nicked state, the linker region, like the N-terminal domain, appears to be involved in slowing DNA rotation and is required for maximal sensitivity to CPT (Losasso et al. 2007; Stewart et al. 1999). A K681A mutation in the linker exhibits a rate of religation that is slower that the WT enzyme, providing further support for the view that the linker communicates with the active site of the enzyme (Fiorani et al. 2009). Although the path of the linker in the crystal structure clearly does not track with the axis of the DNA, the fact that the linker exhibits considerable flexibility and that the DNA proximal surfaces of the coiled-coil structure are rich in basic amino acids suggests a possible direct interaction between the linker and the DNA in solution (Stewart et al. 1998).

2.3 Enzymology of Human Top1

2.3.1 *Reaction Chemistry and Catalysis*

As shown in Fig. 2.2, nucleophilic attack by the O-4 oxygen of the active site Tyr723 on a DNA phosphate leads to a transesterification reaction resulting in the covalent linkage of Top1 to the 3′ end of the broken DNA strand. During the lifetime of this covalent intermediate, strand rotation changes the linking number of the DNA (see Sect. 2.3.2). Religation restores the phosphodiester linkage in the DNA and is the reverse reaction in which the attacking nucleophile is the 5′ oxygen on the broken strand. Addition of denaturants such as alkali or detergents to a Top1 reaction *in vitro* prevents religation and traps the enzyme in the covalent complex on the DNA (Champoux 1976, 1977). The rate of religation is substantially faster than cleavage so that the steady-state level of nicked intermediate is relatively low (Stivers et al. 1994). The pharmacologically important activity of the anticancer drug CPT and many other compounds that target Top1 is to trap the enzyme on the DNA by slowing the religation step of the reaction (Hsiang et al. 1985; Koster et al. 2007; Pommier and Cherfils 2005; Pommier et al. 1998; Porter and Champoux 1989; Staker et al. 2002) (see Chaps. 9 and 10). Certain lesions or DNA modification such as nicks, gaps, base mismatches, abasic sites, and some forms of oxidative

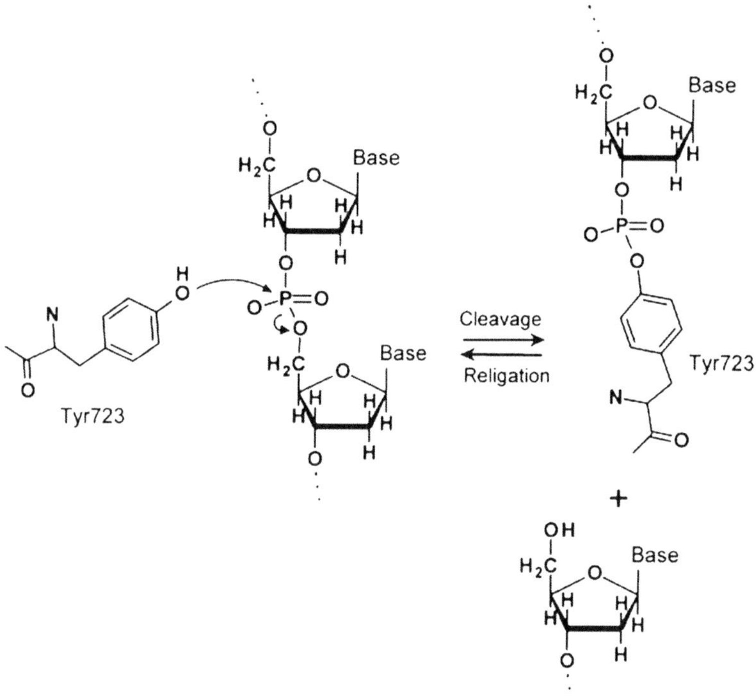

Fig. 2.2 Reaction chemistry for human Top1. In the cleavage reaction, the O-4 atom of the active site Tyr723 is shown as the nucleophile that attacks a phosphodiester bond in DNA to generate a phosphodiester linkage between itself and the 3′ end of the broken strand. The religation reaction involves nucleophilic attack by the free 5′ hydroxyl of the broken strand on the tyrosine-DNA linkage to restore the phosphodiester bond in the DNA and release the active site tyrosine

damage can also lead to Top1-mediated DNA damage by blocking the religation reaction (Lebedeva et al. 2008; Pommier et al. 2003, 2006). Such suicide cleavage reactions can occasionally lead to ligation of the DNA to a new DNA end by the topoisomerase (Been and Champoux 1981; Champoux et al. 1984), a reaction that may cause illegitimate recombination *in vivo* (Bullock et al. 1985; Larsen et al. 1998) and under some conditions may contribute to genetic instability in cancer cells (Larsen and Gobert 1999).

Several co-crystal structures provide insights into the catalytic mechanism of type IB topoisomerases (Davies et al. 2006; Redinbo et al. 2000; Redinbo et al. 1998) as summarized below and described in more detail elsewhere (Champoux 2001; Davies et al. 2006). Transition-state stabilization by human Top1 is achieved by the hydrogen-bonding of Arg488 and Lys532 to the same non-bridging oxygen and the hydrogen-bonding of His632 to the other non-bridging oxygen. In addition, Lys532 acts as a general acid to donate a proton to the leaving 5′ oxygen during cleavage and may facilitate religation by acting as a general base (Interthal et al. 2004). There appears to be no amino acid side chain that acts as a general base to activate Tyr723 for cleavage; instead, the structure shows a water molecule located at a position consistent with it acting as a specific base to accept the proton from the nucleophilic O-4 oxygen of Tyr723. Arg590 is also in close proximity to the O-4 oxygen and may enhance its nucleophilicity by stabilizing the phenolate anion.

2.3.2 Controlled Rotation Mechanism for DNA Relaxation

Although type IA topoisomerases can only relax negative supercoils, all type IB topoisomerases can relax supercoils of both signs with positive supercoils being removed faster than negative supercoils (Frohlich et al. 2007). Modeling studies based on the crystal structure of human Top1 with a 22 base pair oligonucleotide (Stewart et al. 1998) suggested that there was insufficient space within the confines of the closed-clamp configuration to allow free rotation of the duplex DNA downstream of the cleavage site and the term "controlled rotation" was coined to explain how relaxation of both negative and positive supercoiling occurs. By generating a mutant form of human Top1 containing cysteine residues in the opposing loops of the "lips" region (H367C and A499C), it was possible to lock the clamp closed through a disulfide bridge and show that rotation did not require the opening of the protein clamp (Carey et al. 2003). Interestingly, a similar disulfide approach that locked the protein closed through a clamp located closer to the DNA (G365C and S534C) did prevent DNA relaxation (Woo et al. 2003), presumably by constraining domain movements required for the rotation process.

A series of elegant single-molecule experiments have validated the controlled rotation model by showing that the DNA experiences friction during the rotation step of the reaction (Koster et al. 2005). Moreover, these experiments show that DNA rotation is a torque-driven process where the number of supercoils relaxed per cleavage-religation cycle is related to the number of supercoils present in the DNA. The source of the friction is undoubtedly the tightness with which the DNA fits in the enzyme cavity, but as mentioned previously, both the N-terminal domain and the linker domain have also been shown to slow DNA rotation (Frohlich et al. 2004; Stewart et al. 1999). Interestingly, both biochemical and single-molecule measurements indicate that in addition to slowing religation, CPT also inhibits DNA relaxation by retarding DNA rotation (Koster et al. 2007; Stewart et al. 1999).

Simulation studies of the rotation process using molecular dynamics are also consistent with the controlled rotation model and furthermore indicate that the conformational changes in the protein associated with the removal of negative and positive supercoils are different (Sari and Andricioaei 2005). Rotation associated with the relaxation of positive supercoils involves a 10–14 Å opening of the clamp where the two loops meet in the lips region, whereas relaxation of negative supercoils requires the stretching of a loop on the opposite side of the protein near the hinge region by ~12 Å (Fig. 2.1a). In this regard, it is noteworthy that single-molecule experiments show CPT inhibits the relaxation of positive supercoils to a greater extent than the removal of negative supercoils (Koster et al. 2007), suggesting a strong effect of bound CPT on the conformational flexibility of the lips region of the protein. Since Trp205 is located in close proximity to the hinge region, the molecular dynamics simulations are also consistent with the requirement for this amino acid for the inhibitory effects of CPT on the relaxation of negative, but not positive supercoils (Frohlich et al. 2007).

2.3.3 Sequence and Topological Specificity

In the co-crystal structure of human Top1, most protein-DNA interactions involve backbone contacts with both strands of the DNA upstream of the cleavage site, where the cleavage is defined as occurring between the "−1" and "+1" nucleotides (Redinbo et al. 1998). By cataloguing nucleotide frequencies on the scissile strand in the vicinity of a large number of Top1 cleavage sites, a preference was observed for certain nucleotides from positions "−4" to "−1" as follows: 5′-(A/T) (G/C) (A/T) (T)-3′ where covalent attachment is to the "−1" thymine residue (Been et al. 1984; Bonven et al. 1985; Tanizawa et al. 1993). A secondary preference for a cytosine at the "−1" position was also found. When cleavage was examined in the presence of CPT, an additional preference for a +1G was observed (Jaxel et al. 1991).

The only base-specific contact observed in the co-crystal structure involves a hydrogen bond between the side chain of Lys532 and the O−2 atom of the preferred "−1" thymine residue (Redinbo et al. 1998). Since the same interaction is also possible with a cytosine base, but not with an adenine or guanine, it was tempting to attribute the preference for a thymine or a cytosine at the "−1" position to this interaction with Lys532. Although replacement of Lys532 with alanine reduces the catalytic activity of the enzyme as expected for an active site residue (see Sect. 1.3.1), the mutant enzyme exhibited the same nucleotide sequence preference as the WT enzyme when the residual cleavage activity was analyzed (Interthal et al. 2004). This observation indicates that interactions between the enzyme and the DNA other than those involving Lys532 play a dominant role in determining the sequence specificity of the enzyme.

Several studies indicate that human Top1 prefers a supercoiled over a relaxed substrate DNA (Camilloni et al. 1988); Caserta et al. 1989, 1990; Madden et al. 1995; Muller 1985; Zechiedrich and Osheroff 1990). Since Top1 prefers supercoils of both signs, Zeehiedrich and Osheroff (Zechiedrich and Osheroff 1990) proposed that the feature recognized in the supercoiled DNA was a node where two duplex regions of DNA cross. Presumably such node binding would require two DNA binding sites on the enzyme. Although a dimeric form of the enzyme could mediate node binding, a recent study ruled out this possibility and instead showed that several conserved solvent-exposed basic residues in core subdomain III and the linker region are important for the recognition of supercoils (Yang et al. 2009). Since changing pairs of lysines to glutamic acid in core subdomain III significantly reduced the preference for supercoils, it seems likely that these residues are involved in node binding through direct contacts with the DNA backbone. Full manifestation of the preference for supercoiled DNA requires the presence of the linker region in the protein, but reversing the charges on two clusters of basic amino acids in the coiled-coil linker domain had no effect on supercoiled DNA binding. This latter observation suggests that rather than contributing to node binding through a direct interaction between basic amino acid side chains and the DNA, the linker domain plays an indirect structural role in the binding to DNA nodes.

In the cell, DNA is wound into a toroidal supercoil that is constrained by the tight association with histone proteins in the nucleosome (Richmond et al. 1984). These interactions as well as the folding of the nucleosomes into the higher order chromatin structure involve the formation of DNA nodes that resemble those found in purified supercoiled DNA. Thus, while it is tempting to conclude that the preference of Top1 for nodes reflects the mechanism for targeting the enzyme to torsionally-strained supercoils in chromatin, it remains possible that DNA crossings present in chromatin unrelated to torsional stress in the DNA serve as the basis for the observed *in vitro* preference of Top1 for supercoiled plasmid DNA (Madden et al. 1995).

2.4 Biology of Human Top1

2.4.1 Transcription, Replication, and Chromatin Assembly

The movement of a rotationally fixed RNA polymerase along duplex DNA during transcription generates negative supercoils in its wake and positive supercoils in the region ahead of the translocating enzyme (Liu and Wang 1987). The topological dilemma posed by this effect is especially apparent when transcription of adjacent regions on the DNA proceeds in opposite directions. However, even for genes transcribed in the same direction to generate adjoining supercoiled regions of opposite signs, the enormous length of chromosomal DNA and the large distances between adjacent transcription units, combined with the bending and folding induced by bound histones and other chromosomal proteins, present a formidable barrier to the dissipation of such supercoils simply by DNA rotation (Crut et al. 2007; Leng and McMacken 2002; Nelson 1999; Thomen et al. 2002). Strand separation during DNA replication by DNA helicases results in the overwinding of the DNA beyond the advancing replication fork to generate positive supercoils that similarly cannot be resolved by simple rotation of the DNA helix.

In higher eukaryotes, Top1 is an essential enzyme (Lee et al. 1993; Morham et al. 1996) that, in conjunction with Top2, is responsible for relaxing the torsionally-strained supercoils that are generated during both transcription and DNA replication (Avemann et al. 1988; Brill et al. 1987; Champoux 1992, 2001; Fleischmann et al. 1984; Gilmour et al. 1986; Kim and Wang 1989; Kretzschmar et al. 1993; Kroeger and Rowe 1989; Merino et al. 1993; Rose et al. 1988; Salceda et al. 2006; Stewart et al. 1990; Wang 2002; Yang et al. 1987; Zhang et al. 1988). In addition, the wrapping of DNA into negative supercoils in the formation of the nucleosome core

(Richmond et al. 1984) and the formation of right-handed solenoidal supercoils by the SMC family of proteins (Holmes and Cozzarelli 2000; Kimura et al. 1999) generate compensatory positive and negative supercoils, respectively, that are likely relaxed by Top1.

Consistent with the multiple roles for Top1 in maintaining the relaxed topological state in these DNA transactions, the enzyme is expressed constitutively throughout the cell cycle (Baker et al. 1995). Furthermore, although Top1 is distributed throughout the nucleus, it is highly enriched in the nucleolus where it supports a very high rate of rDNA transcription (Christensen et al. 2004; Leppard and Champoux 2005; Muller et al. 1985; Zhang et al. 1988). Consistent with a critical role for Top1 in the nucleolus, the protein is found to directly interact with both nucleolin and RNA polymerase I holoenzyme and these interactions are likely mediated by the N-terminal domain of Top1 (Table 2.1) (Bharti et al. 1996; Christensen et al. 2004; Rose et al. 1988). Similarly, Top1 has been found to be associated with RNA polymerase II and its cofactors, including the TATA binding protein (Carty and Greenleaf 2002; Kretzschmar et al. 1993; Merino et al. 1993; Wu et al. 2010). The interaction with c-jun which regulates the expression of the epidermal growth factor receptor gene may represent a unique example of Top1 acting in conjunction with a transcription factor to activate expression of a specific gene (Mialon et al. 2005). Top1 has also been found in association with cellular DNA replication complexes (Lebel et al. 1999; Wang 1985; Wu et al. 1994) and binds directly to the WRN helicase (Laine et al. 2003; Lebel et al. 1999). Finally, Top1 has been implicated in the replication of papillomavirus and SV40 DNAs (Table 2.1).

A five-fold reduction in the level of human Top1 by siRNA caused defects in DNA replication, a decrease in sensitivity to CPT, nucleolar abnormalities, and a consistent alteration in the transcription of at least 55 genes (Miao et al. 2007). Although the expression of Top2α was unchanged in these cell lines, its association with chromatin was increased, presumably to compensate for the reduction in the level of Top1. The cells also exhibited an unusually high level of chromosome rearrangements, possibly occurring as a result of defects in DNA replication.

2.4.2 Beyond Transcription, Replication, and Chromatin Assembly

Table 2.1 lists a number of proteins that have been shown to directly interact with Top1. In those cases in which the sites of interaction on Top1 have been mapped, the most common region involved is the N-terminal domain of the protein (residues 1–214). In addition to proteins involved in transcription and DNA replication, the interacting proteins have a number of disparate functions that include ubiquitination and sumoylation, DNA repair, RNA splicing, and tumor suppressors. Although many of the partners increase the activity of Top1, a few decrease the activity or target the enzyme for modification. Interacting proteins such as activated PARP-1,

Table 2.1 Proteins that directly interact with human Top1

Interacting protein	Function	Binding site on Top1 (amino acid range)	Effect of interaction on Top1	References
ASF/SF2	RNA splicing factor	?	Decreases cleavage	Andersen et al. (2002); Labourier et al. (1998)
BTBD1	Myogenic differentiation	?	?	Pisani et al. (2004); Xu et al. (2002)
BTBD2	?	215–329	?	Xu et al. (2002)
CK2	Ser/thr protein kinase	?	Increases activity	Kowalska-Loth et al. (2003)
c-jun	Transcription factor	?	?	Mialon et al. (2005)
HMG proteins	Chromatin	?	Increases activity	Javaherian and Liu (1983)
Nucleolin	Ribosome biogenesis	166–210	?	Bharti et al. (1996)
NKX3.1	Tumor suppressor	320–765	Increases activity	Bowen et al. (2007)
Papillomavirus E1/E2 proteins	DNA helicase, viral replication	?	Increases activity	Clower et al. (2006a, b)
Poly (ADP-ribose)-PARP-1	Poly (ADP-ribose) polymerase-1	50–65 and 209–442	Increases religation	Bauer et al. (2001); Malanga and Althaus (2004); Park and Cheng (2005)
p14ARF	Tumor suppressor	215–765	Increases activity	Bandyopadhyay et al. (2007); Karayan et al. (2001)
p53	Tumor suppressor	1–214	Increases activity	Gobert et al. (1996); Mao et al. (2002)
PSF/p54^{nrb}	RNA splicing factor	?	Increases activity	Straub et al. (1998)
RNA pol I	rDNA transcription	1–214	?	Christensen et al. (2004); Rose et al. (1988)
RNA pol II	Transcription	1–114	?	Carty and Greenleaf (2002); Wu et al. (2010)
SV40 T-Ag	DNA helicase, viral replication	1–139 and 383–765	?	Haluska et al. (1998)
TATA binding protein	Transcription factor	1–214	?	Mao et al. (2002); Merino et al. (1993)
HTLV-1 Tax	Transcriptional activator	?	Inhibits activity	Suzuki et al. (2000)
Topors	E3 ligase	2–250	Ubiquitination/ sumoylation	Haluska et al. (1999); Hammer et al. (2007)
UBC9	E2-sumoylation	?	Sumoylation	Mao et al. (2000)
WRN	DNA helicase	?	Enhances religation	Laine et al. (2003)

Those proteins that have been shown to physically interact with human Top1 are listed alphabetically along with their functions and the effects of the interaction on Top1 activity if known. In those cases where the interaction site on Top1 has been mapped, the range of amino acid residues shown to be involved in the interaction are indicated

Topors, UBC9, and possibly WRN likely function to enable to the cell to avoid or repair damage resulting from the aberrant formation of Top1-DNA covalent complexes (see Chap. 13, Topoisomerase-induced DNA damage). Interestingly, the association of Top1 with the tumor suppressor protein p14ARF requires serine phosphorylation and since casein kinase 2 (CK2) which also interacts with Top1 can fulfill this function *in vitro* (Bandyopadhyay et al. 2007), it is likely that mitotic phosphorylation on Ser10 by CK2 is responsible for this modification (Hackbarth et al. 2008). The interaction of Top1 and p53 appears to be related to the activation of p53 at covalent complexes formed when the topoisomerase fails in the religation reaction *in vivo* (Gobert et al. 1999; Humbert et al. 2009; Kohn et al. 2000; Larsen and Gobert 1999; Rockstroh et al. 2007).

In addition to the protein partners discussed above where a direct interaction has been demonstrated, a proteomic analysis using co-immunoprecipitation and affinity chromatography identified a large number of additional proteins that are associated with Top1 (Czubaty et al. 2005), including many of those listed in Table 2.1. Most notably, this study adds to the list of interacting proteins that are RNA splicing factors or are found in complexes containing RNA, such as ribonucleoprotein particles (RNPs). These findings would appear to implicate Top1 as a member of a large group of proteins that are involved in RNA metabolism, but the exact role of the topoisomerase remains obscure.

Acknowledgments The author gratefully acknowledges Sharon Schultz and Zheng Yang for help during the preparation of the manuscript. This work was supported by National Institutes of Health Grant GM049156.

References

Alsner J, Svejstrup JQ, Kjeldsen E, Sorensen BS, Westergaard O (1992) Identification of an N-terminal domain of eukaryotic DNA topoisomerase I dispensable for catalytic activity but essential for in vivo function. *J Biol Chem* **267**(18): 12408–12411

Andersen FF, Tange TO, Sinnathamby T, Olesen JR, Andersen KE, Westergaard O, Kjems J, Knudsen BR (2002) The RNA splicing factor ASF/SF2 inhibits human topoisomerase I mediated DNA relaxation. *J Mol Biol* **322**(4): 677–686

Avemann K, Knippers R, Koller T, Sogo JM (1988) Camptothecin, a specific inhibitor of type I DNA topoisomerase, induces DNA breakage at replication forks. *Mol Cell Biol* **8**(8): 3026–3034

Baker SD, Wadkins RM, Stewart CF, Beck WT, Danks MK (1995) Cell cycle analysis of amount and distribution of nuclear DNA topoisomerase I as determined by fluorescence digital imaging microscopy. *Cytometry* **19**(2): 134–145

Bandyopadhyay K, Lee C, Haghighi A, Baneres JL, Parello J, Gjerset RA (2007) Serine phosphorylation-dependent coregulation of topoisomerase I by the p14ARF tumor suppressor. *Biochemistry* **46**(49): 14325–14334

Bauer PI, Chen HJ, Kenesi E, Kenessey I, Buki KG, Kirsten E, Hakam A, Hwang JI, Kun E (2001) Molecular interactions between poly(ADP-ribose) polymerase (PARP I) and topoisomerase I (Topo I): identification of topology of binding. *FEBS Lett* **506**(3): 239–242

Been MD, Burgess RR, Champoux JJ (1984) Nucleotide sequence preference at rat liver and wheat germ type 1 DNA topoisomerase breakage sites in duplex SV40 DNA. *Nucleic Acids Res* **12**(7): 3097–3114

Been MD, Champoux JJ (1981) DNA breakage and closure by rat liver type 1 topoisomerase: separation of the half-reactions by using a single-stranded DNA substrate. *Proc Natl Acad Sci USA* **78**(5)**:** 2883–2887
Bharti AK, Olson MO, Kufe DW, Rubin EH (1996) Identification of a nucleolin binding site in human topoisomerase I. *Journal Of Biological Chemistry* **271**(4)**:** P 1993–1997
Bonven BJ, Gocke E, Westergaard O (1985) A high affinity topoisomerase I binding sequence is clustered at DNAase I hypersensitive sites in Tetrahymena R-chromatin. *Cell* **41**(2)**:** 541–551
Bowen C, Stuart A, Ju JH, Tuan J, Blonder J, Conrads TP, Veenstra TD, Gelmann EP (2007) NKX3.1 homeodomain protein binds to topoisomerase I and enhances its activity. *Cancer Res* **67**(2)**:** 455–464
Brill SJ, DiNardo S, Voelkel-Meiman K, Sternglanz R (1987) DNA topoisomerase activity is required as a swivel for DNA replication and for ribosomal RNA transcription. *NCI Monogr* **4:** 11–15
Bullock P, Champoux JJ, Botchan M (1985) Association of crossover points with topoisomerase I cleavage sites: a model for nonhomologous recombination. *Science* **230**(4728)**:** 954–958
Camilloni G, Di Martino E, Caserta M, di Mauro E (1988) Eukaryotic DNA topoisomerase I reaction is topology dependent. *Nucleic Acids Res* **16**(14B)**:** 7071–7085
Carey JF, Schultz SJ, Sisson L, Fazzio TG, Champoux JJ (2003) DNA relaxation by human topoisomerase I occurs in the closed clamp conformation of the protein. *Proc Natl Acad Sci USA* **100**(10)**:** 5640–5645
Carty SM, Greenleaf AL (2002) Hyperphosphorylated C-terminal repeat domain-associating proteins in the nuclear proteome link transcription to DNA/chromatin modification and RNA processing. *Mol Cell Proteomics* **1**(8)**:** 598–610
Caserta M, Amadei A, Camilloni G, Di Mauro E (1990) Regulation of the function of eukaryotic DNA topoisomerase I: analysis of the binding step and of the catalytic constants of topoisomerization as a function of DNA topology. *Biochemistry* **29**(35)**:** 8152–8157
Caserta M, Amadei A, Di Mauro E, Camilloni G (1989) In vitro preferential topoisomerization of bent DNA. *Nucleic Acids Res* **17**(21)**:** 8463–8474
Champoux JJ (1976) Evidence for an intermediate with a single-strand break in the reaction catalyzed by the DNA untwisting enzyme. *Proc Natl Acad Sci USA* **73**(10)**:** 3488–3491
Champoux JJ (1977) Strand breakage by the DNA untwisting enzyme results in covalent attachment of the enzyme to DNA. *Proc Natl Acad Sci USA* **74**(9)**:** 3800–3804
Champoux JJ (1992) Topoisomerase I is preferentially associated with normal SV40 replicative intermediates, but is associated with both replicating and nonreplicating SV40 DNAs which are deficient in histones. *Nucleic Acids Res* **20**(13)**:** 3347–3352
Champoux JJ (2001) DNA topoisomerases: structure, function, and mechanism. *Annu Rev Biochem* **70:** 369–413
Champoux JJ, McCoubrey WK, Jr., Been MD (1984) DNA structural features that lead to strand breakage by eukaryotic type-I topoisomerase. *Cold Spring Harb Symp Quant Biol* **49:** 435–442
Christensen MO, Krokowski RM, Barthelmes HU, Hock R, Boege F, Mielke C (2004) Distinct effects of topoisomerase I and RNA polymerase I inhibitors suggest a dual mechanism of nucleolar/nucleoplasmic partitioning of topoisomerase I. *J Biol Chem* **279**(21)**:** 21873–21882
Clower RV, Fisk JC, Melendy T (2006a) Papillomavirus E1 protein binds to and stimulates human topoisomerase I. *J Virol* **80**(3)**:** 1584–1587
Clower RV, Hu Y, Melendy T (2006b) Papillomavirus E2 protein interacts with and stimulates human topoisomerase I. *Virology* **348**(1)**:** 13–18
Crut A, Koster DA, Seidel R, Wiggins CH, Dekker NH (2007) Fast dynamics of supercoiled DNA revealed by single-molecule experiments. *Proc Natl Acad Sci USA* **104**(29)**:** 11957–11962
Czubaty A, Girstun A, Kowalska-Loth B, Trzcinska AM, Purta E, Winczura A, Grajkowski W, Staron K (2005) Proteomic analysis of complexes formed by human topoisomerase I. *Biochim Biophys Acta* **1749**(1)**:** 133–141
Davies DR, Mushtaq A, Interthal H, Champoux JJ, Hol WG (2006) The structure of the transition state of the heterodimeric topoisomerase I of Leishmania donovani as a vanadate complex with nicked DNA. *J Mol Biol* **357**(4)**:** 1202–1210

Fiorani P, Bruselles A, Falconi M, Chillemi G, Desideri A, Benedetti P (2003) Single mutation in the linker domain confers protein flexibility and camptothecin resistance to human topoisomerase I. *J Biol Chem* **278**(44): 43268–43275

Fiorani P, Tesauro C, Mancini G, Chillemi G, D'Annessa I, Graziani G, Tentori L, Muzi A, Desideri A (2009) Evidence of the crucial role of the linker domain on the catalytic activity of human topoisomerase I by experimental and simulative characterization of the Lys681Ala mutant. *Nucleic Acids Res* **37**(20): 6849–6858

Fleischmann G, Pflugfelder G, Steiner EK, Javaherian K, Howard GC, Wang JC, Elgin SC (1984) Drosophila DNA topoisomerase I is associated with transcriptionally active regions of the genome. *Proc Natl Acad Sci USA* **81**(22): 6958–6962

Frohlich RF, Andersen FF, Westergaard O, Andersen AH, Knudsen BR (2004) Regions within the N-terminal domain of human topoisomerase I exert important functions during strand rotation and DNA binding. *J Mol Biol* **336**(1): 93–103

Frohlich RF, Veigaard C, Andersen FF, McClendon AK, Gentry AC, Andersen AH, Osheroff N, Stevnsner T, Knudsen BR (2007) Tryptophane-205 of human topoisomerase I is essential for camptothecin inhibition of negative but not positive supercoil removal. *Nucleic Acids Res* **35**(18): 6170–6180

Gilmour DS, Pflugfelder G, Wang JC, Lis JT (1986) Topoisomerase I interacts with transcribed regions in Drosophila cells. *Cell* **44**(3): 401–407

Gobert C, Bracco L, Rossi F, Olivier M, Tazi J, Lavelle F, Larsen AK, Riou JF (1996) Modulation of DNA topoisomerase I activity by p53. *Biochemistry* **35**(18): 5778–5786

Gobert C, Skladanowski A, Larsen AK (1999) The interaction between p53 and DNA topoisomerase I is regulated differently in cells with wild-type and mutant p53. *Proc Natl Acad Sci USA* **96**(18): 10355–10360

Guex N, Peitsch MC, Schwede T (2009) Automated comparative protein structure modeling with SWISS-MODEL and Swiss-PdbViewer: a historical perspective. *Electrophoresis* **30 Suppl 1**: S162–173

Hackbarth JS, Galvez-Peralta M, Dai NT, Loegering DA, Peterson KL, Meng XW, Karnitz LM, Kaufmann SH (2008) Mitotic phosphorylation stimulates DNA relaxation activity of human topoisomerase I. *J Biol Chem* **283**(24): 16711–16722

Haluska P, Jr., Saleem A, Edwards TK, Rubin EH (1998) Interaction between the N-terminus of human topoisomerase I and SV40 large T antigen. *Nucleic Acids Res* **26**(7): 1841–1847

Haluska P, Jr., Saleem A, Rasheed Z, Ahmed F, Su EW, Liu LF, Rubin EH (1999) Interaction between human topoisomerase I and a novel RING finger/arginine-serine protein. *Nucleic Acids Res* **27**(12): 2538–2544

Hammer E, Heilbronn R, Weger S (2007) The E3 ligase Topors induces the accumulation of polysumoylated forms of DNA topoisomerase I in vitro and in vivo. *FEBS Lett* **581**(28): 5418–5424

Holmes VF, Cozzarelli NR (2000) Closing the ring: links between SMC proteins and chromosome partitioning, condensation, and supercoiling. *Proc Natl Acad Sci USA* **97**(4): 1322–1324

Hsiang YH, Hertzberg R, Hecht S, Liu LF (1985) Camptothecin induces protein-linked DNA breaks via mammalian DNA topoisomerase I. *J Biol Chem* **260**(27): 14873–14878

Humbert N, Martien S, Augert A, Da Costa M, Mauen S, Abbadie C, de Launoit Y, Gil J, Bernard D (2009) A genetic screen identifies topoisomerase 1 as a regulator of senescence. *Cancer Res* **69**(10): 4101–4106

Interthal H, Quigley PM, Hol WG, Champoux JJ (2004) The role of lysine 532 in the catalytic mechanism of human topoisomerase I. *J Biol Chem* **279**(4): 2984–2992

Javaherian K, Liu LF (1983) Association of eukaryotic DNA topoisomerase I with nucleosomes and chromosomal proteins. *Nucleic Acids Res* **11**(2): 461–472

Jaxel C, Capranico G, Kerrigan D, Kohn KW, Pommier Y (1991) Effect of local DNA sequence on topoisomerase I cleavage in the presence or absence of camptothecin. *J Biol Chem* **266**(30): 20418–20423

Karayan L, Riou JF, Seite P, Migeon J, Cantereau A, Larsen CJ (2001) Human ARF protein interacts with topoisomerase I and stimulates its activity. *Oncogene* **20**(7): 836–848

Kim RA, Wang JC (1989) Function of DNA topoisomerases as replication swivels in Saccharomyces cerevisiae. *J Mol Biol* **208**(2): 257–267

Kimura K, Rybenkov VV, Crisona NJ, Hirano T, Cozzarelli NR (1999) 13S condensin actively reconfigures DNA by introducing global positive writhe: implications for chromosome condensation. *Cell* **98**(2): 239–248

Kohn KW, Shao RG, Pommier Y (2000) How do drug-induced topoisomerase I-DNA lesions signal to the molecular interaction network that regulates cell cycle checkpoints, DNA replication, and DNA repair? *Cell Biochem Biophys* **33**(2): 175–180

Koster DA, Croquette V, Dekker C, Shuman S, Dekker NH (2005) Friction and torque govern the relaxation of DNA supercoils by eukaryotic topoisomerase IB. *Nature* **434**(7033): 671–674

Koster DA, Palle K, Bot ES, Bjornsti MA, Dekker NH (2007) Antitumour drugs impede DNA uncoiling by topoisomerase I. *Nature* **448**(7150): 213–217

Kowalska-Loth B, Girstun A, Derlacz R, Staron K (2003) Activation of human topoisomerase I by protein kinase CK2. *Mol Biol Rep* **30**(2): 107–111

Kretzschmar M, Meisterernst M, Roeder RG (1993) Identification of human DNA topoisomerase I as a cofactor for activator-dependent transcription by RNA polymerase II. *Proc Natl Acad Sci USA* **90**(24): 11508–11512

Kroeger PE, Rowe TC (1989) Interaction of topoisomerase 1 with the transcribed region of the Drosophila HSP 70 heat shock gene. *Nucleic Acids Res* **17**(21): 8495–8509

Labourier E, Rossi F, Gallouzi IE, Allemand E, Divita G, Tazi J (1998) Interaction between the N-terminal domain of human DNA topoisomerase I and the arginine-serine domain of its substrate determines phosphorylation of SF2/ASF splicing factor. *Nucleic Acids Res* **26**(12): 2955–2962

Laine JP, Opresko PL, Indig FE, Harrigan JA, von Kobbe C, Bohr VA (2003) Werner protein stimulates topoisomerase I DNA relaxation activity. *Cancer Res* **63**(21): 7136–7146

Larsen AK, Gobert C (1999) DNA topoisomerase I in oncology: Dr Jekyll or Mr Hyde? *Pathol Oncol Res* **5**(3): 171–178

Larsen AK, Gobert C, Gilbert C, Markovits J, Bojanowski K, Skladanowski A (1998) DNA topoisomerases as repair enzymes: mechanism(s) of action and regulation by p53. *Acta Biochim Pol* **45**(2): 535–544

Lebedeva N, Rechkunova N, Boiteux S, Lavrik O (2008) Trapping of human DNA topoisomerase I by DNA structures mimicking intermediates of DNA repair. *IUBMB Life* **60**(2): 130–134

Lebel M, Spillare EA, Harris CC, Leder P (1999) The Werner syndrome gene product co-purifies with the DNA replication complex and interacts with PCNA and topoisomerase I. *J Biol Chem* **274**(53): 37795–37799

Lee MP, Brown SD, Chen A, Hsieh TS (1993) DNA topoisomerase I is essential in Drosophila melanogaster. *Proc Natl Acad Sci USA* **90**(14): 6656–6660

Leng F, McMacken R (2002) Potent stimulation of transcription-coupled DNA supercoiling by sequence-specific DNA-binding proteins. *Proc Natl Acad Sci USA* **99**(14): 9139–9144

Leppard JB, Champoux JJ (2005) Human DNA topoisomerase I: relaxation, roles, and damage control. *Chromosoma* **114**(2): 75–85

Lisby M, Olesen JR, Skouboe C, Krogh BO, Straub T, Boege F, Velmurugan S, Martensen PM, Andersen AH, Jayaram M, Westergaard O, Knudsen BR (2001) Residues within the N-terminal domain of human topoisomerase I play a direct role in relaxation. *J Biol Chem* **276**(23): 20220–20227

Liu LF, Wang JC (1987) Supercoiling of the DNA template during transcription. *Proc Natl Acad Sci USA* **84**(20): 7024–7027

Losasso C, Cretaio E, Palle K, Pattarello L, Bjornsti MA, Benedetti P (2007) Alterations in linker flexibility suppress DNA topoisomerase I mutant-induced cell lethality. *J Biol Chem* **282**(13): 9855–9864

Madden KR, Stewart L, Champoux JJ (1995) Preferential binding of human topoisomerase I to superhelical DNA. *EMBO J* **14**(21): 5399–5409

Malanga M, Althaus FR (2004) Poly(ADP-ribose) reactivates stalled DNA topoisomerase I and Induces DNA strand break resealing. *J Biol Chem* **279**(7): 5244–5248

Mao Y, Mehl IR, Muller MT (2002) Subnuclear distribution of topoisomerase I is linked to ongoing transcription and p53 status. *Proc Natl Acad Sci USA* **99**(3)**:** 1235–1240

Mao Y, Sun M, Desai SD, Liu LF (2000) SUMO-1 conjugation to topoisomerase I: A possible repair response to topoisomerase-mediated DNA damage. *Proc Natl Acad Sci USA* **97**(8)**:** 4046–4051

Merino A, Madden KR, Lane WS, Champoux JJ, Reinberg D (1993) DNA topoisomerase I is involved in both repression and activation of transcription. *Nature* **365**(6443)**:** 227–232

Mialon A, Sankinen M, Soderstrom H, Junttila TT, Holmstrom T, Koivusalo R, Papageorgiou AC, Johnson RS, Hietanen S, Elenius K, Westermarck J (2005) DNA topoisomerase I is a cofactor for c-Jun in the regulation of epidermal growth factor receptor expression and cancer cell proliferation. *Mol Cell Biol* **25**(12)**:** 5040–5051

Miao ZH, Player A, Shankavaram U, Wang YH, Zimonjic DB, Lorenzi PL, Liao ZY, Liu H, Shimura T, Zhang HL, Meng LH, Zhang YW, Kawasaki ES, Popescu NC, Aladjem MI, Goldstein DJ, Weinstein JN, Pommier Y (2007) Nonclassic functions of human topoisomerase I: genome-wide and pharmacologic analyses. *Cancer Res* **67**(18)**:** 8752–8761

Mo YY, Wang C, Beck WT (2000) A novel nuclear localization signal in human DNA topoisomerase I. *J Biol Chem* **275**(52)**:** 41107–41113

Morham SG, Kluckman KD, Voulomanos N, Smithies O (1996) Targeted disruption of the mouse topoisomerase I gene by camptothecin selection. *Mol Cell Biol* **16**(12)**:** 6804–6809

Muller MT (1985) Quantitation of eukaryotic topoisomerase I reactivity with DNA. Preferential cleavage of supercoiled DNA. *Biochim Biophys Acta* **824**(3)**:** 263–267

Muller MT, Pfund WP, Mehta VB, Trask DK (1985) Eukaryotic type I topoisomerase is enriched in the nucleolus and catalytically active on ribosomal DNA. *Embo J* **4**(5)**:** 1237–1243

Nelson P (1999) Transport of torsional stress in DNA. *Proc Natl Acad Sci USA* **96**(25)**:** 14342–14347

Park SY, Cheng YC (2005) Poly(ADP-ribose) polymerase-1 could facilitate the religation of topoisomerase I-linked DNA inhibited by camptothecin. *Cancer Res* **65**(9)**:** 3894–3902

Pisani DF, Cabane C, Derijard B, Dechesne CA (2004) The topoisomerase 1-interacting protein BTBD1 is essential for muscle cell differentiation. *Cell Death Differ* **11**(11)**:** 1157–1165

Pommier Y, Barcelo JM, Rao VA, Sordet O, Jobson AG, Thibaut L, Miao ZH, Seiler JA, Zhang H, Marchand C, Agama K, Nitiss JL, Redon C (2006) Repair of topoisomerase I-mediated DNA damage. *Prog Nucleic Acid Res Mol Biol* **81:** 179–229

Pommier Y, Cherfils J (2005) Interfacial inhibition of macromolecular interactions: nature's paradigm for drug discovery. *Trends Pharmacol Sci* **26**(3)**:** 138–145

Pommier Y, Pourquier P, Fan Y, Strumberg D (1998) Mechanism of action of eukaryotic DNA topoisomerase I and drugs targeted to the enzyme. *Biochim Biophys Acta* **1400**(1–3)**:** 83–105

Pommier Y, Redon C, Rao VA, Seiler JA, Sordet O, Takemura H, Antony S, Meng L, Liao Z, Kohlhagen G, Zhang H, Kohn KW (2003) Repair of and checkpoint response to topoisomerase I-mediated DNA damage. *Mutat Res* **532**(1–2)**:** 173–203

Porter SE, Champoux JJ (1989) The basis for camptothecin enhancement of DNA breakage by eukaryotic topoisomerase I. *Nucleic Acids Res* **17**(21)**:** 8521–8532

Redinbo MR, Champoux JJ, Hol WG (2000) Novel Insights into Catalytic Mechanism from a Crystal Structure of Human Topoisomerase I in Complex with DNA. *Biochemistry* **39**(23)**:** 6832–6840

Redinbo MR, Stewart L, Champoux JJ, Hol WG (1999) Structural flexibility in human topoisomerase I revealed in multiple non-isomorphous crystal structures. *J Mol Biol* **292**(3)**:** 685–696

Redinbo MR, Stewart L, Kuhn P, Champoux JJ, Hol WG (1998) Crystal structures of human topoisomerase I in covalent and noncovalent complexes with DNA. *Science* **279**(5356)**:** 1504–1513

Richmond TJ, Finch JT, Rushton B, Rhodes D, Klug A (1984) Structure of the nucleosome core particle at 7 A resolution. *Nature* **311**(5986)**:** 532–537

Rockstroh A, Kleinert A, Kramer M, Grosse F, Soe K (2007) Cellular stress triggers the human topoisomerase I damage response independently of DNA damage in a p53 controlled manner. *Oncogene* **26**(1)**:** 123–131

Rose KM, Szopa J, Han FS, Cheng YC, Richter A, Scheer U (1988) Association of DNA topoisomerase I and RNA polymerase I: a possible role for topoisomerase I in ribosomal gene transcription. *Chromosoma* **96**(6)**:** 411–416

Salceda J, Fernandez X, Roca J (2006) Topoisomerase II, not topoisomerase I, is the proficient relaxase of nucleosomal DNA. *Embo J* **25**(11)**:** 2575–2583

Sari L, Andricioaei I (2005) Rotation of DNA around intact strand in human topoisomerase I implies distinct mechanisms for positive and negative supercoil relaxation. *Nucleic Acids Res* **33**(20)**:** 6621–6634

Staker BL, Hjerrild K, Feese MD, Behnke CA, Burgin AB, Jr., Stewart L (2002) The mechanism of topoisomerase I poisoning by a camptothecin analog. *Proc Natl Acad Sci USA* **99**(24)**:** 15387–15392

Stewart AF, Herrera RE, Nordheim A (1990) Rapid induction of c-fos transcription reveals quantitative linkage of RNA polymerase II and DNA topoisomerase I enzyme activities. *Cell* **60**(1)**:** 141–149

Stewart L, Ireton GC, Champoux JJ (1996) The domain organization of human topoisomerase I. *J Biol Chem* **271**(13)**:** 7602–7608

Stewart L, Ireton GC, Champoux JJ (1997) Reconstitution of human topoisomerase I by fragment complementation. *J Mol Biol* **269**(3)**:** 355–372

Stewart L, Ireton GC, Champoux JJ (1999) A functional linker in human topoisomerase I is required for maximum sensitivity to camptothecin in a DNA relaxation assay. *J Biol Chem* **274**(46)**:** 32950–32960

Stewart L, Redinbo MR, Qiu X, Hol WG, Champoux JJ (1998) A model for the mechanism of human topoisomerase I. *Science* **279**(5356)**:** 1534–1541

Stivers JT, Shuman S, Mildvan AS (1994) Vaccinia DNA topoisomerase I: single-turnover and steady-state kinetic analysis of the DNA strand cleavage and ligation reactions. *Biochemistry* **33**(1)**:** 327–339

Straub T, Grue P, Uhse A, Lisby M, Knudsen BR, Tange TO, Westergaard O, Boege F (1998) The RNA-splicing factor PSF/p54 controls DNA-topoisomerase I activity by a direct interaction. *J Biol Chem* **273**(41)**:** 26261–26264

Suzuki T, Uchida-Toita M, Andoh T, Yoshida M (2000) HTLV-1 tax oncoprotein binds to DNA topoisomerase I and inhibits its catalytic activity. *Virology* **270**(2)**:** 291–298

Tanizawa A, Kohn KW, Pommier Y (1993) Induction of cleavage in topoisomerase I c-DNA by topoisomerase I enzymes from calf thymus and wheat germ in the presence and absence of camptothecin. *Nucleic Acids Res* **21**(22)**:** 5157–5166

Thomen P, Bockelmann U, Heslot F (2002) Rotational drag on DNA: a single molecule experiment. *Phys Rev Lett* **88**(24)**:** 248102

Wang JC (1985) DNA topoisomerases. *Annu Rev Biochem* **54:** 665–697

Wang JC (1996) DNA Topoisomerases. *Ann Rev Biochem* **65:** 635–692

Wang JC (2002) Cellular roles of DNA topoisomerases: a molecular perspective. *Nat Rev Mol Cell Biol* **3**(6)**:** 430–440

Woo MH, Losasso C, Guo H, Pattarello L, Benedetti P, Bjornsti MA (2003) Locking the DNA topoisomerase I protein clamp inhibits DNA rotation and induces cell lethality. *Proc Natl Acad Sci USA* **100**(24)**:** 13767–13772

Wu J, Phatnani HP, Hsieh TS, Greenleaf AL (2010) The phosphoCTD-interacting domain of Topoisomerase I. *Biochem Biophys Res Commun* **397**(1)**:** 117–119

Wu Y, Hickey R, Lawlor K, Wills P, Yu F, Ozer H, Starr R, Quan JY, Lee M, Malkas L (1994) A 17 S multiprotein form of murine cell DNA polymerase mediates polyomavirus DNA replication in vitro. *J Cell Biochem* **54**(1)**:** 32–46

Xu L, Yang L, Hashimoto K, Anderson M, Kohlhagen G, Pommier Y, D'Arpa P (2002) Characterization of BTBD1 and BTBD2, two similar BTB-domain-containing Kelch-like proteins that interact with Topoisomerase I. *BMC Genomics* **3**(1)**:** 1

Yang L, Wold MS, Li JJ, Kelly TJ, Liu LF (1987) Roles of DNA topoisomerases in simian virus 40 DNA replication in vitro. *Proc Natl Acad Sci USA* **84**(4)**:** 950–954

Yang Z, Carey JF, Champoux JJ (2009) Mutational analysis of the preferential binding of human topoisomerase I to supercoiled DNA. *Febs J* **276**(20)**:** 5906–5919

Yang Z, Champoux JJ (2002) Reconstitution of enzymatic activity by the association of the cap and catalytic domains of human topoisomerase I. *J Biol Chem* **277**(34)**:** 30815–30823

Zechiedrich EL, Osheroff N (1990) Eukaryotic topoisomerases recognize nucleic acid topology by preferentially interacting with DNA crossovers. *Embo J* **9**(13)**:** 4555–4562

Zhang H, Barcelo JM, Lee B, Kohlhagen G, Zimonjic DB, Popescu NC, Pommier Y (2001) Human mitochondrial topoisomerase I. *Proc Natl Acad Sci USA* **98**(19)**:** 10608–10613

Zhang H, Wang JC, Liu LF (1988) Involvement of DNA topoisomerase I in transcription of human ribosomal RNA genes. *Proc Natl Acad Sci USA* **85**(4)**:** 1060–1064

Chapter 3
Mitochondrial Topoisomerases

Ilaria Dalla Rosa, Yves Pommier, and Hongliang Zhang

3.1 Introduction

Mitochondria are essential organelles that play a key role in the energy production and cell death of eukaryotic cells. Mitochondria host the cellular respiratory chain, an electron transport system that converts the energy of nutrients into readily utilizable energy in the form of ATP. Thirteen out of ~150 subunits of the respiratory chain are encoded by the mitochondrial genome (mtDNA) (Fig. 3.1). Although physically separated from the nuclear genome, mtDNA completely relies on the nucleus for its maintenance. All factors of mtDNA metabolism are encoded by nuclear genes and imported into the mitochondria post-translationally.

Like in the nucleus, the topological problems rising from mtDNA transcription and replication require the activity of topoisomerases. Indeed, by now, one representative of each topoisomerase sub-families has been found in mammalian mitochondria: Mitochondrial topoisomerase I (Top1mt) (Zhang et al. 2001b) (a type IB enzyme), topoisomerase III-alpha (Top3α) (Wang et al. 2002b) (a type IA enzyme), and topoisomerase II-beta (Top2β) (Low et al. 2003) (a type IIA enzyme). Top1mt is the only topoisomerase encoded by a nuclear gene whose product is solely devoted to mitochondria. The two other topoisomerases (Top3α and Top2β) are encoded by genes whose products generate both nuclear and mitochondrial products (Low et al. 2003; Wang et al. 2002b).

We will first introduce the general features of mtDNA, its metabolism, and then review the mitochondrial DNA topoisomerases. With few exceptions, we will focus our attention on mammalian cells.

H. Zhang (✉)
Laboratory of Molecular Pharmacology, Center for Cancer Research,
National Cancer Institute, National Institutes of Health, Bethesda, MD, 20892 USA
e-mail: zhangh@pop.nci.nih.gov

Y. Pommier (ed.), *DNA Topoisomerases and Cancer*, Cancer Drug Discovery and Development, DOI 10.1007/978-1-4614-0323-4_3,

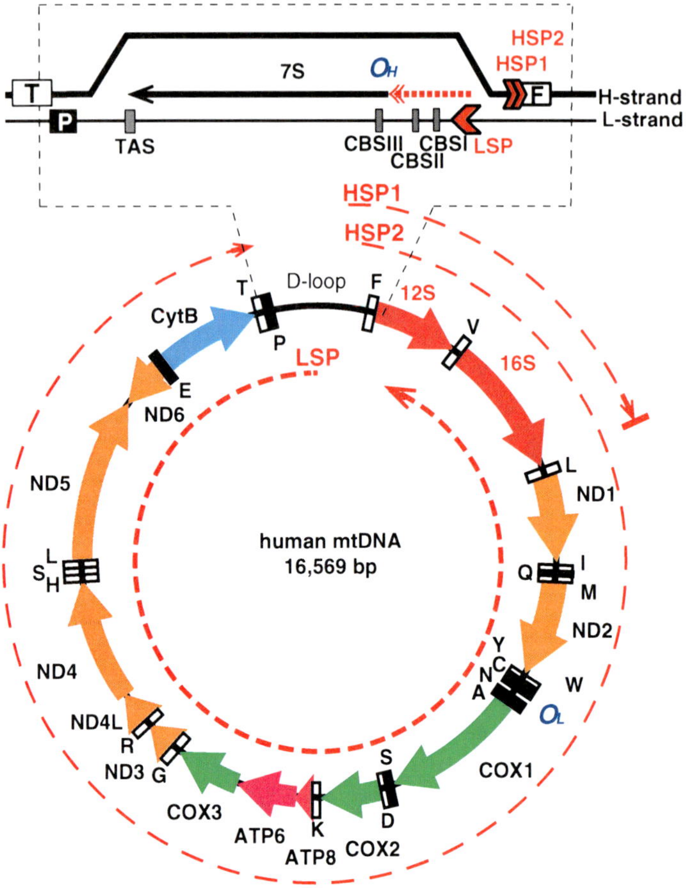

Fig. 3.1 Organization of mammalian mtDNA: Mitochondrial genes coding for subunits of complex I, III, IV and V are represented in orange, blue, green, and magenta, respectively. 12S and 16S rRNAs are in red. tRNAs are shown as *white* and *black boxes* (*white* when encoded on the heavy strand; *black* when on the light strand), and labeled as single-letter amino acid code (outside for the H-strand; inside for L-strand). Dashed *arrows* represent H-strand and L-strand transcripts. The non-coding regulatory region is magnified at the top of the figure: LSP, HSP1 and HSP2 are the L- and H-strand promoters 1 and 2

3.2 Mitochondrial DNA and Its Metabolism

Mammalian mtDNA is a circular double-stranded molecule of approximately 16 kb (Fig. 3.1). The number of mtDNA copies per human cells has been estimated to 10^3–10^4, but this number can vary significantly depending on the cell type and response to different stresses and energy demand (Clay Montier et al. 2009; Hock and Kralli 2009). *In vivo,* the mitochondrial genome is organized in discrete chromosome-like structures, referred to as nucleoids. Each nucleoid consists of 5–7 mtDNA molecules packed together in large nucleoprotein-complexes, which form biosynthetic centers for mtDNA expression and replication (Iborra et al. 2004). Interestingly, Top1mt has been recently identified as a core-component of human nucleoids (Bogenhagen et al. 2008).

MtDNA encodes 13 mRNAs, 2 rRNAs, and 22 tRNAs (Fig. 3.1). All mRNAs produce proteins for respiratory chain complexes whereas rRNAs and tRNAs are components of the mitochondrial translation machinery. The 37 mitochondrial genes lack introns and are tightly packed on both mtDNA strands, denoted as heavy (H) and light (L) strand (Clayton 1982). The only non-coding region of substantial size is the so-called D-loop region that contains three promoters for mtDNA transcription (HSP1, HSP2, and LSP) and the origin of replication for leading-strand synthesis (O_H). The regulatory region of the D-loop (displacement loop) is named after its peculiar triple-stranded structure. Frequently, the replication events initiated at O_H stop prematurely about 600 bp downstream the initiation site, and the nascent DNA chain, known as 7S DNA, displaces the parental H strand generating the D-loop structure (Bogenhagen and Clayton 1978; Gillum and Clayton 1978). In addition to the key elements for mtDNA expression and replication, the D-loop contains several conserved regions with regulatory significance (Sbisà et al. 1997). Three short conserved termination associated sequences (TAS) are involved in the pausing of DNA polymerase and, as a consequence, in the formation of 7 S DNA. Moreover, three conserved sequence blocks termed CBSI, II, and III seem to play a role in the initiation of H-strand synthesis at O_H (see mtDNA replication). The significance as well as the regulation of D-loop formation is still unknown; however, this region is supposed to play a role in mtDNA metabolism and in the assembly of nucleoids.

3.2.1 Transcription of mtDNA

The core machinery for mtDNA transcription consists of mitochondrial RNA polymerase (POLRMT) and two auxiliary cofactors: Mitochondrial transcription factor A (TFAM) and mitochondrial transcription factor B2 (TFB2M) (Falkenberg et al. 2002; Litonin et al.). POLRMT is a single-subunit bacteriophage T7-related RNA polymerase. However, unlike T7 RNA polymerase, it is unable to initiate mtDNA transcription on its own and TFAM and TFB2M are both essential for promoter recognition and transcription initiation. TFAM (h-mtTFA) is a high-mobility-group (HMG)/DNA packaging factor that binds specific sequences upstream mtDNA promoters (Dairaghi et al. 1995; Fisher et al. 1987), whereas TFB2M (h-mt-TFB2) is an rRNA methyltransferase-related transcription factor that forms heterodimeric complexes with POLRMT (Falkenberg et al. 2002). The mechanism of promoter recognition in mammalian mitochondria is not fully understood but it is generally believed that TFB2M recruits POLRMT to the promoter either through a direct interaction with TFAM (McCulloch and Shadel 2003) or recognizing single-stranded DNA regions exposed by TFAM binding [for review see (Bonawitz et al. 2006; Falkenberg et al. 2007)].

MtDNA transcription can initiate from three different promoters located on both strands in the regulatory D-loop region (Fig. 3.1). Transcripts starting from HSP1 stop directly downstream the 16S gene producing only the two mitochondrial rRNAs and two tRNA (V and L; see Fig. 3.1). This termination event involves the mitochondrial transcription termination factor (mTERF), which binds simultaneously to the beginning and the end of the transcription unit, bridging them together to form an rDNA loop. This loop facilitates the recycling of POLRMT from the termination to the initiation site (Martin et al. 2005) and enables the production of high levels of rRNAs that are required for the assembly of mitochondrial ribosomes (Montoya et al. 1983).

Transcription from HSP2 (adjacent to HSP1; Fig. 3.1) proceeds along the entire genome and generates a long polycistronic transcript containing all but one (ND6) mitochondrial proteins, both rRNAs, and 14 out of the 22 tRNAs encoded in the mitochondrial genome. The third mitochondrial transcription unit uses the L strand as template. It starts from a single promoter (LSP) and generates a genome-long polycistronic RNA coding for a single protein (ND6), 8 tRNAs, and RNA primer for mtDNA replication (see below).

The polycistronic RNA precursors produced by POLRMT are processed through excising the tRNAs that flank the majority of mRNAs and rRNAs (Ojala et al. 1981). Processed rRNAs and tRNAs function in the mitochondrial translation machinery. The mitochondrial mRNAs are polyadenylated and translated into essential subunits of the respiratory chain complexes. The mechanism of RNA processing and protein synthesis in mitochondria goes beyond the scope of this chapter [for review see (Shutt and Shadel 2010)].

3.2.2 *Replication of mtDNA*

The minimal mtDNA replisome has been reconstituted *in vitro*. It consists of mitochondrial DNA polymerase γ (POLG), POLRMT, the mitochondrial helicase Twinkle, and the mitochondrial single-strand binding protein mtSSB (Korhonen et al. 2004). On a single-stranded template, POLRMT exhibits low processivity and provides short RNA primers that can be used by POLG to initiate DNA replication (Wanrooij et al. 2008; Gillum and Clayton 1978). For the heavy strand synthesis, the switch from RNA to DNA synthesis occurs in the D-loop region downstream CBSII (see Fig. 3.1). It has been recently shown that this site-specific transition is induced by G-quadrupex structures formed upon transcription of this conserved sequence (Wanrooij et al. 2010). Once DNA replication starts, Twinkle unwinds the DNA duplex ahead of the replication fork, helping the progression of POLG. MtSSB assists probably by enhancing the rate of DNA unwinding (Korhonen et al. 2003), and topoisomerases can deal with the supercoils generated in the process.

The mechanism of mtDNA replication has been under debate for many years and is still an open controversy. Three main models have been proposed. According to the strand-displacement model, mtDNA leading and lagging strands are synthesized asynchronously. Synthesis of the leading strand starts at O_H in the mtDNA regulatory region (Fig. 3.1) and proceeds unidirectionally along approximately two-thirds of the template to reach O_L. The parental H-strand behind the replication fork is displaced as a single stranded DNA and mtSSB binds and protects it from degradation. The displacement of O_L region leads to the formation of a stem-loop structure that promotes the initiation of lagging-strand DNA synthesis in the opposite direction (Clayton 1991; Fuste et al. 2010).

More recently, 2D agarose gel electrophoresis (2D-AGE) data have challenged the asymmetric strand-displacement model, showing the existence of mtDNA replication intermediates resulting from coupled leading and lagging strand synthesis. On the basis of these findings, a strand-coupled model for mtDNA replication was proposed. Similar to classical DNA replication, synthesis of both mtDNA strands proceeds bidirectionally from a broad zone downstream O_H (Holt et al. 2000; Bowmaker 2003). In addition to DNA-duplex replication intermediates, 2D-AGE studies showed further intermediates containing extensive tracts of RNA: DNA hybrids (Yang et al. 2002). This led Holt and coworkers to propose a third model for mtDNA replication, referred to as RITOLS (Ribonucleotide Incorporation ThroughOut the Lagging Strand). This last model for mtDNA replication share most features of the classic strand displacement model with the difference that the lagging strand is initially laid down as RNA and later converted to DNA (Yang et al. 2002; Yasukawa et al. 2006).

Large amounts of data corroborate the strand displacement model for mtDNA replication. On the other hand, stable, partially hybridized RNA has been found throughout the entire mouse mtDNA (Brown et al. 2008). At present, there is no consensus on the mtDNA replication mechanism and it is possible that different mechanisms of mtDNA replication operate in different physiological contexts and/or in different tissues (Yasukawa et al. 2005).

3.3 TOP1mt, a Vertebrate Mitochondrial Topoisomerase

3.3.1 *Discovery of Top1mt*

Mitochondrial topoisomerase activities were first described in the 1980s in mitochondria from human, rat, and bovine cells (Castora and Lazarus 1984; Fairfield et al. 1985; Kosovsky and Soslau 1993; Lin and Castora 1995). However, the first mitochondrial topoisomerase was identified 20 years later with the discovery of a novel gene, *TOP1mt* by systematic analyses of the human genome (Zhang et al. 2001a). The *TOP1mt* cDNA encodes a Top1-like polypeptide containing three of the four domains found in the nuclear Top1 (the core, linker, and C-terminal domains) (Fig. 3.2). The N-terminal domain of nuclear Top1, which contains nuclear localization signals (NLS) and interacts with other proteins (see Chap. 2), is missing from Top1mt. Tagging of Top1mt with green fluorescent protein (GFP) demonstrated its

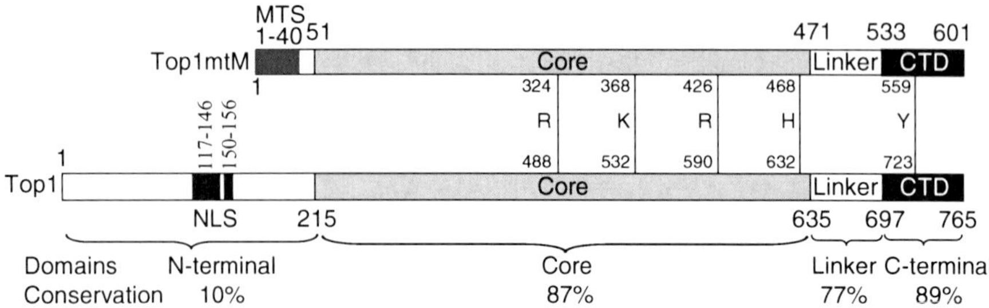

Fig. 3.2 Schematic structure of Top1mt vs. Top1. The conservations (identities and similarities) are indicated for each domain. Positions of critical residues are listed and marked by *vertical lines*

selective localization in mitochondria (Zhang et al. 2001a). Moreover, a mitochondrial targeting signal (MTS) was readily identifiable in the short N-terminal domain of new Top1. To avoid changing the preexisting nomenclature for Top1 and because of its unique mitochondrial localization, we named the new topoisomerase Top1mt. The *TOP1mt* gene maps to chromosome 8q24.3 (Zhang et al. 2001a) in humans and chromosome 15.2 in mice (Zhang et al. 2004b).

Biochemical comparison shows some difference between human mitochondrial and nuclear Top1 enzymes that are consistent with their adaptation to their cellular compartment (Zhang et al. 2001a). The pH of mitochondrial matrix is above 8, and Top1mt works best at pH 8–8.5. The nuclear matrix pH tends to be neutral, within the optimum range for nuclear Top1. Both Top1 and Top1mt can function without divalent cations. However, the optimal catalytic activity of Top1mt is preferentially enhanced by divalent cations (Mg^{2+} or Ca^{2+}), which is consistent with mitochondria as a Ca^{2+} supply for the cell. Camptothecin inhibits both nuclear Top1 and Top1mt activity *in vitro*. However, sequencing of the some camptothecin-resistant cell lines failed to show mutations in Top1mt (Zhang et al. unpublished), suggesting lack of targeting on nuclear Top1 by camptothecin. One reason for the lack of targeting of Top1mt *in vivo* could be the relatively high pH inside mitochondria, which can inactivate CPT by hydrolyzing its hydroxylactone ring (Pommier 2009). It is also not excluded that CPT tends to be excluded from mitochondria because it lacks the positive charge(s) that usually characterize drugs that target mitochondria.

3.3.2 The TOP1B 13-Exon Signature Motif

The human *TOP1mt* gene consists of 14 exons, while the *TOP1* gene contains a total of 21 exons (Zhang et al. 2001a). The last 13 exons of both *TOP1* and *TOP1mt* are highly conserved and have identical structures and sizes (Zhang et al. 2001a).

The *TOP1mt* gene is conserved across vertebrates including chimpanzee, mouse, rat, chicken, and zebra fish, and all the known *TOP1mt* genes possess 14 exons

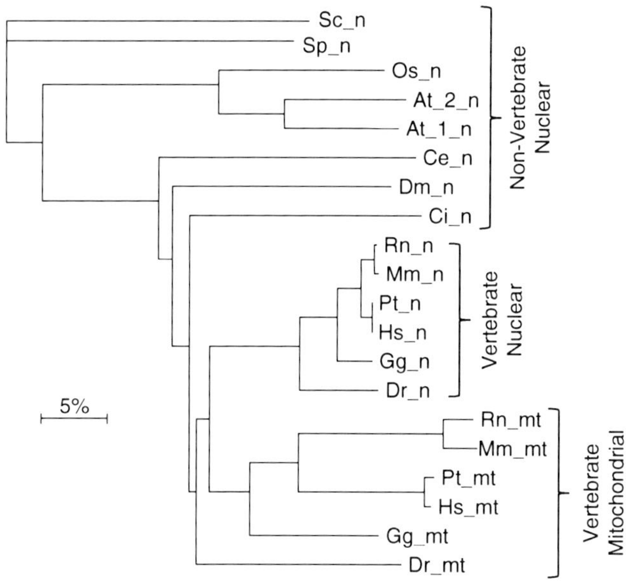

Fig. 3.3 Phylogenic tree of mitochondrial and nuclear Type IB topoisomerases. The comparison is based on the core, linker, and C-terminal region encoded by the last conserved 13 exons from each gene. Hs *Homo sapiens*, Pt *Pan troglodytes*, Rn *Rattus norvegicus*, Mm *Mus musculus*, Gg *Gallus gallus*, Dr *Danio rerio*, Ci *Ciona intestinalis*, Dm *Drosophila melanogaster*, Ce *Caenorhabditis elegans*, Sp *Schizosaccharomyces pombe*, Sc *Saccharomyces cerevisiae*, At *Arabidopsis thaliana*, Os *Oryza sativa*

(Zhang et al. 2004b). The exon sizes of the known *TOP1mt* genes vary for the first exons but are identical for the remaining 13 exons except for the 2nd and 13th exons of the rodent genes that are 3 bp shorter. One amino acid deletion of 2nd and 13th exons from both mouse and rat *TOP1mt* reflects their close genetic relationship. Whether this feature is common to all rodents is yet unknown. The first exons of the *TOP1mt* genes share little homology but all encode a functional MTS.

Using the 13-exon signature motif as a bait, comparative genomic search revealed that *Ciona intestinalis* (a chordate sea squirt and a non-vertebrate evolution neighbor) exhibits a similar exon structure (Zhang et al. 2004a). The corresponding core domain has the same exon structure as the other type IB topoisomerases, suggesting the core domain evolved first, followed by the C-terminal domain, and finally by the linker domain that connects the core and C-terminal domain. Phylogenic analysis of the mitochondrial and nuclear *TOP1* genes (Fig. 3.3) suggests that the 13-exon signature motif appeared in a common ancestor. Following duplication, one gene copy acquired a complex set of exons including a coding sequence for NLS and therefore became a nuclear *TOP1*; the other copy acquired a MTS and thereafter became *TOP1mt*. Because the mitochondrial targeting signals are remarkably different between species, it is plausible that the MTS's were selected based on preexisting genome or environment.

3.3.3 Regulation of TOP1mt Expression

Human *TOP1mt* is regulated by alternative splicing (Zhang et al. 2007). Most alternative splicing happens between exon1 and exon2, with two alternative exons, exon1a and exon1b, which are mutually exclusive. The functions and extent of *TOP1mt* alternative splicing are yet to be understood.

Although little is known regarding the gene regulation of *TOP1mt*, E2F1 has been reported to influence TOP1mt expression. E2F1 knockdown with siRNA results in a significant increase in transcription and replication of mitochondrial DNA as well as the induction of nuclear-encoded *TOP1mt* mRNA. On the contrary, the levels of nuclear-encoded mitochondrial transcription factor A (TFAM) mRNA and protein were unchanged (Goto et al. 2006).

Our ongoing studies using genome-wide analysis of *TOP1mt* expression across the 60 cancer cell lines of the National Cancer Institute (NCI60) are revealing that TOP1mt is coregulated with most other mitochondrial genes encoded in the nucleus (Zoppoli et al. 2011). Moreover, we found that c-myc acts as a positive transcription factor for *TOP1mt* and a large number of other genes involved in mitochondrial biogenesis.

3.3.4 Functional Insights for Top1mt

At this point, the only known biochemical activity of Top1mt is DNA relaxation. The core domain of Top1mt contains the catalytic basic amino acids (RKR) also found in Top1 (Fig. 3.3). The C-terminal domain containing the catalytic tyrosine residue is also highly conserved. The linker domain is slightly less conserved.

To map the cleavage sites of Top1mt in mtDNA, we took advantage of the fact that Top1mt-mtDNA complexes can be trapped in isolated mitochondria treated with CPT (or other anti-Top1 drugs) and sequenced by ligation-mediated PCR (Zhang and Pommier 2008). Analysis of the D-loop region showed a restricted number of Top1mt sites clustering approximately 150 bp in front of the D-loop (Zhang and Pommier 2008).

In spite of its conservation in all vertebrates, *TOP1mt* is not essential in mice. *TOP1mt* knockout mouse are viable and fertile, and their phenotype is under investigation (our ongoing studies). The viability of *TOP1mt* knockout mice was unexpected because knocking out nuclear *TOP1* is early embryonic lethal (Morham et al. 1996) (see Chap. 2) and knocking out other mitochondrial genes involved in mtDNA metabolism (including POLG and TFAM) is uniformly lethal (Tyynismaa and Suomalainen 2009). Thus, lack of Top1mt must be compensated by some other topoisomerase(s). Nuclear Top1 is an unlikely candidate in vertebrates since targeting of nuclear Top1 to mitochondria is toxic to cells, leading to severe disruption of mitochondrial RNA transcription and depletion of mtDNA (Dalla Rosa et al. 2009). Our ongoing studies indicate that a significant fraction of Top2 activity provides sufficient mtDNA relaxation under base line growth conditions (see Sect. 6).

3.4 Mitochondrial Top1 Activity in Yeast

The restriction of Top1mt to vertebrates implies that other eukaryotes employ different mechanisms to provide Top1 activity to mitochondria. The nuclear Top1 of fission yeast (*Schizosaccharomyces pombe*) scores high on MTS computer analysis (Wang et al. 2002a). Therefore, in fission yeast, the single *TOP1* gene likely supplies Top1 to both nuclear and mitochondrial compartments.

Careful analyses failed to reveal a MTS in Top1 from budding yeast (*Saccharomyces cerevisiae*) (Wang et al. 2002a). However, genetic and biochemical evidence support the view that both nuclear and mitochondrial Top1 are related to the same unique *TOP1* gene (Tua et al. 1997; Wang et al. 1995).

Besides yeast, a large number of organisms only have one Type IB topoisomerase gene (see Fig. 3.3). Thus, it is plausible that in these organisms, mitochondria and nuclei share the same Top1 or/and that Top2 activity can perform the functions accomplished by Top1mt in vertebrates.

3.5 Mitochondrial Top3α

As discussed in Chap. 5, the human *TOP3α* gene contains two in-frame initiation codons (Fig. 3.4). Initiation at the first and the 26th AUG generates two different polypeptides of 1,001 and 976 amino acid residues, respectively. The short form of Top3α was initially thought to be the only peptide product until a mitochondrial targeting signal was identified in the long form (Wang et al. 2002a). The short peptide of 976 amino acids exclusively functions in nuclei, while the long form has a dual localization, predominately in the nuclei with a fraction in mitochondria.

Recent studies have shown the importance of the mitochondrial function of Top3 in *Drosophila*. Top3α is required for the maintenance of the mitochondrial genome and male germ-line stem cells (Wu et al. 2010) (see Chap. 5). Like its human counterpart, the fruit fly Top3α polypeptide harbors an in-frame methionine at position 26. The N-terminal region to this methionine contains a MTS. If the methionine at position 26 is mutated to Leucine (M26L), the mutant Top3α is mainly located in mitochondria. On the other hand, if the first methionine is mutated to leucine (M1L), the protein exclusively localizes to the nuclei. Top3α knockout is recessive lethal (Plank et al. 2005) and M26L is sufficient to sustain the essential functions for viability and fertility. M1L flies exhibit fertility defects in both sexes; M1L females are sterile whereas male's fertility is severely impaired and decreases drastically with age. The male sterility is due to the loss of germ-line cells, which is a result of defects in cell proliferation (Wu et al. 2010).

Top3α knockout mice are embryonic lethal, shortly after implantation (Li and Wang 1998). Computer algorithm analyses predict that all available Top3α (mouse, chicken, *C. elegans*, *S. cerevisiae*, and *S. pombe*) have the conserved dual structure allowing their location to both nuclei and mitochondria.

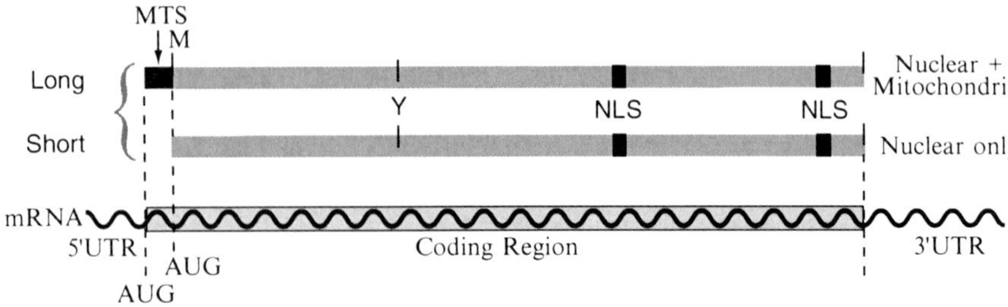

Fig. 3.4 Top3α alternative translation produces two polypeptides targeting the nucleus and mitochondria. *MTS* mitochondrial target signal, *NLS* nuclear localization signal, *UTR* untranslated region, *Y* catalytic tyrosine

3.6 Mitochondrial Topoisomerase II

The nuclear functions of eukaryotic type II topoisomerases, Top2α and Top2β have been well characterized (see Chaps. 1 and 4). However, their potential mitochondrial functions are not well defined. Mitochondrial topoisomerase II activity was first reported 25 years ago in mammalian cells using biochemical assays (Castora et al. 1985; Lin and Castora 1991). Relatively recently, a truncated Top2β polypeptide (~150 instead of the full-length 180 kDa) has been isolated from bovine mitochondria (Low et al. 2003). Judging from MALDI-TOF data, it was proposed that the mitochondrial TopoIIβ is a C-terminal truncated variant of the nuclear enzyme (Low et al. 2003). Our ongoing studies (Zhang et al. in preparation) suggest that not only Top2β, but also Top2α is imported and functions in the mitochondria of vertebrate cells.

3.7 Pending Issues

It is now established that all three types of topoisomerases (IA, IB, and IIA) (see Chap. 1) are present in mitochondria (Table 3.1). However, the division of labor between the mitochondrial topoisomerases is not fully understood and it is likely that the enzymes have only partially overlapping functions in solving the topological issues associated with replication and transcription of mtDNA.

Top3α, the type IA topoisomerase is likely to selectively resolve recombination intermediates and Holliday junctions produced by converging replication forks. Indeed, it is the only topoisomerase that can resolve double-Holliday junctions (Wang 2002). For this, nuclear Top3α is coupled with RecQ helicases such as the Bloom helicase (BLM) in the BTR complex (BLM-Top3α-Rmi1-Rmi2) (Hoadley et al. 2010; Wu and Hickson 2006) (see Chap. 8). Thus, the identification of a RecQ helicase in mitochondria is awaited. Another open question for Top3α

Table 3.1 Mitochondrial topoisomerases

	Type IA	Type IB	Type II	References
Vertebrates	Top3αL	Top1mt	Top2β	Low et al. (2003); Wang et al. (2002b); Zhang et al. (2001b)
Protozoans	TopIAmt	Top1	Top2mt	Bodley and Shapiro (1995); Kulikowicz and Shapiro (2006); Scocca and Shapiro (2008)
Drosophila	Top3αL	?	?	Wang et al. (2002b); Wu et al. (2010)
Schizosaccharomyces pombe	Top3[a]	Top1[a]	?	Wang et al. (2002b)
Saccharomyces cerevisiae	Top3[a]	Top1	?	Tua et al. (1997); Wang et al. (1995); Wang et al. (2002b)

[a]Based on *in silico* analyses

is whether its requirement in mice is related to its long mitochondrial isoform or to the short nuclear isoform. Knock-in experiments are awaited to address this issue.

Top2 but neither Top1 nor Top3 can decatenate the daughter DNA circles formed at the end of mtDNA replication. A recent report indicates that Top2 tends to preferentially act as a decatenase instead of its other function as a DNA relaxation enzyme when catenated DNA is positively supercoiled (Baxter et al. 2011). Thus, it remains to be determined whether positive supercoiling builds up as mtDNA are about to be decatenated. The other pending issue is whether Top2α in addition to Top2β is present in mitochondria and whether partial Top2 proteolysis (Low et al. 2003) is involved in the sequestration of Top2 in mitochondria. Our ongoing studies demonstrate the presence of both full-length Top2α and β in human mitochondria.

Top1's primary biochemical activity, which overlaps with Top2, is to relax supercoils whether they are positive or negative. Because TOP1mt is not essential for murine development under laboratory environment, Top2 must be providing the DNA relaxation activity required for mtDNA transcription and replication. Thus, it remains to be determined why TOP1mt is absolutely conserved in all vertebrates, and for which specific functions. It may be because Top1 does not require ATP and functions well in the presence of millimolar calcium concentrations that are present in mitochondria (Zhang et al. 2001b), whereas high calcium tends to induce abortive cleavage complexes with Top2 (Osheroff and Zechiedrich 1987). More importantly, it is possible that Top1 removes the negative supercoils generated in the wake of transcription complexes more efficiently than Top2 (Brill and Sternglanz 1988; French et al. 2011) thereby avoiding the formation of R-loops (French et al. 2011; Sordet et al. 2009) that are known to be highly lethal to mitochondria (Cerritelli et al. 2003).

Whereas Top1 and Top2 are both validated targets for cancer treatment, there is limited evidence that targeting mitochondrial topoisomerases and more specifically Top1mt would be therapeutically beneficial. The natural marine alkaloid derivatives Top1 inhibitors related to lamellarins have been reported to selectively target human mitochondria (Kluza et al. 2006). However, they are not in clinical development. On the other hand, mitochondrial topoisomerase inhibitors are likely to be valuable as antiparasitic drugs.

Finally, mitochondrial defects are linked not only to neurodegenerative (Alzheimer and Parkinson) and metabolic (diabetes, obesity) diseases, but also increasingly to cancers (Wallace 2005, 2010). mtDNA mutations and polymorphisms, and mitochondrial pathway dysregulations are found in cancer cells (Wallace 2005, 2010). Recently, Top1mt mutations have been identified in patients affected by mitochondrial disorders suggesting a new role of this enzyme in the pathogenesis of mitochondrial diseases (Wang et al. 2010). Systematic search for *TOP1mt* mutations in mitochondrial and metabolic diseases and in cancers will reveal the importance of this enzyme for human health. In parallel, detailed studies on the phenotype of TOP1mt knockout mice and cells are warranted.

References

Baxter J, Sen N, Martinez VL, De Carandini ME, Schvartzman JB, Diffley JF, Aragon L (2011) Positive supercoiling of mitotic DNA drives decatenation by topoisomerase II in eukaryotes. *Science* **331**(6022): 1328–1332

Bodley AL, Shapiro TA (1995) Molecular and cytotoxic effects of camptothecin, a topoisomerase I inhibitor, on trypanosomes and Leishmania. *Proc Natl Acad Sci USA* **92**(9): 3726–3730

Bogenhagen D, Clayton DA (1978) Mechanism of mitochondrial DNA replication in mouse L-cells: kinetics of synthesis and turnover of the initiation sequence. *J Mol Biol* **119**(1): 49–68

Bogenhagen DF, Rousseau D, Burke S (2008) The layered structure of human mitochondrial DNA nucleoids. *J Biol Chem* **283**(6): 3665–3675

Bonawitz ND, Clayton DA, Shadel GS (2006) Initiation and beyond: multiple functions of the human mitochondrial transcription machinery. *Mol Cell* **24**(6): 813–825

Bowmaker M, Yang MY, Yasukawa T, Reyes A, Jacobs HT, Huberman JA, Holt IJ (2003) Mammalian mitochondrial DNA replicates bidirectionally from an initiation zone. *J Biol Chem* **278**(51): 50961–50969

Brill SJ, Sternglanz R (1988) Transcription-dependent DNA supercoiling in yeast DNA topoisomerase mutants. *Cell* **54**(3): 403–411

Brown TA, Tkachuk AN, Clayton DA (2008) Native R-loops persist throughout the mouse mitochondrial DNA genome. *J Biol Chem* **283**(52): 36743–36751

Castora FJ, Lazarus GM (1984) Isolation of a mitochondrial DNA topoisomerase from human leukemia cells. *Biochem Biophys Res Commun* **121**(1): 77–86

Castora FJ, Lazarus GM, Kunes D (1985) The presence of two mitochondrial DNA topoisomerases in human acute leukemia cells. *Biochem Biophys Res Commun* **130**(2): 854–866

Cerritelli SM, Frolova EG, Feng C, Grinberg A, Love PE, Crouch RJ (2003) Failure to produce mitochondrial DNA results in embryonic lethality in Rnaseh1 null mice. *Mol Cell* **11**(3): 807–815

Clay Montier LL, Deng JJ, Bai Y (2009) Number matters: control of mammalian mitochondrial DNA copy number. *J Genet Genomics* **36**(3): 125–131

Clayton DA (1982) Replication of animal mitochondrial DNA. *Cell* **28**(4): 693–705

Clayton DA (1991) Replication and transcription of vertebrate mitochondrial DNA. *Annu Rev Cell Biol* **7**: 453–478

Dairaghi DJ, Shadel GS, Clayton DA (1995) Human mitochondrial transcription factor A and promoter spacing integrity are required for transcription initiation. *Biochim Biophys Acta* **1271**(1): 127–134

Dalla Rosa I, Goffart S, Wurm M, Wiek C, Essmann F, Sobek S, Schroeder P, Zhang H, Krutmann J, Hanenberg H, Schulze-Osthoff K, Mielke C, Pommier Y, Boege F, Christensen MO (2009) Adaptation of topoisomerase I paralogs to nuclear and mitochondrial DNA. *Nucleic Acids Res* **37**(19): 6414–6428

Fairfield FR, Bauer WR, Simpson MV (1985) Studies on mitochondrial type I topoisomerase and on its function. *Biochim Biophys Acta* **824**(1): 45–57

Falkenberg M, Gaspari M, Rantanen A, Trifunovic A, Larsson NG, Gustafsson CM (2002) Mitochondrial transcription factors B1 and B2 activate transcription of human mtDNA. *Nat Genet* **31**(3): 289–294

Falkenberg M, Larsson N-G, Gustafsson CM (2007) DNA replication and transcription in mammalian mitochondria. *Annu Rev Biochem* **76**: 679–699

Fisher RP, Topper JN, Clayton DA (1987) Promoter selection in human mitochondria involves binding of a transcription factor to orientation-independent upstream regulatory elements. *Cell* **50**(2): 247–258

French SL, Sikes ML, Hontz RD, Osheim YN, Lambert TE, El Hage A, Smith MM, Tollervey D, Smith JS, Beyer AL (2011) Distinguishing the roles of Topoisomerases I and II in relief of transcription-induced torsional stress in yeast rRNA genes. *Mol Cell Biol* **31**(3): 482–494

Fuste JM, Wanrooij S, Jemt E, Granycome CE, Cluett TJ, Shi Y, Atanassova N, Holt IJ, Gustafsson CM, Falkenberg M (2010) Mitochondrial RNA polymerase is needed for activation of the origin of light-strand DNA replication. *Mol Cell* **37**(1): 67–78

Gillum AM, Clayton DA (1978) Displacement-loop replication initiation sequence in animal mitochondrial DNA exists as a family of discrete lengths. *Proc Natl Acad Sci USA* **75**(2): 677–681

Goto Y, Hayashi R, Kang D, Yoshida K (2006) Acute loss of transcription factor E2F1 induces mitochondrial biogenesis in HeLa cells. *J Cell Physiol* **209**(3): 923–934

Hoadley KA, Xu D, Xue Y, Satyshur KA, Wang W, Keck JL (2010) Structure and cellular roles of the RMI core complex from the bloom syndrome dissolvasome. *Structure* **18**(9): 1149–1158

Hock MB, Kralli A (2009) Transcriptional control of mitochondrial biogenesis and function. *Annu Rev Physiol* **71**: 177–203

Holt IJ, Lorimer HE, Jacobs HT (2000) Coupled leading- and lagging-strand synthesis of mammalian mitochondrial DNA. *Cell* **100**(5): 515–524

Iborra FJ, Kimura H, Cook PR (2004) The functional organization of mitochondrial genomes in human cells. *BMC Biol* **2**: 9

Kluza J, Gallego MA, Loyens A, Beauvillain JC, Sousa-Faro JM, Cuevas C, Marchetti P, Bailly C (2006) Cancer cell mitochondria are direct proapoptotic targets for the marine antitumor drug lamellarin D. *Cancer Res* **66**(6): 3177–3187

Korhonen JA, Gaspari M, Falkenberg M (2003) TWINKLE Has 5' -3' DNA helicase activity and is specifically stimulated by mitochondrial single-stranded DNA-binding protein. *J Biol Chem* **278**(49): 48627–48632

Korhonen JA, Pham XH, Pellegrini M, Falkenberg M (2004) Reconstitution of a minimal mtDNA replisome in vitro. *EMBO J* **23**(12): 2423–2429

Kosovsky MJ, Soslau G (1993) Immunological identification of human platelet mitochondrial DNA topoisomerase I. *Biochim Biophys Acta* **1164**(1): 101–107

Kulikowicz T, Shapiro TA (2006) Distinct genes encode type II Topoisomerases for the nucleus and mitochondrion in the protozoan parasite *Trypanosoma brucei*. *J Biol Chem* **281**(6): 3048–3056

Li W, Wang JC (1998) Mammalian DNA topoisomerase IIIalpha is essential in early embryogenesis. *Proc Natl Acad Sci USA* **95**(3): 1010–1013

Lin JH, Castora FJ (1991) DNA topoisomerase II from mammalian mitochondria is inhibited by the antitumor drugs, m-AMSA and VM-26. *Biochem Biophys Res Commun* **176**(2): 690–697

Lin JH, Castora FJ (1995) Response of purified mitochondrial DNA topoisomerase I from bovine liver to camptothecin and m-AMSA. *Arch Biochem Biophys* **324**(2): 293–299

Litonin D, Sologub M, Shi Y, Savkina M, Anikin M, Falkenberg M, Gustafsson CM, Temiakov D Human mitochondrial transcription revisited: only TFAM and TFB2M are required for transcription of the mitochondrial genes in vitro. *J Biol Chem* **285**(24): 18129–18133

Low RL, Orton S, Friedman DB (2003) A truncated form of DNA topoisomerase IIbeta associates with the mtDNA genome in mammalian mitochondria. *Eur J Biochem* **270**(20): 4173–4186

Martin M, Cho JY, Cesare AJ, Griffith JD, Attardi G (2005) Termination factor-mediated DNA loop between termination and initiation sites drives mitochondrial rRNA synthesis. *Cell* **123**(7): 1227–1240

McCulloch V, Shadel GS (2003) Human mitochondrial transcription factor B1 interacts with the C-terminal activation region of h-mtTFA and stimulates transcription independently of its RNA methyltransferase activity. *Mol Cell Biol* **23**(16): 5816–5824

Montoya J, Gaines GL, Attardi G (1983) The pattern of transcription of the human mitochondrial rRNA genes reveals two overlapping transcription units. *Cell* **34**(1): 151–159

Morham S, Kluckman KD, Voulomanos N, Smithies O (1996) Targeted disruption of the mouse topoisomerase I gene by camptothecin selection. *Mol Cell Biol* **16:** 6804–6809

Ojala D, Montoya J, Attardi G (1981) tRNA punctuation model of RNA processing in human mitochondria. *Nature* **290**(5806): 470–474

Osheroff N, Zechiedrich EL (1987) Calcium-promoted DNA cleavage by eukaryotic topoisomerase II: trapping the covalent enzyme-DNA complex in an active form. *Biochemistry* **26:** 4303–4309

Plank JL, Chu SH, Pohlhaus JR, Wilson-Sali T, Hsieh TS (2005) Drosophila melanogaster topoisomerase IIIalpha preferentially relaxes a positively or negatively supercoiled bubble substrate and is essential during development. *J Biol Chem* **280**(5): 3564–3573

Pommier Y (2009) DNA topoisomerase I inhibitors: chemistry, biology, and interfacial inhibition. *Chem Rev* **109**(7): 2894–2902

Sbisà E, Tanzariello F, Reyes A, Pesole G, Saccone C (1997) Mammalian mitochondrial D-loop region structural analysis: identification of new conserved sequences and their functional and evolutionary implications. *Gene* **205**(1–2): 125–140

Scocca JR, Shapiro TA (2008) A mitochondrial topoisomerase IA essential for late theta structure resolution in African trypanosomes. *Mol Microbiol* **67**(4): 820–829

Shutt TE, Shadel GS (2010) A compendium of human mitochondrial gene expression machinery with links to disease. *Environ Mol Mutagen* **51**(5): 360–379

Sordet O, Redon CE, Guirouilh-Barbat J, Smith S, Solier S, Douarre C, Conti C, Nakamura AJ, Das BB, Nicolas E, Kohn KW, Bonner WM, Pommier Y (2009) Ataxia telangiectasia mutated activation by transcription- and topoisomerase I-induced DNA double-strand breaks. *EMBO Rep* **10**(8): 887–893

Tua A, Wang J, Kulpa V, Wernette CM (1997) Mitochondrial DNA topoisomerase I of Saccharomyces cerevisiae. *Biochimie* **79**(6): 341–350

Tyynismaa H, Suomalainen A (2009) Mouse models of mitochondrial DNA defects and their relevance for human disease. *EMBO Rep* **10**(2): 137–143

Wallace DC (2005) A mitochondrial paradigm of metabolic and degenerative diseases, aging, and cancer: a dawn for evolutionary medicine. *Annu Rev Genet* **39:** 359–407

Wallace DC (2010) Mitochondrial DNA mutations in disease and aging. *Environ Mol Mutagen* **51**(5): 440–450

Wang J, Kearney K, Derby M, Wernette CM (1995) On the relationship of the ATP-independent, mitochondrial associated DNA topoisomerase of Saccharomyces cerevisiae to the nuclear topoisomerase I. *Biochem Biophys Res Commun* **214**(2): 723–729

Wang JC (2002) Cellular roles of DNA topoisomerases: a molecular perspective. *Nat Rev Mol Cell Biol* **3**(6): 430–440

Wang W, Shen P, Thiyagarajan S, Lin S, Palm C, Horvath R, Klopstock T, Cutler D, Pique L, Schrijver I, Davis RW, Mindrinos M, Speed TP, Scharfe C (2010) Identification of rare DNA variants in mitochondrial disorders with improved array-based sequencing. *Nucleic Acids Res*

Wang Y, Lyu YL, Wang JC (2002a) Dual localization of human DNA topoisomerase IIIalpha to mitochondria and nucleus. *Proc Natl Acad Sci USA* **99**(19): 12114–12119

Wanrooij PH, Uhler JP, Simonsson T, Falkenberg M, Gustafsson CM (2010) G-quadruplex structures in RNA stimulate mitochondrial transcription termination and primer formation. *Proc Natl Acad Sci USA* **107**(37)**:** 16072–16077

Wanrooij S, Fuste JM, Farge G, Shi Y, Gustafsson CM, Falkenberg M (2008) Human mitochondrial RNA polymerase primes lagging-strand DNA synthesis in vitro. *Proc Natl Acad Sci USA* **105**(32)**:** 11122–11127

Wu J, Feng L, Hsieh TS (2010) Drosophila topo IIIalpha is required for the maintenance of mitochondrial genome and male germ-line stem cells. *Proc Natl Acad Sci USA* **107**(14)**:** 6228–6233

Wu L, Hickson ID (2006) DNA helicases required for homologous recombination and repair of damaged replication forks. *Annu Rev Genet* **40:** 279–306

Yang MY, Bowmaker M, Reyes A, Vergani L, Angeli P, Gringeri E, Jacobs HT, Holt IJ (2002) Biased incorporation of ribonucleotides on the mitochondrial L-strand accounts for apparent strand-asymmetric DNA replication. *Cell* **111**(4)**:** 495–505

Yasukawa T, Reyes A, Cluett TJ, Yang M-Y, Bowmaker M, Jacobs HT, Holt IJ (2006) Replication of vertebrate mitochondrial DNA entails transient ribonucleotide incorporation throughout the lagging strand. *EMBO J* **25**(22)**:** 5358–5371

Yasukawa T, Yang M-Y, Jacobs HT, Holt IJ (2005) A bidirectional origin of replication maps to the major noncoding region of human mitochondrial DNA. *Mol Cell* **18**(6)**:** 651–662

Zhang H, Barcelo JM, Lee B, Kohlhagen G, Zimonjic DB, Popescu NC, Pommier Y (2001a) Human mitochondrial topoisomerase I. *Proc Natl Acad Sci USA* **98**(19)**:** 10608–10613

Zhang H, Barceló JM, Lee B, Kohlhagen G, Zimonjic DB, Popescu NC, Pommier Y (2001b) Human mitochondrial topoisomerase I. *Proc Natl Acad Sci USA* **98**(19)**:** 10608–10613

Zhang H, Meng L-H, Zimonjic DB, Popescu NC, Pommier Y (2004a) Thirteen-exon-motif signature for vertebrate nuclear and mitochondrial type IB topoisomerases. *Nucleic Acids Res* **32**(7)**:** 2087–2092

Zhang H, Meng LH, Pommier Y (2007) Mitochondrial topoisomerases and alternative splicing of the human TOP1mt gene. *Biochimie* **89**(4)**:** 474–481

Zhang H, Pommier Y (2008) Mitochondrial topoisomerase I sites in the regulatory D-loop region of mitochondrial DNA. *Biochemistry* **47**(43)**:** 11196–11203

Zoppoli G, Douarre C, Dalla Rosa I, Liu H, Reinhold W, Pommier Y (2011) Coordinated regulation of mitochondrial topoisomerase IB with mitochondrial genes and MYC. *Nucleic Acids Res* : in press.

Chapter 4
Structure and Mechanism of Eukaryotic Type IIA Topoisomerases

James M. Berger and Neil Osheroff

4.1 Introduction

The great length of chromosomes, coupled with the double-helical nature of DNA, leads naturally to topological problems in the genome (Bates and Maxwell 2005; Liu et al. 2009; Wang 2009). For example, any motor protein that transiently unwinds DNA – such as a polymerase or helicase – generates positive supercoils in front of it and negative supercoils in its wake that can affect transcriptional events (Liu and Wang 1987; Pruss and Drlica 1989). Replication and recombination events further lead to DNA entanglements that must be resolved prior to chromosome segregation to prevent the formation of double-stranded DNA breaks (Bates and Maxwell 2005; Liu et al. 2009; Postow et al. 2001; Wang 2009).

To contend with these problems, cells have evolved a specialized class of motor proteins known as topoisomerases (Champoux 2001; Deweese and Osheroff 2009b; Liu et al. 2009; Schoeffler and Berger 2008; Wang 2002). These enzymes manipulate DNA strands through phosphodiester breakage and rejoining events that alter the number of times one DNA strand or duplex wraps around another. Two classes of topoisomerase exist, type I and type II, which differ in their respective abilities to cut either one or two strands of DNA at a time (Champoux 2001; Schoeffler and Berger 2008). Each type is further subdivided into families with distinct specific structural and functional properties. There are presently three groups of type I topoisomerases (IA, IB, and IC) and two groups of type II topoisomerases (IIA and IIB).

J.M. Berger (✉)
Department of Molecular and Cell Biology, QB3 Institute, University of California at Berkeley, 374D Stanley Hall #3220, Berkeley, CA 94720, USA
e-mail: jmberger@berkeley.edu

N. Osheroff (✉)
Departments of Biochemistry and Medicine (Hematology/Oncology), School of Medicine, Vanderbilt University, 654 Robinson Research Building, Nashville, TN 37232-0146, USA
e-mail: neil.osheroff@vanderbilt.edu

Y. Pommier (ed.), *DNA Topoisomerases and Cancer*, Cancer Drug Discovery and Development, DOI 10.1007/978-1-4614-0323-4_4,

All cellular organisms, as well as many viruses, contain a type II topoisomerase; however, the distribution of subtypes varies from one organism to another (Forterre et al. 2007) (see Chap. 1). For example, type IIA enzymes are found in all eukaryotes (Top2), bacteria (topo IV, gyrase), and a few archaeal species. By contrast, type IIB topoisomerases (topo VI) are found predominantly in archaea, as well as in plants, and certain alga. Structural and phylogenetic studies show that the IIA and IIB topoisomerase subtypes share functional elements, but are markedly distinct in their global architecture (Schoeffler and Berger 2008).

The universal use of type II topoisomerases derives from their unique ability to disentangle DNA duplexes (Champoux 2001; Deweese and Osheroff 2009b; Liu et al. 2009; Schoeffler and Berger 2008; Wang 2002). Loss of type II topoisomerase activity is lethal to cells, engendering the formation of double-stranded DNA breaks as intertwined chromosomes are pulled apart and sequestered during cell division (Wang 2002). Aberrant type II topoisomerase function resulting from higher-than-normal levels of enzyme-mediated DNA cleavage, either from genetic or drug-induced means, is also linked to the formation of gross chromosome rearrangements such as DNA translocations (Deweese and Osheroff 2009b). This chapter covers what is known about the structure and mechanism of eukaryotic type IIA topoisomerases. Where appropriate, discussion of bacterial type IIA topoisomerases and type IIB enzymes is also included to highlight specific points, or to draw important contrasts between the different systems.

4.2 Functional Organization

The physical complexity of disentangling two DNA segments necessitates a similarly complicated enzyme reaction. While DNA cleavage and ligation by type IIA topoisomerases require no high-energy cofactor (Goto et al. 1984; Osheroff 1987), these events are stimulated by ATP binding, and the overall topoisomerase reaction proceeds at the expense of nucleotide hydrolysis (Gellert et al. 1976; Liu et al. 1979; Miller et al. 1981). To coordinate all of their necessary enzymatic steps, type IIA topoisomerases use a modular, multifunction architecture to move DNA duplexes through one another.

Each type IIA topoisomerase holoenzyme is formed either by a single, large polypeptide chain (in eukaryotes) (Goto et al. 1984; Miller et al. 1981; Sander and Hsieh 1983), which self-associates to form dimers, or by two subunits (in prokaryotes) that assemble into A_2B_2 tetramers (Mizuuchi et al. 1978; Sugino et al. 1980). The GyrB/ParE and GyrA/ParC subunits of bacterial type II topoisomerases (gyrase and topo IV) are evolutionarily related to the N- and C-terminal domains of their eukaryotic homolog (Top2), respectively (Caron and Wang 1994; Lynn et al. 1986; Uemura et al. 1986). All type IIA topoisomerases consist of two catalytic regions, each of which comprises two distinct domains. An ATPase functionality, formed by both a GHKL and a RNaseP fold, resides in the N-terminus of Top2 (and GyrB/ParE) (Fig. 4.1) (Classen et al. 2003; Lindsley and Wang 1991;

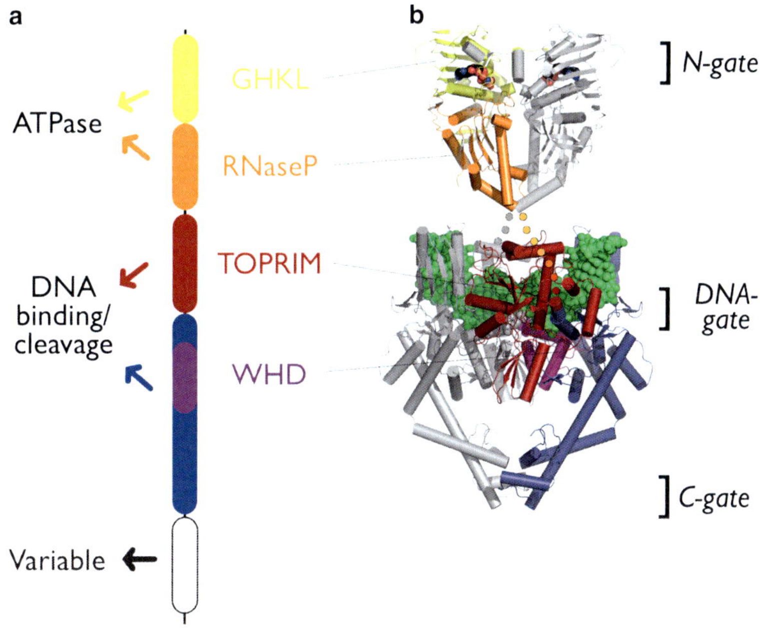

Fig. 4.1 Top2 organization and structure. (**a**) Linear domain map, from N- to C-terminus (*top to bottom*), highlighting the relative position of conserved functional elements. (**b**) Top2 ATPase domain [*top* (Classen et al. 2003)] and DNA binding and cleavage core [*bottom* (Schmidt et al. 2010)] structures, color-coded to match *panel* a. Bound DNA (likely to correspond to a substrate G-segment) is shown as *green spheres*. The positions of various dissociable protein "gates" that control strand passage are demarcated

Staudenbauer and Orr 1981; Tamura and Gellert 1990; Wigley et al. 1991). This composite motor element is found in other macromolecular systems, such as MutL/MLP1 mismatch repair proteins and Hsp90-class chaperones, while the GHKL domain alone is further shared with bacterial histidine-kinases (Bergerat et al. 1997; Corbett and Berger 2004; Dutta and Inouye 2000). DNA binding and cleavage is carried out by the middle third of Top2, which encompasses a composite active site formed by a *TOPRIM* (TOpoisomerase/PRIMase) fold (part of GyrB/ParE) and a Winged-Helix Domain (*WHD*) (resident within GyrA/ParC) (Fig. 4.1) (Aravind et al. 1998; Berger et al. 1998). These two folds are both linked to and embedded within a variety of scaffolding elements that assist with both DNA binding and coordinating the movement of one DNA duplex through another (Berger et al. 1996; Morais Cabral et al. 1997).

The C-terminus of the principle DNA binding and cleavage region is variable among type IIA topoisomerases (Fig. 4.1a). In prokaryotes, this region forms a unique type of all-β domain that binds, and in some cases bends, duplex DNA segments to control topoisomerase function (Corbett et al. 2004; Reece and Maxwell 1991). In some eukaryotic type IIA enzymes (e.g., yeast Top2, human Top2β), this region makes no known contribution to catalytic activity (Caron et al. 1994). However, in human Top2α, it redirects the preference of the catalytic machinery to remove positive (vs. negative) supercoils (McClendon et al. 2008; McClendon et al. 2005). The C-terminal domain of Top2 has no apparent structure and is rich in phosphorylation sites (Corbett et al. 1993; Sahyoun et al. 1986; Shiozaki and Yanagida 1992). The exact purpose of this post-translational modification on Top2 function has been a subject of debate, but at the least it appears to serve as a recruitment signal for phospho-peptide binding proteins such as TopBP1 and 14-3-3ε (Kurz et al. 2000; Yamane et al. 2002). Which biochemical events control phosphorylation status, or the attachment of other post-translation modifications (e.g., sumoylation), are not fully understood.

4.3 General Mechanism

Over the years, a wealth of biochemical and structural studies has converged to produce a general framework for the type II topoisomerase reaction (Fig. 4.2a) (reviewed in (Champoux 2001; Deweese and Osheroff 2009b; Schoeffler and Berger 2008)). The enzyme first binds one substrate duplex (termed the gate- or G-segment), which serves as the site of DNA cleavage. ATP binding, together with the engagement of a

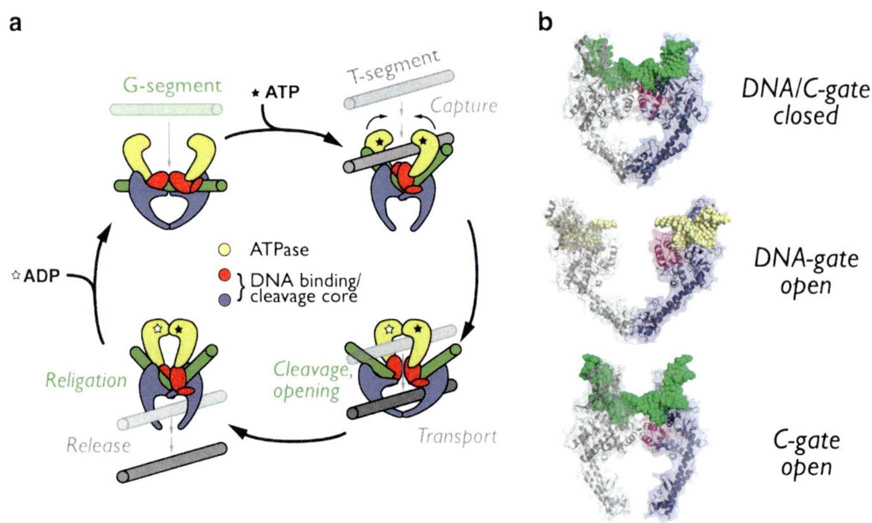

Fig. 4.2 Strand passage and gating. (**a**) General scheme for strand passage for Top2 showing key events in the reaction cycle. (**b**) Comparison of three structures of the DNA binding and cleavage core showing the DNA- and C-gates in different (*open or closed*) association states (Berger et al. 1996; Dong and Berger 2007; Schmidt et al. 2010). G-segment DNAs seen in the crystal structures are shown in *green*; for the middle structure, DNA (*yellow*) was modeled based on its configuration seen in the other two complexes

second duplex (the transport- or T-segment), leads to dimerization of the ATPase regions and produces a functionally competent enzyme-substrate complex in which the G-segment is cleaved (Roca and Wang 1992; Wigley et al. 1991). While the presence of ATP and the T-segment stimulate DNA cleavage (Corbett et al. 1992), they are not required for this event (Mueller-Planitz and Herschlag 2006). At present, the point at which DNA cleavage occurs during the strand passage reaction remains an open issue.

Once the complete enzyme-substrate complex has been established, a series of conformational changes occurs that: (1) opens the G-segment, (2) passes the T-segment through the break, and (3) closes and reseals the G-segment. The T-segment is then believed to be expelled from the enzyme by the transient opening of a dimer interface located C-terminal to the TOPRIM / WHD elements (Roca et al. 1996; Williams and Maxwell 1999b). Once the DNA is released from the enzyme, this interface closes. The hydrolysis of ATP during strand passage serves to dissociate the ATPase domains so that the cycle can repeat.

The action of type II topoisomerases can be likened to a series of canal locks that open and close in a defined sequence to navigate one DNA segment through another. This approach has been considered in terms of a "gating" mechanism, whereby each dissociable protein interface corresponds to a particular gate. The ATPase domains form a portal at the N-terminus of the protein (the "N-gate"), while the C-terminal dimerization domains form the C-gate (Roca and Wang 1992; Roca and Wang 1994; Wigley et al. 1991). Because a T-segment passes through both the gates, as opposed to entering and exiting through only one, type II topoisomerases are said to operate by a "two-gate" mechanism. In actuality, type IIA topoisomerases have at least three gates, with the third formed both by the two halves the broken G-segment, and the active site for DNA cleavage (Figs. 4.1b and 4.2b) (Berger et al. 1996; Williams and Maxwell 1999a, b). Structural studies suggest that the C-terminal, RNaseP-like domains of the ATPase regions might comprise a fourth gate (Classen et al. 2003; Wei et al. 2005; Wigley et al. 1991).

4.4 Role of ATP

The need for ATP in the type II topoisomerase reaction has been amply demonstrated. However, aside from bacterial gyrase, which can actively add DNA supercoils into substrates (Gellert et al. 1976), the underlying reason why chemical energy is required to power reactions that are relatively isoenergetic (e.g., DNA decatenation), or thermodynamically favorable (relaxation of DNA supercoils) has remained enigmatic.

To date, studies into the eukaryotic type IIA topoisomerase ATPase reaction have linked nucleotide binding to closure of the ATPase gate and T-segment entrapment (Classen et al. 2003; Hu et al. 1998; Lindsley and Wang 1993a; Osheroff 1986; Roca and Wang 1992; Wei et al. 2005). ATP binding further stimulates G-segment cleavage within the DNA gate. In this regard, ATP can be viewed as a cofactor that helps restrict DNA scission to stages in the catalytic cycle during which a T-segment

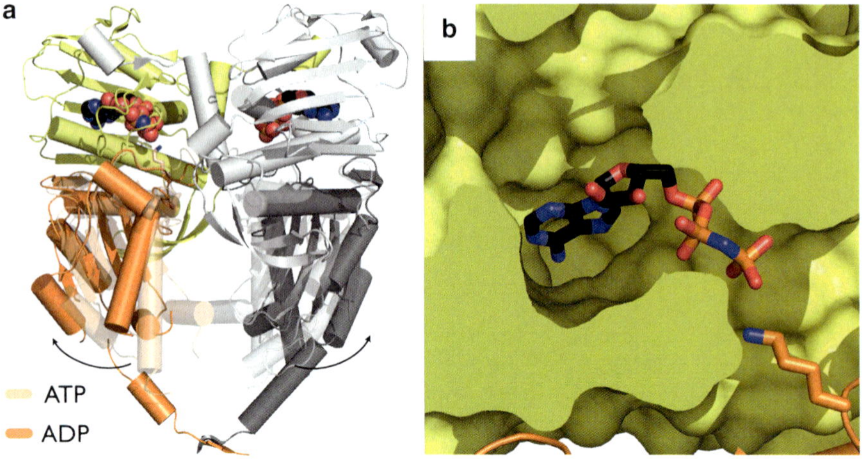

Fig. 4.3 ATPase mechanics. (**a**) Superposition of ATP- and ADP-bound states of the human Top2 ATPase region showing the relative movements between the GHKL and RNaseP (*transducer*) domains (Wei et al. 2005). (**b**) Cutaway of the ATPase active site showing how a lysine from the RNaseP domain protrudes through a narrow tunnel into the catalytic pocket

is likely available for transport, and which helps co-ordinate the opening and closing of additional subunit interfaces to prevent aberrant subunit dissociation and chromosome fragmentation. Consistent with this view, non-hydrolyzable ATP analogs can support a single round of DNA passage in Top2, including T-segment release, but also stabilize closure of the N- and C-gates following strand transport (Osheroff 1986; Roca and Wang 1992). The action of the ATPase regions is also highly cooperative, with the binding of nucleotide to one protomer of the eukaryotic type IIA enzyme being sufficient to drive strand transport through the entire Top2 dimer (Lindsley and Wang 1993b).

Nucleotide hydrolysis is far from a superfluous byproduct of the type II topoisomerase reaction, however. Breakdown of ATP is required for the enzyme to act more than once (Osheroff 1986). Hydrolysis also accelerates the rate of T-segment transport nearly 20-fold, and it appears to be linked to conformational changes that are coupled to the movement of the passed DNA through the DNA gate (Baird et al. 1999). Finally, in the absence of ATP hydrolysis, as demonstrated by the use of non-hydrolyzable ATP analogs or the inclusion of ATPase inhibitors such as ICRF-187, Top2 remains topologically entangled with its DNA substrate, leading it to be described as a protein clamp that engulfs the G-segment (Osheroff 1986; Roca et al. 1994; Roca and Wang 1992).

Structural studies of human Top2 have indicated that hydrolysis unlatches the RNaseP domain of the ATPase region to permit large-scale motions of this domain relative to the GHKL ATP-binding fold (Wei et al. 2005) (Fig. 4.3a). Motions of this type have been seen in other type II topoisomerases (Corbett and Berger 2005; Lamour et al. 2002), and appear to affect the position of a key lysine in and out of the active site (Fig. 4.3b), possibly as a means to coordinate P_i release. Movement of the RNaseP domain has been proposed to help transduce allosteric signals from the ATPase gate to the DNA gate as a means to coordinate G-segment cleavage and opening with T-segment movement through the enzyme (Baird et al. 1999). A small linker region between the ATPase and DNA gate regions appears to be important for this communication (Bjergbaek et al. 2000).

4.5 G-Segment Recognition

Early biochemical studies established that Top2 binds ~28 bp of duplex DNA within a G-segment (Lee et al. 1989). Other studies of Top2, as well as of bacterial type IIA topoisomerases, additionally showed that these enzymes can significantly bend DNA, and that they prefer to bind to highly curved DNA regions and crossovers (Buck and Zechiedrich 2004; Kirchhausen et al. 1985; Moore et al. 1983; Roca et al. 1993; Schultz et al. 1996; Stone et al. 2003; Zechiedrich and Osheroff 1990). Both sets of observations have been confirmed by crystallographic studies of non-covalent topoisomerase-DNA complexes, as well as covalent cleavage complexes (Bax et al. 2010; Dong and Berger 2007; Laponogov et al. 2010; Laponogov et al. 2009; Schmidt et al. 2010). The degree of DNA deformation evident in the crystal structures is significant (~150° bend overall), and in the vicinity of the scissile bonds, the DNA is constrained into an A-form conformation. Bending appears to be enforced, at least in part, by the intercalation of an invariant isoleucine on each subunit between a CpG base-pair step, creating two dyad-opposed bends of ~75° each (Figs 4.1b and 4.2b).

The significance of the ability of type IIA topoisomerases to bend DNA has been the subject of debate. One possible role of bending may be to aid in "topology simplification", an established phenomenological property whereby type IIA topoisomerases reduce or "simplify" the topological complexity of DNA below that produced at thermodynamic equilibrium in the absence of enzyme (e.g., producing a substantially narrower Gaussian distribution of DNA topoisomers during a relaxation reaction than would be obtained from a nicking/religation reaction) (Rybenkov et al. 1997). Modeling studies indicate that DNA bends tend to aid in the capture of secondary DNA segments, either inter- or intra-molecularly, and that a topoisomerase-enforced bend (particularly if coupled with a corresponding T-segment bend) would correspondingly tend to pass DNA strands in a direction biased toward lower topological complexity (Buck and Zechiedrich 2004; Klenin et al. 2002). For their part, the corresponding type IIB topoisomerases of archaea and plants do not appear to substantially alter DNA shape, if at all, nor do they exhibit simplification behavior (Corbett et al. 2007; Stuchinskaya et al. 2009). Thus, although the exact molecular basis for simplification remains to be fully established (Buck and Zechiedrich 2004; Klenin et al. 2002; Trigueros et al. 2004; Yan et al. 1999), the direct visualization of DNA bending by Top2 is consistent with G-segment deformation playing a role in the process.

DNA bending by type IIA topoisomerases may also help to coordinate the single-stranded nicks mediated by each protomer active site to generate the double-stranded DNA break needed for strand passage. Recent studies demonstrate that the introduction of a nick at one scissile bond dramatically enhances cleavage at the opposite scissile bond (Deweese and Osheroff 2009a). It has been proposed that nicks trigger faster rates of scission by introducing flexibility into DNA, thereby allowing it to attain the bent state required for efficient cleavage (Dong and Berger 2007).

Insofar as recognition determinants, the lack of conserved base/side-chain interactions in available type IIA topoisomerase-DNA complexes (outside of the intercalating isoleucine) agrees well with biochemical studies suggesting that G-segment binding is generally structure, rather than sequence, dependent. In Top2, one exception for this trend is a preference for pyrimidine/purine steps (particularly CpG) at the "+8"/"+9" positions of a DNA sequence with respect to the site of cleavage (Dong and Berger 2007; Mueller-Planitz and Herschlag 2007). Nonetheless, alterations that can aid duplex deformability, such as abasic sites, nicks, or mismatches, have a strongly potentiating effect on binding affinity and cleavage propensity (Deweese and Osheroff 2009a; Kingma et al. 1995; Kingma and Osheroff 1997). These findings raise the possibility that naturally-occurring DNA lesions may act as poisons for type II topoisomerases, leading to stable cleavage complexes that necessitate repair.

4.6 G-Segment Cleavage

Shortly after the discovery of type IIA topoisomerases and their ability to cleave DNA, it became clear that these proteins form a transient, covalent attachment to target G-segments (Liu et al. 1983; Sander and Hsieh 1983; Sugino et al. 1980). Strand scission is mediated by a tyrosine nucleophile resident on the Top2 WHD (Horowitz and Wang 1987; Worland and Wang 1989), along with divalent metal ions that are liganded by the associated, N-terminal TOPRIM domain (Deweese et al. 2009; Noble and Maxwell 2002; Sissi et al. 2008; West et al. 2000). Although many divalent metal ions (e.g., Mn^{2+} or Ca^{2+}) can support DNA cleavage in Top2, Mg^{2+} is required for full activity (Goto et al. 1984; Osheroff 1987). Upon cleavage, the two cut sites are staggered four-base pairs apart from one another across the major groove, which generates transient, enzyme-linked 5′ DNA overhangs (Morrison and Cozzarelli 1979; Sander and Hsieh 1983).

Exactly how type II topoisomerases cleave DNA has been an outstanding question for more than two decades. Structural and bioinformatic studies have suggested that the functional elements used in the type IIA topoisomerase cleavage reaction, including the metal dependence of this event, is broadly shared by both type IIB and type IA enzymes (Aravind et al. 1998; Berger et al. 1998). Biochemical, enzymatic, and mutagenesis studies have highlighted the need for conserved acidic amino acids in metal coordination and cleavage (Deweese et al. 2009; Noble and Maxwell 2002; Sissi et al. 2008; West et al. 2000). They also have indicated that type IIA topoisomerases utilize a two-metal-ion mechanism for DNA cleavage.

Recently, imaging of a covalent Top2/DNA cleavage complex revealed a possible mechanism for strand scission (Fig. 4.4) (Schmidt et al. 2010). In this structure, which was trapped using a bridging phosphorothiolate as a suicide substrate, the active-site tyrosine is covalently attached to the 5′ DNA end, coordinated by both invariant active-site amino acids and divalent metal ions. The divalent metals further

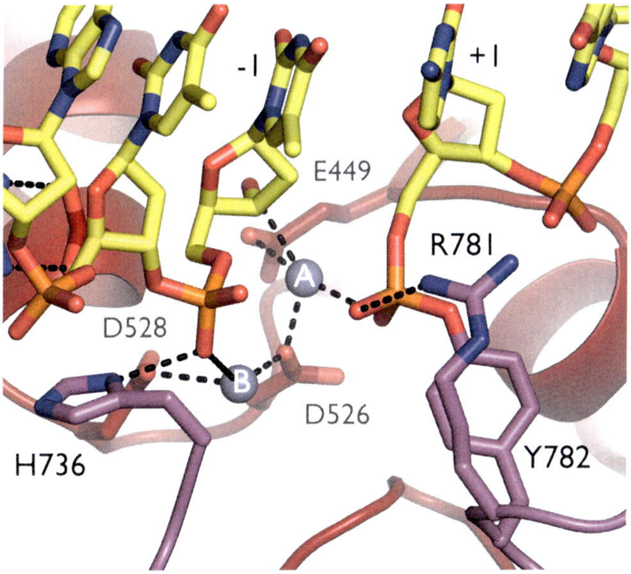

Fig. 4.4 Close-up of the Top2 active site covalently attached to DNA, showing associated metals (*gray spheres*) and liganding interactions (*dashed lines*) (Schmidt et al. 2010). Labels refer to the amino acid numbering for yeast Top2

associate with the free 3′ DNA end, but also surprisingly with the non-scissile phosphate immediately upstream of the cleavage site. This configuration differs significantly from other phospho-transferase/hydrolase enzymes that also rely on a pair of metal ions for function. In these reactions, two metals straddle the reactive phosphodiester species, stabilizing a pentavalent phosphorane transition state (Steitz and Steitz 1993; Yang et al. 2006). With the topoisomerases, it appears that an arginine replaces the metal ion that would otherwise reside near the catalytic tyrosine (Schmidt et al. 2010); the position of this amino acid both would allow it to participate in transition state chemistry and/or to depress the pK_a of the tyrosine to make it more nucleophilic. Notably, this same type of coordination has been seen in cleavage complexes with bacterial type IIA topoisomerases, though there is some debate as to whether two metals occupy the active site at the same time, or if one metal hops between two different sites depending on the state of the cleavage reaction (Bax et al. 2010; Laponogov et al. 2010).

4.7 G-Segment Opening and T-Segment Release

Following DNA cleavage, the two halves of the G-segment must separate by 25–30 Å to permit T-segment passage. Structures of the DNA- and C-gate regions of Top2 have revealed that these motions are accommodated by a swiveling of the primary DNA binding lobes, and the WHDs resident therein, about a pair of coiled-coil lever arms that extend from the protein (Berger et al. 1996; Corbett et al. 2005; Fass et al. 1999; Morais Cabral et al. 1997). The C-gate is itself formed by two small globular domains, one on each protomer, which reside at the tips of coiled-coil arms. This interface can remain closed while the DNA undergoes large, *en bloc* movements that drive G-segment opening and closure (Berger et al. 1996; Fass et al. 1999).

T-segment release from the enzyme is accomplished by transient opening of the C-gate. Initial evidence for C-gate opening was originally obtained from experiments showing that yeast Top2 can support a single round of T-segment transport even in when the ATPase-gate is irreversibly closed by the presence of AMPPNP (Roca and Wang 1992). Subsequent studies of eukaryotic and bacterial type IIA topoisomerases using a C-gate mutant that could be locked by engineered disulfide bonds provided further support for this model (Roca et al. 1996; Williams and Maxwell 1999b). More recently, some structures of the Top2 and gyrase DNA binding, and cleavage cores bound non-covalently to duplex DNA have captured a state of the protein in which the C-gate interface has separated (Dong and Berger 2007; Wohlkonig et al. 2010), demonstrating that the association status of this interface can indeed toggle between open and closed intermediates.

4.8 Concluding Remarks

Although a generally accepted molecular picture of Top2 activity is now available, there still exist many unanswered questions surrounding its detailed mechanisms of action. For example, the timing and synchronization of gate opening/closure events with the ATPase cycle remains to be established, as does the effect of inhibitors on actuation of the various topoisomerase interfaces. How Top2 engages a T-segment prior to and during strand passage, and how this DNA element impacts the various stages of the topoisomerase cycle is similarly unresolved. Such gaps fundamentally impede our understanding of the mechanics underlying nucleotide-dependent, DNA strand transport.

Broader biological issues also remain. The regulatory role of various post-translational modifications on activity is unclear, as are the effects of known protein/protein interactions between Top2 and exogenous factors. From a therapeutic perspective, how various poisons act on eukaryotic Top2 to stabilize DNA cleavage, and the extent to which the mechanisms of myriad classes of inhibitors overlap with each other or with bacterial type II topoisomerase poisons is unknown. Answering these and other long-standing questions will require significant efforts in the future.

Acknowledgements The authors thank Karl Drlica for critical reading and helpful comments on this chapter. This work was supported by the NCI (CA077373, to JMB) and NIGMS (GM033944, to NO).

References

Aravind, L., Leipe, D.D., and Koonin, E.V. (1998). Toprim--a conserved catalytic domain in type IA and II topoisomerases, DnaG-type primases, OLD family nucleases and RecR proteins. Nucleic Acids Res *26*, 4205–4213.

Baird, C.L., Harkins, T.T., Morris, S.K., and Lindsley, J.E. (1999). Topoisomerase II drives DNA transport by hydrolyzing one ATP. Proc Natl Acad Sci USA *96*, 13685–13690.

Bates, A.D., and Maxwell, A. (2005). DNA topology, 2nd edn (Oxford ; New York, Oxford University Press).

Bax, B.D., Chan, P.F., Eggleston, D.S., Fosberry, A., Gentry, D.R., Gorrec, F., Giordano, I., Hann, M.M., Hennessy, A., Hibbs, M., *et al.* (2010). Type IIA topoisomerase inhibition by a new class of antibacterial agents. Nature *466*, 935–940.

Berger, J.M., Fass, D., Wang, J.C., and Harrison, S.C. (1998). Structural similarities between topoisomerases that cleave one or both DNA strands. Proc Natl Acad Sci USA *95*, 7876–7881.

Berger, J.M., Gamblin, S.J., Harrison, S.C., and Wang, J.C. (1996). Structure and mechanism of DNA topoisomerase II. Nature *379*, 225–232.

Bergerat, A., de Massy, B., Gadelle, D., Varoutas, P.C., Nicolas, A., and Forterre, P. (1997). An atypical topoisomerase II from Archaea with implications for meiotic recombination. Nature *386*, 414–417.

Bjergbaek, L., Kingma, P., Nielsen, I.S., Wang, Y., Westergaard, O., Osheroff, N., and Andersen, A.H. (2000). Communication between the ATPase and cleavage/religation domains of human topoisomerase IIalpha. J Biol Chem *275*, 13041–13048.

Buck, G.R., and Zechiedrich, E.L. (2004). DNA disentangling by type-2 topoisomerases. J Mol Biol *340*, 933–939.

Caron, P., and Wang, J.C. (1994). Alignment of Primary Sequences of DNA Topoisomerases. In Advances in Pharmacology, L.F. Liu, ed. (Academic Press), pp. 271–291.

Caron, P.R., Watt, P., and Wang, J.C. (1994). The C-terminal domain of Saccharomyces cerevisiae DNA topoisomerase II. Mol Cell Biol *14*, 3197–3207.

Champoux, J.J. (2001). DNA topoisomerases: structure, function, and mechanism. Annu Rev Biochem *70*, 369–413.

Classen, S., Olland, S., and Berger, J.M. (2003). Structure of the topoisomerase II ATPase region and its mechanism of inhibition by the chemotherapeutic agent ICRF-187. Proc Natl Acad Sci USA *100*, 10629–10634.

Corbett, A.H., Fernald, A.W., and Osheroff, N. (1993). Protein kinase C modulates the catalytic activity of topoisomerase II by enhancing the rate of ATP hydrolysis: evidence for a common mechanism of regulation by phosphorylation. Biochemistry *32*, 2090–2097.

Corbett, A.H., Zechiedrich, E.L., and Osheroff, N. (1992). A role for the passage helix in the DNA cleavage reaction of eukaryotic topoisomerase II. A two-site model for enzyme-mediated DNA cleavage. J Biol Chem *267*, 683–686.

Corbett, K.D., Benedetti, P., and Berger, J.M. (2007). Holoenzyme assembly and ATP-mediated conformational dynamics of topoisomerase VI. Nat Struct Mol Biol *14*, 611–619.

Corbett, K.D., and Berger, J.M. (2004). Structure, molecular mechanisms, and evolutionary relationships in DNA topoisomerases. Annu Rev Biophys Biomol Struct *33*, 95–118.

Corbett, K.D., and Berger, J.M. (2005). Structural dissection of ATP turnover in the prototypical GHL ATPase TopoVI. Structure *13*, 873–882.

Corbett, K.D., Schoeffler, A.J., Thomsen, N.D., and Berger, J.M. (2005). The structural basis for substrate specificity in DNA topoisomerase IV. J Mol Biol *351*, 545–561.

Corbett, K.D., Shultzaberger, R.K., and Berger, J.M. (2004). The C-terminal domain of DNA gyrase A adopts a DNA-bending beta-pinwheel fold. Proc Natl Acad Sci USA *101*, 7293–7298.

Deweese, J.E., Guengerich, F.P., Burgin, A.B., and Osheroff, N. (2009). Metal ion interactions in the DNA cleavage/ligation active site of human topoisomerase IIalpha. Biochemistry *48*, 8940–8947.

Deweese, J.E., and Osheroff, N. (2009a). Coordinating the two protomer active sites of human topoisomerase IIalpha: nicks as topoisomerase II poisons. Biochemistry *48*, 1439–1441.

Deweese, J.E., and Osheroff, N. (2009b). The DNA cleavage reaction of topoisomerase II: wolf in sheep's clothing. Nucleic Acids Res *37*, 738–748.

Dong, K.C., and Berger, J.M. (2007). Structural basis for gate-DNA recognition and bending by type IIA topoisomerases. Nature *450*, 1201–1205.

Dutta, R., and Inouye, M. (2000). GHKL, an emergent ATPase/kinase superfamily. Trends Biochem Sci *25*, 24–28.

Fass, D., Bogden, C.E., and Berger, J.M. (1999). Quaternary changes in topoisomerase II may direct orthogonal movement of two DNA strands. Nat Struct Biol *6*, 322–326.

Forterre, P., Gribaldo, S., Gadelle, D., and Serre, M.C. (2007). Origin and evolution of DNA topoisomerases. Biochimie *89*, 427–446.

Gellert, M., Mizuuchi, K., O'Dea, M.H., and Nash, H.A. (1976). DNA gyrase: an enzyme that introduces superhelical turns into DNA. Proc Natl Acad Sci USA *73*, 3872–3876.

Goto, T., Laipis, P., and Wang, J.C. (1984). The purification and characterization of DNA topoisomerases I and II of the yeast Saccharomyces cerevisiae. J Biol Chem *259*, 10422–10429.

Horowitz, D.S., and Wang, J.C. (1987). Mapping the active site tyrosine of Escherichia coli DNA gyrase. J Biol Chem *262*, 5339–5344.

Hu, T., Chang, S., and Hsieh, T. (1998). Identifying Lys359 as a critical residue for the ATP-dependent reactions of Drosophila DNA topoisomerase II. J Biol Chem *273*, 9586–9592.

Kingma, P.S., Corbett, A.H., Burcham, P.C., Marnett, L.J., and Osheroff, N. (1995). Abasic sites stimulate double-stranded DNA cleavage mediated by topoisomerase II. DNA lesions as endogenous topoisomerase II poisons. J Biol Chem *270*, 21441–21444.

Kingma, P.S., and Osheroff, N. (1997). Spontaneous DNA damage stimulates topoisomerase II-mediated DNA cleavage. J Biol Chem *272*, 7488–7493.

Kirchhausen, T., Wang, J.C., and Harrison, S.C. (1985). DNA gyrase and its complexes with DNA: direct observation by electron microscopy. Cell *41*, 933–943.

Klenin, K., Langowski, J., and Vologodskii, A. (2002). Computational analysis of the chiral action of type II DNA topoisomerases. J Mol Biol *320*, 359–367.

Kurz, E.U., Leader, K.B., Kroll, D.J., Clark, M., and Gieseler, F. (2000). Modulation of human DNA topoisomerase IIalpha function by interaction with 14-3-3epsilon. J Biol Chem *275*, 13948–13954.

Lamour, V., Hoermann, L., Jeltsch, J.M., Oudet, P., and Moras, D. (2002). An open conformation of the Thermus thermophilus gyrase B ATP-binding domain. J Biol Chem *277*, 18947–18953.

Laponogov, I., Pan, X.S., Veselkov, D.A., McAuley, K.E., Fisher, L.M., and Sanderson, M.R. (2010). Structural basis of gate-DNA breakage and resealing by type II topoisomerases. PLoS ONE *5*, e11338.

Laponogov, I., Sohi, M.K., Veselkov, D.A., Pan, X.S., Sawhney, R., Thompson, A.W., McAuley, K.E., Fisher, L.M., and Sanderson, M.R. (2009). Structural insight into the quinolone-DNA cleavage complex of type IIA topoisomerases. Nat Struct Mol Biol *16*, 667–669.

Lee, M.P., Sander, M., and Hsieh, T. (1989). Nuclease protection by Drosophila DNA topoisomerase II. Enzyme/DNA contacts at the strong topoisomerase II cleavage sites. J Biol Chem *264*, 21779–21787.

Lindsley, J.E., and Wang, J.C. (1991). Proteolysis patterns of epitopically labeled yeast DNA topoisomerase II suggest an allosteric transition in the enzyme induced by ATP binding. Proc Natl Acad Sci USA *88*, 10485–10489.

Lindsley, J.E., and Wang, J.C. (1993a). On the coupling between ATP usage and DNA transport by yeast DNA topoisomerase II. J Biol Chem *268*, 8096–8104.

Lindsley, J.E., and Wang, J.C. (1993b). Study of Allosteric Communication Between Protomers by Immunotagging. Nature *361*, 749–750.

Liu, L.F., Liu, C.C., and Alberts, B.M. (1979). T4 DNA topoisomerase: a new ATP-dependent enzyme essential for initiation of T4 bacteriophage DNA replication. Nature *281*, 456–461.

Liu, L.F., Rowe, T.C., Yang, L., Tewey, K.M., and Chen, G.L. (1983). Cleavage of DNA by mammalian DNA topoisomerase II. J Biol Chem *258*, 15365–15370.

Liu, L.F., and Wang, J.C. (1987). Supercoiling of the DNA template during transcription. Proc Natl Acad Sci USA *84*, 7024–7027.

Liu, Z., Deibler, R.W., Chan, H.S., and Zechiedrich, L. (2009). The why and how of DNA unlinking. Nucleic Acids Res *37*, 661–671.

Lynn, R., Giaever, G., Swanberg, S.L., and Wang, J.C. (1986). Tandem regions of yeast DNA topoisomerase II share homology with different subunits of bacterial gyrase. Science *233*, 647–649.

McClendon, A.K., Gentry, A.C., Dickey, J.S., Brinch, M., Bendsen, S., Andersen, A.H., and Osheroff, N. (2008). Bimodal recognition of DNA geometry by human topoisomerase II alpha: preferential relaxation of positively supercoiled DNA requires elements in the C-terminal domain. Biochemistry *47*, 13169–13178.

McClendon, A.K., Rodriguez, A.C., and Osheroff, N. (2005). Human topoisomerase IIalpha rapidly relaxes positively supercoiled DNA: implications for enzyme action ahead of replication forks. J Biol Chem *280*, 39337–39345.

Miller, K.G., Liu, L.F., and Englund, P.T. (1981). A homogeneous type II DNA topoisomerase from HeLa cell nuclei. J Biol Chem *256*, 9334–9339.

Mizuuchi, K., O'Dea, M.H., and Gellert, M. (1978). DNA gyrase: subunit structure and ATPase activity of the purified enzyme. Proc Natl Acad Sci USA *75*, 5960–5963.

Moore, C.L., Klevan, L., Wang, J.C., and Griffith, J.D. (1983). Gyrase:DNA Complexes Visualized as Looped Structures by Electron Microscopy. J Biol Chem *258*, 4612–4617.

Morais Cabral, J.H., Jackson, A.P., Smith, C.V., Shikotra, N., Maxwell, A., and Liddington, R.C. (1997). Crystal structure of the breakage-reunion domain of DNA gyrase. Nature *388*, 903–906.

Morrison, A., and Cozzarelli, N.R. (1979). Site-specific cleavage of DNA by E. coli DNA gyrase. Cell *17*, 175–184.

Mueller-Planitz, F., and Herschlag, D. (2006). Interdomain communication in DNA topoisomerase II. DNA binding and enzyme activation. J Biol Chem *281*, 23395–23404.

Mueller-Planitz, F., and Herschlag, D. (2007). DNA topoisomerase II selects DNA cleavage sites based on reactivity rather than binding affinity. Nucleic Acids Res *35*, 3764–3773.

Noble, C.G., and Maxwell, A. (2002). The role of GyrB in the DNA cleavage-religation reaction of DNA gyrase: a proposed two metal-ion mechanism. J Mol Biol *318*, 361–371.

Osheroff, N. (1986). Eukaryotic topoisomerase II. Characterization of enzyme turnover. J Biol Chem *261*, 9944–9950.

Osheroff, N. (1987). Role of the divalent cation in topoisomerase II mediated reactions. Biochemistry *26*, 6402–6406.

Postow, L., Crisona, N.J., Peter, B.J., Hardy, C.D., and Cozzarelli, N.R. (2001). Topological challenges to DNA replication: conformations at the fork. Proc Natl Acad Sci USA *98*, 8219–8226.

Pruss, G.J., and Drlica, K. (1989). DNA supercoiling and prokaryotic transcription. Cell *56*, 521–523.

Reece, R.J., and Maxwell, A. (1991). The C-terminal domain of the Escherichia coli DNA gyrase A subunit is a DNA-binding protein. Nucleic Acids Res *19*, 1399–1405.

Roca, J., Berger, J.M., Harrison, S.C., and Wang, J.C. (1996). DNA transport by a type II topoisomerase: direct evidence for a two-gate mechanism. Proc Natl Acad Sci USA *93*, 4057–4062.

Roca, J., Berger, J.M., and Wang, J.C. (1993). On the simultaneous binding of eukaryotic DNA topoisomerase II to a pair of double-stranded DNA helices. J Biol Chem *268*, 14250–14255.

Roca, J., Ishida, R., Berger, J.M., Andoh, T., and Wang, J.C. (1994). Antitumor bisdioxopiperazines inhibit yeast DNA topoisomerase II by trapping the enzyme in the form of a closed protein clamp. Proc Natl Acad Sci USA *91*, 1781–1785.

Roca, J., and Wang, J.C. (1992). The capture of a DNA double helix by an ATP-dependent protein clamp: a key step in DNA transport by type II DNA topoisomerases. Cell *71*, 833–840.

Roca, J., and Wang, J.C. (1994). DNA transport by a type II DNA topoisomerase: evidence in favor of a two gate mechanism. Cell *77*, 609–616.

Rybenkov, V.V., Ullsperger, C., Vologodskii, A.V., and Cozzarelli, N.R. (1997). Simplification of DNA topology below equilibrium values by type II topoisomerases. Science *277*, 690–693.

Sahyoun, N., Wolf, M., Besterman, J., Hsieh, T., Sander, M., LeVine, H., 3 rd, Chang, K.J., and Cuatrecasas, P. (1986). Protein kinase C phosphorylates topoisomerase II: topoisomerase activation and its possible role in phorbol ester-induced differentiation of HL-60 cells. Proc Natl Acad Sci USA *83*, 1603–1607.

Sander, M., and Hsieh, T. (1983). Double strand DNA cleavage by type II DNA topoisomerase from Drosophila melanogaster. J Biol Chem *258*, 8421–8428.

Schmidt, B.H., Burgin, A.B., Deweese, J.E., Osheroff, N., and Berger, J.M. (2010). A novel and unified two-metal mechanism for DNA cleavage by type II and IA topoisomerases. Nature *465*, 641–644.

Schoeffler, A.J., and Berger, J.M. (2008). DNA topoisomerases: harnessing and constraining energy to govern chromosome topology. Q Rev Biophys *41*, 41–101.

Schultz, P., Olland, S., Oudet, P., and Hancock, R. (1996). Structure and conformational changes of DNA topoisomerase II visualized by electron microscopy. Proc Natl Acad Sci *93*, 5936–5940.

Shiozaki, K., and Yanagida, M. (1992). Functional dissection of the phosphorylated termini of fission yeast DNA topoisomerase II. J Cell Biol *119*, 1023–1036.

Sissi, C., Chemello, A., Vazquez, E., Mitchenall, L.A., Maxwell, A., and Palumbo, M. (2008). DNA gyrase requires DNA for effective two-site coordination of divalent metal ions: further insight into the mechanism of enzyme action. Biochemistry *47*, 8538–8545.

Staudenbauer, W.L., and Orr, E. (1981). DNA gyrase: affinity chromatography on novobiocin-Sepharose and catalytic properties. Nucleic Acids Res *9*, 3589–3603.

Steitz, T.A., and Steitz, J.A. (1993). A general two-metal-ion mechanism for catalytic RNA. Proc Natl Acad Sci USA *90*, 6498–6502.

Stone, M.D., Bryant, Z., Crisona, N.J., Smith, S.B., Vologodskii, A., Bustamante, C., and Cozzarelli, N.R. (2003). Chirality sensing by Escherichia coli topoisomerase IV and the mechanism of type II topoisomerases. Proc Natl Acad Sci USA *100*, 8654–8659.

Stuchinskaya, T., Mitchenall, L.A., Schoeffler, A.J., Corbett, K.D., Berger, J.M., Bates, A.D., and Maxwell, A. (2009). How do type II topoisomerases use ATP hydrolysis to simplify DNA topology beyond equilibrium? Investigating the relaxation reaction of nonsupercoiling type II topoisomerases. J Mol Biol *385*, 1397–1408.

Sugino, A., Higgins, N.P., and Cozzarelli, N.R. (1980). DNA gyrase subunit stoichiometry and the covalent attachment of subunit A to DNA during DNA cleavage. Nucleic Acids Res *8*, 3865–3874.

Tamura, J.K., and Gellert, M. (1990). Characterization of the ATP binding site on Escherichia coli DNA gyrase. Affinity labeling of Lys-103 and Lys-110 of the B subunit by pyridoxal 5′-diphospho-5′-adenosine. J Biol Chem *265*, 21342–21349.

Trigueros, S., Salceda, J., Bermudez, I., Fernandez, X., and Roca, J. (2004). Asymmetric removal of supercoils suggests how topoisomerase II simplifies DNA topology. J Mol Biol *335*, 723–731.

Uemura, T., Morikawa, K., and Yanagida, M. (1986). The nucleotide sequence of the fission yeast DNA topoisomerase II gene: structural and functional relationships to other DNA topoisomerases. Embo J *5*, 2355–2361.

Wang, J.C. (2002). Cellular roles of DNA topoisomerases: a molecular perspective. Nat Rev Mol Cell Biol *3*, 430–440.

Wang, J.C. (2009). Untangling the double helix : DNA entanglement and the action of the DNA topoisomerases (Cold Spring Harbor, N.Y., Cold Spring Harbor Laboratory Press).

Wei, H., Ruthenburg, A.J., Bechis, S.K., and Verdine, G.L. (2005). Nucleotide-dependent domain movement in the ATPase domain of a human type IIA DNA topoisomerase. J Biol Chem *280*, 37041–37047.

West, K.L., Meczes, E.L., Thorn, R., Turnbull, R.M., Marshall, R., and Austin, C.A. (2000). Mutagenesis of E477 or K505 in the B’ domain of human topoisomerase II beta increases the requirement for magnesium ions during strand passage. Biochemistry *39*, 1223–1233.

Wigley, D.B., Davies, G.J., Dodson, E.J., Maxwell, A., and Dodson, G. (1991). Crystal structure of an N-terminal fragment of the DNA gyrase B protein. Nature *351*, 624–629.

Williams, N.L., and Maxwell, A. (1999a). Locking the DNA gate of DNA gyrase: investigating the effects on DNA cleavage and ATP hydrolysis. Biochemistry *38*, 14157–14164.

Williams, N.L., and Maxwell, A. (1999b). Probing the two-gate mechanism of DNA gyrase using cysteine cross-linking. Biochemistry *38*, 13502–13511.

Wohlkonig, A., Chan, P.F., Fosberry, A.P., Homes, P., Huang, J., Kranz, M., Leydon, V.R., Miles, T.J., Pearson, N.D., Perera, R.L., *et al.* (2010). Structural basis of quinolone inhibition of type IIA topoisomerases and target-mediated resistance. Nat Struct Mol Biol *17*, 1152–1153.

Worland, S.T., and Wang, J.C. (1989). Inducible overexpression, purification, and active site mapping of DNA topoisomerase II from the yeast Saccharomyces cerevisiae. J Biol Chem *264*, 4412–4416.

Yamane, K., Wu, X., and Chen, J. (2002). A DNA damage-regulated BRCT-containing protein, TopBP1, is required for cell survival. Mol Cell Biol *22*, 555–566.

Yan, J., Magnasco, M.O., and Marko, J.F. (1999). A kinetic proofreading mechanism for disentanglement of DNA by topoisomerases. Nature *401*, 932–935.

Yang, W., Lee, J.Y., and Nowotny, M. (2006). Making and breaking nucleic acids: two-Mg2+–ion catalysis and substrate specificity. Mol Cell *22*, 5–13.

Zechiedrich, E.L., and Osheroff, N. (1990). Eukaryotic topoisomerases recognize nucleic acid topology by preferentially interacting with DNA crossovers. Embo J *9*, 4555–4562.

Chapter 5
Essential Functions of Topoisomerase IIIα in the Nucleus and Mitochondria

Stefanie Hartman Chen*, Jianhong Wu*, and Tao-shih Hsieh

5.1 Introduction

DNA topoisomerases are the enzymes that manage the topological states of the DNA during replication, transcription, recombination, and chromatin remodeling. DNA topoisomerases fall into two main categories: type I and type II (Champoux 2001; Wang 2002). The type I monomeric enzymes transiently cleave one strand of DNA at a time; for the type II enzymes, both strands in a DNA double helix are simultaneously transiently cleaved by the homodimeric enzyme. Type I topoisomerases can be further grouped into two subfamilies: type IA, which attaches to the 5′ phosphate of the broken strand and performs strand exchange, and type IB, which covalently links to the 3′ phosphate of the broken strand and uses a swiveling mechanism to relieve topological stress. All organisms examined, with the exception of viruses, possess at least one type IA DNA topoisomerase. The presence of a type IA enzyme in mitochondria, which replicate their own genome, has also been shown (Wang et al. 2002; Wu et al. 2010). The ubiquitous presence of type IA DNA topoisomerases reflects their indispensable role in DNA transactions. Top3 is a member of the type IA subfamily that is conserved from bacteria to humans. In this chapter, we outline the contributions of a eukaryotic isozyme of Top3, Top3α, in DNA segregation of late replication intermediates, and its function in preventing unruly recombination by resolving intermediates together with its interaction partner, the Bloom syndrome helicase (Blm).

---

*These authors contributed equally to this work.

T.-s. Hsieh (✉)
Department of Biochemistry, Duke University Medical Center,
Durham, NC 27710, USA
e-mail: thsieh@duke.edu

Y. Pommier (ed.), *DNA Topoisomerases and Cancer*, Cancer Drug Discovery and Development, DOI 10.1007/978-1-4614-0323-4_5,

5.2 Discovery of Eukaryotic Type IA Topoisomerases

The first eukaryotic type IA topoisomerase was discovered in yeast as part of a screen for gene deletions that created hyperrecombination phenotypes (Wallis et al. 1989). In addition to hyperrecombination, the deletion strain exhibited an increase in chromosome nondisjunction, smaller cell sizes, and decreased formation of diploids and spores. Named topoisomerase 3 (Top3), as the third topoisomerase discovered in yeast, this enzyme showed homology to and could be complemented by *E. coli* topoisomerase I, suggesting that Top3 belonged in the type IA family.

Kim and Wang provided further evidence that Top3 was indeed a type IA topoisomerase by purifying and characterizing the yeast protein (Kim and Wang 1992). Top3 could weakly relax negatively, but not positively, supercoiled substrates, and relaxation was increased at a higher temperature, indicating a preference for single-stranded regions. As further evidence, denatured DNA was an effective competitor for the relaxation activity of Top3, and Top3 could efficiently relax a negatively supercoiled DNA plasmid containing a 29-nucleotide single-stranded region on one strand. Using a 3′-radiolabeled DNA substrate, Top3 was shown to covalently attach to the 5′ end of the DNA backbone. These traits are consistent with the type IA family.

A human homolog of this protein was subsequently discovered with enzymatic activities similar to the yeast Top3 (Hanai et al. 1996). Sequence data mining revealed that metazoans express a second homolog with the same relaxation activity, dubbed Top3β (Seki et al. 1998). The original metazoan type IA then became known as Top3α. The two enzymes share homology in their N-terminal regions, including the catalytic active site region, but diverge in their C-terminal "tail" regions (Fig. 5.1).

As type IA topoisomerases, both isozymes are able to relax DNA with single-stranded regions in steps of one linking number. They are able to partially relax highly negatively supercoiled DNA in the presence of divalent cations (Hanai et al. 1996; Goulaouic et al. 1999; Wilson et al. 2000; Plank et al. 2005). Top3β was shown to preferentially cleave the single-stranded side of an R- or D-loop (Wilson-Sali and Hsieh 2002a), a biochemical function which is as yet untested for Top3α. However, Top3α was shown to relax bubble substrates, or plasmids with permanently single-stranded regions (Plank et al. 2005).

5.3 Differential Cellular Roles of Top3α and Top3β

Despite the similarity of the two isozymes, distinct cellular phenotypes were soon established. Top3α is essential for embryonic development. Mice lacking Top3α died during gestation. Cultured embryos from the mutant mice showed poor proliferation and an unidentifiable inner cell mass (Li and Wang 1998). Flies with an insertional mutation in *top3α* either die as embryos or pupate but never eclose (Plank et al. 2005). With *top3α* knocked out, mitotic tissues like imaginal discs are absent, while endoreplication in salivary glands and fat bodies are unaffected (Wu et al. 2010).

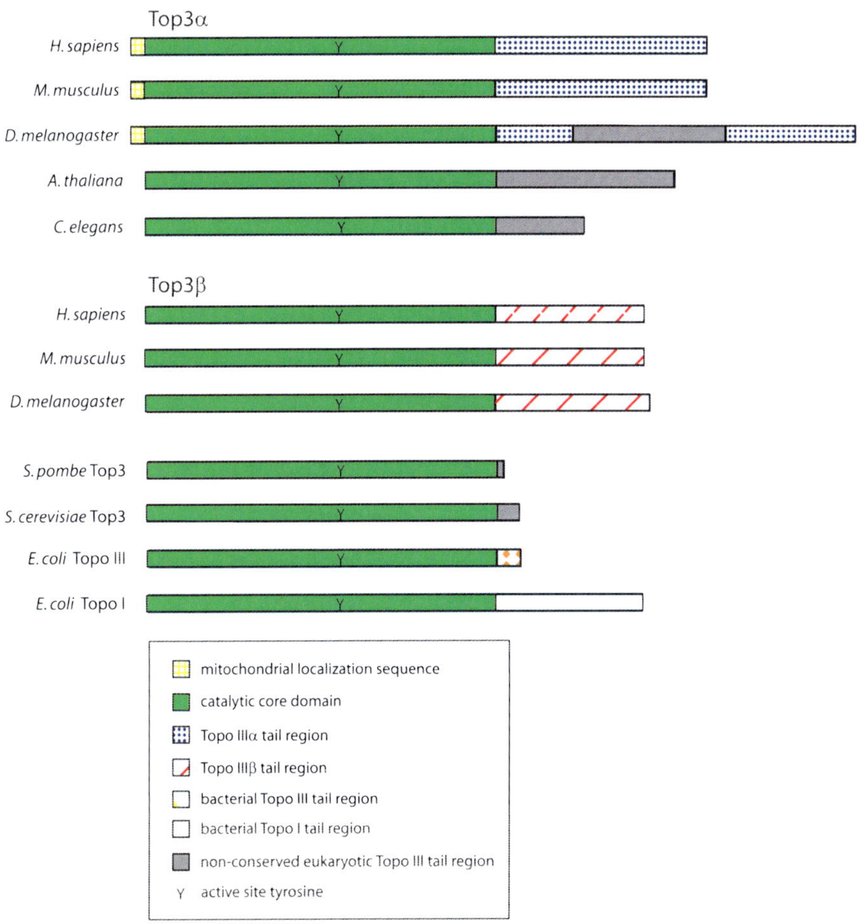

Fig. 5.1 Alignment of members of the type IA family of topoisomerases. While all share a conserved catalytic domain, including the active site tyrosine, the members differ in their C-terminal regions

These phenotypes indicate a critical role for Top3α in developmental processes, especially for mitotic growth, for which Top3β cannot substitute.

In contrast, mice lacking Top3β develop to maturity without apparent defects, although their lifespan is reduced (Kwan and Wang 2001). In addition, the litter size of mutant mice is reduced both over time and through successive generations; increased genome instability, including aneuploidy, is also observed in the cells of these animals (Kwan et al. 2003). The shorter lifespan appears to be linked to autoimmunity caused by an increase in apoptosis, possibly related to the occurrence of aneuploidy (Kwan et al. 2007). Although an intriguing effect, Top3β does not appear to be involved in development or essential for survival. Flies with *top3β* deleted also have no apparent defect observed (Wu et al. 2006a).

To further explore the cellular defects in the absence of Top3α, a DT40 cell line with inducible repression of the enzyme was produced (Seki et al. 2006). Top3α-depleted cells stopped growing within three days, exhibiting an accumulation of cells arrested in G_2 phase. These cells also had highly aberrant karyotypes, with some so fragmented that they were unscorable. In contrast, cells depleted of Top3β resembled wild type.

Together, these studies indicate that, despite having similar enzymatic activities in isolation, the differing regions of Top3α and Top3β direct them to separate cellular functions. In addition to having a distinct C-terminal domain, Top3α also differs from its isozyme by the presence of an N-terminal mitochondrial localization signal, as discussed in the following section.

5.4 Functions of Top3α in Mitochondria

Human Top3α mRNA has been shown to have two potential translation initiation codons. Initiation at the first AUG produces a peptide of 1,001 amino acids, while initiation at the second gives rise to a 976-amino-acid peptide (Wang et al. 2002). The second codon appears to be preferred for translation based on the sequence context (Hanai et al. 1996); hence, the shorter form of Top3α is the major product. Sequence analysis has revealed the presence of a mitochondrial import signal in the first 25 amino acids of the 1001-amino-acid form of human Top3α, and in many other metazoan Top3α (Wang et al. 2002). Since the longer form possesses both nuclear and mitochondrial import sequences, the resulting protein can target to both nuclei and mitochondria.

In *Drosophila*, Top3α has been shown to localize to both nuclei and mitochondria (Fig. 5.2. and (Wu et al. 2010)). When the first AUG is altered to UUG so that translation initiates exclusively from the second AUG, a protein, deprived of the mitochondrial import sequence but retaining the nuclear localization signal at the carboxyl

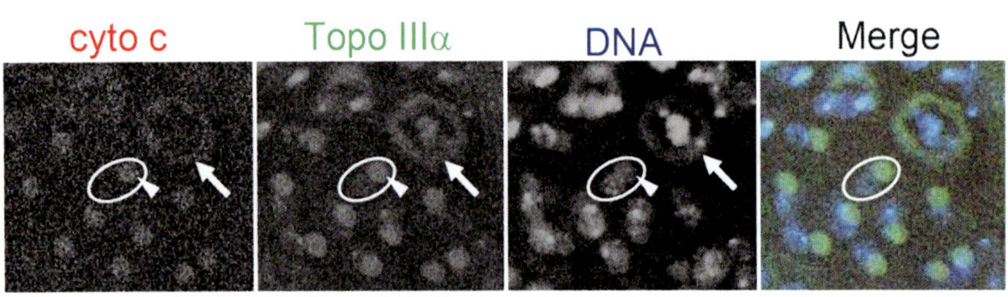

Fig. 5.2 Top3α is localized in both nuclei and mitochondria. Testes of Oregon-R were dissected, fixed with 6% formaldehyde and stained with cytochrome c and Top3α antibodies, and DAPI to visualize DNA. The *arrow* indicates a spermatocyte with highly condensed chromatin which is surrounded by clustered mitochondria. Spermatids at onion stage exhibit a characteristic pattern of a nucleus neighboring a mitochondrial derivative (nebenkern). A typical pair of nucleus and nebenkern (*arrowhead*) is *circled*

portion, is encoded. As expected, this protein is exclusively localized in nuclei. When the second AUG is changed to UUG, translation is exclusively from the first AUG, giving rise to a protein with a mitochondrial import sequence at its N-terminus and a nuclear localization signal in its C-terminus. This protein predominantly localizes in the mitochondria, with a detectable fraction in the nuclei. These data thus indicate that the second AUG in wildtype Top3α is used as an alternative translation initiation codon to produce the major nuclear form of Top3α (Wu et al. 2010).

In the absence of mitochondrial Top3α, though they can survive to adulthood, the flies have been shown to have a 4- to 15-fold decrease in mtDNA copy number and a 2- to 3-fold decrease in ATP content, indicating that Top3α plays a key role in mitochondrial DNA (mtDNA) maintenance (Wu et al. 2010). *Drosophila* mtDNA is a circular molecule of about 20 kb, and its maintenance seems to be impossible in the absence of topoisomerases. Among all the topoisomerases present in *Drosophila*, which include Top3α and Top3β (type IA), Topo I (type IB), and Topo II (type IIA) (Wyckoff and Hsieh 1988; Lee et al. 1993; Wilson-Sali and Hsieh 2002b; Plank et al. 2005), it appears that only Top3α can be imported into both the nuclei and the mitochondria. Although it has been reported that the human nuclear genome encodes a mitochondria-specific type IB topoisomerase, Top1mt (Zhang et al. 2001), which is not essential for viability (Zhang et al. 2007), no such enzyme is predicted from the *Drosophila* genome sequence. Since the sole type II topoisomerase in *Drosophila* appears to be exclusively localized in the nuclei, this suggests that the type II topoisomerase may be dispensable for the segregation of mtDNA. A plausible mechanism of Top3α in mtDNA segregation will be discussed in the following section.

5.5 Functions of Top3 in the Segregation of Late Replication Intermediates

E. coli Top3 is very efficient in the decatenation of gapped, interlinked DNA dimers and DNA replication intermediates *in vitro* (DiGate and Marians 1988). The decatenation activity is strongly dependent on the presence of a single-stranded region, which provides a binding site for the Top3. This observation leads to the idea that Top3 may play a role in bacterial chromosome segregation. It has been considered that Top3-RecQ duo activities may play a key role in the segregation process since the association between Top3 and RecQ was established in budding yeast (Gangloff et al. 1994).

Suski and Marians (Suski and Marians 2008) have demonstrated that *E. coli* Top3-RecQ can resolve stalled, converging replication forks generated *in vitro* by the replication of *oriC* plasmid DNA using the Tus-Ter system. These authors showed that the late replication intermediate, two nearly replicated daughter molecules linked via the unreplicated parental DNA region (Fig. 5.3A, a), can be resolved by a process of two sequential steps. First, RecQ DNA helicase unwinds the DNA duplex between the converging replication forks (Fig. 5.3A, a and b). Top3 then unlinks the two gapped, entangled daughter molecules at the single-stranded region (Fig. 5.3A, b), giving rise to two gapped daughter DNA circles (Fig. 5.3A, c).

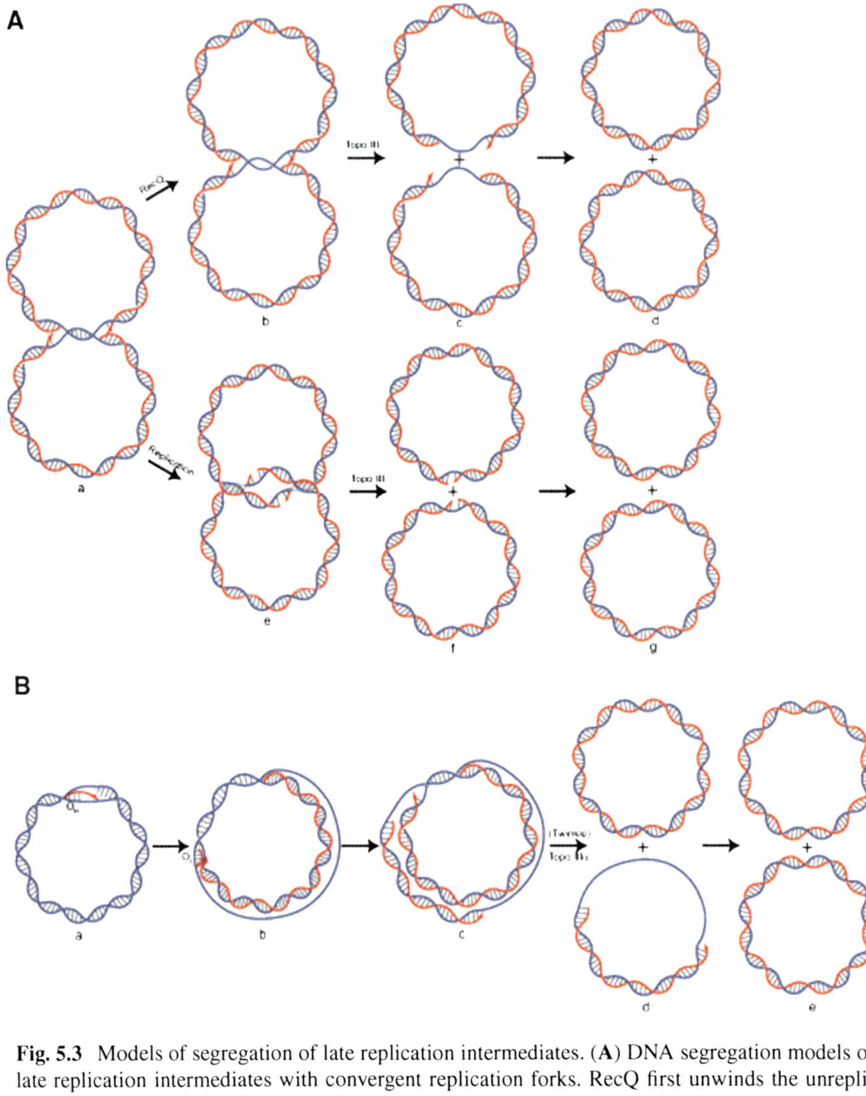

Fig. 5.3 Models of segregation of late replication intermediates. (**A**) DNA segregation models of late replication intermediates with convergent replication forks. RecQ first unwinds the unreplicated parental stands (**a**, **b**), then Top3 segregates the conjoined gapped circles (**b**, **c**). The gapped molecules complete replication (**c**, **d**).Alternatively, the conjoined gapped circles will be generated after the parental duplex is completely unwound, but before the gaps between the 3′-end of the leading strand and 5′-end of the last Okazaki fragments of the lagging strands are sealed (**e**). Top3 unlinks the conjoined gapped circles (**e**, **f**). Gaps are sealed to give rise to two daughter molecules (**f**, **g**). (**B**) The strand displacement model of mitochondrial DNA replication. Replication of leading strand initiates at the origin of heavy strand synthesis (O_H) and proceeds unidirectionally, displacing the parental heavy strand as single-stranded DNA (**a**, **b**). When the synthesis of the heavy strand proceeds two thirds of the DNA circle, the origin of light strand synthesis (O_L) is exposed, and synthesis of the daughter light strand proceeds in the opposite direction relative to the synthesis direction of daughter heavy strand (**b**, **c**). The daughter molecule with the new light strand lags in completion of DNA replication, leading to a gapped circle. The mitochondrial DNA helicase Twinkle may first unwinds the unreplicated duplex region and Top3α carries out strand passage to segregate the circles (**c**, **d**). Finally, the unlinked molecules complete DNA replication (**d**, **e**)

It is also plausible that the prerequisite unwinding by RecQ helicase is not required for the chromosome segregation. In this model (Fig. 5.3A, a, e, f, g), Top3 unlinks the daughter chromosomes after the last parental DNA duplex turn is unwound, but before the gaps in the lagging strands are replicated and sealed. In this process, Top3 may bind to a single-stranded region on the lagging strand's template (Nurse et al. 2003).

Animal mitochondrial genomes typically exist as circular, covalently closed molecules ranging from 15–20 kb (Boore 1999). It has been proposed that mtDNA replicates itself via a strand displacement mechanism [(Brown et al. 2005); Fig. 5.3B]. In *Drosophila*, in the absence of the mitochondrial import sequence of Top3α, and consequently no mitochondrial entry of Top3α, the mtDNA copy number will be decreased (Wu et al. 2010), suggesting that Top3α is required for the maintenance of the mitochondrial genome. The mtDNA may utilize a mechanism similar to the bacteria genome to segregate daughter chromosomes via Top3-DNA helicase, specifically Top3α-Twinkle (Fig. 5.3B). The leading strand starts to replicate at the origin of heavy strand synthesis (O_H) and proceeds unidirectionally (Fig. 5.3B, a). When the synthesis of the heavy strand proceeds around two-thirds of the circle, the origin of light strand synthesis (O_L) is exposed, and synthesis of the daughter light strand initiates (Fig. 5.3B, b). Consequently, the daughter molecule with the new light strand being synthesized lags in completion of DNA replication, leading to gapped, conjoined circles (Fig. 5.3B, c), which is essentially a late replication intermediate similar to the one discussed above (Fig. 5.3A). In one of the plausible pathways of segregation, the mitochondrial DNA helicase Twinkle may first unwind the unreplicated duplex region with Top3α then carrying out strand passage to segregate the circles (Fig. 5.3B, c, d).

While the above discussion focuses on the potential function of Top3α in the segregation of replication intermediates in mitochondria, similar functions could be required during mitotic growth in nucleus as well. In this case, Top3α may collaborate with its partner helicase, Bloom syndrome helicase (Blm), to segregate intertwined hemicatenanes that are present as intermediates during DNA replication. The presence of Top3α and Bloom helicase in anaphase bridges during mitotic divisions (Chan et al. 2007), also discussed in a later section) may indeed be related to such a function. Furthermore, genetic analysis has indeed implicated a function of chromosome segregation for Top3 in *Schizosaccharomyces pombe* (Goodwin et al. 1999).

5.6 Partnership with Bloom Syndrome Helicase

5.6.1 Interaction with the RecQ Family

While clearly involved in maintaining genomic integrity, the functional role of Top3α in the cell was further elucidated by the discovery of an interacting partner. The yeast RecQ family helicase, Sgs1, was discovered as a suppressor of the slow growth induced by deletion of Top3 (Gangloff et al. 1994). Although deleting Top3 causes a huge increase in recombination rate, the slight increase in recombination caused by deleting Sgs1 alone did not increase when Top3 was also deleted, indicating an epistatic effect.

Higher eukaryotes have more members of the RecQ family, with *Drosophila* containing Blm, RecQ4 and RecQ5, while humans have RecQ1, Blm, Werner syndrome helicase, RecQ4 and RecQ5 (see Chap. 8). The RecQ family helicases, named after their bacterial homolog, are 3′–5′ helicases involved in supporting genomic stability. Although RecQ5β was shown to interact with both Top3α and Top3β (Shimamoto et al. 2000), a functional relationship has only been established for Top3α and Blm. Blm preferentially works on recombination structures, such as Holliday junctions and G-quadruplexes, and mutations in Blm, like mutations in RecQ4 and Werner syndrome helicase, cause predisposition to cancers (Chu and Hickson 2009).

The interaction between Top3α and the RecQ helicase Blm was first shown by cellular co-localization and co-immunoprecipitation in both somatic and meiotic cells (Johnson et al. 2000; Wu et al. 2000). Blm-Top3α interactions can be shown by other techniques including Far Western, and Blm was found to have two independent binding domains for Top3α, one at each terminal end of the protein (Wu et al. 2000). Blm was also able to stimulate the relaxation activity of Top3α in the presence of a single-stranded binding protein and to recruit Top3α to single-stranded regions (Wu and Hickson 2002).

Further evidence of the interaction between these two proteins was shown through a series of *in vitro* and *in vivo* studies. In *Xenopus* egg extracts, Xblm was able to bind Xtop3α, with this interaction increasing upon induction of DNA checkpoint kinases or addition of Y- or fork-shaped DNA structures, which mimic DNA damage (Li et al. 2004). Xblm required the presence of Xtop3α to bind chromatin, regardless of replication blockage, whereas Xtop3α was able to itself bind chromatin when replication blockage was induced, indicating a role for Top3α in recruiting Blm to sites of damage. Association with Xtop3α was also necessary for the phosphorylation of Xblm in response to DNA damage.

In yeast, Sgs1 mutants with defective helicase activity but retaining the ability to bind Top3 were better at rescuing MMS sensitivity than those with full helicase activity but no ability to bind Top3 (Ui et al. 2005). In contrast, the binding of Sgs1 to Top3 and its helicase activity were both required for the suppression of sister chromatid recombination. The critical role of the interactions between Top3 and Sgs1 in their genetic functions can be further demonstrated with the functionality of the fusion proteins of Top3/Sgs1 (Bennett and Wang 2001). These studies indicate that the interaction between the two proteins is an important component of the genomic stability maintenance system employed in this process.

5.6.2 Double Holliday Junction Resolution

While these studies provided clear evidence of a Blm-Top3α functional complex, with Blm seemingly creating a toxic intermediate that was processed by Top3α, the exact target structure or pathway of action was yet to be elucidated. Starting with the

Szostak model of double-strand break repair (Szostak et al. 1983), the observed increase in sister chromatid exchange in Blm-deficient cells and the enzymatic activities of the two proteins in the complex, led to the proposal that they may act on a double Holliday junction structure, a recombination intermediate (Wang 2002). Using yeast as a powerful genetic system, it was demonstrated that the double Holliday junction structure present during meiotic recombination can be dissolved by Top3 and Sgs1, generating non-crossover recombination products (Ira et al. 2003).

Biochemical evidence for this model was first shown on a substrate of linked oligonucleotides, creating two Holliday junctions that were separated by 14 base pairs with annealed single-stranded loops on the end of each strand. Top3α and Blm were able to separate the two single-stranded circles by unlinking the connections between the junctions, in a process termed "dissolution" (Wu and Hickson 2003).

This process was further elucidated by a more complex double Holliday junction structure, involving double-stranded circles with junctions that were 165 base pairs apart. The junction migration process was shown to be convergent, and dissolution was specific to Top3α, since neither Top1 nor Top3β were able to substitute (Plank et al. 2006). However, there is clear evidence that the function of dissolution of Holliday junctions by human Top3α can be substituted with other type IA enzymes (Wu et al. 2006b). It remains a possibility that the specificity of Top3α may be dependent on the particular system.

The dissolution of double Holliday junctions into solely non-crossover products involves complex topological maneuvering from a combined action of Top3α and Blm. Despite being well accepted, the exact mechanism of this reaction remains quite puzzling. While Blm alone can easily migrate single Holliday junctions (HJs), the convergence of two HJs necessitates the action of a type IA topoisomerase, which requires single-stranded DNA (ssDNA), to act to relieve the topological linkages in the region between the junctions, where positive supercoils will accumulate.

Two models have recently been proposed to explain this reaction (Plank and Hsieh 2009). The Unravel & Unlink model proposes a sequential reaction, in which a region of ssDNA is first created, followed by coordinated separation of the strands and renaturation (Fig. 5.4a). In the HJ Migration model, the two enzymes are arranged in a complex such that Top3α is able to perform strand passage as the helicase is migrating the junctions to separate the two entangled dsDNA strands (Fig. 5.4b).

The Unravel & Unlink model has precedent in the Suski & Marians experiment discussed above (Fig. 5.3A) (Suski and Marians 2008), in which *E. coli* RecQ first separates the strands of stalled converging replication forks, followed by Top3 separating the single-stranded region of the two gapped circles. Similarly, in metazoan systems, the RecQ helicase Blm may forge ahead to create a ssDNA region, with the help of ssDNA binding proteins (such as RPA) to secure the region and possibly Top3α to eliminate supercoiling resistance. Top3α could then bind to the ssDNA region and perform strand passage, possibly with the help of Blm to re-anneal the DNA or eliminate secondary structures. How the enzymes can coordinate their activities and why they would act differently at the different sites is unclear, but may be related to which enzyme binds first (Blm to the HJ or Top3α to the ssDNA region).

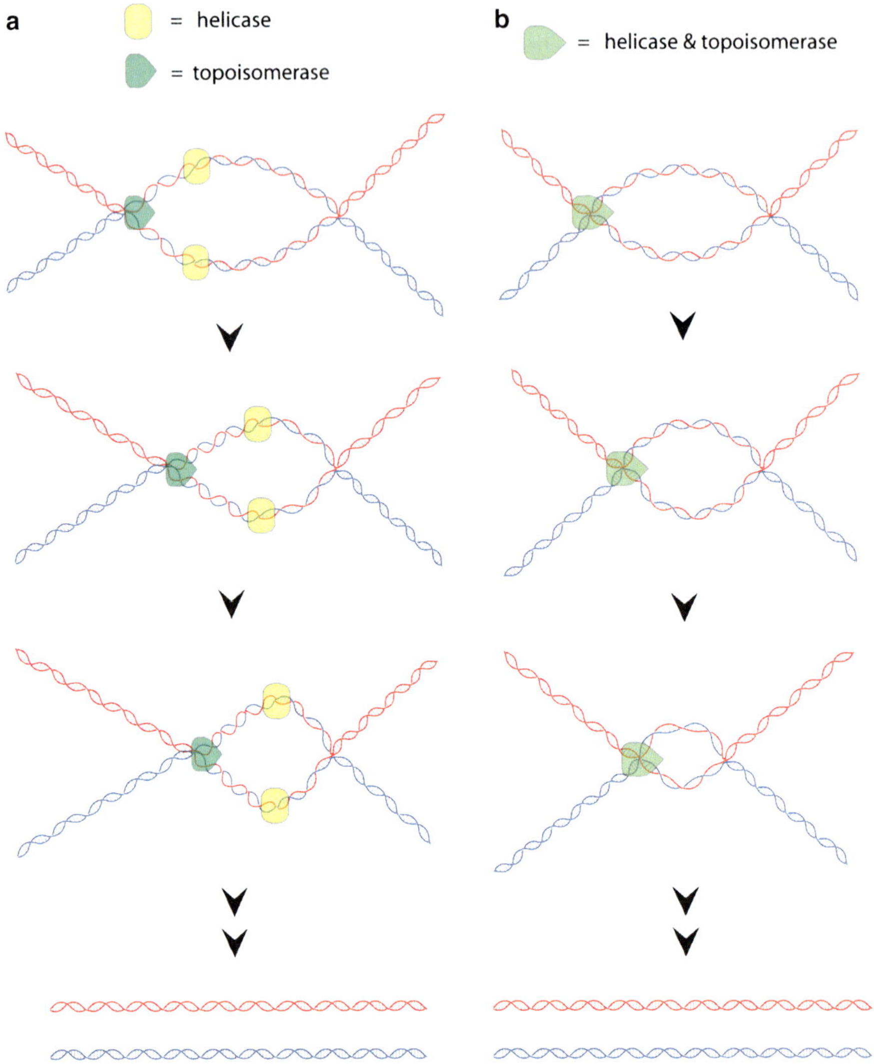

Fig. 5.4 (**a**) The Unravel & Unlink model. A region of DNA between the junctions is first separated to ssDNA before being segregated by the topoisomerase and re-annealed into non-crossover products. In this model, enzyme coordination is unclear, but the DNA bending could be less inhibitory. (**b**) The HJ Migration model. Top3α and Blm form a complex such that HJ migration and strand passage are concomitant. While protein coordination is clear, the stiffness of the intervening dsDNA may impede DNA bending as the junctions approach each other. In each case, only one junction is shown migrating for simplicity

The HJ migration model proposes that a single complex of Top3α and Blm can migrate each junction by the HJ migration action of Blm concomitant with strand passage by Top3α, which would both eliminate the build-up of supercoiling and separate the dsDNA strands. A limited region of ssDNA is still likely to allow Top3α to act, but the strands would be unwound and rewound as the complex progresses to largely maintain dsDNA. This model is consistent with a tight coupling of Top3α and Blm activities, but has the problem of requiring a sharp bend in the interlying dsDNA, well below persistence length, as the junctions approach each other.

Some combination of the two models may also be taking place. Perhaps, HJ migration occurs until the migration is stalled by the energetics of dsDNA bending, at which point the interlying DNA region must first be unraveled followed by unlinking. Whether there is any regulation in convergent versus divergent migration of the two HJs remains to be determined. More information about the structure and stoichiometry of the Blm-Top3α complex as well as the order of events will help to elucidate the exact mechanism in the future.

5.7 RMI Proteins

5.7.1 Rmi1 Is a Part of the Complex

In addition to Top3α and Blm, which were established as the necessary and sufficient components for double Holliday junction dissolution *in vitro*, recent screens have found a number of non-enzymatic additions to the complex. These small associating proteins have been termed Rmi, for Rec-Q mediated genome instability (Chang et al. 2005; Mullen et al. 2005).

Rmi1 is an OB (oligonucleotide or oligosaccharide binding)-fold protein shown to co-immunoprecipitate with the Blm complex. The human version, originally called BLAP75 (for Bloom-associated protein, 75 kDa), was shown to stabilize the Blm-Top3α interaction. In addition, it was required for phosphorylation of Blm, recruited Blm to foci after DNA damage, and its absence led to an increase in sister chromatid exchange, the hallmark of a Blm defect (Yin et al. 2005). The yeast Rmi1 mutant showed defects more closely associated with the function of Top3, with deletion of Rmi1 resembling deletion of Top3, which were both rescued, in part, by Sgs1 (Chang et al. 2005; Mullen et al. 2005).

It was soon discovered that when Rmi1 was added to the Blm-Top3α complex *in vitro*, double Holliday junction dissolution activity was increased several fold (Raynard et al. 2006; Wu et al. 2006b), indicating a functional aspect to the binding protein. In yeast, this effect appears to be due to Rmi1 stimulating the ssDNA binding activities of Top3 and Sgs1 (Chen and Brill 2007). In humans, a genetic variant of Rmi1 causes increased cancer susceptibility, resembling the phenotype of mutations in Blm (Broberg et al. 2007). Taken together, it appears that Rmi1 is important for the proper functioning of the Blm-Top3α complex in living organisms.

5.7.2 Rmi2 and Beyond

In 2008, two groups simultaneously identified another structural member of the complex, a small protein dubbed Rmi2 (Singh et al. 2008; Xu et al. 2008).

This polypeptide co-purified and co-immunoprecipitated with Blm, Top3α, and Rmi1. Rmi2 appears to form a complex with Rmi1, rendering it more soluble, through the interaction of Rmi1's second and Rmi2's only OB-fold domain. Unlike Rmi1, however, sequence homology indicates that Rmi2 exists only in vertebrates and plants, perhaps explaining the absence of the second OB-fold in yeast Rmi1. The OB-fold containing complex of Rmi1 and Rmi2 stabilizes the Blm-Top3α complex, but cannot bind ssDNA. The two Rmi proteins also appear to form a subcomplex with Top3α, as seen with Rmi1 alone.

The exact components involved in the *in vivo* reaction are still unclear. In reporting Rmi2, another small protein was also discovered in the pulldown, suggesting more structural proteins may be involved (Singh et al 2008). Because these proteins lack enzymatic activity, their function is likely stabilization and localization of the main components, as the studies above suggest. Whether Top3α is permanently or temporarily bound to Rmi proteins in the cell will be interesting to observe.

5.8 Top3α and Anaphase Bridges

Recently, a role for Blm and Top3α was observed in chromosome segregation during mitosis (Chan et al. 2007). Blm is localized to anaphase bridges between separating chromatin, including a class of ultrafine bridges not readily detectable by DNA staining. The presence of these structures was reduced as anaphase proceeded, but increased in the absence of Blm or Topo II. Top3α and Rmi1 were also shown to localize to the bridges in a Blm-dependent manner, indicating an important role for the complex in chromatin separation. Presumably, a DNA structure similar to a recombination intermediate is occurring during segregation, requiring a similar mechanism to untangle. Proper segregation is also an important component of maintaining chromosomal stability, which may also be maintained by Blm and Top3α.

5.9 Conclusions

Most of what is known about the functional role of Top3α in the cell is based on its intimate partnership with the RecQ helicase Blm. Together these proteins play an important role in properly maintaining the cell's genetic information. The actions of the complex appear to be specific to Top3α and Blm and are assisted by the structural Rmi proteins. In addition to recombination intermediates, the two may also function to ensure faithful chromosomal segregation.

However, the lethality of cells lacking Top3α compared to the relative viability of cells lacking Blm indicates that not all of the topoisomerase's roles can be defined through this partnership. Indeed, Blm has been shown to have a variety of functions outside of the complex, including histone phosphorylation and restart of stalled replication forks. One clue to an additional role for Top3α may lie in the N-terminal region of the protein sequence, which contains the mitochondrial localization domain. The distinct functions of Top3α in specific subcellular compartments will be an interesting area for future study.

References

Bennett RJ, and Wang JC (2001) Association of yeast DNA topoisomerase III and Sgs1 DNA helicase: Studies of fusion proteins. PNAS 98, 11108–11113

Boore JL (1999) Animal mitochondrial genomes. Nucl. Acids Res. 27, 1767–1780

Broberg K, Hoglund M, Gustafsson C, Bjork J, Ingvar C, Albin M, and Olsson H (2007) Genetic variant of the human homologous recombination-associated gene RMI1 (S455N) impacts the risk of AML/MDS and malignant melanoma. Cancer Letters 258, 38–44

Brown TA, Cecconi C, Tkachuk AN, Bustamante C, and Clayton DA (2005) Replication of mitochondrial DNA occurs by strand displacement with alternative light-strand origins, not via a strand-coupled mechanism. Genes Dev 19, 2466–2476

Champoux JJ (2001) DNA topoisomerases: structure, function, and mechanism. Annu Rev Biochem 70, 369–413

Chan KL, North PS, and Hickson ID (2007) BLM is required for faithful chromosome segregation and its localization defines a class of ultrafine anaphase bridges. Embo J 26, 3397–3409

Chang M, Bellaoui M, Zhang C, Desai R, Morozov P, Delgado-Cruzata L, Rothstein R, Freyer GA, Boone C, and Brown GW (2005) RMI1/NCE4, a suppressor of genome instability, encodes a member of the RecQ helicase/Topo III complex. Embo J 24, 2024–2033

Chen CF, and Brill SJ (2007) Binding and activation of DNA topoisomerase III by the Rmi1 subunit. J Biol Chem

Chu WK, and Hickson ID (2009) RecQ helicases: multifunctional genome caretakers. Nature Reviews Cancer 9, 644–654

DiGate RJ, and Marians KJ (1988) Identification of a potent decatenating enzyme from Escherichia coli. J Biol Chem 263, 13366–13373

Gangloff S, McDonald JP, Bendixen C, Arthur L, and Rothstein R (1994) The yeast type I topoisomerase Top3 interacts with Sgs1, a DNA helicase homolog: a potential eukaryotic reverse gyrase. Mol. Cell. Biol. 14, 8391–8398

Goodwin A, Wang SW, Toda T, Norbury C, and Hickson ID (1999) Topoisomerase III is essential for accurate nuclear division in Schizosaccharomyces pombe. Nucl. Acids Res. 27, 4050–4058

Goulaouic H, Roulon T, Flamand O, Grondard L, Lavelle F, and Riou JF (1999) Purification and characterization of human DNA topoisomerase IIIalpha. Nucl. Acids Res. 27, 2443–2450

Hanai R, Caron PR, and Wang JC (1996) Human TOP3: a single-copy gene encoding DNA topoisomerase III. PNAS 93, 3653–3657

Ira G, Malkova A, Liberi G, Foiani M, and Haber JE (2003) Srs2 and Sgs1-Top3 suppress crossovers during double-strand break repair in yeast. Cell 115, 401–411

Johnson FB, Lombard DB, Neff NF, Mastrangelo M-A, Dewolf W, Ellis NA, Marciniak RA, Yin Y, Jaenisch R, and Guarente L (2000) Association of the Bloom Syndrome Protein with Topoisomerase III{{alpha}} in Somatic and Meiotic Cells. Cancer Res 60, 1162–1167

Kim RA, and Wang JC (1992) Identification of yeast TOP3 gene product as a single strand-specific DNA topoisomerase. J Biol Chem 267, 17178–17185

Kwan KY, and Wang JC (2001) Mice lacking DNA topoisomerase IIIbeta develop to maturity but show a reduced mean lifespan. PNAS 98, 5717–5721

Kwan KY, Moens PB, and Wang JC (2003) Infertility and aneuploidy in mice lacking a type IA DNA topoisomerase IIIbeta. PNAS 100, 2526–2531

Kwan KY, Greenwald RJ, Mohanty S, Sharpe AH, Shaw AC, and Wang JC (2007) Development of autoimmunity in mice lacking DNA topoisomerase 3-beta. PNAS 104, 9242–9247

Lee MP, Brown SD, Chen A, and Hsieh TS (1993) DNA topoisomerase I is essential in Drosophila melanogaster. PNAS 90, 6656–6660

Li W, and Wang JC (1998) Mammalian DNA topoisomerase IIIalpha is essential in early embryogenesis. Proc Natl Acad Sci USA 95, 1010–1013

Li W, Kim S-M, Lee J, and Dunphy WG (2004) Absence of BLM leads to accumulation of chromosomal DNA breaks during both unperturbed and disrupted S phases. J. Cell Biol. 165, 801–812

Mullen JR, Nallaseth FS, Lan YQ, Slagle CE, and Brill SJ (2005) Yeast Rmi1/Nce4 Controls Genome Stability as a Subunit of the Sgs1-Top3 Complex. Mol. Cell. Biol. 25, 4476–4487

Nurse P, Levine C, Hassing H, and Marians KJ (2003) Topoisomerase III can serve as the cellular decatenase in Escherichia coli. J Biol Chem 278, 8653–8660

Plank JL, Chu SH, Pohlhaus JR, Wilson-Sali T, and Hsieh TS (2005) Drosophila melanogaster topoisomerase IIIalpha preferentially relaxes a positively or negatively supercoiled bubble substrate and is essential during development. J Biol Chem 280, 3564–3573

Plank JL, Wu J, and Hsieh T-s (2006) Topoisomerase III{alpha} and Bloom's helicase can resolve a mobile double Holliday junction substrate through convergent branch migration. PNAS 103, 11118–11123

Plank JL, and Hsieh TS (2009) Helicase-appended Topoisomerases: New Insight into the Mechanism of Directional Strand-transfer. J Biol Chem 284, 30737–30741

Raynard S, Bussen W, and Sung P (2006) A double Holliday junction dissolvasome comprising BLM, topoisomerase IIIalpha, and BLAP75. J Biol Chem 281, 13861–13864

Seki M, Nakagawa T, Seki T, Kato G, Tada S, Takahashi Y, Yoshimura A, Kobayashi T, Aoki A, Otsuki M, Habermann FA, Tanabe H, Ishii Y, and Enomoto T (2006) Bloom helicase and DNA topoisomerase IIIalpha are involved in the dissolution of sister chromatids. Mol Cell Biol 26, 6299–6307

Seki T, Seki M, Onodera R, Katada T, and Enomoto T (1998) Cloning of cDNA Encoding a Novel Mouse DNA Topoisomerase III (Topo IIIbeta) Possessing Negatively Supercoiled DNA Relaxing Activity, Whose Message Is Highly Expressed in the Testis. J. Biol. Chem. 273, 28553–28556

Shimamoto A, Nishikawa K, Kitao S, and Furuichi Y (2000) Human RecQ5beta, a large isomer of RecQ5 DNA helicase, localizes in the nucleoplasm and interacts with topoisomerases 3alpha and 3beta. Nucleic Acids Res 28, 1647–1655

Singh TR, Ali AM, Busygina V, Raynard S, Fan Q, Du C, Andreassen PR, Sung P, and Meetei AR (2008) BLAP18/RMI2, a novel OB-fold containing protein, is an essential component of the Bloom helicase-double Holliday junction dissolvasome. Genes & Development, 2856–2868

Suski C, and Marians KJ (2008) Resolution of converging replication forks by RecQ and topoisomerase III. Mol Cell 30, 779–789

Szostak JW, Orr-Weaver TL, Rothstein RJ, and Stahl FW (1983) The double-strand-break repair model for recombination. Cell 33, 25–35

Ui A, Seki M, Ogiwara H, Onodera R, Fukushige S, Onoda F, and Enomoto T (2005) The ability of Sgs1 to interact with DNA topoisomerase III is essential for damage-induced recombination. DNA Repair (Amst) 4, 191–201

Wallis JW, Chrebet G, Brodsky G, Rolfe M, and Rothstein R (1989) A hyper-recombination mutation in S. cerevisiae identifies a novel eukaryotic topoisomerase. Cell 58, 409–419

Wang JC (2002) Cellular roles of DNA topoisomerases: a molecular perspective. Nat Rev Mol Cell Biol 3, 430–440

Wang Y, Lyu YL, and Wang JC (2002) Dual localization of human DNA topoisomerase IIIalpha to mitochondria and nucleus. Proc Natl Acad Sci USA 99, 12114–12119

Wilson-Sali T, and Hsieh T-s (2002a) Preferential cleavage of plasmid-based R-loops and D-loops by Drosophila topoisomerase III{beta}. PNAS 99, 7974–7979

Wilson-Sali T, and Hsieh TS (2002b) Generation of double-stranded breaks in hypernegatively supercoiled DNA by Drosophila topoisomerase IIIbeta, a type IA enzyme. J Biol Chem 277, 26865–26871

Wilson TM, Chen AD, and Hsieh T (2000) Cloning and characterization of Drosophila topoisomerase IIIbeta. Relaxation of hypernegatively supercoiled DNA. J Biol Chem 275, 1533–1540

Wu J, Hou JH, and Hsieh TS (2006a) A new Drosophila gene wh (wuho) with WD40 repeats is essential for spermatogenesis and has maximal expression in hub cells. Dev Biol 296, 219–230

Wu J, Feng L, and Hsieh TS (2010) Drosophila topo III{alpha} is required for the maintenance of mitochondrial genome and male germ-line stem cells. PNAS Epub ahead of print

Wu L, Davies SL, North PS, Goulaouic H, Riou JF, Turley H, Gatter KC, and Hickson ID (2000) The Bloom's syndrome gene product interacts with topoisomerase III. J Biol Chem 275, 9636–9644

Wu L, and Hickson ID (2002) The Bloom's syndrome helicase stimulates the activity of human topoisomerase III{alpha}. Nucl. Acids Res. 30, 4823–4829

Wu L, and Hickson ID (2003) The Bloom's syndrome helicase suppresses crossing over during homologous recombination. Nature 426, 870–874

Wu L, Bachrati CZ, Ou J, Xu C, Yin J, Chang M, Wang W, Li L, Brown GW, and Hickson ID (2006b) BLAP75/RMI1 promotes the BLM-dependent dissolution of homologous recombination intermediates. Proc Natl Acad Sci USA 103, 4068–4073

Wyckoff E, and Hsieh TS (1988) Functional expression of a Drosophila gene in yeast: genetic complementation of DNA topoisomerase II. PNAS 85, 6272–6276

Xu D, Guo R, Sobeck A, Bachrati CZ, Yang J, Enomoto T, Brown GW, Hoatlin ME, Hickson ID, and Wang W (2008) RMI, a new OB-fold complex essential for Bloom syndrome protein to maintain genome stability. Genes & Development 22, 2843–2855

Yin J, Sobeck A, Xu C, Meetei AR, Hoatlin M, Li L, and Wang W (2005) BLAP75, an essential component of Bloom's syndrome protein complexes that maintain genome integrity. Embo J 24, 1465–1476

Zhang H, Barcelo JM, Lee B, Kohlhagen G, Zimonjic DB, Popescu NC, and Pommier Y (2001) Human mitochondrial topoisomerase I. Proc Natl Acad Sci USA 98, 10608–10613

Zhang H, Meng LH, and Pommier Y (2007) Mitochondrial topoisomerases and alternative splicing of the human TOP1mt gene. Biochimie 89, 474–481

Chapter 6
DNA Topoisomerase I and Illegitimate Recombination

Céline Auzanneau and Philippe Pourquier

6.1 Introduction

DNA topoisomerases are ubiquitous enzymes that are essential for cell proliferation in higher eukaryotes (Leppard and Champoux 2005; Pommier 2006; Wang 2002). They remove DNA supercoils that are generated during elongation of newly replicated and/or transcribed strands. They also suppress torsional constraints associated with chromosome condensation and decondensation during cell division (Leppard and Champoux 2005; Pommier 2006; Wang 2002). These functions rely on their capability to introduce transient breaks in the DNA where the catalytic tyrosine of the topoisomerase remains covalently attached to the cleaved strand by a tyrosyl-phosphodiester bond (Champoux 1981). The DNA-Topoisomerase complexes are generally referred to as "cleavable" or "cleavage" complexes. There are seven topoisomerases encoded by the human genome [reviewed in (Leppard and Champoux 2005; Wang 2002)]. They are classified in two groups, type I and type II enzymes (Fig. 6.1a). Type II enzymes include the α and β isoforms of Top2 and spo11, a topoisomerase specifically expressed in germ cells. They usually act as heterodimers and cleave both strands of the DNA, allowing the passage of a duplex DNA through the double-strand break, leading to the decatenation of daughter chromatids during mitosis.

Type I enzymes act as monomers and cleave one strand of the duplex DNA [reviewed in (Leppard and Champoux 2005; Li and Liu 2001; Pommier 2006; Wang 2002) and Chaps. 1–5. They are divided in two subgroups, depending on the polarity of DNA cleavage (Fig. 6.1a). The type IA enzymes remain covalently bound to the 5′-end of the broken strand. They include top3α and top3β isoforms which are

P. Pourquier (✉)
INSERM U916 VINCO, Institut Bergonié & University of Bordeaux,
229 cours de l'Argonne, 33076, Bordeaux cedex, France
e-mail: pourquier@bergonie.org

Y. Pommier (ed.), *DNA Topoisomerases and Cancer*, Cancer Drug Discovery and Development, DOI 10.1007/978-1-4614-0323-4_6,

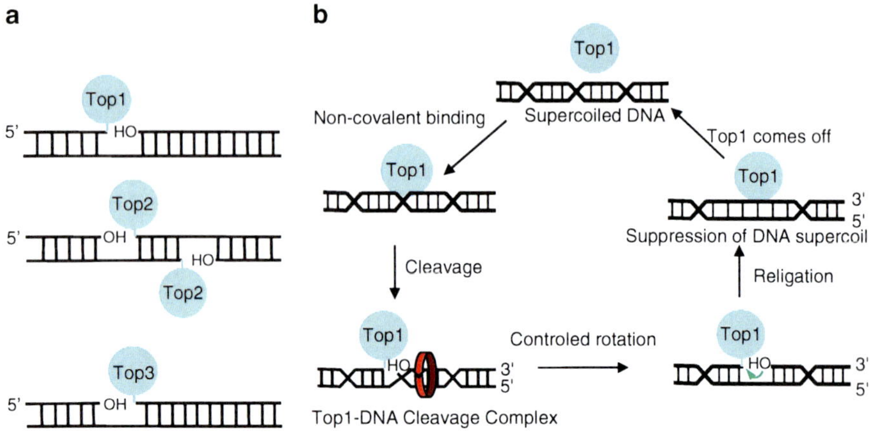

Fig. 6.1 (**a**) The three types of human DNA topoisomerases. Topoisomerase I and III act as monomers, cleave one strand of duplex DNA and remain covalently attached to the 3′ end, or the 5′-end of the cleaved strand, respectively. Topoisomerase II act as dimers and cleave both strands of the DNA duplex. They remain covalently attached to the 5′-end of the cleaved strands. (**b**) Catalytic cycle of human Top1. See text for details

predominantly involved in the resolution of crossovers during homologous recombination, in association with the BLM helicase, RMI1, and RMI2 proteins which form the "resolvasome" complex (Chu and Hickson 2009) (see Chap. 8). Type IB enzymes on the other hand, remain covalently attached to the 3′-end of the broken strand (Fig. 6.1a). They include mitochondrial (Top1mt) and nuclear topoisomerases I, which will be referred to as Top1 for simplicity. Top1 knockout is lethal in higher eukaryotes such as flies or mice (Lee et al. 1993; Morham et al. 1996) but is dispensable in yeast where Top1 activity is compensated by other topoisomerases (Thrash et al. 1984; Uemura and Yanagida 1984). Besides its essential role in DNA relaxation, a growing number of studies suggest that Top1 could also regulate other DNA processes such as apoptosis (see Chap. 19), transcription regulation, RNA splicing, DNA repair, or DNA recombination, indicating that it may also contribute to the maintenance of genomic integrity. In this chapter, we will review the experimental evidence suggesting the potential role of Top1 in illegitimate recombination either directly *via* its strand transferase activity, or indirectly *via* the regulation of other cellular mechanisms.

6.2 The Top1 Catalytic Cycle

As mentioned earlier, the main role of Top1 is to ensure the removal of positive and negative supercoils that form during replication or transcription forks' progression. The mechanism by which Top1 removes DNA supercoils is modeled in Fig. 6.1b with four consecutive steps. Step 1 corresponds to the non-covalent binding of the enzyme to the double-stranded DNA molecule (Fig. 6.1b). Conversely to classical restriction enzymes, eukaryotic Top1 does not recognize specific sequences but has a loose preference for binding at following base motifs: 5′-(A/T) (G/C) (A/T) T-3′ where the last T corresponds to the base that is involved in the covalent bond with the enzyme and is referred to as position "−1" relative to the enzyme cleavage site (Jaxel et al. 1991) (Fig. 6.1b). It is interesting to note that this sequence is somehow relatively conserved across eukaryotes (Andersen et al. 1985; Been et al. 1984; Porter and Champoux 1989; Tanizawa et al. 1993). Moreover, Top1 has a preference for bent or supercoiled DNA substrate (Camilloni et al. 1988; Caserta et al. 1989; Krogh et al. 1991) even though it could also accommodate linear DNA substrates in vitro (see below). A series of in vitro biochemical studies demonstrated that binding of Top1 required a bipartite mode of interaction which defined two specific regions of interaction with the duplex DNA: Region A (from position "−7" up to the cleavage site) and region B further downstream from the Top1 site (position "+6" to "+11") (Christiansen et al. 1993; Svejstrup et al. 1990). This was in accordance with crystal structures data of Top1-DNA complexes showing that Top1 binds to the duplex DNA with a clamp conformation that fully encompasses the DNA duplex (Leppard and Champoux 2005; Redinbo et al. 1998; Staker et al. 2002; Stewart et al. 1998). In step 2, Top1 cleaves one strand of the duplex DNA *via* a transesterification reaction, which results in the formation of a covalent link between the catalytic tyrosine of the enzyme (Tyr 723 in human, Tyr 727 in yeast S. cerevisiae, Tyr 274 in vaccinia) and the 3′-end of the DNA backbone (Champoux 1981; Lynn et al. 1989; Shuman et al. 1989) (Fig. 6.1b). This step leads to the formation of cleavage complexes that can be isolated upon rapid denaturation of Top1 by a detergent, proteinase K digestion, or simple heating. Suppression of DNA supercoils is performed in step 3 by a "controlled rotation" of the cleaved strand around the intact strand within the active site of the enzyme-DNA complex (Koster et al. 2005; Stewart et al. 1998). In the last step, religation (resealing) of the broken strand restores the continuity of the DNA backbone and allows Top1 to detach from its substrate. This reverse transesterification reaction relies on the nucleophilic attack of the Top1-DNA 3′-tyrosyl phosphodiester bond by the free 5′-hydroxyl residue of the cleaved strand (Fig. 6.1b). In normal conditions, Top1 cleavage and religation reactions are in equilibrium and the religation step is favored, which translates into the fact that very few Top1-DNA cleavage complexes can be detected at any given time (Stivers et al. 1994).

Optimal religation requires a perfect alignment of the 5′-hydroxyl terminus of the broken strand with the scissile tyrosyl-phosphodiester bond. As described in more details below, misalignment of the 5′-hydroxyl terminus by drugs or the presence of DNA modifications results in the accumulation of Top1-DNA complexes that increase the probability that improper DNA species bearing a free 5′-hydroxyl terminus could be religated in place of the normal strand, leading to the formation of illegitimate products. Such recombination events are easily detectable in vitro or indirectly in cells and are favored when Top1-DNA cleavage complexes half-life is prolonged.

6.3 DNA Recombination Linked to Top1 Cleavage and Religation Activities

6.3.1 *The Different Models for Top1-Mediated DNA Recombination*

The first study suggesting a potential role of Top1 in recombination was published more than 30 years ago by J. J. Champoux and his coworkers, when the enzyme was still referred to as DNA untwisting enzyme (Champoux 1977). It was hypothesized that recombination was essentially linked to the relaxation activity of Top1. In the accompanying model, this process was initiated by the unwinding of two homologous regions of duplex DNAs, followed by strand invasion and rewinding of the complementary strands to form a DNA structure equivalent to a Holliday recombination intermediate (Fig. 6.2). This was in accordance with the fact that single-strand breaks induced by Top1 would facilitate the opening of homologous regions. However, it also implied that unpairing would occur systematically in the same regions of both double-stranded DNAs which may be unlikely, despite the existence of recombination hotspots (McMilin et al. 1974). Also, this model could not explain

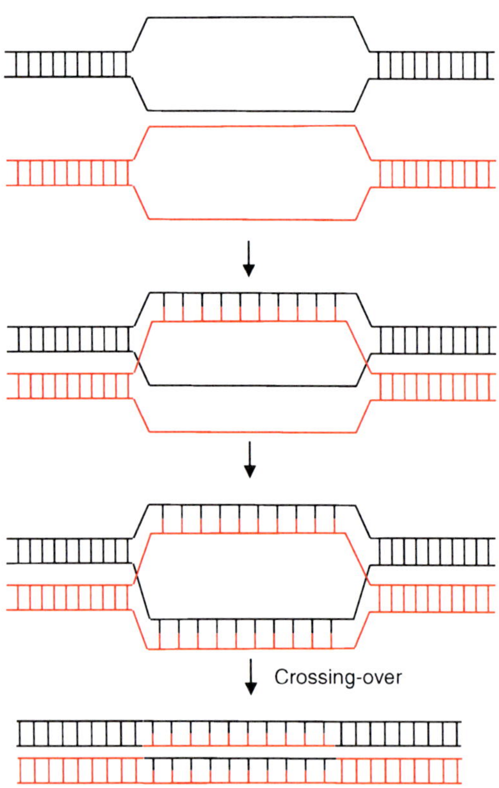

Fig. 6.2 The initial model describing the hypothetical implication of Top1 in DNA recombination (adapted from Champoux (1977)). Top1 unwinds the two homologous regions of duplex DNA, which facilitates strand invasion and base pairing. This is followed by rewinding of complementary strands to form a variant of the Holliday recombination intermediate which is further resolved by the cellular machinery leading to recombination

Top1-mediated recombination between non-homologous DNA substrates. It was further reconsidered shortly after L. F. Liu et al. reported the key finding that Top1, purified to homogeneity from HeLa cells' nuclei, could form covalent complexes with DNA substrates in which the enzyme remained attached to the 3′-end of the cleaved strand (Halligan et al. 1982). These complexes were referred to as "donor" molecules (donors). When donors were incubated with double-stranded DNA species bearing a 5′-hydroxyl (referred to as acceptors), one could detect the formation of recombinant products resulting from the joining of donors with acceptors (Halligan et al. 1982). Conversely to the initial model, this process did not necessarily require a sequence homology between donors and acceptors. Even though the exact nature of the donors was not precisely defined in that study, it was interesting to note that recombination was independent of the 5′-termini of the acceptors since ligation was observed with either blunt, 5′-protrusive or 5′-recessed ends (Halligan et al. 1982). Nevertheless, those results provided the first evidence that eukaryotic Top1 can act as a strand-transferase and generate illegitimate recombination products in vitro via its DNA religation activity. Shortly after, the first indirect evidence that Top1 could mediate illegitimate recombination was reported in a cellular context (Bullock et al. 1985). The authors showed that sequences immediately flanking SV40 excisional recombination crossovers were similar to the in vitro cleavage sites of SV40 DNA by purified rat liver Top1. This finding led to a new model (Fig. 6.3) in which DNA cleavage by Top1 on preferred sites would generate a double-strand break in which Top1 remains covalently linked to the 3′-protrusive ends. These intermediates (donors) could then ligate DNA strands bearing a free 5′-hydroxyl terminus, this step being favored by the base pairing of small regions of homology at the junction sites. This model was in accordance with the fact that preferred Top1 sequences were only found on one side of the junctions and that recombination only relied on Top1 catalytic activity of DNA cleavage. However, it also implied that Top1 cleavage occurred in the vicinity of a DNA break (or gap) in the opposite (non-scissile) strand to form the donor molecule (Bullock et al. 1985) (Fig. 6.3). Additional studies using other cellular models further strengthened this hypothesis. In murine cells infected with the parvovirus minute virus of mice (MVM), integration sites of foreign DNA were enriched for preferred eukaryotic Top1 cleavage sites and recombination was enhanced by the presence of a DNA sequence motif corresponding to Top1 consensus cleavage sites in viral DNA (Hogan and Faust 1986).

Similar observations were made in two clones of human hepatocarcinoma cells infected by the duck hepatitis DNA virus (DHBV) (Hino et al. 1989). DHBV has an open circular genome in which a three-strand flap region is formed by the S positive strand and the overlap of the L minus strand termini. This overlap is located opposite to a region encompassing nucleotides 2,519 and 2,535 of the S positive strand and is a highly preferred integration region (Hino et al. 1989). Interestingly, this region also included a potential Top1 consensus sequence (where Top1 would cleave at nucleotide 2,528) that was found in the proximity of virus-cellular DNA junctions (Hino et al. 1989; Wang and Rogler 1991). It was therefore proposed that cleavage at nucleotide 2,528 by cellular Top1 would linearize the open circular form of DHBV and contribute to viral integration by religation of cellular 5′-hydroxy DNA

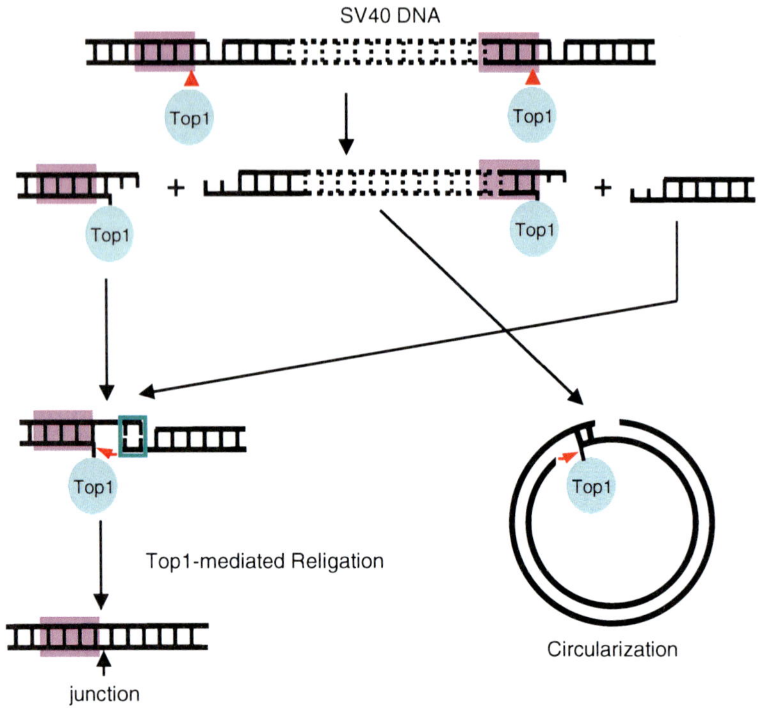

Fig. 6.3 Hypothetical mechanism of human Top1-mediated excisional recombination: the deletion model (adapted from Bullock et al. (1985)). Cellular Top1 would perform cleavage in preferred sequences (*pink boxes*) in the vicinity of crossover regions opposite to a nick or a gap. This would lead to a chromosome break and the release of a linear viral SV40 DNA molecule. Then, Top1 covalently linked to the 3′-end of DNA extremities would catalyze the circularization of the viral SV40 DNA and the ligation of chromosomal ends leading to a deletion. End-joining would be facilitated by the presence of base pairing at the junction sites (*blue box*)

ends (Wang and Rogler 1991). It was subsequently verified that purified human Top1 could indeed cleave oligonucleotides mimicking the three-strand flap region of DHBV at position 2,528 and mimic both linearization of the DHBV and the linkage of virus DNA to a 5′-hydroxyl end of a heterologous DNA in vitro (Pourquier et al. 1999).

The strand transferase activity of type IB topoisomerase was also revealed in other organisms. In yeast *S. cerevisiae*, transformation of DNA fragments with no homology to the yeast genome led to a ≈10-fold-increase of illegitimate recombination when Top1 was overexpressed (Zhu and Schiestl 1996). Even though overexpression of Top1 could indirectly affect the expression of genes involved in DNA recombination, the fact that sequences of the flanking regions of integration sites were highly homologous to the consensus sequence of DNA cleavage by various eukaryotic Top1, argued against an indirect effect of Top1. Moreover, the frequency of integration was dramatically reduced in Top1-deficient yeasts, confirming that this recombinogenic activity was related to Top1 catalytic activity and further strengthened the active role of Top1 in illegitimate recombination in vivo (Zhu and Schiestl 1996).

The role of vaccinia virus Top1 in DNA recombination was extensively studied by S. Shuman's group and provided key evidences on the implication of Top1 in DNA recombination (Shuman 1998). Vaccinia Top1 is a small type IB topoisomerase (Pommier et al. 2010). In contrast to the eukaryotic enzyme, vaccinia Top1 cleaves duplex DNA at a specific recognition sequence 5′-C/TCCTT↓-3′ (where the arrow indicates the cleavage site) (Shuman and Prescott 1990) and is resistant to camptothecins (Shuman et al. 1988). It was shown that expression of vaccinia Top1 in *Escherichia coli* enhances by >200-fold the titer of infection of bacteriophage λ, by promoting integrase-independent prophage excision (Shuman 1989). Sequencing of five excision sites revealed in all cases the presence of a Top1 cleavage consensus sequence on one strand of both recombining partners (Shuman 1991). In three cases, direct repeats were present at the target sites which extended beyond the Top1 cleavage site, and no deletion could be detected at 3′ to the Top1 cleavage sites. These data led to a different model than the one proposed by Champoux (Fig. 6.4a) in which, physical interaction of the Top1 molecules bound to each site would be required to promote a strand transfer leading to the formation of a Holliday junction. This hypothesis was strengthened by electron microscopy observations of filamentous structures resulting from the incubation of duplex DNA with purified vaccinia Top1. Analyses of these intramolecular filaments suggested that protein-protein interaction between two DNA-bound Top1 molecules, rather than interactions between two DNA duplexes, were responsible for the geometric organization of these stem-loop structures (Shuman et al. 1997). In this model, it was also hypothesized that resolution of Holliday junctions would be achieved by cellular nucleases independently of Top1 (Fig. 6.4a) (Shuman 1991). However, it was further demonstrated that vaccinia Top1 itself could perform this task, since it could process synthetic Holliday junctions in vitro by a mechanism involving concerted transesterification reactions at two Top1 cleavage sites opposite to the crossover (Fig. 6.4b) (Sekiguchi et al. 1996, 2000). Systematic site-directed mutagenesis studies of vaccinia Top1 allowed the identification of six amino-acids, including the active tyrosine, which are essential for this transesterification reaction (Shuman 1998). Interestingly, the crystal structure of a vaccinia Top1 fragment compared to those of site-specific recombinases such as HP1 integrase or Cre-recombinase, revealed that despite their weak primary sequence homology, the spatial positioning of these residues was highly conserved (Cheng et al. 1998). Because these amino-acids are conserved in all members of the type IB topoisomerase family, it was surmised that type IB topoisomerases and nucleases from the recombinases family derived from a common ancestral enzyme (Cheng et al. 1998). In addition, recombinases such as λ integrase, Tn3 family of transposons, Cre-recombinase, XerC and XerD proteins, as well as the Flp-recombinase also possess a topoisomerase activity in vitro (Abremski et al. 1986; Cornet et al. 1997; Kikuchi and Nash 1979; Landy 1989; Xu et al. 1998).

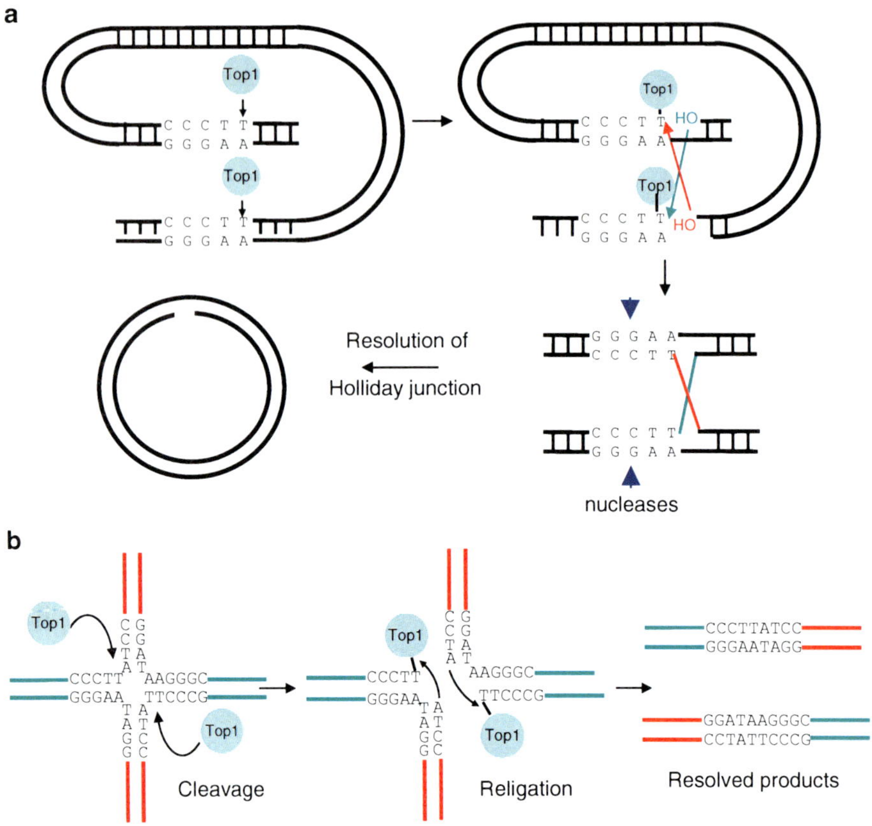

Fig. 6.4 (**a**) Mechanistic model for vaccinia Top1-mediated DNA recombination (adapted from Shuman (1991)). Two vaccinia Top1 molecules cleave duplex DNA at two CCCTT sites and liberate two 5′-hydroxyl ends (*red* and *blue*). Because of the sequence homology between the two regions upstream from the cleavage sites, crossover could occur prior to religation by Top1, leading to the formation of Holliday junctions that would be resolved by cellular nucleases. (**b**) Hypothetical model for the resolution of Holliday junctions by vacinia Top1 (adapted from Sekiguchi et al. (1996)). Synthetic Holliday junctions are formed by the crossing over of two DNA entities (*red* and *blue*). When concerted cleavage of two Top1 molecules occurs at two CCCTT cleavage sites opposite to the crossover, it results in the separation of two chimeric entities that are resealed by Top1 to restore the continuity of recombinant products

6.3.2 Top1-DNA Complexes as Key Determinants for Top1-Mediated Illegitimate Recombination

Even though the two models proposed by Champoux and Shuman are mechanistically different, probably because of the inherent specificities of each Top1 enzyme, they both rely on the initial formation of Top1-DNA cleavage complexes to serve as donor molecules that would in turn catalyze the religation of non homologous acceptors. As such, they represent key intermediates in Top1-mediated illegitimate

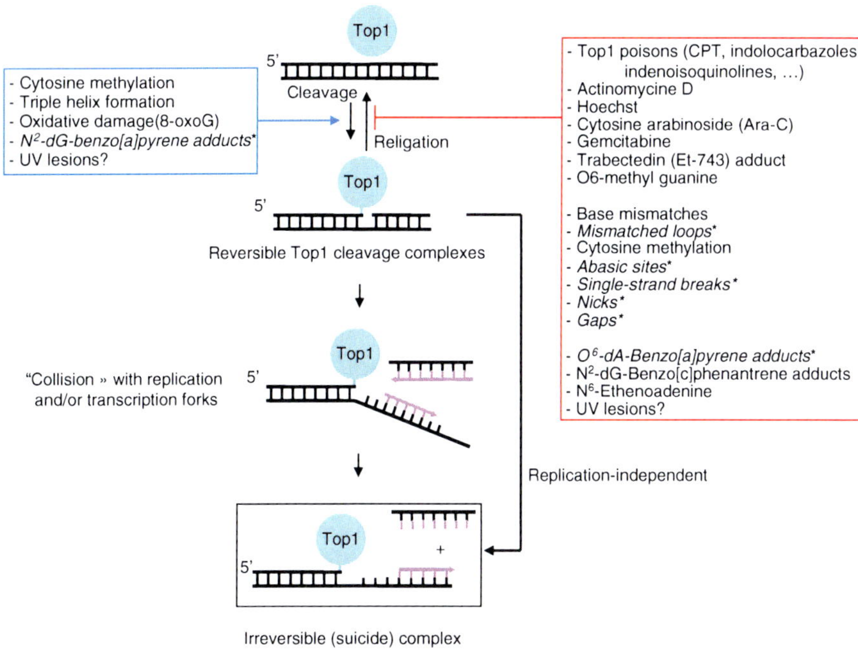

Fig. 6.5 The different modes of Top1 poisoning. Drugs and DNA modifications that impair the DNA cleavage and/or the religation steps of the Top1 reaction are shown inside the *blue* and *red boxes*, respectively. Modifications shown in *italic* induce irreversible Top1 complexes when they are adjacent to a Top1 cleavage site. Top1 trapping can lead to double-strand breaks via the collision of advancing replication forks with stabilized cleavage complexes. Irreversible Top1 cleavage complexes can also lead to DSBs independently of replication

recombination and it is likely that prolonged half-life of these complexes would greatly enhance this process. Stabilization of Top1-cleavage complexes has been observed in various experimental conditions including the presence of Top1 inhibitors such as camptothecins (CPT) or the presence of DNA modifications in the vicinity of the enzyme cleavage site (Fig. 6.5).

6.3.2.1 CPT-Induced Replication Mediated Breaks and Recombination

CPT derivatives are Top1 poisons that are widely used in the treatment of solid tumors (Pommier 2009) (see Chap. 12). They selectively interact and reversibly "stabilize" the Top1-DNA complexes by inhibiting the religation step of the Top1 reaction (Bjornsti et al. 1989; Hsiang et al. 1985; Hsiang and Liu 1988; Jaxel et al. 1988; Tanizawa et al. 1993) (see Chap. 9). Such stabilization is sufficient to induce replication-mediated DNA double-strand breaks (DSBs) either by direct collision of advancing replication forks with stabilized complexes (D'Arpa et al. 1990; Holm et al. 1989; Hsiang et al. 1989; Kaufmann et al. 1991; Strumberg et al. 2000) or by the accumulation of positive supercoils ahead of the replication machinery that promote replication fork stalling and breakage (Koster et al. 2007). Transcription has also been involved in the conversion of Top1-DNA complexes into cytotoxic lesions following CPT treatment (Desai et al. 2003; Sordet et al. 2008, 2009, 2010; Wu and Liu 1997), which can explain the replication-independent cytotoxicity of Top1 poisons (Barrows et al. 1998; Morris and Geller 1996; O'Connor et al. 1991; Stefanis et al. 1999). In both cases, Top1 poisoning by CPT leads to unique asymmetrical DNA lesions which include one free-end DSB resulting from replication run-off (Strumberg et al. 2000), and a Top1-DNA intermediate in which the enzyme remains irreversibly attached to the 3′-end of the scissile strand (Fig. 6.5).

Top1-mediated double-strand breaks are thought to be responsible for CPT cytotoxicity. Even though the precise mechanism is still unknown (Pommier et al. 2003), it is suggested that these lesions which are mainly S-phase dependent, are primarily repaired by homologous recombination (HR) (Arnaudeau et al. 2001; Saleh-Gohari et al. 2005), an error-free mechanism that uses the undamaged homologous chromosome as a template. The use of HR normally prevents chromosome rearrangements, but it was reported that inappropriate template usage, which is often due to HR genes dysfunction, could potentially lead to DNA rearrangements such as deletions, translocations, or loss of heterozygocity (LOH), which are known to be mutagenic (Lengauer et al. 1998; Natarajan and Palitti 2008; Reliene et al. 2007). Alternatively, DSBs could be processed by the non-homologous end-joining (NHEJ) pathway. It is therefore possible that DBSs that are formed by fork collapse following CPT treatment or in the presence of preexisting DNA lesions, could participate to the onset of carcinogenesis if left unrepaired. Several studies show indirect evidence consistent with this hypothesis. Cells treated with CPT exhibit increased levels of gene deletions and DNA rearrangements such as sister chromatid exchanges (Chatterjee et al. 1989; Degrassi et al. 1989; Hashimoto et al. 1995; Ribas et al. 1996; Ryan et al. 1994). CHO cells treated with high dose of CPT have a 50-fold higher rate of mutations in the *hprt* locus as compared to control cells (Balestrieri et al. 2001). These mutations consist of large deletions or complex rearrangements rather than single base mutations. Identical results were obtained in Drosophila using in vivo assays such as the recombination test, the wing spot assay, or the somatic w/w$^+$ eye assay. The latter assay has the advantage to separately evaluate the effect of LOH by homologous mitotic recombination (interchromosomal), unequal sister strand recombination (intrachromosomal), and structural chromosomal aberrations on a quantitative basis (Vogel and Nivard 1999). It was clear from these studies that CPT can induce primarily homologous mitotic recombinations (Cunha et al. 2002; Sortibran et al. 2006; Torres et al. 1998).

6.3.2.2 Irreversible Top1 Cleavage Complexes Are Recombinogenic

Irreversible Top1-DNA cleavage complexes that are commonly referred to as "suicide" complexes are prone to generate recombinant products in vitro and potentially in vivo. As mentioned earlier, these suicide complexes can be formed in the presence of CPT following replication or eventually transcription (Fig. 6.5). They could form when the DNA structure is altered in the vicinity of a Top1 cleavage site. A variety of DNA modifications from endogenous or environmental sources can shift the Top1 cleavage/religation equilibrium and result in Top1 trapping (Fig. 6.5) [see also (Pommier et al. 2003, 2006; Pourquier and Pommier 2001) for detailed reviews]. It is generally accepted that their presence alters hydrogen bonding and/or local helical twist. The effects of such modifications on Top1 activity have been studied in vitro using synthetic oligonucleotides. Globally, and regardless to their chemical structures, these lesions either prevent Top1 binding to the DNA when they are located immediately upstream to the Top1 cleavage site on the scissile strand, or increase Top1 cleavage complexes formation when they are located elsewhere (Pourquier and Pommier 2001). Most of them inhibit the religation step of the Top1 reaction such as in the case of CPT (Fig. 6.5, box outlined in red). They can be classified in three groups. One group includes the DNA lesions produced by anticancer agents such as nucleoside analogs (ara-C or gemcitabine) or alkylating agents such as MNNG, MNU, BCNU, or temozolomide (leading to O6-methylguanine) or ecteinascidin 743 (leading to N2-adducts). The second group includes common endogenous lesions such as base mismatches or short mispaired loops (due to replicative errors), and abasic sites which arise spontaneously by hydrolysis of the glycosidic bond primarily to purine bases. Abasic sites can also be produced during the course of excision repair of base damage from cell metabolism, or during excision of exogenous damage (Friedberg et al. 1995; Lindahl and Wood 1999). It is estimated that approximately 10,000 abasic sites are formed per human genome per day (Lindahl 1993). This group also includes single-strand breaks, nicks or base gaps which result from the processing of abasic sites, base damage, or uracil misincorporation by the base excision repair system (Friedberg et al. 1995; Lindahl and Wood 1999). The third group includes all "bulky" DNA adducts which are produced by carcinogens from environmental sources such as polyaromatic hydrocarbons leading to benzo[a] pyrene adducts or vinyl adducts (ethenoadenine). There are only few instances where the increase in Top1 cleavage complexes is due to an enhancement of the enzyme binding to its substrate and/or to an increase in the DNA cleavage rate (Fig. 6.2, box outlined in blue). The most representative lesion in this category is 8-oxoguanine, which is produced at an estimated rate of 100–500 lesions per cell per day (Lindahl 1993; Sokhansanj and Wilson 2004). 8-Oxoguanines result from the attack of guanines by oxygen radicals that are generated by various forms of oxidative stresses such as lipid peroxidation, inflammation, cellular respiration, and near-ultraviolet light (Friedberg et al. 1995; Lindahl 1993; Sokhansanj and Wilson 2004).

UV-induced DNA lesions such as cyclopyrimidine dimers and 6,4-photoproducts can also trap Top1-DNA complexes in vitro (Lanza et al. 1996) and in cells (Mielke et al. 2007; Subramanian et al. 1998). However, it is still unclear whether UV-mediated Top1 poisoning is due to an increase in DNA cleavage or to an inhibition of religation.

Despite their chemical diversity, most DNA modifications trap Top1 in a reversible manner, and the enhancement of enzyme-DNA covalent complexes is only transient. This is sufficient to generate replication-mediated cytotoxic DNA double-strand

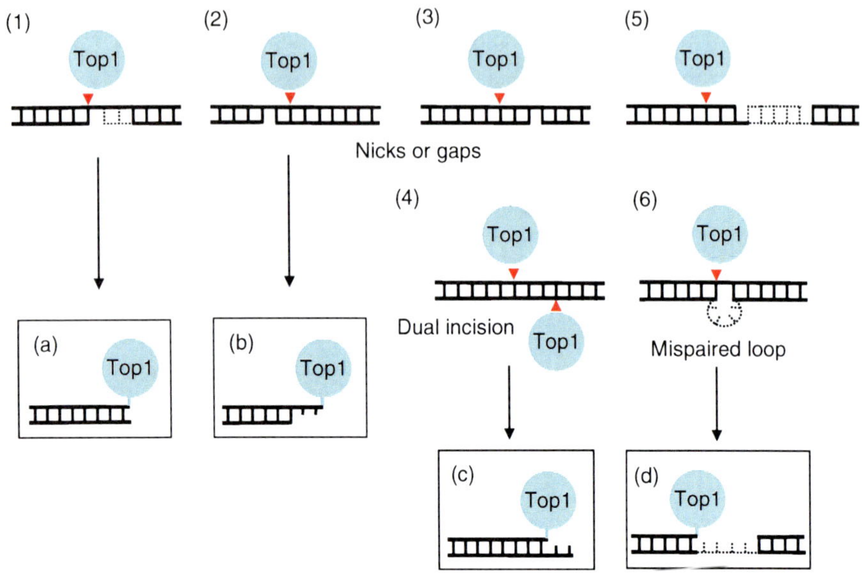

Fig. 6.6 DNA modifications leading to recombinogenic and irreversible Top1 cleavage. Top1-mediated DNA cleavage with nicks or gaps in the non-scissile strand downstream (*1*, *3*) or upstream (*2*) of the enzyme cleavage site lead to the formation of suicide products (donor molecules). Top1 remains irreversibly attached to blunt (**a**), 3′-protrusive (**b**), or 3′-recessed (**c**) ends. 3′-recessed suicide products can be obtained following dual incision on two vicinal sites on both strands (*4*). Presence of nicks or small gaps in the scissile strand downstream from the Top1 site (*5*) or the presence of mispaired loop opposite to this site (*6*), leads to the formation of an extended gap that prevents religation

breaks if they are left unrepaired. In this respect, these lesions are mimicking CPT effects. Irreversible Top1 trapping can be detected independently of replication, when DNA base pairing is profoundly altered on both strands of the DNA substrate immediately downstream from the Top1 site, or immediately upstream of this site on the non-scissile strand (Pommier et al. 2003; Pourquier and Pommier 2001) (Fig. 6.6). Hydrogen bonding defects in these locations prevents a proper alignment of the 5′-hydroxyl DNA end with the scissile phospho-tyrosine bond which is normally required for optimal religation. The modifications which lead to such irreversible complexes include primarily strand interruptions such as mispaired loops, strand breaks, nicks or gaps, but also bulky adducts such as O^6-dA- or N^2-dG-benzo[a]pyrene adducts (Fig. 6.5). Nicked or gapped substrates have first been used in vitro to produce suicide complexes as a tool to uncouple cleavage and religation and separately study the effects of CPT on each of these reactions (Svejstrup et al. 1991). Depending on the localization of the strand breakage, various types of suicide products (donors) can be generated, Top1 being irreversibly bound to either 3′-recessed, 3′-protrusive, or blunt ends (Fig. 6.6). It is interesting to note that irreversible trapping could be detected even when nicks are located as far as 10 bases from the Top1 site (Christiansen and Westergaard 1994). Blunt end donors are formed when Top1 cleaves DNA substrates in which the non-scissile strand is nicked directly opposite to the Top1 site (Fig. 6.6, panels 1 and a). This leads to the formation of a double-strand break (Andersen et al. 2003; Cheng and Shuman 2000a; Christiansen and Westergaard 1994; Pourquier et al. 1997; Shuman 1992b). When nicks are located few bases upstream of the Top1 site on the non-scissile strand, Top1 cleavage results in 3′-protrusive suicide products (Fig. 6.6, panels 2 and b) (Cheng and Shuman 2000a). Conversely, when nicks or gaps are located few nucleotides downstream from the cleavage site, or eventually when concerted cleavage of two Top1 monomers occurs in two proximal sites (one in each strand), Top1 remains irreversibly trapped on 3′-recessed ends (Fig. 6.6, panels 3, 4 and c) (Andersen et al. 2003; Christiansen and Westergaard 1994; Henningfeld and Hecht 1995; Pommier et al. 1995; Shuman 1992b). Irreversible trapping of Top1 on 3′-recessed could also be obtained when nicks or gaps are present on the scissile strand downstream of the enzyme cleavage site, or when Top1 cleaves opposite to a mismatched loop on the non-scissile strand. In that case, religation is prevented by the presence of a single-stranded region of variable length which moves the free 5′-hydroxyl of the acceptor strand away from the 3′-DNA phosphotyrosyl linkage (Fig. 6.6, panels 5, 6 and d) (Henningfeld and Hecht 1995). These suicide complexes are biologically relevant since they mimic irreversible Top1 complexes that are formed following replication fork collapse.

6.3.3 Intra and Intermolecular Religation, Two Mechanisms for Top1-Mediated Illegitimate Recombination

In vitro, a variety of donor molecules have been used to investigate the recombinogenic potential of Top1 when it is irreversibly trapped on its cleavage site (Christiansen et al. 1993; Christiansen and Westergaard 1994; Henningfeld and Hecht 1995; Pommier et al. 1995; Pourquier et al. 1997; Shuman 1992a, b; Svejstrup et al. 1990, 1991). These studies allowed the identification of two classes of end-joining reactions catalyzed by Top1: Intramolecular and intermolecular DNA ligation. They differ in their requirements for both sequence homologies between donors and acceptors and interaction of Top1 with the acceptor (Christiansen and Westergaard 1994; Shuman 1992b).

Intramolecular DNA ligation requires homology of the incoming acceptor to the non-scissile strand of the donor. This was demonstrated, in vitro, when Top1 bound to a 3′-recessed end catalyzes strand transfer only if the acceptor can base-pair to the single-stranded region immediately flanking the Top1 site (Shuman 1992a; Svejstrup et al. 1991). This mechanism is in accordance with the fact that in vivo recombination sites conserved several bases of sequence identity 3′ of the parental cleavage site (Shuman 1991). For the vaccinia enzyme, it was shown that a minimal of 4 base pairs homology was required, and that the efficiency of strand transfer was enhanced with the extent of base pairing (Shuman 1992a). In the case of human Top1, intramolecular religation of a complementary single-strand substrate required at least a

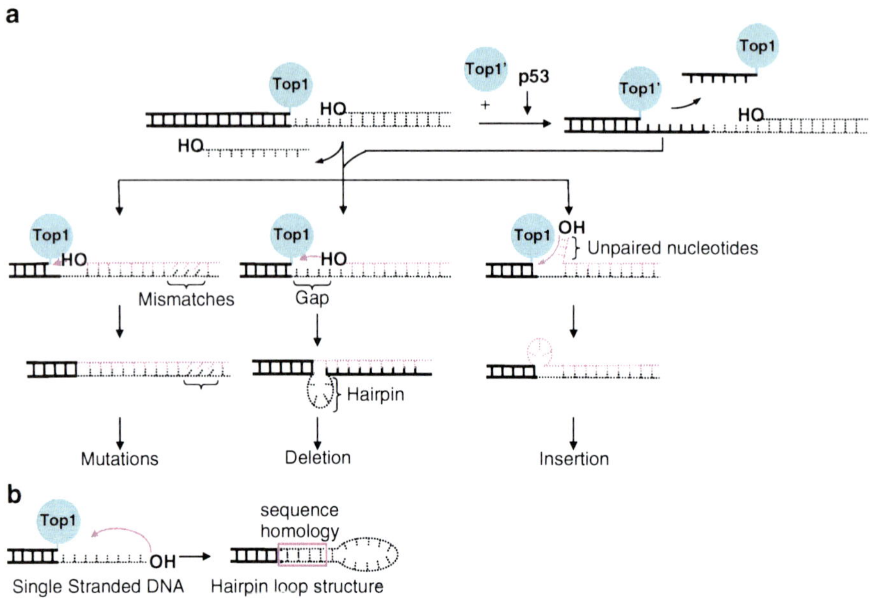

Fig. 6.7 Intramolecular ligation catalyzed by Top1. (**a**) Top1 suicide products can religate single-stranded acceptor molecules that display sequence homologies downstream from the Top1 cleavage site. Imperfect annealing of the acceptor downstream from the Top1 cleavage resulting in mismatches, base gaps or unpaired nucleotides could respectively result in the formation of point mutations, deletions or insertions following religation. Alternatively, suicide products can be cleaved by a second Top1 molecule (Top1′) and generate a gaped substrate which further stimulates recombination repair. This double Top1 cleavage is stimulated by p53 (**b**) Intramolecular ligation could also occur when the downstream part of the non-scissile strand forms a loop and can base pair (even partially) to itself. Religation would result in the formation of a hairpin structure

two nucleotide homology (Christiansen and Westergaard 1994). This indicates that the extent of base pairing rather than the interaction of Top1 with the acceptor downstream from the Top1 site (region B) is critical for efficient intramolecular strand transfer. It was also shown that acceptors that retain a potential to base-pair 3′ to the Top1 site, but do not fully hybridize to the non-scissile strand, leading to mismatches gaps or extrahelical bases, can still be religated by this mechanism but lead to mutations, deletions, or insertions, respectively (see Fig. 6.7a) (Christiansen and Westergaard 1992; Henningfeld and Hecht 1995; Shuman 1992a). Top1-mediated deletions of fragments as large as 18 nucleotides could be observed, but required the formation of a hairpin structure in order to physically bring the two DNA ends in close proximity for ligation (Henningfeld and Hecht 1995). It was also shown that suicide complexes could be recognized by a second Top1 molecule inducing a second cleavage immediately upstream of the original suicide cleavage site (Soe et al. 2001) (Fig. 6.7a). This mechanism referred as Top1-induced recombination repair (TIRR) was also described in cells (Soe et al. 2002) and is stimulated by the presence of p53 in vitro (Stephan et al. 2002). Mechanistically, it is however

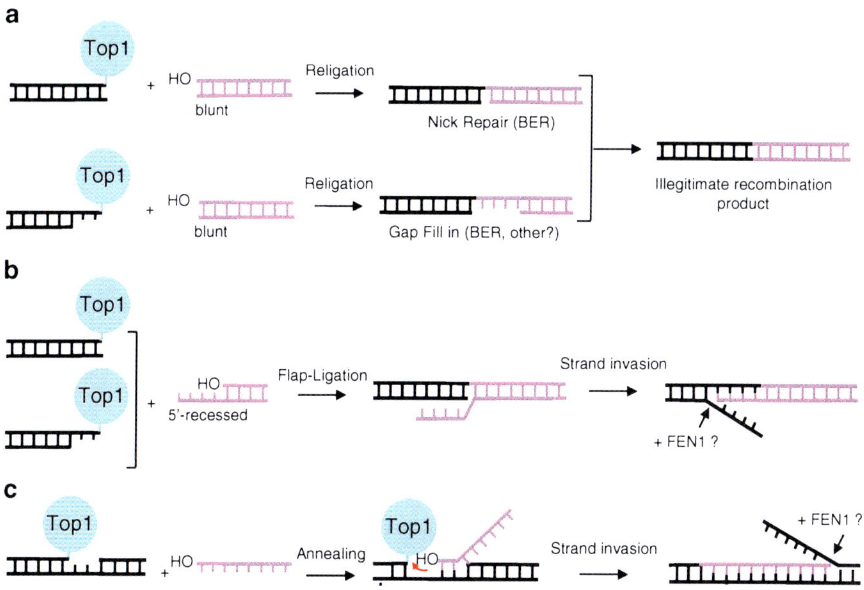

Fig. 6.8 Intermolecular ligation catalyzed by topoisomerase I. (**a**) Suicide Top1-clevage complexes (donors) can ligate double-stranded heterologous acceptors (in *pink*) independently of sequence homology. Depending on the structure of the donor, nicked or gapped recombinant products are formed and it is hypothesized that DNA continuity can be restored by specific DNA repair pathways such as BER. (**b**) The Flap ligation pathway. This intermolecular ligation pathway requires that donor molecules with 3′-protrusive or blunt ends share small sequence homologies with 5′-recessed ends of duplex acceptors. These homologies facilitate base pairing and strand invasion of the complementary strand of the acceptor. Subsequent religation by Top1 leads to recombinant products with a flap that can be eliminated by specialized enzymes from BER such as flap endonuclease 1 (*FEN1*). (**c**) Similar flapped recombinant products could also arise from the ligation of single-stranded acceptors sharing partial homology to a single-stranded region of the donor in the vicinity of the Top1 site

impossible to distinguish double-cleavage TIRR from conventional intramolecular ligation. Several studies also reported intramolecular strand transfer in the absence of "exogenous" acceptors. In that case, the 5′-tail of the non-scissile strand served as an acceptor, given that it was bearing a 5′-hydroxyl end and could partially base pair to itself 3′ to the Top1 site (Fig. 6.7b) (Pommier et al. 1995; Shuman 1992a). These recombinant products are reminiscent of the hairpin structures that are generated *via* the Top1 activity of λ-integrase (Nash and Robertson 1989; Nunes-Duby et al. 1989).

In contrast with intramolecular ligation, intermolecular strand transfer does not require sequence homology between the donor and the acceptor, which is consistent for a role of Top1 in the generation of chromosomal translocations. This potential was demonstrated in vitro using model substrates in which Top1 was irreversibly bound to the 3′-terminus of blunt or 3′-protrusive ends of DNA duplexes (Fig. 6.8a) (Andersen et al. 2003; Christiansen and Westergaard 1994; Pourquier et al. 1997; Shuman 1992b).

These complexes could ligate heterologous acceptors regardless of their sequence, provided they have double-stranded 5′-hydroxyl termini, since no ligation of 5′-staggered end duplexes or single-stranded DNAs could be observed (Christiansen and Westergaard 1994; Shuman 1992b). This process would result in the formation of nicked or gaped intermediates which are known to be good substrates for the short patch base excision repair pathway (BER) (Fig. 6.8a) (Friedberg et al. 1995). Conversely to intramolecular ligation in which the correct alignment of the 5′-hydroxyl terminus results from complementary base pairing, optimal intermolecular strand transfer is ensured by a non-covalent interaction between Top1 and the acceptor within region B (Christiansen and Westergaard 1994). This is in accordance with the fact that intermolecular strand transfer is inhibited by high salt concentrations which disrupts Top1 binding to its substrate (Christiansen and Westergaard 1994).

More recently, flap-ligation has been identified as a new pathway for intermolecular strand transfer (Fig. 6.8b & c). The efficiency of such a mechanism relies on sequence homology between the 3′-tail of the acceptor molecule and a region of the scissile strand upstream of the phosphotyrosyl linkage. This homology would facilitate strand invasion and subsequent base pairing of the 3′-tail that is necessary for ligation of the 5′-hydroxyl terminus (Fig. 6.8c). Single-strand flaps formed by such a process can eventually be recognized and removed by specific endonucleases such as FEN-1 (Flap Endonuclease 1), which belongs to the long patch BER pathway (Friedberg et al. 1995). Flap ligation was first described for vaccinia Top1 which required a minimum of 6 nt homology for efficient strand transfer (Cheng and Shuman 2000b). Because the acceptors were similar to 5′-recessed DNA intermediates that are formed during homologous recombination, it was proposed that Top1-mediated flap ligation could be involved in double-strand break repair (Cheng and Shuman 2000b). Human Top1 can also mediate flap-ligation in vitro but this reaction is highly sensitive to the length of the duplex region of the donor upstream of the cleavage site. It is striking to observe that 6 bp increase of this duplex region could lead to a complete abrogation of flap-ligation (Andersen et al. 2003). In addition, flap ligation was stimulated when human Top1 was deleted from its N-terminal domain, suggesting that in normal conditions, Top1 would rather prevent invasion of illegitimate acceptors, further implying that factors other than Top1 would be required for efficient repair of DNA breaks *via* this mechanism (Andersen et al. 2003).

6.4 Top1-Mediated DNA Recombination Independent from Cleavage and Religation

Besides DNA relaxation, Top1 can regulate other functions independently of its DNA cleavage/religation activity, especially transcription and RNA splicing, and potentially DNA repair. These roles are often related to the ability of the enzyme to interact with other cellular proteins (Leppard and Champoux 2005; Pourquier and

Pommier 2001) (see Chap. 2). For example, modulation of transcription by the human Top1 is due to its direct interaction with the TATA binding protein (TBP), which increases transcription initiation (but not the elongation) by stimulating the formation of the TFIID-TFIIA complexes in promoter regions (Kretzschmar et al. 1993; Merino et al. 1993; Shykind et al. 1997). This effect is still observed for the catalytically inactive Top1 mutant (Y723F) (Shykind et al. 1997). Top1 also has a specific kinase activity, independent of the catalytic tyrosine, which is involved in RNA splicing (Rossi et al. 1998). Top1 directly interacts and phosphorylates the RS domain of the splicing factor ASF/SF2 (from the SR-family) (Rossi et al. 1996), which is necessary for the onset of spliceosome assembly (Xiao and Manley 1997, 1998; Yeakley et al. 1999). Top1 can also bind to the late splicing factor PSF/p54(nrb), which results in increased Top1-mediated DNA relaxation in vitro (Straub et al. 1998, 2000).

Top1 could also be involved in DNA repair, though its precise mechanism is not well documented. First, Top1 can interact with the tumor suppressor p53 protein in vitro and in cells. This interaction enhances Top1 activity (Albor et al. 1998; Gobert et al. 1996, 1999; Mao et al. 2000) and increases Top1 cleavage complexes in p53 wild-type, but not p53-deficient or NER-defective cells following UV irradiation (Mao et al. 2000; Subramanian et al. 1998). Another study reported that wild-type p53 is associated with Top1 in untreated B-lymphoblastoid cells (Smith and Grosovsky 1999). This cooperation between Top1 and p53 could serve to recruit DNA repair factors to the damaged sites. Top1 is also known to associate with PARP-1, another key protein involved in the repair of single-strand breaks *via* the Base Excision Repair pathway (Drew and Plummer 2009). PARP-1 destabilizes the Top1 cleavage complexes and promote religation either by direct interaction with Top1 or by the poly-(ADP) ribosylation of Top1 in the presence of NAD (Park and Cheng 2005).

How these additional functions of Top1 could affect genomic stability independently of Top1's strand transferase activity? This question can be addressed with Top1-deficient cells, where DNA rearrangements have been observed. Top1-deficient yeasts have a high frequency of mitotic recombination within the rDNA cluster (Christman et al. 1988) and inhibition of yeast Top1 by CPT leads to the accumulation of aberrant DNA structures resembling either recombination intermediates or aberrant replication termination late Cairns structures (Levac and Moss 1996). These aberrations probably contribute to the chromatin reorganization that is observed in Top1−/− yeasts (Uemura and Yanagida 1984). Similar observations were made in two human cancer cell lines (HCT116 and MCF7) in which Top1 levels are stably downregulated by small interfering RNA (Miao et al. 2007). Both cell lines exhibit an approximately five-fold reduction of Top1 level compared to their respective normal counterparts. Reduction of Top1 levels in HCT116 cells is accompanied by a three-fold increase in numerical aberrations and a 17-fold increase in the number of deletions, translocations, and inversions (Miao et al. 2007). Moreover, Top1 downregulation is associated with increased nuclear size and higher number of nucleoli. Comparative expression profiling between cells with reduced levels of Top1 and their normal counterparts identified a list of 55 genes differentially expressed with no corresponding alteration at the genomic level, suggesting that Top1 downregulation-induced nuclear rearrangements were related to a change in transcription regulation (Miao et al. 2007).

Together these studies indicate that Top1 plays a role in the maintenance of genomic integrity. It is now clear that absence or reduced levels of Top1 are associated with the formation of DNA breaks (Miao et al. 2007; Tuduri et al. 2009) that constitute a prerequisite for recombination. It was also recently shown that Top1-deficient cells accumulate stalled replication forks and chromosome breaks in S phase and that this phenotype was reversed by the suppression of R-loops formation during transcription in an ASF/SF2-dependent manner (Tuduri et al. 2009). In this context, Top1 could prevent genomic instability by preventing collisions between replication and transcription factories by inhibiting R-loop formation via the removal of DNA supercoiling and/or via its functional interaction with ASF/SF2 splicing factor (Sordet et al. 2009, 2010; Tuduri et al. 2009). Alternatively, reduction of Top1 levels could have transcription-mediated effects on the expression of specific genes or set of genes which are important for the maintenance of genomic integrity, including DNA repair genes (Miao et al. 2007). Another possibility is that reduction of Top1 levels might directly impact DNA repair efficacy and/or damage recognition, leading to increased levels of breaks and increased genomic instability. Indeed, cells with reduced levels of Top1 show a reduction in the repair of UV-induced DNA lesions associated with reduced formation of repair patches as evidenced by PCNA staining in treated cells (Mao and Muller 2003). Also, mutant p53, which is transcriptionally inactive, is constitutively associated with Top1 in HT29 cells and still able to stimulate Top1, including its recombinase activity (Gobert et al. 1999), leading to genomic instability. This is in accordance with gene amplification induced by CPT that is observed in cells expressing a "gain of function" mutant of p53 (El-Hizawi et al. 2002).

6.5 Conclusions

This chapter stresses the similarities between Top1 and DNA recombinases and demonstrates how Top1 can mediate heterologous strand transfer with various efficiencies depending on the origin of the enzyme and on the nature of both donor and acceptors molecules. The recombinogenic potential of Top1 is primarily linked to its religation activity and is favored when the Top1-DNA cleavage complexes half-life is prolonged. It is also possible to distinguish between intramolecular and intermolecular religation, two mechanisms which differ in their requirements for sequence homology between donors and acceptors and for the non-covalent interaction of Top1 with the incoming acceptor.

One major consequence of the recombinase activity of Top1 was certainly the development of ligation systems relying on vaccinia Top1 strand transferase activity. Indeed, vaccinia Top1 cleaves at CCCTT↓ sites of various DNA structures and accommodates a large spectrum of heterologous substrates, including duplex DNAs containing a 3'A overhang (Cheng and Shuman 2000a). This strategy is particularly adapted to the direct cloning of PCR products that can hybridize to the last unpaired T of a unique CCCTT sequence and is commercialized as TOPO-TA cloning kits (Invitrogen, Carlsbad, CA) (Cheng and Shuman 2000a; Shuman 1994).

Although the experimental evidences suggesting a role of Top1 in illegitimate recombination in vivo are indirect, they all converge towards a functional link between the enzyme activity and the level of cellular DNA rearrangements. Moreover, it is clear that different mechanisms can account for Top1-mediated DNA recombinations. One could directly involve the strand transferase activity of Top1. This mechanism relies on the level of Top1-DNA complexes and could explain the increased levels of DNA rearrangements observed in cells treated with CPT, but also in cells with high levels of endogenous DNA lesions. Alternatively, DNA recombinations could be due to the alteration of other cellular processes (such as transcription or DNA repair) that are regulated by Top1, but are indirectly related to Top1's religation activity. This would explain the chromosomal alterations and replication alterations observed in cells with reduced levels of Top1 (Miao et al. 2007; Tuduri et al. 2009). Identification of the pathways that are specifically altered following Top1 downregulation and lead to DNA recombination would be of critical interest to better understand the role of Top1 in genomic instability.

References

Abremski K, Wierzbicki A, Frommer B, Hoess RH (1986) Bacteriophage P1 Cre-loxP site-specific recombination. Site-specific DNA topoisomerase activity of the Cre recombination protein. *J Biol Chem* **261**(1): 391–396.

Albor A, Kaku S, Kulesz-Martin M (1998) Wild-type and mutant forms of p53 activate human topoisomerase I: a possible mechanism for gain of function in mutants. *Cancer Res* **58**(10): 2091–2094.

Andersen AH, Gocke E, Bonven BJ, Nielsen OF, Westergaard O (1985) Topoisomerase I has a strong binding preference for a conserved hexadecameric sequence in the promoter region of the rRNA gene from Tetrahymena pyriformis. *Nucleic Acids Res* **13**(5): 1543–1557.

Andersen FF, Andersen KE, Kusk M, Frohlich RF, Westergaard O, Andersen AH, Knudsen BR (2003) Recombinogenic flap ligation mediated by human topoisomerase I. *J Mol Biol* **330**(2): 235–246.

Arnaudeau C, Lundin C, Helleday T (2001) DNA double-strand breaks associated with replication forks are predominantly repaired by homologous recombination involving an exchange mechanism in mammalian cells. *J Mol Biol* **307**(5): 1235–1245.

Balestrieri E, Zanier R, Degrassi F (2001) Molecular characterisation of camptothecin-induced mutations at the hprt locus in Chinese hamster cells. *Mutat Res* **476**(1–2): 63–69.

Barrows LR, Holden JA, Anderson M, D'Arpa P (1998) The CHO XRCC1 mutant, EM9, deficient in DNA ligase III activity, exhibits hypersensitivity to camptothecin independent of DNA replication. *Mutat Res* **408**(2): 103–110.

Been MD, Burgess RR, Champoux JJ (1984) Nucleotide sequence preference at rat liver and wheat germ type 1 DNA topoisomerase breakage sites in duplex SV40 DNA. *Nucleic Acids Res* **12**(7): 3097–3114.

Bjornsti MA, Benedetti P, Viglianti GA, Wang JC (1989) Expression of human DNA topoisomerase I in yeast cells lacking yeast DNA topoisomerase I: restoration of sensitivity of the cells to the antitumor drug camptothecin. *Cancer Res* **49**(22): 6318–6323.

Bullock P, Champoux JJ, Botchan M (1985) Association of crossover points with topoisomerase I cleavage sites: a model for nonhomologous recombination. *Science* **230**(4728): 954–958.

Camilloni G, Di Martino E, Caserta M, di Mauro E (1988) Eukaryotic DNA topoisomerase I reaction is topology dependent. *Nucleic Acids Res* **16**(14): 7071–7085.

Caserta M, Amadei A, Di Mauro E, Camilloni G (1989) In vitro preferential topoisomerization of bent DNA. *Nucleic Acids Res* **17**(21): 8463–8474.

Champoux JJ (1977) Renaturation of complementary single-stranded DNA circles: complete rewinding facilitated by the DNA untwisting enzyme. *Proc Natl Acad Sci USA* **74**(12): 5328–5332.

Champoux JJ (1981) DNA is linked to the rat liver DNA nicking-closing enzyme by a phosphodiester bond to tyrosine. *J Biol Chem* **256**(10): 4805–4809.

Chatterjee S, Cheng MF, Trivedi D, Petzold SJ, Berger NA (1989) Camptothecin hypersensitivity in poly(adenosine diphosphate-ribose) polymerase-deficient cell lines. *Cancer Commun* **1**(6): 389–394.

Cheng C, Kussie P, Pavletich N, Shuman S (1998) Conservation of structure and mechanism between eukaryotic topoisomerase I and site-specific recombinases. *Cell* **92**(6): 841–850.

Cheng C, Shuman S (2000a) DNA strand transfer catalyzed by vaccinia topoisomerase: ligation of DNAs containing a 3′ mononucleotide overhang. *Nucleic Acids Res* **28**(9): 1893–1898.

Cheng C, Shuman S (2000b) Recombinogenic flap ligation pathway for intrinsic repair of topoisomerase IB-induced double-strand breaks. *Mol Cell Biol* **20**(21): 8059–8068.

Christiansen K, Svejstrup BD, Andersen AH, Westergaard O (1993) Eukaryotic topoisomerase I-mediated cleavage requires bipartite DNA interaction. *J Biol Chem* **268:** 9690–9701.

Christiansen K, Westergaard O (1992) *DNA Repair Mechanisms, Alfred Benzon Symposium 35*, Copenhagen.

Christiansen K, Westergaard O (1994) Characterization of intra- and intermolecular DNA ligation mediated by eukaryotic topoisomerase I. *J Biol Chem* **269:** 721–729.

Christman MF, Dietrich FS, Fink GR (1988) Mitotic recombination in the rDNA of S. cerevisiae is suppressed by the combined action of DNA topoisomerases I and II. *Cell* **55**(3): 413–425.

Chu WK, Hickson ID (2009) RecQ helicases: multifunctional genome caretakers. *Nat Rev Cancer* **9**(9): 644–654.

Cornet F, Hallet B, Sherratt DJ (1997) Xer recombination in Escherichia coli. Site-specific DNA topoisomerase activity of the XerC and XerD recombinases. *J Biol Chem* **272**(35): 21927–21931.

Cunha KS, Reguly ML, Graf U, Rodrigues de Andrade HH (2002) Comparison of camptothecin derivatives presently in clinical trials: genotoxic potency and mitotic recombination. *Mutagenesis* **17**(2): 141–147.

D'Arpa P, Beardmore C, Liu LF (1990) Involvement of nucleic acid synthesis in cell killing mechanisms of topoisomerase poisons. *Cancer Res* **50**(21): 6919–6924.

Degrassi F, De Salvia R, Tanzarella C, Palitti F (1989) Induction of chromosomal aberrations and SCE by camptothecin, an inhibitor of mammalian topoisomerase I. *Mutat Res* **211**(1): 125–130.

Desai SD, Zhang H, Rodriguez-Bauman A, Yang JM, Wu X, Gounder MK, Rubin EH, Liu LF (2003) Transcription-dependent degradation of topoisomerase I-DNA covalent complexes. *Mol Cell Biol* **23**(7): 2341–2350.

Drew Y, Plummer R (2009) PARP inhibitors in cancer therapy: two modes of attack on the cancer cell widening the clinical applications. *Drug Resist Updat* **12**(6): 153–156.

El-Hizawi S, Lagowski JP, Kulesz-Martin M, Albor A (2002) Induction of gene amplification as a gain-of-function phenotype of mutant p53 proteins. *Cancer Res* **62**(11): 3264–3270.

Friedberg EC, Walker GC, Siede W (1995) *DNA repair and mutagenesis*, Washington, DC: ASM Press.

Gobert C, Bracco L, Rossi F, Olivier M, Tazi J, Lavelle F, Larsen AK, Riou JF (1996) Modulation of DNA topoisomerase I activity by p53. *Biochemistry* **35**(18): 5778–5786.

Gobert C, Skladanowski A, Larsen AK (1999) The interaction between p53 and DNA topoisomerase I is regulated differently in cells with wild-type and mutant p53. *Proc Natl Acad Sci USA* **96**(18): 10355–10360

Halligan BD, Davis JL, Edwards KA, Liu LF (1982) Intra- and intermolecular strand transfer by HeLa DNA topoisomerase I. *J Biol Chem* **257**(7)**:** 3995–4000.

Hashimoto H, Chatterjee S, Berger NA (1995) Mutagenic activity of topoisomerase I inhibitors. *Clin Cancer Res* **1**(4)**:** 369–376.

Henningfeld KA, Hecht SM (1995) A model for topoisomerase I-mediated insertions and deletions with duplex DNA substrates containing branches, nicks, and gaps. *Biochemistry* **34:** 6120–6129.

Hino O, Ohtake K, Rogler CE (1989) Features of two hepatitis B virus (HBV) DNA integrations suggest mechanisms of HBV integration. *J Virol* **63**(6)**:** 2638–2643.

Hogan A, Faust EA (1986) Nonhomologous recombination in the parvovirus chromosome: role for a CTATTTCT motif. *Mol Cell Biol* **6**(8)**:** 3005–3009.

Holm C, Covey JM, Kerrigan D, Pommier Y (1989) Differential requirement of DNA replication for the cytotoxicity of DNA topoisomerase I and II inhibitors in Chinese hamster DC3F cells. *Cancer Res* **49**(22)**:** 6365–6368.

Hsiang YH, Hertzberg R, Hecht S, Liu LF (1985) Camptothecin induces protein-linked DNA breaks via mammalian DNA topoisomerase I. *J Biol Chem* **260**(27)**:** 14873–14878.

Hsiang YH, Lihou MG, Liu LF (1989) Arrest of replication forks by drug-stabilized topoisomerase I-DNA cleavable complexes as a mechanism of cell killing by camptothecin. *Cancer Res* **49**(18)**:** 5077–5082.

Hsiang YH, Liu LF (1988) Identification of mammalian DNA topoisomerase I as an intracellular target of the anticancer drug camptothecin. *Cancer Res* **48**(7)**:** 1722–1726.

Jaxel C, Capranico G, Kerrigan D, Kohn KW, Pommier Y (1991) Effect of local DNA sequence on topoisomerase I cleavage in the presence or absence of camptothecin. *J Biol Chem* **266**(30)**:** 20418–20423.

Jaxel C, Kohn KW, Pommier Y (1988) Topoisomerase I interaction with SV40 DNA in the presence and absence of camptothecin. *Nucleic Acids Res* **16:** 11157–11170.

Kaufmann WK, Boyer JC, Estabrooks LL, Wilson SJ (1991) Inhibition of replicon initiation in human cells following stabilization of topoisomerase-DNA cleavable complexes. *Mol Cell Biol* **11**(7)**:** 3711–3718.

Kikuchi Y, Nash HA (1979) Nicking-closing activity associated with bacteriophage lambda int gene product. *Proc Natl Acad Sci USA* **76**(8)**:** 3760–3764.

Koster DA, Croquette V, Dekker C, Shuman S, Dekker NH (2005) Friction and torque govern the relaxation of DNA supercoils by eukaryotic topoisomerase IB. *Nature* **434**(7033)**:** 671–674

Koster DA, Palle K, Bot ES, Bjornsti MA, Dekker NH (2007) Antitumour drugs impede DNA uncoiling by topoisomerase I. *Nature* **448**(7150)**:** 213–217.

Kretzschmar M, Meisterernst M, Roeder RG (1993) Identification of human DNA topoisomerase I as a cofactor for activator- dependent transcription by RNA polymerase II. *Proc Natl Acad Sci USA* **90**(24)**:** 11508–11512.

Krogh S, Mortensen UH, Westergaard O, Bonven BJ (1991) Eukaryotic topoisomerase I-DNA interaction is stabilized by helix curvature. *Nucleic Acids Res* **19**(6)**:** 1235–1241.

Landy A (1989) Dynamic, structural, and regulatory aspects of lambda site-specific recombination. *Annu Rev Biochem* **58:** 913–949.

Lanza A, Tornaletti S, Rodolfo C, Scanavini MC, Pedrini AM (1996) Human DNA topoisomerase I-mediated cleavages stimulated by ultraviolet light-induced DNA damage. *J Biol Chem* **271**(12)**:** 6978–6986.

Lee MP, Brown SD, Chen A, Hsieh TS (1993) DNA topoisomerase I is essential in Drosophila melanogaster. *Proc Natl Acad Sci USA* **90**(14)**:** 6656–6660.

Lengauer C, Kinzler KW, Vogelstein B (1998) Genetic instabilities in human cancers. *Nature* **396**(6712)**:** 643–649.

Leppard JB, Champoux JJ (2005) Human DNA topoisomerase I: relaxation, roles, and damage control. *Chromosoma* **114**(2)**:** 75–85.

Levac P, Moss T (1996) Inactivation of topoisomerase I or II may lead to recombination or to aberrant replication termination on both SV40 and yeast 2 micron DNA. *Chromosoma* **105**(4)**:** 250–260.

Li TK, Liu LF (2001) Tumor cell death induced by topoisomerase-targeting drugs. *Annu Rev Pharmacol Toxicol* **41:** 53–77.

Lindahl T (1993) Instability and decay of the primary structure of DNA [see comments]. *Nature* **362**(6422): 709–715.

Lindahl T, Wood RD (1999) Quality control by DNA repair. *Science* **286**(5446): 1897–1905.

Lynn RM, Bjornsti MA, Caron PR, Wang JC (1989) Peptide sequencing and site-directed mutagenesis identify tyrosine-727 as the active site tyrosine of Saccharomyces cerevisiae DNA topoisomerase I. *Proc Natl Acad Sci USA* **86**(10): 3559–3563.

Mao Y, Muller MT (2003) Down modulation of topoisomerase I affects DNA repair efficiency. *DNA Repair (Amst)* **2**(10): 1115–1126.

Mao Y, Okada S, Chang LS, Muller MT (2000) p53 dependence of topoisomerase I recruitment in vivo. *Cancer Res* **60**(16): 4538–4543.

McMilin KD, Stahl MM, Stahl FW (1974) Rec-mediated recombinational hot spot activity in bacteriophage lambda. I. Hot spot activity associated with spi-deletions and bio substitutions. *Genetics* **77**(3): 409–423.

Merino A, Madden KR, Lane WS, Champoux JJ, Reinberg D (1993) DNA topoisomerase I is involved in both repression and activation of transcription. *Nature* **365**(6443): 227–232.

Miao ZH, Player A, Shankavaram U, Wang YH, Zimonjic DB, Lorenzi PL, Liao ZY, Liu H, Shimura T, Zhang HL, Meng LH, Zhang YW, Kawasaki ES, Popescu NC, Aladjem MI, Goldstein DJ, Weinstein JN, Pommier Y (2007) Nonclassic functions of human topoisomerase I: genome-wide and pharmacologic analyses. *Cancer Res* **67**(18): 8752–8761.

Mielke C, Kalfalah FM, Christensen MO, Boege F (2007) Rapid and prolonged stalling of human DNA topoisomerase I in UVA-irradiated genomic areas. *DNA Repair (Amst)* **6**(12): 1757–1763.

Morham SG, Kluckman KD, Voulomanos N, Smithies O (1996) Targeted disruption of the mouse topoisomerase I gene by camptothecin selection. *Mol Cell Biol* **16**(12): 6804–6809.

Morris EJ, Geller HM (1996) Induction of neuronal apoptosis by camptothecin, an inhibitor of DNA topoisomerase-I: evidence for cell cycle-independent toxicity. *J Cell Biol* **134**(3): 757–770.

Nash HA, Robertson CA (1989) Heteroduplex substrates for bacteriophage lambda site-specific recombination: cleavage and strand transfer products. *Embo J* **8**(11): 3523–3533.

Natarajan AT, Palitti F (2008) DNA repair and chromosomal alterations. *Mutat Res* **657**(1): 3–7.

Nunes-Duby SE, Matsumoto L, Landy A (1989) Half-att site substrates reveal the homology independence and minimal protein requirements for productive synapsis in lambda excisive recombination. *Cell* **59**(1): 197–206.

O'Connor PM, Nieves-Neira W, Kerrigan D, Bertrand R, Goldman J, Kohn KW, Pommier Y (1991) S-phase population analysis does not correlate with the cytotoxicity of camptothecin and 10,11-methylenedioxycamptothecin in human colon carcinoma HT-29 cells. *Cancer Commun* **3**(8): 233–240.

Park SY, Cheng YC (2005) Poly(ADP-ribose) polymerase-1 could facilitate the religation of topoisomerase I-linked DNA inhibited by camptothecin. *Cancer Res* **65**(9): 3894–3902.

Pommier Y (2006) Topoisomerase I inhibitors: camptothecins and beyond. *Nat Rev Cancer* **6**(10): 789–802.

Pommier Y (2009) DNA topoisomerase I inhibitors: chemistry, biology, and interfacial inhibition. *Chem Rev* **109**(7): 2894–2902.

Pommier Y, Barcelo JM, Rao VA, Sordet O, Jobson AG, Thibaut L, Miao ZH, Seiler JA, Zhang H, Marchand C, Agama K, Nitiss JL, Redon C (2006) Repair of topoisomerase I-mediated DNA damage. *Prog Nucleic Acid Res Mol Biol* **81:** 179–229.

Pommier Y, Jenkins J, Kohlhagen G, Leteurtre F (1995) DNA recombinase activity of eukaryotic DNA topoisomerase I; Effects of camptothecin and other inhibitors. *Mutat Res* **337:** 135–145.

Pommier Y, Leo E, Zhang H, Marchand C (2010) DNA topoisomerases and their poisoning by anticancer and antibacterial drugs. *Chem Biol* **17**(5): 421–433.

Pommier Y, Redon C, Rao VA, Seiler JA, Sordet O, Takemura H, Antony S, Meng L, Liao Z, Kohlhagen G, Zhang H, Kohn KW (2003) Repair of and checkpoint response to topoisomerase I-mediated DNA damage. *Mutat Res* **532**(1–2): 173–203.

Porter SE, Champoux JJ (1989) Mapping in vivo topoisomerase I sites on simian virus 40 DNA: asymmetric distribution of sites on replicating molecules. *Mol Cell Biol* **9**(2): 541–550.

Pourquier P, Jensen AD, Gong SS, Pommier Y, Rogler CE (1999) Human DNA topoisomerase I-mediated cleavage and recombination of duck hepatitis B virus DNA in vitro. *Nucleic Acids Res* **27**(8): 1919–1925.

Pourquier P, Pilon AA, Kohlhagen G, Mazumder A, Sharma A, Pommier Y (1997) Trapping of mammalian topoisomerase I and recombinations induced by damaged DNA containing nicks or gaps. Importance of DNA end phosphorylation and camptothecin effects. *J Biol Chem* **272**(42): 26441–26447.

Pourquier P, Pommier Y (2001) Topoisomerase I-mediated DNA damage. *Adv Cancer Res* **80:** 189–216.

Redinbo MR, Stewart L, Kuhn P, Champoux JJ, Hol WG (1998) Crystal structures of human topoisomerase I in covalent and noncovalent complexes with DNA [see comments]. *Science* **279**(5356): 1504–1513.

Reliene R, Bishop AJ, Schiestl RH (2007) Involvement of homologous recombination in carcinogenesis. *Adv Genet* **58:** 67–87.

Ribas G, Xamena N, Creus A, Marcos R (1996) Sister-chromatid exchanges (SCE) induction by inhibitors of DNA topoisomerases in cultured human lymphocytes. *Mutat Res* **368**(3–4): 205–211.

Rossi F, Labourier E, Gallouzi IE, Derancourt J, Allemand E, Divita G, Tazi J (1998) The C-terminal domain but not the tyrosine 723 of human DNA topoisomerase I active site contributes to kinase activity. *Nucleic Acids Res* **26**(12): 2963–2970.

Rossi F, Labourier E, Forne T, Divita G, Derancourt J, Riou JF, Antoine E, Cathala G, Brunel C, Tazi J (1996) Specific phosphorylation of SR proteins by mammalian DNA topoisomerase I. *Nature* **381:** 80–82.

Ryan AJ, Squires S, Strutt HL, Evans A, Johnson RT (1994) Different fates of camptothecin-induced replication fork-associated double-strand DNA breaks in mammalian cells. *Carcinogenesis* **15**(5): 823–828.

Saleh-Gohari N, Bryant HE, Schultz N, Parker KM, Cassel TN, Helleday T (2005) Spontaneous homologous recombination is induced by collapsed replication forks that are caused by endogenous DNA single-strand breaks. *Mol Cell Biol* **25**(16): 7158–7169.

Sekiguchi J, Cheng C, Shuman S (2000) Resolution of a Holliday junction by vaccinia topoisomerase requires a spacer DNA segment 3′ of the CCCTT/cleavage sites. *Nucleic Acids Res* **28**(14): 2658–2663.

Sekiguchi J, Seeman NC, Shuman S (1996) Resolution of Holliday junctions by eukaryotic DNA topoisomerase I. *Proc Natl Acad Sci USA* **93**(2): 785–789.

Shuman S (1989) Vaccinia DNA topoisomerase I promotes illegitimate recombination in Escherichia coli. *Proc Natl Acad Sci USA* **86**(10): 3489–3493.

Shuman S (1991) Recombination mediated by vaccinia virus DNA topoisomerase I in Escherichia coli is sequence specific. *Proc Natl Acad Sci USA* **88**(22): 10104–10108.

Shuman S (1992a) DNA strand transfer reactions catalyzed by vaccinia topoisomerase I. *J Biol Chem* **267**(12): 8620–8627.

Shuman S (1992b) Two classes of DNA end-joining reactions catalyzed by vaccinia topoisomerase I. *J Biol Chem* **267:** 16755–16758.

Shuman S (1994) Novel approach to molecular cloning and polynucleotide synthesis using vaccinia DNA topoisomerase. *J Biol Chem* **269**(51): 32678–32684.

Shuman S (1998) Vaccinia virus DNA topoisomerase: a model eukaryotic type IB enzyme. *Biochim Biophys Acta* **1400**(1–3): 321–337.

Shuman S, Bear DG, Sekiguchi J (1997) Intramolecular synapsis of duplex DNA by vaccinia topoisomerase. *Embo J* **16**(21): 6584–6589.

Shuman S, Golder M, Moss B (1988) Characterization of vaccinia virus DNA topoisomerase I expressed in Escherichia coli. *J Biol Chem* **263**(31): 16401–16407.

Shuman S, Kane EM, Morham SG (1989) Mapping the active-site tyrosine of vaccinia virus DNA topoisomerase I. *Proc Natl Acad Sci USA* **86**(24): 9793–9797.

Shuman S, Prescott J (1990) Specific DNA cleavage and binding by vaccinia virus DNA topoisomerase I. *J Biol Chem* **265**(29): 17826–17836.

Shykind BM, Kim J, Stewart L, Champoux JJ, Sharp PA (1997) Topoisomerase I enhances TFIID-TFIIA complex assembly during activation of transcription. *Genes Dev* **11**(3): 397–407.

Smith HM, Grosovsky AJ (1999) PolyADP-ribose-mediated regulation of p53 complexed with topoisomerase I following ionizing radiation. *Carcinogenesis* **20**(8): 1439–1443.
Soe K, Dianov G, Nasheuer HP, Bohr VA, Grosse F, Stevnsner T (2001) A human topoisomerase I cleavage complex is recognized by an additional human topisomerase I molecule in vitro. *Nucleic Acids Res* **29**(15): 3195–3203.
Soe K, Hartmann H, Schlott B, Stevnsner T, Grosse F (2002) The tumor suppressor protein p53 stimulates the formation of the human topoisomerase I double cleavage complex in vitro. *Oncogene* **21**(43): 6614–6623.
Sokhansanj BA, Wilson DM, 3 rd (2004) Oxidative DNA damage background estimated by a system model of base excision repair. *Free Radic Biol Med* **37**(3): 422–427.
Sordet O, Larochelle S, Nicolas E, Stevens EV, Zhang C, Shokat KM, Fisher RP, Pommier Y (2008) Hyperphosphorylation of RNA polymerase II in response to topoisomerase I cleavage complexes and its association with transcription- and BRCA1-dependent degradation of topoisomerase I. *J Mol Biol* **381**(3): 540–549.
Sordet O, Nakamura AJ, Redon CE, Pommier Y (2010) DNA double-strand breaks and ATM activation by transcription-blocking DNA lesions. *Cell Cycle* **9**(2): 274–278.
Sordet O, Redon CE, Guirouilh-Barbat J, Smith S, Solier S, Douarre C, Conti C, Nakamura AJ, Das BB, Nicolas E, Kohn KW, Bonner WM, Pommier Y (2009) Ataxia telangiectasia mutated activation by transcription- and topoisomerase I-induced DNA double-strand breaks. *EMBO Rep* **10**(8): 887–893.
Sortibran AN, Tellez MG, Rodriguez-Arnaiz R (2006) Genotoxic profile of inhibitors of topoisomerases I (camptothecin) and II (etoposide) in a mitotic recombination and sex-chromosome loss somatic eye assay of Drosophila melanogaster. *Mutat Res* **604**(1–2): 83–90.
Staker BL, Hjerrild K, Feese MD, Behnke CA, Burgin AB, Jr., Stewart L (2002) The mechanism of topoisomerase I poisoning by a camptothecin analog. *Proc Natl Acad Sci USA* **99**(24): 15387–15392.
Stefanis L, Park DS, Friedman WJ, Greene LA (1999) Caspase-dependent and -independent death of camptothecin-treated embryonic cortical neurons. *J Neurosci* **19**(15): 6235–6247.
Stephan H, Grosse F, Soe K (2002) Human topoisomerase I cleavage complexes are repaired by a p53-stimulated recombination-like reaction in vitro. *Nucleic Acids Res* **30**(23): 5087–5093.
Stewart L, Redinbo MR, Qiu X, Hol WG, Champoux JJ (1998) A model for the mechanism of human topoisomerase I see comments. *Science* **279**(5356): 1534–1541.
Stivers JT, Shuman S, Mildvan AS (1994) Vaccinia DNA topoisomerase I: single-turnover and steady-state kinetic analysis of the DNA strand cleavage and ligation reactions. *Biochemistry* **33**(1): 327–339.
Straub T, Grue P, Uhse A, Lisby M, Knudsen BR, Tange TO, Westergaard O, Boege F (1998) The RNA-splicing factor PSF/p54 controls DNA-topoisomerase I activity by a direct interaction. *J Biol Chem* **273**(41): 26261–26264.
Straub T, Knudsen BR, Boege F (2000) PSF/p54(nrb) stimulates "jumping" of DNA topoisomerase I between separate DNA helices. *Biochemistry* **39**(25): 7552–7558.
Strumberg D, Pilon AA, Smith M, Hickey R, Malkas L, Pommier Y (2000) Conversion of topoisomerase I cleavage complexes on the leading strand of ribosomal DNA into 5′-phosphorylated DNA double-strand breaks by replication runoff. *Mol Cell Biol* **20**(11): 3977–3987.
Subramanian D, Rosenstein BS, Muller MT (1998) Ultraviolet-induced DNA damage stimulates topoisomerase I-DNA complex formation in vivo: possible relationship with DNA repair. *Cancer Res* **58**(5): 976–984.
Svejstrup JQ, Christiansen K, Andersen AH, Lund K, Westergaard O (1990) Minimal DNA duplex requirements for topoisomerase I-mediated cleavage in vitro. *J Biol Chem* **265**(21): 12529–12535.
Svejstrup JQ, Christiansen K, Gromova II, Andersen AH, Westergaard O (1991) New technique for uncoupling the cleavage and religation reactions of eukaryotic topoisomerase I. The mode of action of camptothecin at a specific recognition site. *J Mol Biol* **222:** 669–678.
Tanizawa A, Kohn KW, Pommier Y (1993) Induction of cleavage in topoisomerase I c-DNA by topoisomerase I enzymes from calf thymus and wheat germ in the presence and absence of camptothecin. *Nucleic Acids Res* **21**(22): 5157–5166.

Thrash C, Voelkel K, DiNardo S, Sternglanz R (1984) Identification of Saccharomyces cerevisiae mutants deficient in DNA topoisomerase I activity. *J Biol Chem* **259**(3): 1375–1377.

Torres C, Creus A, Marcos R (1998) Genotoxic activity of four inhibitors of DNA topoisomerases in larval cells of Drosophila melanogaster as measured in the wing spot assay. *Mutat Res* **413**(2): 191–203.

Tuduri S, Crabbe L, Conti C, Tourriere H, Holtgreve-Grez H, Jauch A, Pantesco V, De Vos J, Thomas A, Theillet C, Pommier Y, Tazi J, Coquelle A, Pasero P (2009) Topoisomerase I suppresses genomic instability by preventing interference between replication and transcription. *Nat Cell Biol* **11**(11): 1315–1324.

Uemura T, Yanagida M (1984) Isolation of type I and II DNA topoisomerase mutants from fission yeast: single and double mutants show different phenotypes in cell growth and chromatin organization. *Embo J* **3**(8): 1737–1744.

Vogel EW, Nivard MJ (1999) A novel method for the parallel monitoring of mitotic recombination and clastogenicity in somatic cells in vivo. *Mutat Res* **431**(1): 141–153.

Wang HP, Rogler CE (1991) Topoisomerase I-mediated integration of hepadnavirus DNA in vitro. *J Virol* **65**(5): 2381–2392.

Wang JC (2002) Cellular roles of DNA topoisomerases: a molecular perspective. *Nat Rev Mol Cell Biol* **3**(6): 430–440.

Wu J, Liu LF (1997) Processing of topoisomerase I cleavable complexes into DNA damage by transcription. *Nucleic Acids Res* **25**(21): 4181–4186.

Xiao SH, Manley JL (1997) Phosphorylation of the ASF/SF2 RS domain affects both protein-protein and protein-RNA interactions and is necessary for splicing. *Genes Dev* **11**(3): 334–344.

Xiao SH, Manley JL (1998) Phosphorylation-dephosphorylation differentially affects activities of splicing factor ASF/SF2. *Embo J* **17**(21): 6359–6367.

Xu CJ, Grainge I, Lee J, Harshey RM, Jayaram M (1998) Unveiling two distinct ribonuclease activities and a topoisomerase activity in a site-specific DNA recombinase. *Mol Cell* **1**(5): 729–739.

Yeakley JM, Tronchere H, Olesen J, Dyck JA, Wang HY, Fu XD (1999) Phosphorylation regulates in vivo interaction and molecular targeting of serine/arginine-rich pre-mRNA splicing factors. *J Cell Biol* **145**(3): 447–455.

Zhu J, Schiestl RH (1996) Topoisomerase I involvement in illegitimate recombination in Saccharomyces cerevisiae. *Mol Cell Biol* **16**(4): 1805–1812.

Chapter 7
Topoisomerase-Induced DNA Damage

Yves Pommier and Neil Osheroff

7.1 Introduction

The remarkable efficiency of topoisomerases is related to the large number of DNA transactions that these enzymes have to carry out within milliseconds with an exquisite accuracy. The fast catalytic cycles of topoisomerases I (Top1) and II (Top2) have in common a two-step transesterification mechanism. First, topoisomerases cleave the DNA by covalent linkage of their catalytic nucleophilic tyrosine to one end of the break; and secondly, they religate the DNA as the enzymes are released from the DNA end by a second transesterification where the nucleophile is the sugar hydroxyl end (see Chaps. 1–4). These transient cleavage complexes (Top1cc and Top2cc for Top1 and Top2, respectively) allow changes in DNA topology that are characteristic of each class of enzyme. In the case of Top1, the single-strand break allows the swiveling of the broken 5′-end around the intact opposite backbone. Multiple rounds of controlled rotation occur in one catalytic step (i.e., before Top1 religates the DNA) and Top1 acts as a highly processive DNA "untwisting enzyme" (Champoux and Dulbecco 1972). The reaction is highly efficient, does not require cofactor, and operates effectively even at ice-temperature (Koster et al. 2005; Stewart et al. 1998) (see Chap. 2). In the case of Top2, the enzyme works as homodimers (Top2α and Top2β). Each monomer cleaves the opposite strands of the DNA to allow the passage of another strand through the double-strand break while maintaining a strong dimer interface throughout the reaction (see Chap. 4). In contrast to Top1, the Top2 catalytic cycle requires cofactors (Mg^{2+} and ATP) and proceeds one step at a time (see Chap. 4). Also, the Top2 catalytic tyrosine forms a covalent intermediate with the 5′-end of the DNA, whereas Top1 attaches covalently to the 3′-end.

Y. Pommier (✉)
Laboratory of Molecular Pharmacology, Center for Cancer Research,
National Cancer Institute, National Institutes of Health, Bethesda, MD, USA
e-mail: pommier@nih.gov

Y. Pommier (ed.), *DNA Topoisomerases and Cancer*, Cancer Drug Discovery and Development, DOI 10.1007/978-1-4614-0323-4_7,

The genome is a highly dynamic and extremely long polymer susceptible to endogenous damage and base misincorporations. Table 7.1 summarizes the most frequent lesions and their estimated frequencies per genome per day. Oxidative base lesions, abasic sites, and DNA nicks are among the most common endogenous lesions, with thousands per human cell per day (Barnes and Lindahl 2004; Beckman and Ames 1997; Lindahl 1993; Vilenchik and Knudson 2003).

7.2 Trapping of Top1 By Endogenous and Carcinogenic DNA Lesions

Because of Top1's abundance and its widespread distribution throughout the genome (Baranello et al. 2010; Bermejo et al. 2007; Pommier et al. 1994; Porter and Champoux 1989), it is likely that Top1 encounters endogenous DNA lesions and alternative DNA structures with a relatively high frequency. Systematic analyses of such effects are summarized in Table 7.2 and specific examples shown in Fig. 7.1. In general, the accumulation of Top1cc is due to an inhibition of the religation step. This is because religation requires the 5′-sugar hydroxyl to be precisely positioned to attack and release the 3′-phosphotyrosyl bond [see Chap. 2 and (Pommier et al. 2006; Pourquier and Pommier 2001)]. The normal stacking of the 5′-base is critical for such alignment, which explains why the presence of abasic sites and mismatches interfere with the religation of Top1cc (Pourquier et al. 1997a, b). Notably, biochemical fractionation of human cell extracts reveal that Top1 has prominent DNA nicking activity against mismatches (Yeh et al. 1994).

The religation activity of Top1 can also be altered by carcinogenic adducts and oxidative DNA damages (Table 7.1). DNA backbone alterations and secondary DNA structures, which by themselves do not interfere with Top1's cleavage activity,

Table 7.1 Estimated frequencies of DNA lesions normally occurring in mammalian cells

Damage	Events per cell per day	References
Oxidative DNA lesions	150,000	Barnes and Lindahl (2004); Beckman and Ames (1997); Lindahl (1993); Vilenchik and Knudson (2003)
Hydrolytic depurinations	2,000–10, 000	
Cytosine deamination to uracil	100–500	
Guanine-O6 methylation	3,100	
Guanine-8 oxydation	100–500	
Adenine-3 methylation	600	
Hydroxymethyluracils	600	
Thymine and thymidine glycols	300	
Single-strand breaks (SSBs)	5,000	
Double-strand breaks (DSBs)	10–50	
Interstrand crosslinks (ISCs)	10	
DNA-protein crosslinks	Unknown	

Table 7.2 Exogenous and endogenous factors producing Top1 cleavage complexes

Endogenous DNA lesions				Pourquier and Pommier (2001); Sordet et al. (2004b)
Single base mismatches	T	r	Polymerase and mismatch defects	Pourquier and Pommier (2001); Pourquier et al. (1997b)
Mismatched loops	T	ir	Mismatch deficiencies	Pourquier et al. (1997b)
Abasic sites	T	ir	AP sites; base excision repair	Pourquier et al. (1997b)
8-oxoguanosine	B	r	Free radicals	Lesher et al. (2002)
5-hydroxycytosine	?	r	Free radicals	Lesher et al. (2002)
Single-strand breaks	T	ir	Free radicals; base excision repair	Pourquier et al. (1997a); Wang et al. (1998)
Cytosine methylation	F+T	r	Physiological	Leteurtre et al. (1994)
Triple helix formation	F+T	r	?	Antony et al. (2004a)
Apoptotic chromatin fragmentation	B+T	ir	Appears ubiquitous during apoptosis	Sordet et al. (2003, 2004a, b, c)
Exogenous DNA lesions				Pourquier and Pommier (2001)
UV lesions	?	?	Dimers and 6,4-photoproducts	Lanza et al. (1996); Subramanian et al. (1998)
IR-induced DNA breaks	T	ir	Both single- and double-strand breaks	Pourquier et al. (1997a)
O^6-methylguanine	T	r	Produced by alkylating drugs (MNNG)	Pourquier et al. (2001)
O^6-dA-benzo[*a*]pyrene adducts	T	r	Intercalated carcinogenic adducts	Pommier et al. (2000b)
N^2-dG-benzo[*a*]pyrene adducts	F	ir	Minor groove carcinogenic adducts	Pommier et al. (2000a, 2002)
N^2-dG-benzo[*c*]phenanthrene adducts	T	r	Intercalated carcinogenic adducts	Pommier et al. (2002)
N^6-Ethenoadenine	T	r	Carcinogenic vinyl adduct	Pourquier et al. (1998)
N^2-dG-ethyl adducts	T	r	Produced by acetaldehyde (alcohol)	Antony et al. (2004b)
N^2-dG-crotonaldehyde adducts	T	ir	Exogenous carcinogens and endogenous	Dexheimer et al. (2008b)

can also have irreversible effects on Top1cc (Henningfeld et al. 1996; Henningfeld and Hecht 1995; Pourquier et al. 1999) (see Table 7.2). Two examples are shown in Fig. 7.1, where a Top1cc is converted into an irreversible Top1-DNA adduct with a gap by a preexisting nick on the scissile strand (c), or a hairpin loop on the non-scissile strand (e) (Henningfeld et al. 1996; Henningfeld and Hecht 1995; Pourquier et al. 1997a, 1999). When the nick is on the non-scissile strand, Top1cc can be converted into a DSB (Pourquier et al. 1997a; Pourquier and Pommier, 2001) (see Chap. 6).

Top1 suicide complexes such as those shown in Fig. 7.1 are highly mutagenic and can lead to recombination after a single-stranded DNA bearing a 5′-hydroxyl end attacks the Top1-tyrosyl-DNA bond even in the absence of tight complementarity (Christiansen and Westergaard 1994; Pommier et al. 1995; Shuman 1989) (see Chap. 6).

The ubiquitous nature of Top1cc generated by DNA alterations under normal conditions probably explains why all eukaryotic cells contain a tyrosyl-DNA-phosphodiesterase (TDP1) activity that excises stalled Top1 from the 3′-ends of DNA (Dexheimer et al. 2008a; Pouliot et al. 1999; Yang et al. 1996) (see Chap. 16).

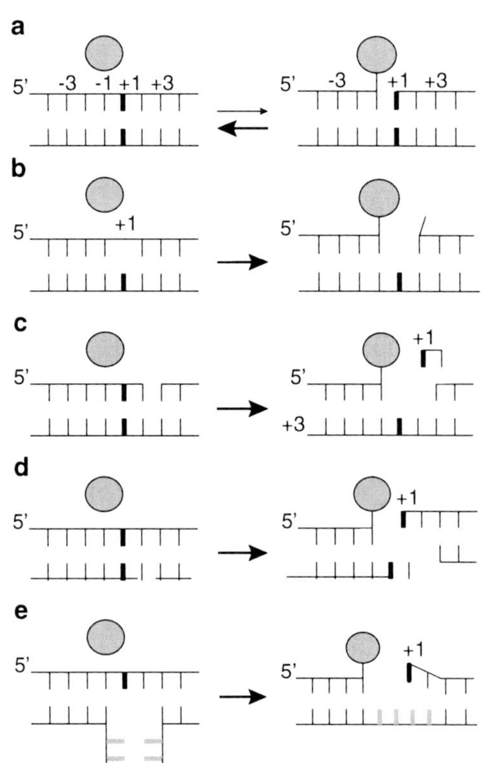

Fig. 7.1 Examples of DNA alterations that convert Top1cc into irreversible Top1 suicide complexes. (**a**) In a normal cleavage complex religation is faster than cleavage; (**b**) Presence of an abasic site at the +1 position interfere with the realignment of the +1 base and its religation; (**c**) A nick 3′-from the Top1cc lead to loss of the +1 base and the attached DNA segment (here a dinucleotide); (**d**) A nick on the non-scissile strand converts the Top1cc into an irreversible Top1 suicide complex with a double-strand break; (**e**) A hairpin loop on the non-scissile strand converts the Top1-mediated nick into an irreversible gap. Top1 is shown as *gray circle*

7.3 Trapping of Top2 by Endogenous and Carcinogenic DNA Lesions

Like Top1, Top2 is widely distributed throughout the genome and therefore is likely to encounter different forms of DNA damage (Berrios et al. 1985; Earnshaw and Heck 1985). A number of DNA lesions have been shown to alter the DNA cleavage/religation equilibrium of type II topoisomerases that lead to an increase in the concentration of Top2cc (see Table 7.3) (Deweese and Osheroff 2009b; Kingma and Osheroff 1998; Sabourin and Osheroff 2000; Velez-Cruz et al. 2005). The type II enzyme is particularly sensitive to abasic sites, alkylated bases that contain exocyclic rings, and other lesions that distort the double helix. Top2 is able to locate DNA damage even within a high background of normal bases. For example, the random inclusion of 4–5 abasic sites in a plasmid that is ~4,400 bp in length increased the concentration of Top2cc ~four- to six-fold (Kingma et al. 1995; Sabourin and Osheroff 2000). Thus, the potency of DNA lesions is ~2,000–fold higher than that of the anticancer drug etoposide. In addition, the generation of ethano-DNA lesions in human leukemia cells raises the concentration of Top2cc ~four-fold (Velez-Cruz et al. 2005).

Although DNA lesions poison both Top1 and Top2, the mechanisms by which nucleic acid damage increases levels of cleavage complexes are quite different for the two enzymes. In contrast to Top1, DNA lesions that poison Top2 increase levels of cleavage complexes primarily by stimulating the forward rate of DNA scission (Deweese et al. 2008; Kingma and Osheroff 1998). In fact, rates of religation of lesion-containing substrates are generally faster than seen with wild-type DNA sequences (Kingma et al. 1995, 1997; Kingma and Osheroff 1997a, b; Sabourin and Osheroff 2000; Velez-Cruz et al. 2005).

The effects of DNA damage on Top2 are position-specific (Kingma et al. 1997; Kingma and Osheroff 1997a, b; Sabourin and Osheroff 2000; Velez-Cruz et al. 2005; Wang et al. 1999, 2000). In general, lesions increase cleavage at naturally occurring sites of Top2 action. Furthermore, in order to enhance cleavage, lesions must be located within the four-base stagger that separates the two scissile bonds. Lesions located immediately outside of the scissile bonds generally inhibit rates of scission.

As described above, the mechanism by which damage interferes with Top1-mediated DNA religation is conceptually straightforward. In contrast, the effects of lesions on the forward rate of Top2-mediated DNA scission are less obvious and probably are related to DNA structure. Structural and enzymological studies indicate that the DNA segment that is cleaved by Top2 contains a sharp (~150°) bend (Dong and Berger 2007; Hardin et al. 2011; Schmidt et al. 2010). This bend appears to be a prerequisite for cleavage and is believed to play an important role in coordinating the two protomer subunits of the type II enzyme (Deweese et al. 2008; Deweese and Osheroff 2009a). Lesions that increase DNA flexibility or induce kinks or distortions in the double helix likely facilitate DNA bending and thus increase the rate of

Table 7.3 Exogenous and endogenous factors producing Top2 cleavage complexes

Endogenous DNA lesions	Mech[a]	Rev[b]	Notes	References (Kingma and Osheroff 1998)
Abasic sites	F	r	Apurinic and apyrimidinic sites; base excision repair	Kingma et al. (1997, 1999); Sabourin and Osheroff (2000); Velez-Cruz et al. (2005)
Processed abasic sites	F/T	r/ir	Base excision repair intermediates	Wilstermann and Osheroff (2001)
8-oxoguanine/8-oxoadenine	F	r	Free radicals; weak topoisomerase II poison	Sabourin and Osheroff (2000)
O^6-methylguanine	F	r	Free radicals; weak topoisomerase II poison	Sabourin and Osheroff (2000)
Deoxyuracil	F	r	Cytosine deamination	Kingma and Osheroff (1997b)
Base mismatches	F	r	DNA replication	Bigioni et al. (1994); Kingma and Osheroff (1997b)
Ribonucleotides	F	r	DNA replication	Wang et al. (1999, 2000)
1,N^6-ethenodeoxyadenine	F	r	Lipid peroxidation; industrial chemicals	Sabourin and Osheroff (2000); Velez-Cruz et al. (2005)
1,N^2-ethenodeoxyguanosine	F	r	Lipid peroxidation; industrial chemicals	Velez-Cruz et al. (2005)
3,N^4-ethenodeoxycytidine	F	r	Lipid peroxidation; industrial chemicals	Velez-Cruz et al. (2005)
3,N^4-ethenodeoxycytidine	F	r	Lipid peroxidation; industrial chemicals	Velez-Cruz et al. (2005)
M_1dG	F	r	Lipid peroxidation; industrial chemicals	Velez-Cruz et al. (2005)
Single-stranded DNA breaks	F, T	R, ir	Free radicals; cellular processes	Deweese et al. (2008); Deweese and Osheroff (2009a)
Exogenous DNA lesions				
UV lesions	N	r	Cyclobutane dimers	Corbett et al. (1991)
Cytosine arabinoside	F	r	AraC-induced DNA lesions	Cline and Osheroff (1999)
Ethenobase adducts	F	r	Chloracetaldehyde treatment of cells	Velez-Cruz et al. (2005)
benzo[*a*]pyrene 7,8-diol 9,10-epoxide deoxyadenosine	NA	NA	Intercalated carcinogenic adducts	Khan et al. (2003)

[a]Mechanism for Top1 cleavage complex production: T, trapping of the Top1 cleavage complexes (i.e., inhibition of religation); B, enhancement of binding; F, enhancement of the forward (cleavage) reaction; *ND* not determined; N, no effect on levels of DNA cleavage, but inhibits DNA strand passage

[b]Reversibility of the Top1 cleavage complexes: *r* reversible, *ir* irreversible

scission. This proposed mechanism accounts for the required positional specificity (i.e., between the scissile bonds) of lesions for DNA cleavage enhancement. Conversely, since lesion located outside of the scissile bonds likely induce a bend in the wrong position, they impair DNA scission at the normal site. The model also accounts for the finding that lesions that induce the largest distortion or flexibility in the double helix act as the most effective Top2 poisons.

The one group of lesions that varies from the positional requirement discussed above are DNA nicks (Deweese et al. 2008; Deweese and Osheroff 2009a). If located in the vicinity of a scissile bond, a nick can act as suicide substrates as described above for Top1 (Deweese et al. 2008; Deweese and Osheroff 2009a). In this case, non-covalently attached DNA can dissociate from the active site of Top2 following cleavage and result in an irreversible Top2cc. However, if a nick is located at one of the scissile bonds, it does not act as a suicide substrate. Rather, it increases the rate of scission at the opposite scissile bond by ~ten-fold (Deweese et al. 2008; Deweese and Osheroff 2009a). This is most likely because the presence of a nick alleviates some of the strain on the double helix in the enzyme-DNA complex and (as discussed above) allows the double helix to attain the bent transition state more readily. This process appears to be so efficient that the presence of a nick anywhere on one nucleic acid strand is sufficient to generate a Top2 DNA cleavage site four bases away on the opposite strand.

The physiological benefits of DNA lesions poisoning Top2 are unclear. However, human type II topoisomerases appear to play roles in releasing chromosomal loops during apoptosis (Belyaev 2005; Solovyan et al. 2002). It has been suggested that the apoptotic activities of Top2 are enhanced (or perhaps triggered) by DNA lesions that are generated following the release of oxidative radicals from permeable mitochondria in apoptotic cells (Belyaev 2005; Solovyan et al. 2002) (see Chap. 19). Many oxidative lesions induce little distortion in the double helix and (consequently) are poor Top2 poisons. However, most of these lesions are converted to abasic sites by the base excision repair pathway, which in turn are excellent Top2 poisons (Barnes and Lindahl 2004).

References

Antony S, Arimondo PB, Sun JS, Pommier Y (2004a) Position- and orientation-specific enhancement of topoisomerase I cleavage complexes by triplex DNA structures. *Nucleic Acids Res* **32**(17): 5163–5173

Antony S, Theruvathu JA, Brooks PJ, Lesher DT, Redinbo M, Pommier Y (2004b) Enhancement of camptothecin-induced topoisomerase I cleavage complexes by the acetaldehyde adduct N2-ethyl-2'-deoxyguanosine. *Nucleic Acids Res* **32**(18): 5685–5692

Baranello L, Bertozzi D, Fogli MV, Pommier Y, Capranico G (2010) DNA topoisomerase I inhibition by camptothecin induces escape of RNA polymerase II from promoter-proximal pause site, antisense transcription and histone acetylation at the human HIF-1alpha gene locus. *Nucleic Acids Res* **38**(1): 159–171

Barnes DE, Lindahl T (2004) Repair and genetic consequences of endogenous DNA base damage in mammalian cells. *Annu Rev Genet* **38**: 445–476

Beckman KB, Ames BN (1997) Oxidative decay of DNA. *J Biol Chem* **272**(32): 19633–19636

Belyaev IY (2005) DNA loop organization and DNA fragmentation during radiation-induced apoptosis in human lymphocytes. *Radiats Biol Radioecol* **45**(5): 541–548

Bermejo R, Doksani Y, Capra T, Katou YM, Tanaka H, Shirahige K, Foiani M (2007) Top1- and Top2-mediated topological transitions at replication forks ensure fork progression and stability and prevent DNA damage checkpoint activation. *Genes Dev* **21**(15): 1921–1936

Berrios M, Osheroff N, Fisher PA (1985) In situ localization of DNA topoisomerase II, a major polypeptide component of the Drosophila nuclear matrix fraction. *Proc Natl Acad Sci USA* **82**(12): 4142–4146

Bigioni M, Zunino F, Capranico G (1994) Base mutation analysis of topoisomerase II-idarubicin-DNA ternary complex formation. Evidence for enzyme subunit cooperativity in DNA cleavage. *Nucleic Acids Res* **22**(12): 2274–2281

Champoux JJ, Dulbecco R (1972) An activity from mammalian cells that untwists superhelical DNA--a possible swivel for DNA replication (polyoma-ethidium bromide-mouse-embryo cells-dye binding assay). *Proc Natl Acad Sci USA* **69**: 143–146

Christiansen K, Westergaard O (1994) Characterization of intra- and intermolecular DNA ligation mediated by eukaryotic topoisomerase I. *J Biol Chem* **269**: 721–729

Cline SD, Osheroff N (1999) Cytosine arabinoside (araC) lesions are position-specific topoisomerase II poisons and stimulate DNA cleavage mediated by the human type II enzymes. *J Biol Chem* **274**: 29740–29743

Corbett AH, Zechiedrich EL, Lloyd RS, Osheroff N (1991) Inhibition of eukaryotic topoisomerase II by ultraviolet-induced cyclobutane pyrimidine dimers. *J Biol Chem* **266**(29): 19666–19671

Deweese JE, Burgin AB, Osheroff N (2008) Using 3'-bridging phosphorothiolates to isolate the forward DNA cleavage reaction of human topoisomerase IIalpha. *Biochemistry* **47**(13): 4129–4140

Deweese JE, Osheroff N (2009a) Coordinating the two protomer active sites of human topoisomerase IIalpha: nicks as topoisomerase II poisons. *Biochemistry* **48**(7): 1439–1441

Deweese JE, Osheroff N (2009b) The DNA cleavage reaction of topoisomerase II: wolf in sheep's clothing. *Nucleic Acids Res* **37**(3): 738–748

Dexheimer TS, Antony S, Marchand C, Pommier Y (2008a) Tyrosyl-DNA phosphodiesterase as a target for anticancer therapy. *Anticancer Agents Med Chem* **8**(4): 381–389

Dexheimer TS, Kozekova A, Rizzo CJ, Stone MP, Pommier Y (2008b) The modulation of topoisomerase I-mediated DNA cleavage and the induction of DNA-topoisomerase I crosslinks by crotonaldehyde-derived DNA adducts. *Nucleic Acids Res* **36**(12): 4128–4136

Dong KC, Berger JM (2007) Structural basis for gate-DNA recognition and bending by type IIA topoisomerases. *Nature* **450**(7173): 1201–1205

Earnshaw WC, Heck MM (1985) Localization of topoisomerase II in mitotic chromosomes. *J Cell Biol* **100**(5): 1716–1725

Hardin AH, Sarkar SK, Seol Y, Liou GF, Osheroff N, Neuman KC (2011) Direct measurement of DNA bending by type IIA topoisomerases: implications for non-equilibrium topology simplification. *Nucleic Acids Res*

Henningfeld KA, Arslan T, Hecht SM (1996) Alteration of DNA primary structure by topoisomerase I. Isolation of the covalent topoisomerase I-DNA binary complex in enzymatically competent form. *J Am Chem Soc* **47**: 11701–11714

Henningfeld KA, Hecht S (1995) A model for topoisomerase I-mediated insertions and deletions with duplex DNA substrates containing branches, nicks, and gaps. *Biochemistry* **34**: 6120–6129

Khan QA, Kohlhagen G, Marshall R, Austin CA, Kalena GP, Kroth H, Sayer JM, Jerina DM, Pommier Y (2003) Position-specific trapping of topoisomerase II by benzo[a]pyrene diol epoxide adducts: implications for interactions with intercalating anticancer agents. *Proc Natl Acad Sci USA* **100**(21): 12498–12503

Kingma PS, Burden DA, Osheroff N (1999) Binding of etoposide to topoisomerase II in the absence of DNA: decreased affinity as a mechanism of drug resistance. *Biochemistry* **38**: 3457–3461

Kingma PS, Corbett AH, Burcham PC, Marnett LJ, Osheroff N (1995) Abasic sites stimulate double-stranded DNA cleavage mediated by topoisomerase II: anticancer drugs mimic endogenous DNA lesions. *J Biol Chem* **270**: 21441–21444

Kingma PS, Greider CA, Osheroff N (1997) Spontaneous DNA lesions poison human topoisomerase IIα and stimulate cleavage proximal to leukemic 11q23 chromosomal breakpoints. *Biochemistry* **36:** 5934–5939

Kingma PS, Osheroff N (1997a) Apurinic sites are position-specific topoisomerase II poisons. *J Biol Chem* **272**(2)**:** 1148–1155

Kingma PS, Osheroff N (1997b) Spontaneous DNA damage stimulates topoisomerase II-mediated DNA cleavage. *J Biol Chem* **272**(11)**:** 7488–7493

Kingma PS, Osheroff N (1998) The response of eukaryotic topoisomerases to DNA damage. *Biochim Biophys Acta* **1400:** 223–232

Koster DA, Croquette V, Dekker C, Shuman S, Dekker NH (2005) Friction and torque govern the relaxation of DNA supercoils by eukaryotic topoisomerase IB. *Nature* **434**(7033)**:** 671–674

Lanza A, Tornatelli S, Rodolfo C, Scanavini MC, Pedrini AM (1996) Human DNA topoisomerase I-mediated cleavages stimulated by ultraviolet light-induced DNA damage. *J Biol Chem* **271:** 6978–6986

Lesher DT, Pommier Y, Stewart L, Redinbo MR (2002) 8-Oxoguanine rearranges the active site of human topoisomerase I. *Proc Natl Acad Sci USA* **99**(19)**:** 12102–12107

Leteurtre F, Kohlhagen G, Fesen MR, Tanizawa A, Kohn KW, Pommier Y (1994) Effects of DNA methylation on topoisomerase I and II cleavage activities. *J Biol Chem* **269:** 7893–7900

Lindahl T (1993) Instability and decay of the primary structure of DNA. *Nature* **362:** 709–715

Pommier Y, Barcelo JM, Rao VA, Sordet O, Jobson AG, Thibaut L, Miao ZH, Seiler JA, Zhang H, Marchand C, Agama K, Nitiss JL, Redon C (2006) Repair of topoisomerase I-mediated DNA damage. *Prog Nucleic Acid Res Mol Biol* **81:** 179–229

Pommier Y, Jenkins J, Kohlhagen G, Leteurtre F (1995) DNA recombinase activity of eukaryotic DNA topoisomerase I; effects of camptothecin and other inhibitors. *Mutat Res* **337**(2)**:** 135–145

Pommier Y, Kohlhagen G, Laco GS, Kroth H, Sayer JM, Jerina DM (2002) Different effects on human topoisomerase I by minor groove and intercalated deoxyguanosine adducts derived from two polycyclic aromatic hydrocarbon diol epoxides at or near a normal cleavage site. *J Biol Chem* **277**(16)**:** 13666–13672

Pommier Y, Kohlhagen G, Pourquier P, Sayer JM, Kroth H, Jerina DM (2000a) Benzo[a]pyrene epoxide adducts in DNA are potent inhibitors of a normal topoisomerase I cleavage site and powerful inducers of other topoisomerase I cleavages. *Proc Natl Acad Sci USA* **97:** 2040–2045

Pommier Y, Laco GS, Kohlhagen G, Sayer JM, Kroth H, Jerina DM (2000b) Position-specific trapping of topoisomerase I-DNA cleavage complexes by intercalated benzo[a]-pyrene diol epoxide adducts at the 6-amino group of adenine. *Proc Natl Acad Sci USA* **97**(20)**:** 10739–10744

Pommier Y, Poddevin B, Gupta M, Jenkins J (1994) DNA topoisomerases I & II cleavage sites in the type 1 human immunodeficiency virus (HIV-1) DNA promoter region. *Biochem Biophys Res Commun* **205**(3)**:** 1601–1609

Porter SE, Champoux JJ (1989) Mapping in vivo topoisomerase I sites on simian virus 40 DNA: asymmetric distribution of sites on replicating molecules. *Mol Cell Biol* **9**(2)**:** 541–550

Pouliot JJ, Yao KC, Robertson CA, Nash HA (1999) Yeast gene for a Tyr-DNA phosphodiesterase that repairs topo I covalent complexes. *Science* **286:** 552–555

Pourquier P, Bjornsti M-A, Pommier Y (1998) Induction of topoisomerase I cleavage complexes by the vinyl chloride adduct, 1,*N*6-ethenoadenine. *J Biol Chem* **273:** 27245–27249

Pourquier P, Jensen AD, Gong SS, Pommier Y, Rogler CE (1999) Human DNA topoisomerase I-mediated cleavage and recombination of duck hepatitis B virus DNA in vitro. *Nucleic Acids Res* **27**(8)**:** 1919–1925

Pourquier P, Pilon A, Kohlhagen G, Mazumder A, Sharma A, Pommier Y (1997a) Trapping of mammalian topoisomerase I and recombinations induced by damaged DNA containing nicks or gaps: importance of DNA end phosphorylation and camptothecin effects. *J Biol Chem* **272:** 26441–26447

Pourquier P, Pommier Y (2001) Topoisomerase I-mediated DNA damage. *Adv Cancer Res* **80:** 189–216

Pourquier P, Ueng L-M, Kohlhagen G, Mazumder A, Gupta M, Kohn KW, Pommier Y (1997b) Effects of uracil incorporation, DNA mismatches, and abasic sites on cleavage and religation activities of mammalian topoisomerase I. *J Biol Chem* **272:** 7792–7796

Pourquier P, Waltman JL, Urasaki Y, Loktionova NA, Pegg AE, Nitiss JL, Pommier Y (2001) Topoisomerase I-mediated cytotoxicity of N-methyl-N'-nitro-N- nitrosoguanidine: trapping of topoisomerase I by the O6-methylguanine. *Cancer Res* **61**(1): 53–58

Sabourin M, Osheroff N (2000) Sensitivity of human type II topoisomerases to DNA damage: stimulation of enzyme-mediated DNA cleavage by abasic, oxidized and alkylated lesions. *Nucleic Acids Res* **28**(9): 1947–1954

Schmidt BH, Burgin AB, Deweese JE, Osheroff N, Berger JM (2010) A novel and unified two-metal mechanism for DNA cleavage by type II and IA topoisomerases. *Nature* **465**(7298): 641–644

Shuman S (1989) Vaccinia DNA topoisomerase I promotes illegitimate recombination in Eschrichia coli. *Proceedings of the National Academy of Sciences, USA* **86**: 3489–3493

Solovyan VT, Bezvenyuk ZA, Salminen A, Austin CA, Courtney MJ (2002) The role of topoisomerase II in the excision of DNA loop domains during apoptosis. *J Biol Chem* **277**(24): 21458–21467

Sordet O, Khan Q, Kohn KW, Pommier Y (2003) Apoptosis induced by topoisomerase inhibitors. *Curr Med Chem Anticancer Agents* **3**: 271–290

Sordet O, Khan QA, Plo I, Pourquier P, Urasaki Y, Yoshida A, Antony S, Kohlhagen G, Solary E, Saparbaev M, Laval J, Pommier Y (2004a) Apoptotic Topoisomerase I-DNA Complexes Induced by Staurosporine-mediated Oxygen Radicals. *J Biol Chem* **279**(48): 50499–50504

Sordet O, Khan QA, Pommier Y (2004b) Apoptotic Topoisomerase I-DNA Complexes Induced by Oxygen Radicals and Mitochondrial Dysfunction. *Cell Cycle* **3**(9): 1095–1097

Sordet O, Liao Z, Liu H, Antony S, Stevens EV, Kohlhagen G, Fu H, Pommier Y (2004c) Topoisomerase I-DNA complexes contribute to arsenic trioxide-induced apoptosis. *J Biol Chem* **279**(32): 33968–33975

Stewart L, Redinbo MR, Qiu X, Hol WG, Champoux JJ (1998) A model for the mechanism of human topoisomerase I. *Science* **279**(5356): 1534–1541

Subramanian D, Rosenstein BS, Muller MT (1998) Ultraviolet-induced DNA damage stimulates topoisomerase I-DNA complex formation in vivo: possible relationship with DNA repair. *Cancer Res* **58**: 976–984

Velez-Cruz R, Riggins JN, Daniels JS, Cai H, Guengerich FP, Marnett LJ, Osheroff N (2005) Exocyclic DNA lesions stimulate DNA cleavage mediated by human topoisomerase II alpha in vitro and in cultured cells. *Biochemistry* **44**(10): 3972–3981

Vilenchik MM, Knudson AG (2003) Endogenous DNA double-strand breaks: production, fidelity of repair, and induction of cancer. *Proc Natl Acad Sci USA* **100**(22): 12871–12876

Wang X, Henningfeld KA, Hecht SM (1998) DNA topoisomerase I-mediated formation of structurally modified DNA duplexes. Effects of metal ions and topoisomerase I inhibitors. *Biochemistry* **37**(8): 2691–2700

Wang Y, Knudsen BR, Bjergbaek L, Westergaard O, Andersen AH (1999) Stimulated activity of human topoisomerases IIalpha and IIbeta on RNA-containing substrates. *J Biol Chem* **274**(32): 22839–22846

Wang Y, Thyssen A, Westergaard O, Andersen AH (2000) Position-specific effect of ribonucleotides on the cleavage activity of human topoisomerase II. *Nucleic Acids Res* **28**(24): 4815–4821

Wilstermann AM, Osheroff N (2001) Base excision repair intermediates as topoisomerase II poisons. *J Biol Chem* **276**(49): 46290–46296

Yang S-W, Burgin AB, Huizenga BN, Robertson CA, Yao KC, Nash HA (1996) A eukaryotic enzyme that can disjoin dead-end covalent complexes between DNA and type I topoisomerases. *Proc Natl Acad Sci USA* **93**: 11534–11539

Yeh Y-C, Liu H-F, Ellis CA, Lu A-L (1994) Mammalian topoisomerase I has a mismatch nicking activity. *J Biol Chem* **269**: 15498–15504

Chapter 8
Topoisomerases and Carcinogenesis: Topoisomerase IIIα and BLM

Mounira Amor-Guéret and Jean-François Riou

8.1 Introduction

DNA topoisomerases are enzymes that modulate DNA topology through a smart "3 in 1" mechanism that includes successive cleavage, strand passing, and resealing of DNA. This mechanism allows the resolution of all the topological constraints on DNA that occur during replication and transcription. DNA topoisomerases are divided into two categories, type I and type II; these types transiently cleave one or two DNA strands, respectively, at a time. The two types are further divided into four subfamilies: IA, IB, IIA, and IIB (Wang 2002) (see Chap. 1). Enzymes from each subfamily share sequence homology and common features in their reaction mechanism. The type IA subfamily includes bacterial DNA topoisomerase I (the first discovered DNA topoisomerase called *ω protein*), and also bacterial topoisomerase III, archaeal reverse gyrase, yeast topoisomerase III, human topoisomerase IIIα, and human topoisomerase IIIβ (the most recently discovered enzyme). At least one type IA DNA topoisomerase is found in all organisms, excepted viruses. In contrast, type IB is not generally found in prokaryotes. *E. coli* DNA topoisomerase I represents the major activity for relaxation of negative supercoils in this organism, but the discovery of *S. cerevisiae* DNA topoisomerase III association with Sgs1 helicase (Gangloff et al. 1994) together with the coupling of a type IA topoisomerase with a helicase in the same polypeptide (Confalonieri et al. 1993) has altered the definition of the catalytic and biological functions of this class of enzymes (Duguet 1997).

M. Amor-Guéret (✉)
Institut Curie, Centre de Recherche, CNRS UMR 3348, Centre Universitaire, Batiment 110, Orsay 91405, France
e-mail: mounira.amor@curie.fr

J.-F. Riou (✉)
Régulation et Dynamique des Génomes, INSERM U565, CNRS UMR 7196, Muséum National d'Histoire Naturelle, 43 rue Cuvier, CP 26, 75005 Paris, France
e-mail: riou@mnhn.fr

Y. Pommier (ed.), *DNA Topoisomerases and Cancer*, Cancer Drug Discovery and Development, DOI 10.1007/978-1-4614-0323-4_8,

The purpose of this review is to provide a perspective of the physiological function of human topoisomerase IIIα (Top3α) and its associated helicase BLM to explain the cellular requirement for these enzymes to maintain genomic integrity and to prevent cancer.

8.2 Historical Background

The DNA topoisomerase III gene (*TOP3*) was first identified in yeast; this gene complemented a hyper-recombination mutation phenotype and presented homology to bacterial type I topoisomerase (Wallis et al. 1989). *S. cerevisiae Top3* mutants have a complex phenotype, including hyper-recombination at repetitive loci, a slow-growth phenotype with a cell cycle delay in late S/G2, hypersensitivity to DNA damaging agents, and meiotic defects. In contrast to *S. cerevisiae*, *S. pombe Top3* nulls mutants induced a loss of viability (Goodwin et al. 1999; Maftahi et al. 1999).

The Sgs1 helicase was originally discovered in a genetic screen. A mutant allele of SGS1 was identified as a suppressor of the slow-growth phenotype of *S. cerevisiae Top3* mutants and biochemical evidence demonstrated a physical interaction between Sgs1 and Top3 (Gangloff et al. 1994). Sgs1 was also identified as a protein that interacts with topoisomerase II (Watt et al. 1995) and was annotated in databases as a gene presenting genetic interactions with topoisomerase I (GENEMB7870). Sgs1 belongs to the RecQ family of DNA helicases (Umezu et al. 1990); all members studied to date are important for genomic integrity [reviewed in (Sharma et al. 2006)] and its mutant phenotype in yeast resembles that of *Top3* mutants but to a milder degree (Gangloff et al. 1994, 1999; Watt et al. 1995).

The close relationship between RecQ helicase and Top3 is maintained in higher eukaryotes. Higher eukaryotic cells have two enzymes, Top3α and Top3β (Wang 2002). Knocking out of the Top3α gene in mice results in embryonic lethality (Li and Wang 1998), whereas Top3β knock out does not affect development but reduces the life span (Kwan et al. 2003). Humans have five RecQ homologues: RECQ1, BLM, WRN, RECQ4, and RECQ5. Mutations in three of them have been implicated in genetic instability disorders. Bloom syndrome (BS) and Werner syndrome (WS) are caused by mutations in the BLM and WRN genes, respectively, whereas mutations in the RECQ4 gene are responsible of three syndromes – Rothmund Thompson, RAPADALINO, and Baller-Gerold syndrome (Kitao et al. 1999; Sharma et al. 2006; Siitonen et al. 2003; Van Maldergem et al. 2006; Yu et al. 1996). BLM and RECQ1 (RECQL) interact with Top3α (Johnson et al. 2000; Otsuki et al. 2008; Wu et al. 2000). RECQ5β, a splicing isoform of RECQ5, can interact with both Top3α and β (Shimamoto et al. 2000). In contrast, RECQ4 and WRN do not appear to interact with Top3α; the interaction with Top3β has not yet been tested. Recently, a third member of the Sgs1-Top3 complex, Rmi1, was discovered (Chang et al. 2005; Mullen et al. 2005) that is also conserved in humans (also called BLAP75) (Yin et al. 2005); Rmi1 is part of a larger complex that will be described below (for a review see (Liu and West 2008)).

8.3 The Bloom's Syndrome Protein

The BLM protein is a member of the DExH box-containing RecQ helicase subfamily (Ellis et al. 1995) displaying ATP- and Mg^{2+}-dependent 3′–5′-DNA helicase activity (Karow et al. 1997). *BLM* is the causative gene for Bloom's syndrome (Karow et al. 1997). Bloom's syndrome (BS) is a rare human autosomal recessive disorder associated with growth retardation, immunodeficiency, and early predisposition to develop all kinds of cancers that affect the general population at relatively late age. Cells from BS patients have a complex phenotype associating spontaneous hypermutability, several cytogenetic abnormalities, including an increase in the frequency of chromosome breaks, sister chromatid reunions (telomeres associations), symmetric quadriradial chromatid interchanges between homologous chromosomes, SCEs (Fig. 8.1) [reviewed in (Amor-Gueret 2004; German 1993; German et al. 1965)], and mitotic abnormalities (Fig. 8.2) (German 1969). BS cells also

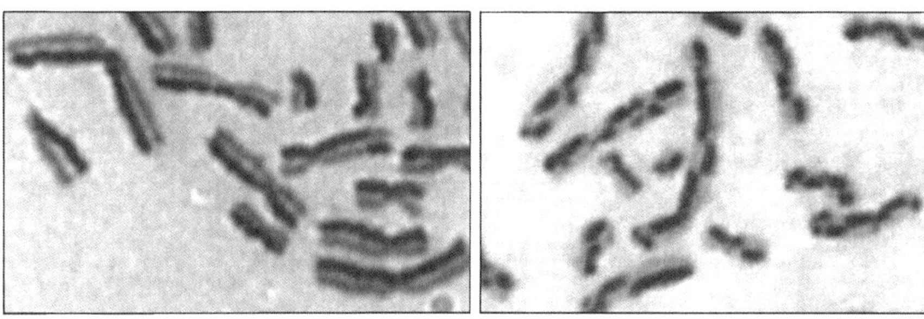

Fig. 8.1 Increased sister chromatid exchanges (SCEs) in Bloom Syndrome cells. The sister chromatids in the images are differentially labelled so that regions of chromatid exchange can be seen as regions of light and dark staining. Little chromatid exchange is seen in normal cell metaphase (*left panel*), whereas most of the chromosomes in a Bloom Syndrome cell metaphase (*right panel*) show chromatid exchange (Photos by Géraldine Buhagiar-Labarchède)

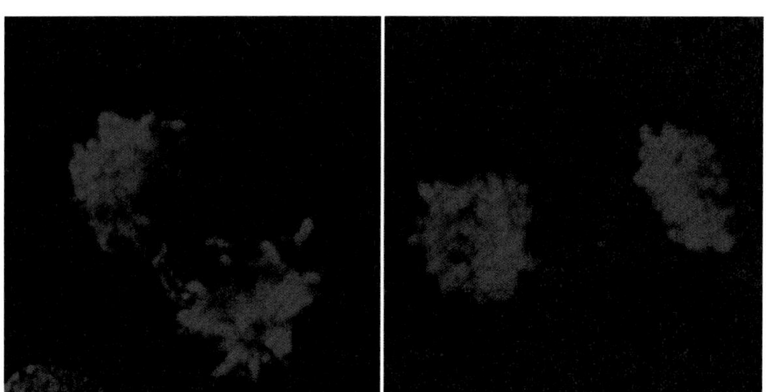

Fig. 8.2 Representative images of BLM-deficient cells presenting an anaphase bridge (*left panel*) or a lagging chromosome (*right panel*). Scale bars, 10 μm (Photos by Sébastien Rouzeau)

display a reduced average fork velocity and an increased frequency of origin firing and of stalled replication forks (Davies et al. 2007; Rao et al. 2007). The preferred substrates for recombinant BLM are G-quadruplex DNA (Mohaghegh et al. 2001; Sun et al. 1998), D-loop structures (Bachrati et al. 2006; van Brabant et al. 2000), and X-junctions (Karow et al. 2000). *In vitro*, BLM unwinds DNA structures that mimic replication forks and HR intermediates, such as D-loops, and catalyzes the branch migration of Holliday junctions (Bachrati et al. 2006; Karow et al. 2000; van Brabant et al. 2000). BLM inhibits the D-loop formation catalyzed by RAD51 by displacing RAD51 from single-stranded DNA, thereby disrupting nucleoprotein filaments (Bugreev et al. 2007). BLM resolves double Holliday junctions (dHJ) together with Top3α, Rmi1/BLAP75, and Rmi2 (Raynard et al. 2006; Wu et al. 2006) and catalyzes the regression of replication forks (Machwe et al. 2006; Ralf et al. 2006). BLM has been proposed to play a major role in the response to genotoxic stresses and in restarting stalled replication forks in association with Top3α (reviewed in (Amor-Gueret 2006; Chu and Hickson 2009). However, the specific functions of BLM remain unknown and the physiological relevance of the interaction between BLM and Top3α within the cell remains unclear.

8.4 Physical and Functional Interactions Between BLM and Topoisomerase IIIα

BLM interacts with Top3α and this interaction was reported to be mediated by its N-terminal (residues 1–212) and C-terminal (residues 1266–1417) domains (Wu et al. 2000). Both BLM and Top3α localize to promyelocytic leukemia protein nuclear bodies (PML-NBs, also referred to as ND10s or PODs) in somatic and meiotic human cells. Top3α localization is disrupted in BS cells, indicating that BLM is required for proper localization of Top3α to PML-NBs (Johnson et al. 2000). More recently, it was reported that only the first 133 amino acids of BLM are necessary and sufficient for its interaction with Top3α. This Top3α-interaction domain of BLM is not required for BLM's localization to the PML nuclear bodies, whereas it is necessary for Top3α recruitment, confirming that Top3α is recruited to the PML nuclear bodies via its interaction with BLM (Hu et al. 2001).

BLM stimulates the ability of Top3α to act upon negatively supercoiled DNA. This stimulation requires the Top3α interaction domain of BLM and the presence of either replication protein A (RPA) or single-strand binding protein (SSB), suggesting that BLM recruits Top3α to single-stranded DNA (Wu and Hickson 2002). This is further supported by the data showing that Top3α fails to show co-localization with replicating single-strand DNA sites in BLM-deficient cells, whereas the few single-strand DNA replication foci in BLM-proficient cells are associated with Top3α (Rao et al. 2007). Interestingly, greater number of Top1 and Top2 cleavage complexes are observed in transformed BS cell lines, suggesting enhanced accessibility of chromatin to topoisomerases or reduced removal rates in BLM-deficient cells (Rao et al. 2005).

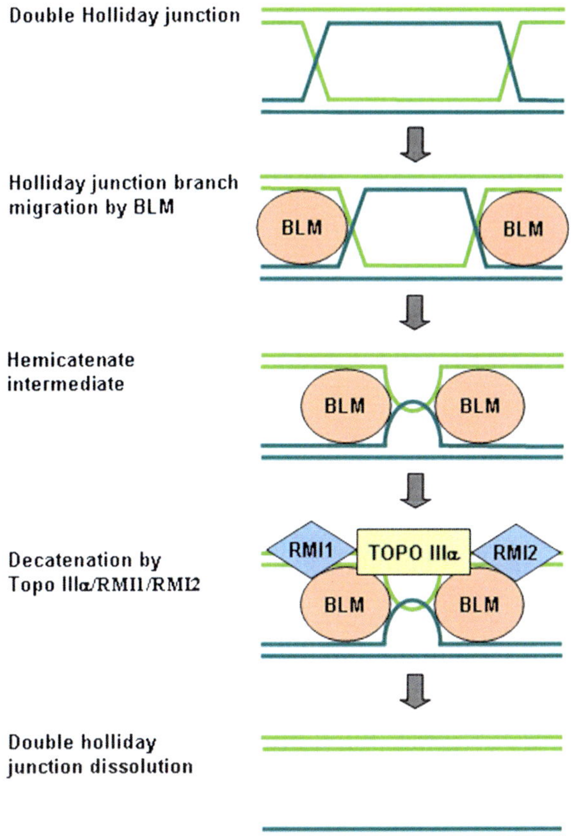

Fig. 8.3 Proposed role of the BLM/Top3α complex in the dissolution of a dHJ (modified from Mankouri and Hickson (2007)) by Sébastien Rouzeau. BLM-mediated convergent branch migration of each of the Holliday junction creates a hemicatenane intermediate that is decatenated by Topα, in association with RMI1 and RMI2

BLM cooperates specifically with Top3α to catalyze the resolution of the dHJs intermediates (that mimic converged replication forks) to generate exclusively non-crossover recombinant products in a process called "dissolution of dHJ" – to distinguish it from Holliday junction "resolution" catalyzed by resolvases (Wu and Hickson 2003). Indeed, the combination of BLM and Top3α can disentangle unlinked DNA molecules containing two adjacent Holliday junctions through BLM-mediated Holliday junction convergent branch migration followed by a Top3α-mediated decatenation of the resulting hemicatenane (Plank et al. 2006; Wu and Hickson 2003) (Fig. 8.3). Such a mechanism avoids crossover products, where the DNA flanking the original sites of the junctions is exchanged, which could be deleterious to the cell. The aberrant processing of dHJs in the absence of BLM or Top3α could account for the elevation of SCE frequency.

Importantly, the BLM-Top3α complex is tightly associated with at least one other protein called BLAP75 or RMI1 (see section "BLM-Top3α complex and the FANC pathway"). Down-regulation of BLAP75/RMI1 expression destabilizes both BLM and Top3α and results in an increase in the level of sister chromatid exchanges (SCEs), similar to that of cells depleted of BLM by siRNA

(Meetei et al. 2003; Yin et al. 2005). BLAP75/RMI1 induces a strong enhancement of the BLM-Top3α-mediated dHJ dissolution reaction (Raynard et al. 2006; Wu et al. 2006). Moreover, although BLM alone is able to unwind Holliday junctions *in vitro*, this activity is significantly enhanced by the combination of Top3α and RMI1/BLAP75 (Bussen et al. 2007).

8.5 The BLM-Top3α Complex and SCE Formation

The hallmark of BS cells and the only criterion for BS diagnosis is a high rate of SCEs (Chaganti et al. 1974). SCEs are generally thought to be the consequence of replication-dependent double-strand breaks (DSBs) and are mediated by homologous recombination dependent on RAD54 or RAD51 in human BLM-deficient cells (Lahkim Bennani-Belhaj et al. 2010; Srivastava et al. 2009). Expression of a full-length BLM in BS cells returns the number of SCEs to normal levels, whereas expression of a BLM fragment lacking the Top3α interaction domain (amino acids 133–1417) results in intermediate SCE levels. The failure of the truncated BLM protein (133–1417) to reverse SCEs to wild-type level is not due to a defect in DNA helicase activity, because immunoprecipitated 133–1417 protein has a four-fold higher activity than wild-type BLM. The BLM-Top3α complex is implicated in the regulation of recombination in somatic cells (Hu et al. 2001). This is supported by recent data showing that siRNA-mediated depletion of Top3α in normal fibroblasts increases SCEs to levels similar to those observed in response to siRNA-mediated BLM depletion (Hemphill et al. 2009).

8.6 The BLM-Topoisomerase IIIα Complex in Mitosis

8.6.1 BLM Protein

BLM production is regulated during the cell cycle; BLM protein accumulates in large amounts in S phase, persists in G2/M, and sharply decreases in amount in G1 (Dutertre et al. 2000; Sanz et al. 2000). BLM also undergoes mitosis-specific phosphorylation that strongly reduces its electrophoretic mobility. BLM phosphorylated during mitosis is excluded from the nuclear matrix and is not degraded via the ubiquitin-proteasome pathway. However, mitotic BLM phosphorylation affects neither 3′–5′ DNA helicase activity nor interaction with Top3α (Dutertre et al. 2002). Mitotic BLM is phosphorylated by ATM kinase at Thr-99 and Thr-122 (Beamish et al. 2002), by Cdc2 at Ser-714 and Thr-766 and at multiple sites not identified so far (Bayart et al. 2006), and by MPS1 at Ser-144 (Leng et al. 2006). MPS1-dependent BLM phosphorylation is required to prevent mitotic exit (Leng et al. 2006).

8.6.2 BS Cells

The BS phenotype includes a significant increase in the frequency of anaphase bridges and lagging chromosomes during cell division, indicating a defect in sister chromatid separation during mitosis (Chan et al. 2007; German 1969). BLM localizes to anaphase bridges and is required for their elimination, suggesting that BLM helps to resolve aberrant chromosome structures generated during DNA replication. Moreover, BLM is associated with DAPI-negative ultrafine DNA bridges that do not appear to contain histones (UFBs). More than half of these bridges are from centromeric origin, likely representing DNA that has been replicated but not fully decatenated (Chan et al. 2007). The frequency of centromeric UFBs is strongly increased by catalytic inhibitors of Top2. The physiological function of these bridges could be to hold sister centromeres together during metaphase in conjunction with cohesin proteins (Wang et al. 2008). UFBs of non-centromeric origin were revealed by the detection of FANCD2 and FANCI proteins as further described in the next section. The Plk-interacting checkpoint helicase (PICH) protein is also associated with UFBs (Baumann et al. 2007). PICH localization to UFBs is independent of BLM and a significant increase in the frequency of PICH-positive bridges is observed in BS cells, indicating that BLM is required for the suppression of these bridges during anaphase (Chan et al. 2007). Top3α and RMI1 also localize to anaphase bridges and their staining pattern in anaphase cells is identical to that of BLM (Chan et al. 2007). This co-localization of Top3α and RMI1 with BLM is detected in both conventional chromosomal bridges and in the BLM-DNA ultrafine bridges and is strictly dependent on BLM expression. In contrast, depletion of Top3α does not prevent BLM association with anaphase bridges (Chan et al. 2007). These data implicate the BLM-Top3α complex in regulating ploidy through a role in anaphase bridge resolution.

8.7 The BLM-Top3 α Complex and the FANC Pathway

8.7.1 FANC Proteins

Fanconi anemia (FA) is a rare autosomal recessive or X-linked disorder resulting from mutations in genes regulating replication-dependent removal of interstrand DNA crosslinks (ICL); thirteen FA complementation groups have been identified so far (subtypes A, B, C, D1 (BRCA2), D2, E, F, G, I, J (BRIP1, BACH1, Rtel), L, M, N (PALB2)). Eight of the 13 FANC proteins form a large nuclear complex, called the FANC core complex [reviewed in (Moldovan and D'Andrea 2009)]. The first connection between the BLM-Top3α complex and the FANC pathway was established when a BLM-containing complex immunopurified from HeLa nuclear extracts was found to contain RPA and Top3α, both known to interact independently with BLM (Brosh et al. 2000; Dutertre et al. 2002; Hu et al. 2001; Wu et al. 2000), several novel polypeptides termed BLAPs (for BLM-associated polypeptides), and five of the FA complementation group proteins (FANCA, FANCG, FANCC, FANCE, and FANCF). This complex has been named BRAFT (for BLM, RPA, FA, and Top3α) (Meetei et al. 2003). Subsequent studies confirmed the physical and functional relationship between BLM-Top3α and FANC pathways in both exponentially growing cells and mitotic cells.

8.7.2 Function of BLM-Top3α Complex and FA Proteins in Response to ICL

The mono-ubiquitinated isoform of FANCD2 co-localizes and interacts with BLM in response to crosslinked DNA and stalled replication forks. ICL-dependent phosphorylation of BLM is dependent upon the FA core complex: ICL-dependent phosphorylation is abolished in FA-G and FA-C cells, and restored after re-introduction of the wild-type FANCC or FANCG in the corresponding FA cell line. However, BLM is not required for the FANCA, FANCC, or FANCD2 translocation to chromatin in response to either crosslinked DNA or UVC-mediated replication arrest, indicating that the FA core complex is an upstream regulator of BLM function in response to ICL (Pichierri et al. 2004). ICL damage results in an increased number of radial chromosomal structures in BLM or Top3α-depleted cells, whereas depletion of Top3α in BS cells does not increase radials, indicating that BLM and Top3α are epistatic for suppression of radial formation. In contrast, neither depleting BLM nor Top3α in FANCD2-deficient, FANCC-deficient, or FANCA-deficient cell lines nor depleting FANCA in BS cells increases radial formation in response to crosslinked DNA, indicating that BLM and Top3α are epistatic to the FA pathway in response to ICL formation (Hemphill et al. 2009).

8.7.3 Function of BLM-Top3α and FA Proteins in Mitosis

BLM and Top3α co-localize on UFBs of centromeric origin or those associated with FA proteins (Chan and Hickson 2009). FANCD2 and FANCI form a focus at each terminus of non-centromeric bridges, marking the extremities of the so-called FA-associated UFBs (Chan et al. 2009; Naim and Rosselli 2009). The formation of FANCD2/FANCI sister foci is induced by the DNA crosslinker mitomycin C and by the replication inhibitor aphidicolin, but not by inhibition of Top2. Top2 inhibitors increase the frequency of centromeric UFBs. This indicates that mitotic FANCD2/FANCI sister foci represent sites of sister chromatid linkages, which probably derive from unresolved replication intermediates. Aphidicolin-induced FAND2 sister foci localize specifically to fragile sites, with FRA16D being a hotspot, indicating that

BLM-Top3α, RMI1, and RMI2 are required for the resolution of fragile site-associated UFBs (Chan and Hickson 2009; Chan et al. 2009; Chu and Hickson 2009). Chan et al. proposed that fragile DNA sites sometimes fail to be fully replicated before cells enter mitosis, leading to the formation of late-replication intermediates which are equivalent to sites in which two replication forks converge without the completion of the replication (Chan et al. 2009). BLM-Top3α, RMI1, and RMI2 may serve either to decatenate such unreplicated regions in late S/G2, which would suppress UFB formation, or to process the UFB DNA after it has formed in anaphase [reviewed in (Chan and Hickson 2009)].

8.8 Role of Top3α/BLM at Telomeres

8.8.1 Role of Top3α in Telomere Maintenance

Telomeres are repeated DNA sequences associated with proteins that cap chromosome ends. Telomeres are shortened at each round of cell division and two mechanisms are involved in the maintenance of telomeres. The first involves the ribonucleic telomerase complex that adds telomeric repeats at the 3′ end of chromosomes (McEachern et al. 2000). The second mechanism involves recombination between telomeres, a mechanism known in mammalian cells as Alternative Lengthening of Telomeres (ALT), which was initially identified in yeast (Cesare and Reddel 2008).

In *S. cerevisiae*, most cells that lack the genes for telomerase components enter cell cycle arrest with a low rate of survivors; survival requires RAD52-dependent homologous recombination (Lundblad and Blackburn 1993; Teng and Zakian 1999). The majority of survivors have multiple copies of the subtelomeric Y′ element and very short telomeric repeats (type I survivors), while a minor fraction of the survivors present an heterogeneous lengthening of telomeric repeats from 0.5 kb to more than 10 kb (type II survivors) (Chen et al. 2001). The generation of type II survivors was shown to depend on the presence of Sgs1p helicase; WRN or BLM can partially substitute for Sgs1p in this pathway (Cohen and Sinclair 2001; Johnson et al. 2001; Lillard-Wetherell et al. 2005).

Approximately 15% of human tumor cells display an ALT phenotype (Colgin and Reddel 1999). ALT cells are characterized by the absence of telomerase activity, heterogeneous telomere length, and the presence of nuclear foci termed ALT-associated PML bodies (APBs) that contain telomeric DNA, telomeric associated proteins such as TRF1, TRF2, and POT1, extra-chromosomal circular telomeric DNA (t-circles), and DNA recombination/repair proteins (Cesare and Reddel 2008). The latter include the MRE11/RAD50/NBS1 complex proteins and the RecQ helicases WRN and BLM that interact with TRF1 and TRF2 (Yeager et al. 1999; Grobelny et al. 2000; Stavropoulos et al. 2002; Lillard-Wetherell et al. 2004). Although the exact function of APBs is not completely understood, a close linkage among the formation of APBs, the presence of telomeric proteins, and telomere maintenance by recombination has been suggested (Jiang et al. 2005, 2007; Zhong et al. 2007). Recent evidence indicates that APBs provide a platform (called telomere clusters) where post-replicative telomere recombination intermediates are resolved (Draskovic et al. 2009). These structures maintain a spatio-temporal organisation of telomeres needed for the completion of telomere-telomere recombination reactions. Top3α associates with TRF2 and co-localizes with APBs in ALT cells (Temime-Smaali et al. 2008). Proteomic analysis of telomeric chromatin also indicated that ALT cells have a specific protein composition, which includes Top3α and BLM as specific ALT factors that differs from that of telomerase-positive cells (Dejardin and Kingston 2009).

siRNA-mediated depletion studies have indicated that Top3α is an important telomere-associated factor, essential for telomere maintenance and TRF2 stability in ALT cells (Temime-Smaali et al. 2008). In ALT cell clones with down-regulated Top3α expression, the ALT phenotype disappears and telomerase activity is reactivated (Tsai et al. 2006). A dramatic decrease in telomere length was also observed in ALT cells where BLM was depleted by shRNA (Bhattacharyya et al. 2009). In contrast, both acute and long-term depletion of Top3α or BLM in telomerase-positive cells did not induce detectable alteration of telomere length or stability (Bhattacharyya et al. 2009; Temime-Smaali et al. 2008; Tsai et al. 2006). Conversely, the capacity of over-expressed BLM to lengthen telomeres in ALT cells provides another argument that BLM can function at telomeres (Stavropoulos et al. 2002).

8.8.2 T-Loop Processing by Top3α and BLM

One of the characteristics of mammalian telomeric DNA is the presence of a 3′ single-stranded G-rich overhang. This G-overhang can invade the duplex telomere repeats, forming a D-loop structure. This telomeric structure is called a t-loop; its formation means that telomere ends are not recognized as DNA strand breaks by the DNA damage machinery (Griffith et al. 1999). The t-loop thus protects telomeres but also represents a challenge for telomere replication since the G-overhang must be both accessible to telomerase and protected from the DNA damage machinery (Wang et al. 2004). In telomerase-positive cells, the telomeric protein TRF2 is critical for repression of homologous recombination at telomeric ends (Poulet et al. 2009; Wang et al. 2004). *In vitro*, TRF2 is involved in the topological process of t-loop formation and its N-terminal basic domain induces positive supercoiling in plasmid DNA containing telomeric repeats, thus favoring G-overhang invasion into duplex telomeric sequences (Amiard et al. 2007). In contrast to TRF2, purified Top3α is able to disrupt *in vitro* strand invasion in telomeric sequences, suggesting that it may resolve t-loops at the onset of telomere replication (Riou, J.F., unpublished results). Unwinding of the telomeric D-loop is also catalyzed *in vitro* by BLM and WRN (Opresko et al. 2002). The redundancy of activities that resolve t-loops may explain why Top3α or BLM depletion in telomerase-positive cells does not affect telomere structure or length.

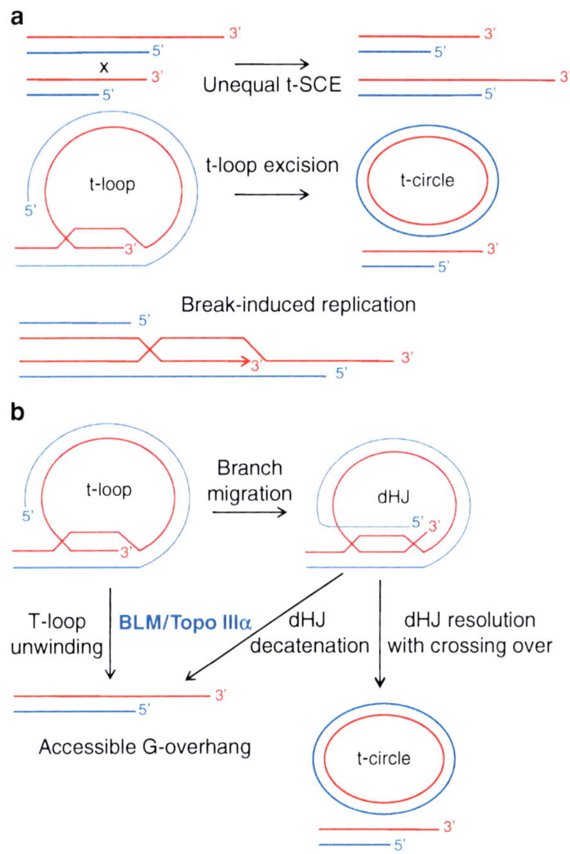

Fig. 8.4 Recombination activities at telomere and t-loop resolution (modified from Chavez et al. (2009); Royle et al. (2009)). (**a**) Recombination activities at telomeres in ALT cells: unequal t-SCE, t-loop excision, and telomere extension by BIR. (**b**) t-loop processing at telomeres and generation of t-circles: a t-loop might be unwound by BLM or Top3α or other helicases to generate a G-overhang accessible for telomere replication. In ALT cells, t-loops may branch migrate to generate a substrate with dHJ that is resolved with crossing over to form t-circles or that is processed (branch migration or dHJ decatenation/dissolution by Top3α/BLM) to generate an accessible G-overhang

In ALT cells, recombination between telomeres has been demonstrated (Cesare and Reddel 2008). Several mechanisms could account for these recombination events, including break-induced replication (BIR), unequal sister chromatid exchange (t-SCE), or a rolling t-circle amplification [for a review see (Royle et al. 2009)] (Fig. 8.4a). ALT cells have increased t-SCEs relative to normal cells, but this mechanism is thought to contribute to the observed heterogeneous length of telomeres in these cells rather than telomere length maintenance. Interestingly, the expression of a mutant form of TRF2 lacking its basic domain ($TRF2_{\Delta B}$) in telomerase-positive cells leads to stochastic loss of telomeric ends and the generation of t-circles by homologous recombination (Wang et al. 2004). The presence of t-circles is one of the hallmarks of ALT cells, suggesting that the anti-recombinogenic function of Top3α/BLM is altered in these cells. The formation of t-circles may be explained by the transformation of a t-loop into a dHJ that is further resolved by crossing over to form a t-circle (Chavez et al. 2009) (Fig. 8.4b). The direct involvement of Top3α and BLM in these processes remains to be established.

8.8.3 G-Quadruplex Regulation at Telomeres

Evidence is accumulating that non-canonical four-stranded DNA structures called G-quadruplexes can form among telomere repeats during lagging strand DNA replication and at the 3′ telomeric G-overhang (De Cian et al. 2008). A failure to resolve G-quadruplexes may lead to replication fork collapse or to uncapping of the telomeric tail (Folini et al. 2009). The use of small molecule ligands that specifically bind to the telomeric G-quadruplexes revealed that the formation of G-quadruplexes is deleterious for the stability of telomeres in both telomerase-positive and ALT cell lines (De Cian et al. 2008; Gomez et al. 2004; Riou 2004; Riou et al. 2002; Rodriguez et al. 2008; Temime-Smaali et al. 2009). Stabilization of G-quadruplexes by specific ligands impairs the binding of essential proteins such as POT1, TRF2, and Top3α to telomeres and inhibits the catalytic activity of BLM (Gomez et al. 2006; Li et al. 2001; Salvati et al. 2007; Tahara et al. 2006; Temime-Smaali et al. 2009). In ALT cells, G-quadruplex ligands induce a disruption of APBs and a depletion of the Top3/TRF2/BLM complex that mimics the phenotype induced by the siRNA depletion of Top3α (Temime-Smaali et al. 2008, 2009).

8.9 BLM-Top3α and Cancer

A program of surveillance referred to as Bloom's Syndrome Registry was established in 1960 and data on 168 BS patients (93 males, 75 females) obtained through 1991 was reported (German et al. 1977, 1979; German and Passarge 1989). One hundred types of cancers had arisen in 71 of the 168 BS patients by that time and the distribution of sites and types of cancers were similar to those found in the general population (German and Ellis 1997; German 1997). Nearly half of the registered BS patients (71/168) had at least one cancer at a mean age of 24.7; 40% of these patients had more than one primary cancer (29/71). Acute leukemias, lymphomas, and rare tumors (medulloblastoma, Wilm's tumor, osteogenic sarcoma) represented 21%, 23%, and 5% of the cancers, respectively, and predominated in the first two decades of life, whereas carcinomas represented 51% of the cancers and generally appeared late in the second decade (Amor-Gueret 2004).

Some genetic variants of *BLM* and of its interacting partners *Top3α* and *RMI1* are reported to have an impact on cancer risk in the general population (Broberg et al. 2009). In *BLM*, the single nucleotide polymorphism (SNP) rs401549 is associated with increased risk for bladder cancer but not for malignant melanoma, whereas patients with rs2532105 have increased risk for malignant melanoma, bladder cancer, and breast cancer but not for acute myeloid leukemia/myelodysplastic syndrome (AML/MDS). In AML/MDS, *BLM* rs393974 and rs6496724 are also associated with cancer risk. In the *Top3α* gene, rs12945597 is associated with increased risk for AML/MDS and malignant melanoma but not for bladder cancer, whereas the rs12945597 is associated with increased breast cancer risk. In *RMI1*, the SNP rs296887 is associated with increased risk for AML/MDS and malignant melanoma but not for bladder cancer. An allele-dosage effect was reported for the combination of rs12945597 (*Top3α*) and rs2532105 (*BLM*) for AML/MDS, bladder and breast cancer. However, except for the *TOP3α* rs12945597 and *BLM* rs2532105 for which the association was significant, the authors indicate that the results need to be validated in a larger cohort (Broberg et al. 2009).

8.10 Conclusions

Collectively, genetic, cellular, and biochemical evidence supports a major role for the BLM/Top3α complex in preventing the formation of SCEs during S phase. BLM, in association with Top3α, is located at both UFBs and conventional anaphase bridges during mitosis, thus these proteins have a structural function necessary during chromosome segregation and the late decatenation processes. Despite the lack of genome wide studies, it is clear that BLM/Top3α substrates are found in parts of the genome where non-canonical DNA structures are present, including telomeres where t-loop and G-quadruplexes structures are present. These findings suggest that BLM/Top3α may represent potential therapeutic targets for manipulating telomere functions especially in cancers characterized by the ALT phenotype.

Acknowledgments Supported by the «Ligue Nationale contre le Cancer, Equipes Labellisées» (J.F.R.), Cancéropôle/Région Ile-de-France (J.F.R. and M.A.G.) and by the "Institut Curie" and CNRS (M.A.G.).

References

Amiard, S., Doudeau, M., Pinte, S., Poulet, A., Lenain, C., Faivre-Moskalenko, C., Angelov, D., Hug, N., Vindigni, A., Bouvet, P., *et al.* (2007). A topological mechanism for TRF2-enhanced strand invasion. Nat Struct Mol Biol *14*, 147–154.

Amor-Gueret, M. (2004). Bloom's syndrome. Orphanet Encyclopedia http://www.orpha.net/data/patho/GB/uk-Bloomsyndrome.pdf.

Amor-Gueret, M. (2006). Bloom syndrome, genomic instability and cancer: the SOS-like hypothesis. Cancer Lett *236*, 1–12.

Bachrati, C.Z., Borts, R.H., and Hickson, I.D. (2006). Mobile D-loops are a preferred substrate for the Bloom's syndrome helicase. Nucleic Acids Res *34*, 2269–2279.

Baumann, C., Korner, R., Hofmann, K., and Nigg, E.A. (2007). PICH, a centromere-associated SNF2 family ATPase, is regulated by Plk1 and required for the spindle checkpoint. Cell *128*, 101–114.

Bayart, E., Dutertre, S., Jaulin, C., Guo, R.B., Xi, X.G., and Amor-Gueret, M. (2006). The Bloom syndrome helicase is a substrate of the mitotic Cdc2 kinase. Cell Cycle *5*, 1681–1686.

Beamish, H., Kedar, P., Kaneko, H., Chen, P., Fukao, T., Peng, C., Beresten, S., Gueven, N., Purdie, D., Lees-Miller, S., *et al.* (2002). Functional link between BLM defective in Bloom's syndrome and the ataxia-telangiectasia-mutated protein, ATM. J Biol Chem *277*, 30515–30523.

Bhattacharyya, S., Keirsey, J., Russell, B., Kavecansky, J., Lillard-Wetherell, K., Tahmaseb, K., Turchi, J.J., and Groden, J. (2009). Telomerase-associated protein 1, HSP90, and topoisomerase

IIalpha associate directly with the BLM helicase in immortalized cells using ALT and modulate its helicase activity using telomeric DNA substrates. J Biol Chem *284*, 14966–14977.

Broberg, K., Huynh, E., Schlawicke Engstrom, K., Bjork, J., Albin, M., Ingvar, C., Olsson, H., and Hoglund, M. (2009). Association between polymorphisms in RMI1, TOP3A, and BLM and risk of cancer, a case-control study. BMC Cancer *9*, 140.

Brosh, R.M., Jr., Li, J.L., Kenny, M.K., Karow, J.K., Cooper, M.P., Kureekattil, R.P., Hickson, I.D., and Bohr, V.A. (2000). Replication protein A physically interacts with the Bloom's syndrome protein and stimulates its helicase activity. J Biol Chem *275*, 23500–23508.

Bugreev, D.V., Yu, X., Egelman, E.H., and Mazin, A.V. (2007). Novel pro- and anti-recombination activities of the Bloom's syndrome helicase. Genes Dev *21*, 3085–3094.

Bussen, W., Raynard, S., Busygina, V., Singh, A.K., and Sung, P. (2007). Holliday junction processing activity of the BLM-Topo IIIalpha-BLAP75 complex. J Biol Chem *282*, 31484–31492.

Cesare, A.J., and Reddel, R.R. (2008). Telomere uncapping and alternative lengthening of telomeres. Mech Ageing Dev *129*, 99–108.

Chaganti, R.S., Schonberg, S., and German, J. (1974). A manyfold increase in sister chromatid exchanges in Bloom's syndrome lymphocytes. Proc Natl Acad Sci USA *71*, 4508–4512.

Chan, K.L., and Hickson, I.D. (2009). On the origins of ultra-fine anaphase bridges. Cell Cycle *8*, 3065–3066.

Chan, K.L., North, P.S., and Hickson, I.D. (2007). BLM is required for faithful chromosome segregation and its localization defines a class of ultrafine anaphase bridges. EMBO J *26*, 3397–3409.

Chan, K.L., Palmai-Pallag, T., Ying, S., and Hickson, I.D. (2009). Replication stress induces sister-chromatid bridging at fragile site loci in mitosis. Nat Cell Biol *11*, 753–760.

Chang, M., Bellaoui, M., Zhang, C., Desai, R., Morozov, P., Delgado-Cruzata, L., Rothstein, R., Freyer, G.A., Boone, C., and Brown, G.W. (2005). RMI1/NCE4, a suppressor of genome instability, encodes a member of the RecQ helicase/Topo III complex. Embo J *24*, 2024–2033.

Chavez, A., Tsou, A.M., and Johnson, F.B. (2009). Telomeres do the (un)twist: helicase actions at chromosome termini. Biochim Biophys Acta *1792*, 329–340.

Chen, Q., Ijpma, A., and Greider, C.W. (2001). Two survivor pathways that allow growth in the absence of telomerase are generated by distinct telomere recombination events. Mol Cell Biol *21*, 1819–1827.

Chu, W.K., and Hickson, I.D. (2009). RecQ helicases: multifunctional genome caretakers. Nat Rev Cancer *9*, 644–654.

Cohen, H., and Sinclair, D.A. (2001). Recombination-mediated lengthening of terminal telomeric repeats requires the Sgs1 DNA helicase. Proc Natl Acad Sci USA *98*, 3174–3179.

Colgin, L.M., and Reddel, R.R. (1999). Telomere maintenance mechanisms and cellular immortalization. Curr Opin Genet Dev *9*, 97–103.

Confalonieri, F., Elie, C., Nadal, M., de La Tour, C., Forterre, P., and Duguet, M. (1993). Reverse gyrase: a helicase-like domain and a type I topoisomerase in the same polypeptide. Proc Natl Acad Sci USA *90*, 4753–4757.

Davies, S.L., North, P.S., and Hickson, I.D. (2007). Role for BLM in replication-fork restart and suppression of origin firing after replicative stress. Nat Struct Mol Biol *14*, 677–679.

De Cian, A., Lacroix, L., Douarre, C., Temime-Smaali, N., Trentesaux, C., Riou, J.F., and Mergny, J.L. (2008). Targeting telomeres and telomerase. Biochimie *90*, 131–155.

Dejardin, J., and Kingston, R.E. (2009). Purification of proteins associated with specific genomic Loci. Cell *136*, 175–186.

Draskovic, I., Arnoult, N., Steiner, V., Bacchetti, S., Lomonte, P., and Londono-Vallejo, A. (2009). Probing PML body function in ALT cells reveals spatiotemporal requirements for telomere recombination. Proc Natl Acad Sci USA *106*, 15726–15731.

Duguet, M. (1997). When helicase and topoisomerase meet! J Cell Sci *110 (Pt 12)*, 1345–1350.

Dutertre, S., Ababou, M., Onclercq, R., Delic, J., Chatton, B., Jaulin, C., and Amor-Gueret, M. (2000). Cell cycle regulation of the endogenous wild type Bloom's syndrome DNA helicase. Oncogene *19*, 2731–2738.

Dutertre, S., Sekhri, R., Tintignac, L.A., Onclercq-Delic, R., Chatton, B., Jaulin, C., and Amor-Gueret, M. (2002). Dephosphorylation and Subcellular Compartment Change of the Mitotic Bloom's Syndrome DNA Helicase in Response to Ionizing Radiation. J Biol Chem *277*, 6280–6286.

Ellis, N.A., Groden, J., Ye, T.Z., Straughen, J., Lennon, D.J., Ciocci, S., Proytcheva, M., and German, J. (1995). The Bloom's syndrome gene product is homologous to RecQ helicases. Cell *83*, 655–666.

Folini, M., Gandellini, P., and Zaffaroni, N. (2009). Targeting the telosome: therapeutic implications. Biochim Biophys Acta *1792*, 309–316.

Gangloff, S., de Massy, B., Arthur, L., Rothstein, R., and Fabre, F. (1999). The essential role of yeast topoisomerase III in meiosis depends on recombination. Embo J *18*, 1701–1711.

Gangloff, S., McDonald, J.P., Bendixen, C., Arthur, L., and Rothstein, R. (1994). The yeast type I topoisomerase Top3 interacts with Sgs1, a DNA helicase homolog: a potential eukaryotic reverse gyrase. Mol Cell Biol *14*, 8391–8398.

German, D.C., and Ellis, A. (1997). Bloom syndrome. In *The genetic basis of human cancer*, D.C.a.E. German, A., ed. (Vogelstein B., Kinzler K.W.), pp. 733–751.

German, J. (1969). Bloom's syndrome. I. Genetical and clinical observations in the first twenty-seven patients. Am J Hum Genet *21*, 196–227.

German, J. (1993). Bloom syndrome: a mendelian prototype of somatic mutational disease. Medicine (Baltimore) *72*, 393–406.

German, J. (1997). Bloom's syndrome. XX. The first 100 cancers. Cancer Genet Cytogenet *93*, 100–106.

German, J., Archibald, R., and Bloom, D. (1965). Chromosomal Breakage in a Rare and Probably Genetically Determined Syndrome of Man. Science *148*, 506–507.

German, J., Bloom, D., and Passarge, E. (1977). Bloom's syndrome. V. Surveillance for cancer in affected families. Clin Genet *12*, 162–168.

German, J., Bloom, D., and Passarge, E. (1979). Bloom's syndrome. VII. Progress report for 1978. Clin Genet *15*, 361–367.

German, J., and Passarge, E. (1989). Bloom's syndrome. XII. Report from the Registry for 1987. Clin Genet *35*, 57–69.

Gomez, D., Paterski, R., Lemarteleur, T., Shin-Ya, K., Mergny, J.L., and Riou, J.F. (2004). Interaction of telomestatin with the telomeric single-strand overhang. J Biol Chem *279*, 41487–41494.

Gomez, D., Wenner, T., Brassart, B., Douarre, C., O'Donohue, M.F., El Khoury, V., Shin-Ya, K., Morjani, H., Trentesaux, C., and Riou, J.F. (2006). Telomestatin-induced telomere uncapping is modulated by POT1 through G-overhang extension in HT1080 human tumor cells. J Biol Chem *281*, 38721–38729.

Goodwin, A., Wang, S.W., Toda, T., Norbury, C., and Hickson, I.D. (1999). Topoisomerase III is essential for accurate nuclear division in Schizosaccharomyces pombe. Nucleic Acids Res *27*, 4050–4058.

Griffith, J.D., Comeau, L., Rosenfield, S., Stansel, R.M., Bianchi, A., Moss, H., and de Lange, T. (1999). Mammalian telomeres end in a large duplex loop. Cell *97*, 503–514.

Grobelny, J.V., Godwin, A.K., and Broccoli, D. (2000). ALT-associated PML bodies are present in viable cells and are enriched in cells in the G(2)/M phase of the cell cycle. J Cell Sci *113*, 4577–4585.

Hemphill, A.W., Akkari, Y., Newell, A.H., Schultz, R.A., Grompe, M., North, P.S., Hickson, I.D., Jakobs, P.M., Rennie, S., Pauw, D., *et al.* (2009). Topo IIIalpha and BLM act within the Fanconi anemia pathway in response to DNA-crosslinking agents. Cytogenet Genome Res *125*, 165–175.

Hu, P., Beresten, S.F., van Brabant, A.J., Ye, T.Z., Pandolfi, P.P., Johnson, F.B., Guarente, L., and Ellis, N.A. (2001). Evidence for BLM and Topoisomerase IIIalpha interaction in genomic stability. Hum Mol Genet *10*, 1287–1298.

Jiang, W.Q., Zhong, Z.H., Henson, J.D., Neumann, A.A., Chang, A.C., and Reddel, R.R. (2005). Suppression of alternative lengthening of telomeres by Sp100-mediated sequestration of the MRE11/RAD50/NBS1 complex. Mol Cell Biol *25*, 2708–2721.

Jiang, W.Q., Zhong, Z.H., Henson, J.D., and Reddel, R.R. (2007). Identification of candidate alternative lengthening of telomeres genes by methionine restriction and RNA interference. Oncogene.

Johnson, F.B., Lombard, D.B., Neff, N.F., Mastrangelo, M.A., Dewolf, W., Ellis, N.A., Marciniak, R.A., Yin, Y., Jaenisch, R., and Guarente, L. (2000). Association of the Bloom syndrome protein with topoisomerase IIIalpha in somatic and meiotic cells. Cancer Res *60*, 1162–1167.

Johnson, F.B., Marciniak, R.A., McVey, M., Stewart, S.A., Hahn, W.C., and Guarente, L. (2001). The Saccharomyces cerevisiae WRN homolog Sgs1p participates in telomere maintenance in cells lacking telomerase. Embo J *20*, 905–913.

Karow, J.K., Chakraverty, R.K., and Hickson, I.D. (1997). The Bloom's syndrome gene product is a 3'-5' DNA helicase. J Biol Chem *272*, 30611–30614.

Karow, J.K., Constantinou, A., Li, J.L., West, S.C., and Hickson, I.D. (2000). The Bloom's syndrome gene product promotes branch migration of holliday junctions. Proc Natl Acad Sci USA *97*, 6504–6508.

Kitao, S., Shimamoto, A., Goto, M., Miller, R.W., Smithson, W.A., Lindor, N.M., and Furuichi, Y. (1999). Mutations in RECQL4 cause a subset of cases of Rothmund-Thomson syndrome. Nat Genet *22*, 82–84.

Kwan, K.Y., Moens, P.B., and Wang, J.C. (2003). Infertility and aneuploidy in mice lacking a type IA DNA topoisomerase III beta. Proc Natl Acad Sci USA *100*, 2526–2531.

Lahkim Bennani-Belhaj, K., Rouzeau, S., Buhagiar-Labarchede, G., Chabosseau, P., Onclercq-Delic, R., Bayart, E., Cordelieres, F., Couturier, J., and Amor-Gueret, M. (2010). The Bloom syndrome protein limits the lethality associated with RAD51 deficiency. Mol Cancer Res *8*, 385–394.

Leng, M., Chan, D.W., Luo, H., Zhu, C., Qin, J., and Wang, Y. (2006). MPS1-dependent mitotic BLM phosphorylation is important for chromosome stability. Proc Natl Acad Sci USA *103*, 11485–11490.

Li, J.L., Harrison, R.J., Reszka, A.P., Brosh, R.M., Jr., Bohr, V.A., Neidle, S., and Hickson, I.D. (2001). Inhibition of the Bloom's and Werner's syndrome helicases by G-quadruplex interacting ligands. Biochemistry *40*, 15194–15202.

Li, W., and Wang, J.C. (1998). Mammalian DNA topoisomerase IIIalpha is essential in early embryogenesis. Proc Natl Acad Sci USA *95*, 1010–1013.

Lillard-Wetherell, K., Combs, K.A., and Groden, J. (2005). BLM helicase complements disrupted type II telomere lengthening in telomerase-negative sgs1 yeast. Cancer Res *65*, 5520–5522.

Lillard-Wetherell, K., Machwe, A., Langland, G.T., Combs, K.A., Behbehani, G.K., Schonberg, S.A., German, J., Turchi, J.J., Orren, D.K., and Groden, J. (2004). Association and regulation of the BLM helicase by the telomere proteins TRF1 and TRF2. Hum Mol Genet *13*, 1919–1932.

Liu, Y., and West, S.C. (2008). More complexity to the Bloom's syndrome complex. Genes Dev *22*, 2737–2742.

Lundblad, V., and Blackburn, E.H. (1993). An alternative pathway for yeast telomere maintenance rescues est1- senescence. Cell *73*, 347–360.

Machwe, A., Xiao, L., Groden, J., and Orren, D.K. (2006). The Werner and Bloom syndrome proteins catalyze regression of a model replication fork. Biochemistry *45*, 13939–13946.

Maftahi, M., Han, C.S., Langston, L.D., Hope, J.C., Zigouras, N., and Freyer, G.A. (1999). The top3(+) gene is essential in Schizosaccharomyces pombe and the lethality associated with its loss is caused by Rad12 helicase activity. Nucleic Acids Res *27*, 4715–4724.

Mankouri, H.W., and Hickson, I.D. (2007). The RecQ helicase-topoisomerase III-Rmi1 complex: a DNA structure-specific 'dissolvasome'? Trends Biochem Sci *32*, 538–546.

McEachern, M.J., Krauskopf, A., and Blackburn, E.H. (2000). Telomeres and their control. Annu Rev Genet *34*, 331–358.

Meetei, A.R., Sechi, S., Wallisch, M., Yang, D., Young, M.K., Joenje, H., Hoatlin, M.E., and Wang, W. (2003). A multiprotein nuclear complex connects Fanconi anemia and Bloom syndrome. Mol Cell Biol *23*, 3417–3426.

Mohaghegh, P., Karow, J.K., Brosh Jr, R.M., Jr., Bohr, V.A., and Hickson, I.D. (2001). The Bloom's and Werner's syndrome proteins are DNA structure-specific helicases. Nucleic Acids Res *29*, 2843–2849.

Moldovan, G.L., and D'Andrea, A.D. (2009). How the fanconi anemia pathway guards the genome. Annu Rev Genet *43*, 223–249.

Mullen, J.R., Nallaseth, F.S., Lan, Y.Q., Slagle, C.E., and Brill, S.J. (2005). Yeast Rmi1/Nce4 controls genome stability as a subunit of the Sgs1-Top3 complex. Mol Cell Biol *25*, 4476–4487.

Naim, V., and Rosselli, F. (2009). The FANC pathway and BLM collaborate during mitosis to prevent micro-nucleation and chromosome abnormalities. Nat Cell Biol *11*, 761–768.

Opresko, P.L., von Kobbe, C., Laine, J.P., Harrigan, J., Hickson, I.D., and Bohr, V.A. (2002). Telomere-binding protein TRF2 binds to and stimulates the Werner and Bloom syndrome helicases. J Biol Chem *277*, 41110–41119.

Otsuki, M., Seki, M., Inoue, E., Abe, T., Narita, Y., Yoshimura, A., Tada, S., Ishii, Y., and Enomoto, T. (2008). Analyses of functional interaction between RECQL1, RECQL5, and BLM which physically interact with DNA topoisomerase IIIalpha. Biochim Biophys Acta *1782*, 75–81.

Pichierri, P., Franchitto, A., and Rosselli, F. (2004). BLM and the FANC proteins collaborate in a common pathway in response to stalled replication forks. EMBO J *23*, 3154–3163.

Plank, J.L., Wu, J., and Hsieh, T.S. (2006). Topoisomerase IIIalpha and Bloom's helicase can resolve a mobile double Holliday junction substrate through convergent branch migration. Proc Natl Acad Sci USA *103*, 11118–11123.

Poulet, A., Buisson, R., Faivre-Moskalenko, C., Koelblen, M., Amiard, S., Montel, F., Cuesta-Lopez, S., Bornet, O., Guerlesquin, F., Godet, T., *et al.* (2009). TRF2 promotes, remodels and protects telomeric Holliday junctions. EMBO J *28*, 641–651.

Ralf, C., Hickson, I.D., and Wu, L. (2006). The Bloom's syndrome helicase can promote the regression of a model replication fork. J Biol Chem *281*, 22839–22846.

Rao, V.A., Conti, C., Guirouilh-Barbat, J., Nakamura, A., Miao, Z.H., Davies, S.L., Sacca, B., Hickson, I.D., Bensimon, A., and Pommier, Y. (2007). Endogenous gamma-H2AX-ATM-Chk2 checkpoint activation in Bloom's syndrome helicase deficient cells is related to DNA replication arrested forks. Mol Cancer Res *5*, 713–724.

Rao, V.A., Fan, A.M., Meng, L., Doe, C.F., North, P.S., Hickson, I.D., and Pommier, Y. (2005). Phosphorylation of BLM, dissociation from topoisomerase IIIalpha, and colocalization with gamma-H2AX after topoisomerase I-induced replication damage. Mol Cell Biol *25*, 8925–8937.

Raynard, S., Bussen, W., and Sung, P. (2006). A double Holliday junction dissolvasome comprising BLM, topoisomerase IIIalpha, and BLAP75. J Biol Chem *281*, 13861–13864.

Riou, J.F. (2004). G-quadruplex interacting agents targeting the telomeric G-overhang are more than simple telomerase inhibitors. Curr Med Chem Anticancer Agents *4*, 439–443.

Riou, J.F., Guittat, L., Mailliet, P., Laoui, A., Renou, E., Petitgenet, O., Megnin-Chanet, F., Helene, C., and Mergny, J.L. (2002). Cell senescence and telomere shortening induced by a new series of specific G-quadruplex DNA ligands. Proc Natl Acad Sci USA *99*, 2672–2677.

Rodriguez, R., Muller, S., Yeoman, J.A., Trentesaux, C., Riou, J.F., and Balasubramanian, S. (2008). A novel small molecule that alters shelterin integrity and triggers a DNA-damage response at telomeres. J Am Chem Soc *130*, 15758–15759.

Royle, N.J., Mendez-Bermudez, A., Gravani, A., Novo, C., Foxon, J., Williams, J., Cotton, V., and Hidalgo, A. (2009). The role of recombination in telomere length maintenance. Biochem Soc Trans *37*, 589–595.

Salvati, E., Leonetti, C., Rizzo, A., Scarsella, M., Mottolese, M., Galati, R., Sperduti, I., Stevens, M.F., D'Incalci, M., Blasco, M., *et al.* (2007). Telomere damage induced by the G-quadruplex ligand RHPS4 has an antitumor effect. J Clin Invest *117*, 3236–3247.

Sanz, M.M., Proytcheva, M., Ellis, N.A., Holloman, W.K., and German, J. (2000). BLM, the Bloom's syndrome protein, varies during the cell cycle in its amount, distribution, and co-localization with other nuclear proteins. Cytogenet Cell Genet *91*, 217–223.

Sharma, S., Doherty, K.M., and Brosh, R.M., Jr. (2006). Mechanisms of RecQ helicases in pathways of DNA metabolism and maintenance of genomic stability. Biochem J *398*, 319–337.

Shimamoto, A., Nishikawa, K., Kitao, S., and Furuichi, Y. (2000). Human RecQ5beta, a large isomer of RecQ5 DNA helicase, localizes in the nucleoplasm and interacts with topoisomerases 3alpha and 3beta. Nucleic Acids Res *28*, 1647–1655.

Siitonen, H.A., Kopra, O., Kaariainen, H., Haravuori, H., Winter, R.M., Saamanen, A.M., Peltonen, L., and Kestila, M. (2003). Molecular defect of RAPADILINO syndrome expands the phenotype spectrum of RECQL diseases. Hum Mol Genet *12*, 2837–2844.

Srivastava, V., Modi, P., Tripathi, V., Mudgal, R., De, S., and Sengupta, S. (2009). BLM helicase stimulates the ATPase and chromatin-remodeling activities of RAD54. J Cell Sci.

Stavropoulos, D.J., Bradshaw, P.S., Li, X., Pasic, I., Truong, K., Ikura, M., Ungrin, M., and Meyn, M.S. (2002). The Bloom syndrome helicase BLM interacts with TRF2 in ALT cells and promotes telomeric DNA synthesis. Hum Mol Genet *11*, 3135–3144.

Sun, H., Karow, J.K., Hickson, I.D., and Maizels, N. (1998). The Bloom's syndrome helicase unwinds G4 DNA. J Biol Chem *273*, 27587–27592.

Tahara, H., Shin-Ya, K., Seimiya, H., Yamada, H., Tsuruo, T., and Ide, T. (2006). G-Quadruplex stabilization by telomestatin induces TRF2 protein dissociation from telomeres and anaphase bridge formation accompanied by loss of the 3′ telomeric overhang in cancer cells. Oncogene *25*, 1955–1966.

Temime-Smaali, N., Guittat, L., Sidibe, A., Shin-ya, K., Trentesaux, C., and Riou, J.F. (2009). The G-quadruplex ligand telomestatin impairs binding of topoisomerase IIIalpha to G quadruplex-forming oligonucleotides and uncaps telomeres in ALT cells. PLoS One *4*, e6919.

Temime Smaali, N., Guittat, L., Wenner, T., Bayart, E., Douarre, C., Gomez, D., Giraud-Panis, M.J., Londono-Vallejo, A., Gilson, E., Amor-Gueret, M., *et al.* (2008). Topoisomerase IIIalpha is required for normal proliferation and telomere stability in alternative lengthening of telomeres. EMBO J *27*, 1513–1524.

Teng, S.C., and Zakian, V.A. (1999). Telomere-telomere recombination is an efficient bypass pathway for telomere maintenance in Saccharomyces cerevisiae. Mol Cell Biol *19*, 8083–8093.

Tsai, H.J., Huang, W.H., Li, T.K., Tsai, Y.L., Wu, K.J., Tseng, S.F., and Teng, S.C. (2006). Involvement of topoisomerase III in telomere-telomere recombination. J Biol Chem *281*, 13717–13723.

Umezu, K., Nakayama, K., and Nakayama, H. (1990). Escherichia coli RecQ protein is a DNA helicase. Proc Natl Acad Sci USA *87*, 5363–5367.

van Brabant, A.J., Ye, T., Sanz, M., German, I.J., Ellis, N.A., and Holloman, W.K. (2000). Binding and melting of D-loops by the Bloom syndrome helicase. Biochemistry *39*, 14617–14625.

Van Maldergem, L., Siitonen, H.A., Jalkh, N., Chouery, E., De Roy, M., Delague, V., Muenke, M., Jabs, E.W., Cai, J., Wang, L.L., *et al.* (2006). Revisiting the craniosynostosis-radial ray hypoplasia association: Baller-Gerold syndrome caused by mutations in the RECQL4 gene. J Med Genet *43*, 148–152.

Wallis, J.W., Chrebet, G., Brodsky, G., Rolfe, M., and Rothstein, R. (1989). A hyper-recombination mutation in S. cerevisiae identifies a novel eukaryotic topoisomerase. Cell *58*, 409–419.

Wang, J.C. (2002). Cellular roles of DNA topoisomerases: a molecular perspective. Nat Rev Mol Cell Biol *3*, 430–440.

Wang, L.H., Schwarzbraun, T., Speicher, M.R., and Nigg, E.A. (2008). Persistence of DNA threads in human anaphase cells suggests late completion of sister chromatid decatenation. Chromosoma *117*, 123–135.

Wang, R.C., Smogorzewska, A., and de Lange, T. (2004). Homologous recombination generates T-loop-sized deletions at human telomeres. Cell *119*, 355–368.

Watt, P.M., Louis, E.J., Borts, R.H., and Hickson, I.D. (1995). Sgs1: a eukaryotic homolog of E. coli RecQ that interacts with topoisomerase II in vivo and is required for faithful chromosome segregation. Cell *81*, 253–260.

Wu, L., Bachrati, C.Z., Ou, J., Xu, C., Yin, J., Chang, M., Wang, W., Li, L., Brown, G.W., and Hickson, I.D. (2006). BLAP75/RMI1 promotes the BLM-dependent dissolution of homologous recombination intermediates. Proc Natl Acad Sci USA *103*, 4068–4073.

Wu, L., Davies, S.L., North, P.S., Goulaouic, H., Riou, J.F., Turley, H., Gatter, K.C., and Hickson, I.D. (2000). The Bloom's syndrome gene product interacts with topoisomerase III. J Biol Chem *275*, 9636–9644.

Wu, L., and Hickson, I.D. (2002). The Bloom's syndrome helicase stimulates the activity of human topoisomerase IIIalpha. Nucleic Acids Res *30*, 4823–4829.

Wu, L., and Hickson, I.D. (2003). The Bloom's syndrome helicase suppresses crossing over during homologous recombination. Nature *426*, 870–874.

Yeager, T.R., Neumann, A.A., Englezou, A., Huschtscha, L.I., Noble, J.R., and Reddel, R.R. (1999). Telomerase-negative immortalized human cells contain a novel type of promyelocytic leukemia (PML) body. Cancer Res *59*, 4175–4179.

Yin, J., Sobeck, A., Xu, C., Meetei, A.R., Hoatlin, M., Li, L., and Wang, W. (2005). BLAP75, an essential component of Bloom's syndrome protein complexes that maintain genome integrity. Embo J *24*, 1465–1476.

Yu, C.E., Oshima, J., Fu, Y.H., Wijsman, E.M., Hisama, F., Alisch, R., Matthews, S., Nakura, J., Miki, T., Ouais, S., *et al.* (1996). Positional cloning of the Werner's syndrome gene. Science *272*, 258–262.

Zhong, Z.H., Jiang, W.Q., Cesare, A.J., Neumann, A.A., Wadhwa, R., and Reddel, R.R. (2007). Disruption of telomere maintenance by depletion of the MRE11/RAD50/NBS1 complex in cells that use alternative lengthening of telomeres. J Biol Chem *282*, 29314–29322.

Chapter 9
Topoisomerases Inhibitors: A Paradigm for Interfacial Inhibition

Christophe Marchand and Yves Pommier

9.1 Interfacial Versus Orthosteric and Allosteric Inhibition

For several decades, drug development has been based on the discovery and development of pharmacological inhibitors that block biological processes by preventing the binding of a natural ligand to a particular receptor site. These competitive inhibitors belong to the category of ligands described by Paul Ehrlich in his "key and lock" theory 100 years ago and are often referred to as orthosteric inhibitors to differentiate them from allosteric inhibitors. Allostery has been conceptualized by Monod, Changeux, and Jacob (Monod et al. 1963). Allosteric inhibition applies to inhibitors that bind to a site topologically distinct from the receptor site, which results in a distant propagating effect that remotely affects the ligand affinity for its receptor site. An allosteric effect can also be generated by positive regulators that results in the stimulation of the receptor (Christopoulos 2002).

Interfacial inhibitors differ from orthosteric and allosteric inhibitors because they bind at the interface of two or more macromolecules as the multimeric complex undergoes a structural transition. These macromolecules may or may not exhibit catalytic activities and may be formed by proteins such as tubulin dimer inhibited by colchicines and paclitaxel [Taxol®] (Pommier and Cherfils 2005), or by a combination of proteins and nucleic acids such as topoisomerases trapped on DNA by their respective poisons (Pommier and Marchand 2005).

C. Marchand (✉)
Laboratory of Molecular Pharmacology, Center for Cancer Research,
National Cancer Institute, National Institutes of Health, Bethesda, MD 20892, USA
e-mail: marchanc@mail.nih.gov

Y. Pommier (ed.), *DNA Topoisomerases and Cancer*, Cancer Drug Discovery and Development, DOI 10.1007/978-1-4614-0323-4_9,

9.2 Camptothecin Derivatives: First Example of Interfacial Inhibitors

Camptothecin (CPT, Fig. 9.1f) is an alkaloid first isolated from the bark of the Chinese tree *Camptotheca acuminata* as a potent anticancer drug. CPT was discovered and initially studied in the 1960s by Wall, Wani, and colleagues under contract for the National Cancer Institute (Kepler et al. 1969) well before it was found to target Top1 (Hsiang et al. 1985). The same group also discovered the tubulin inhibitor taxol (paclitaxel) (Wall and Wani 1995). CPT derivatives are now widely used in cancer therapy. The FDA approved the use of two water-soluble CPT derivatives for cancer treatment approximately 10 years ago. Irinitotecan (CPT-11, Camptosar®) is used for the treatment of colorectal carcinomas and topotecan (Hycamtin®, Fig. 9.1f) for the treatment of ovarian and small cell lung cancers (see Chaps. 10 and 12).

CPT is a heterocyclic planar compound with several critical characteristics (Fig. 9.1f). First, only the natural enantiomer (20S) inhibits Top1 but not the synthetic 20R (Hsiang et al. 1989; Jaxel et al. 1989; Wall and Wani 1995). Second, CPT traps Top1 transiently and cleavage complexes reverse rapidly upon drug washout, heating a 65°C or addition of salt (Fig. 9.1a–c) (Covey et al. 1989; Hsiang et al. 1985; Jaxel et al. 1988; Porter and Champoux 1989; Tanizawa et al. 1994). Finally, CPT does not bind to DNA nor to Top1 by itself, it requires the presence of both

Fig. 9.1 Structure of the topoisomerase I cleavage complex trapped by CPT. (**a**, **b**) Top1 nicking-closing reaction. (**a**) Top1 is generally bound non-covalently to DNA. The Top1 catalytic tyrosine (Y723 for human nuclear Top1) is represented in *red* (*Y*). (**a–b**) Top1 cleaves one strand of the duplex as it forms a covalent phosphodiester bond between the catalytic tyrosine and the 3′-DNA terminus. The other DNA terminus is a 5′-hydroxyl (OH). (**b**) The Top1 cleavage complex allows rotation of the 5′-terminus around the intact strand, which relaxes DNA supercoiling (*purple dotted circle with arrowhead*). (**b–a**) Following DNA relaxation, Top1 religates the DNA. Under normal conditions, the religation (closing) reaction rate constant is much higher than the cleavage (nicking) rate constant. More than 90% of the Top1-DNA complexes are non-covalent. (**c**) CPT traps the Top1 cleavage complex by binding at the enzyme-DNA interface between the base pairs flanking the Top1-mediated DNA cleavage site (by convention positions −1 and +1). The colors for the base pairs −2 (*pink*), −1 (*green*), +1 (*blue*) and +2 (*orange*) are the same as in Fig. 9.2. (**d**, **e**) Lateral views of a Top1-DNA complex trapped by CPT (shown in *cyan* with nitrogen and oxygen atoms in *blue and red*, respectively, PDB ID code 1T8I (Staker et al. 2005)). (**d**) Top1 (*orange*) is shown in a surface view to represent the depth of the CPT binding pocket (PDB ID code 1T8I (Staker et al. 2005)). (**e**) Top1 is represented in ribbon diagram to allow visualization of the catalytic tyrosine (*Y*; *red*) and to show the drug intercalation between the −1 and +1 base pairs. (**f**) Chemical structure of CPT. (**g**) Stacking of CPT between two base pairs flanking the Top1 cleavage complex is a common mechanism for other Top1 poisons (Marchand et al. 2006). The left view is oriented as in panels (**d**, **e**) with the DNA viewed from the minor groove. The right view is rotated 90° and show the +1 base pair covering the drug molecule. The catalytic Top1 tyrosine is shown in *red* (*Y*) at the top of the left view. The −1 and +1 base pairs are marked by *dashed arrows*. In the right view, the colored numbers correspond to the drug atoms numbered in panel F. (**h**) Hydrogen bond networks between CPT and Top1 amino acid residues in the drug-Top1-DNA ternary complexes. CPT forms three hydrogen bonds with Asp533, Asn722 and Arg364 (Staker et al. 2005)

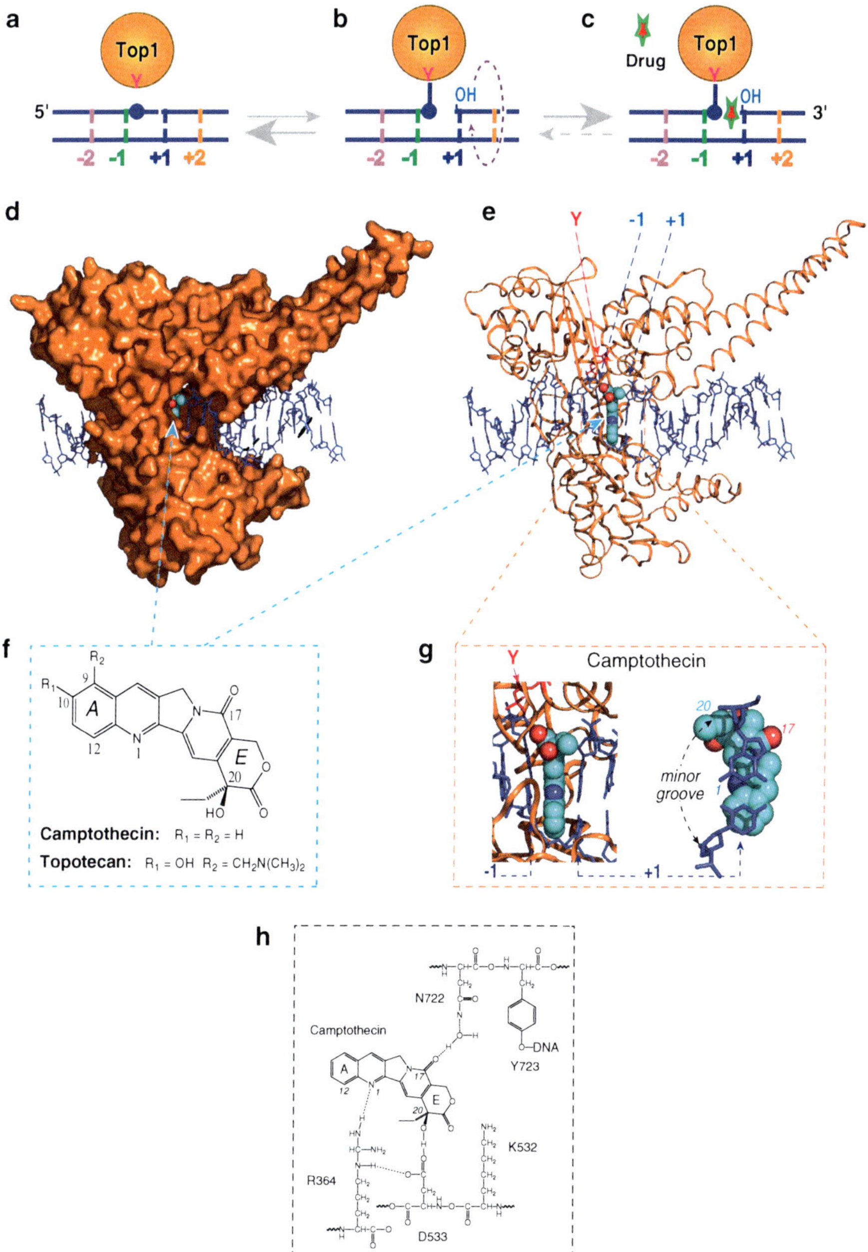
a
Top1
Y
5'
-2 -1 +1 +2
b
Top1
Y
OH
-2 -1 +1
c
Drug
Top1
Y
OH
3'
-2 -1 +1 +2
d
e
Y
-1
+1
f
Camptothecin: R1 = R2 = H
Topotecan: R1 = OH R2 = CH2N(CH3)2
g
Camptothecin
Y
20
17
minor groove
1
-1
+1
h
N722
Camptothecin
O–DNA
Y723
K532
R364
D533

Top1 and DNA associated in a cleavage complex (Hertzberg et al. 1989, 1990; Hsiang et al. 1985; Jaxel et al. 1991; Leteurtre et al. 1993; Pommier et al. 1995). This observation led to the hypothesis that CPT binds at the interface of both Top1 and DNA in a ternary complex (Jaxel et al. 1991). This hypothesis was confirmed 13 years later by the determination of the crystal structure of a ternary Top1 cleavage complex with topotecan, the clinical CPT analog (Staker et al. 2002).

The X-ray structure of CPT in the Top1-DNA complex later revealed that CPT binding is superimposable with the one of topotecan (Fig. 9.1d and e) (Ioanoviciu et al. 2005; Marchand et al. 2006; Staker et al. 2005). This particular binding mode is also common among other non-CPT Top1 inhibitors such as the indenoisoquinolines, norindenoisoquinolines, and indolocarbazoles (Ioanoviciu et al. 2005; Marchand et al. 2006; Staker et al. 2005). The co-crystal structure of CPT bound to the cleavage complex reveals that the drug is deeply bound inside the cleavage site of Top1 (Fig. 9.1d), and intercalated between the base pairs flanking the cleavage site (positions −1 and +1, Fig. 9.1e and g). Moreover, analysis of the contacts between CPT and Top1 residues revealed that CPT also binds Top1 by a network of hydrogen bonds involving residues N722 (adjacent to the catalytic Y723), D533, and R364 (Fig. 9.1h). Mutation of any of these residues leads to CPT resistance (Pommier et al. 1999) although it does not prevent the formation of crystal structures with CPT in a ternary complex with the mutated enzyme (Chrencik et al. 2004). Also, very informative was the recent finding that the mutation N722S, which was identified in a human leukemia cell lines selected for resistance to CPT (Fujimori et al. 1995) is present in plants that synthesize CPT (Sirikantaramas et al. 2008) and makes those plants immune to the camptothecin derivative they produce.

Both the −1 and +1 base pairs stack against the entire surface of CPT (Fig. 9.1g) and their twist angle is reduced from the normal 37° (Fig. 9.2a, the theoretical twist angle is 36°) to approximately 20° (Fig. 9.2d). In contrast with the trapping of Top1 by norindenoisoquinoline (Marchand et al. 2006), this reduction of DNA twist angle at the cleavage site is not compensated by an overwinding of the adjacent +1 and +2 base pairs. In the case of CPT, these +1 and +2 adjacent base pairs are also unwound with a twist angle of 25° (Fig. 9.2e). The entire cleavage site seems unwound with a twist angle of only 84° between −2 and +2 base pairs (Fig. 9.2b) as compared to a theoretical twist angle of 108°. This underwinding is not compensated by the −2 and −1 base pair that have a normal, twist angle of 39° (Fig. 9.2c). This may explain why camptothecin binds more tightly and inhibit better Top1 cleavage complexes in positively supercoiled DNA (Gentry et al. 2011; Koster et al. 2007).

9.3 Generalization of the Interfacial Inhibition Paradigm to Topoisomerase II-Targeted Drugs

In fact, the concept of planar drug binding in the topoisomerase cleavage site was first proposed around 1990 (Capranico et al. 1990a; Pommier et al. 1991) to explain the drug-specific base-sequence selectivity of various anticancer topoisomerase II (Top2) inhibitors [for recent reviews see (Capranico and Binaschi 1998;

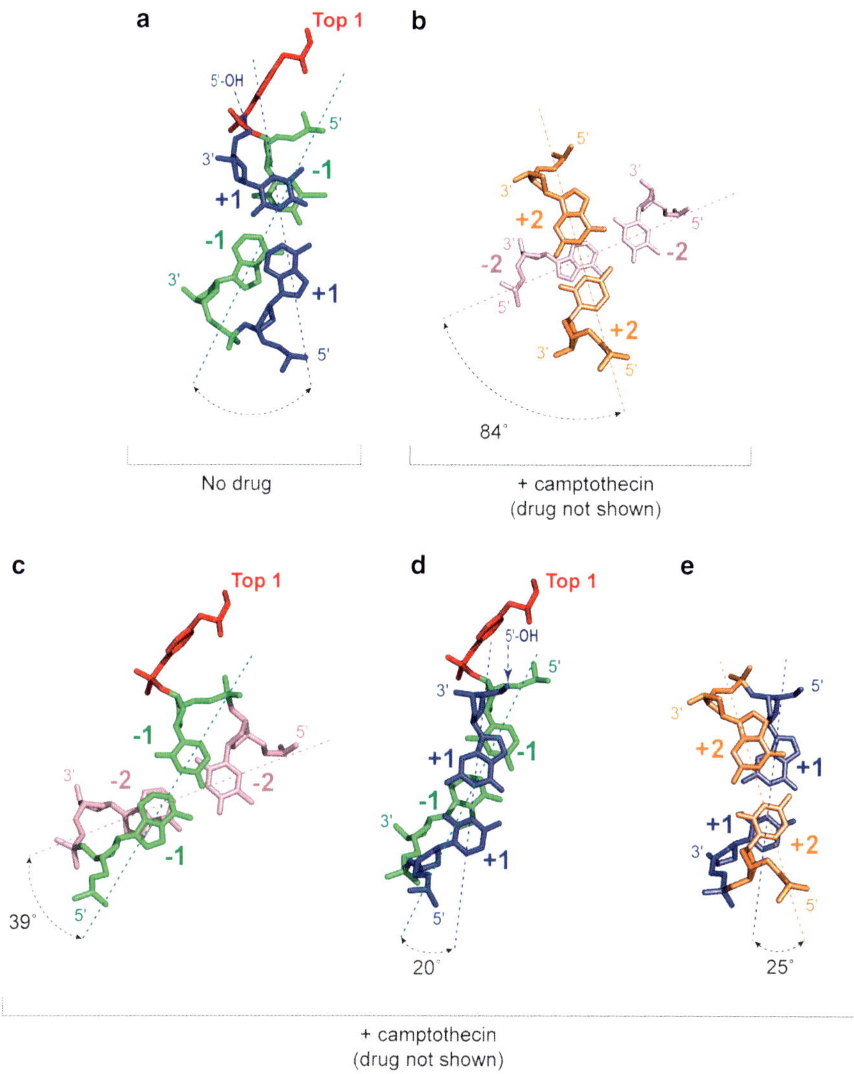

Fig. 9.2 DNA unwinding by CPT at the topoisomerase I cleavage complex. The color code is the same as in Fig. 9.1a–c. (**a**) Twist angle between the base pairs flanking the Top1 cleavage site in the absence of inhibitor (PDB ID Code 1A31 (Redinbo et al. 1998)). The *thin dashed lines* correspond to the base pair long axes. The +1 base pair is colored *dark blue* and the −1 base pair *green*. (**b**) Twist angle between the −2 and +2 base pairs flanking the Top1 cleavage site trapped by CPT (PDB ID code 1T8I (Staker et al. 2005)). The drug has been removed to only show the −2 and +2 nucleotides. The nucleotides are positioned similarly to *panel A*. The *thin dashed lines* correspond to the base pair long axes. (**c**) Twist angle between the −1 and −2 base pairs. (**d**) Twist angle between the −1 and +1 base pairs. (**e**) Twist angle between the +1 and +2 base pairs

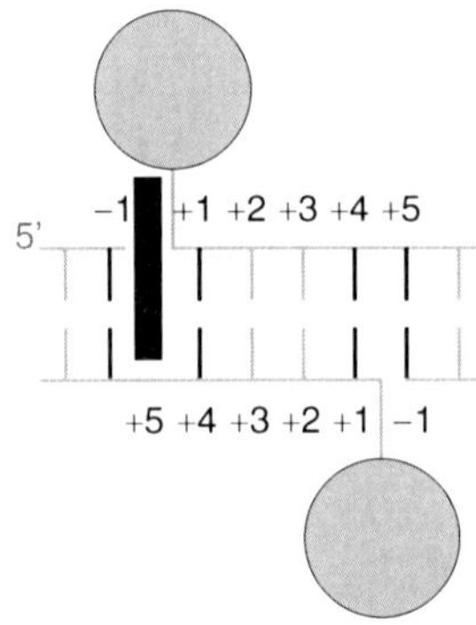

Drug	Base −1	Base +1
Doxorubicin	A	
Amsacrine		A
Etoposide	C	
Mitoxanthrone	C/T	
Ellipticine	T	
Bisanthrene		A
Genistein	T	

Fig. 9.3 Interfacial inhibition by anticancer Top2-targeted drugs. The left scheme shows a schematic representation of the Top2 cleavage complex. Each monomer is shown as *gray circle* and the base pairs are numbered according to their position from the cleavage sites. Top2 poisons have been proposed to bind at the interface of the DNA break (between bases −1 and +1) and Top2. Base sequence preferences are summarized at right. Original information on base sequences preferences can be found in (Capranico and Binaschi 1998; Capranico et al. 1990a, b, 1993; De Isabella et al. 1993, 1995; Leteurtre et al. 1994; Pommier et al. 1991, 2010; Sissi et al. 1998)

Pommier et al. 2010)]. Human Top2 is inhibited by a variety of anticancer agents (see Chaps. 11 and 13) that have been proposed to bind in an interfacial manner (Fig. 9.3). These anticancer agents include the epipodophyllotoxins (teniposide and etoposide) (Pommier et al. 1991), anthracyclines (doxorubicin, daunorubicin, epirubicin) (Capranico et al. 1990a), mitoxantrone (Leteurtre et al. 1994), or ellipticines (Capranico and Binaschi 1998) (see Chap. 11).

Another type of interfacial inhibition has been described for the catalytic inhibitors of Top2 represented by the bisdioxopiperazines ICRF-193 and its chemotherapeutic derivative dexrazoxane (ICRF-187) (Andoh 1998; Classen et al. 2003; Ishida et al. 1994) (see Chap. 11). In this complex, Top2 does not cleave DNA and the enzyme homodimer is trapped encircling both DNA double helices after religation of the passing strand (Pommier et al. 2010). Dexrazoxane binds to a site at the interface of the ATP domains of two Top2 molecules and therefore stabilizes Top2 in this trapped intermediate (Classen et al. 2003).

Bacterial Type II topoisomerases such as gyrase and Topo IV are also the targets of interfacial inhibitors [recently reviewed in (Pommier et al. 2010)]. Because Type II bacterial topoisomerases are essential for bacterial replication, these topoisomerases are prime targets for antibiotics. This approach offers several advantages. First, accumulation of cleavage complexes has a bactericidal effect. Second, antibacterial topoisomerase-targeted therapy does not interfere with the host human topoisomerases. Finally, antibacterial topoisomerase inhibitors usually target both gyrase and Topo IV due to their high level of structural similarities. Quinolone antibiotics represent the best example of bacterial Type II topoisomerase poisons. Quinolone antibiotics were originally limited to Gram-negative bacteria but the introduction of fluorine in their structure broadened their antibacterial spectrum. Several generations of fluoroquinolone antibiotics have now been developed to provide some of the most potent antibiotics available to date such as ciprofloxacin (Fig. 9.4e)

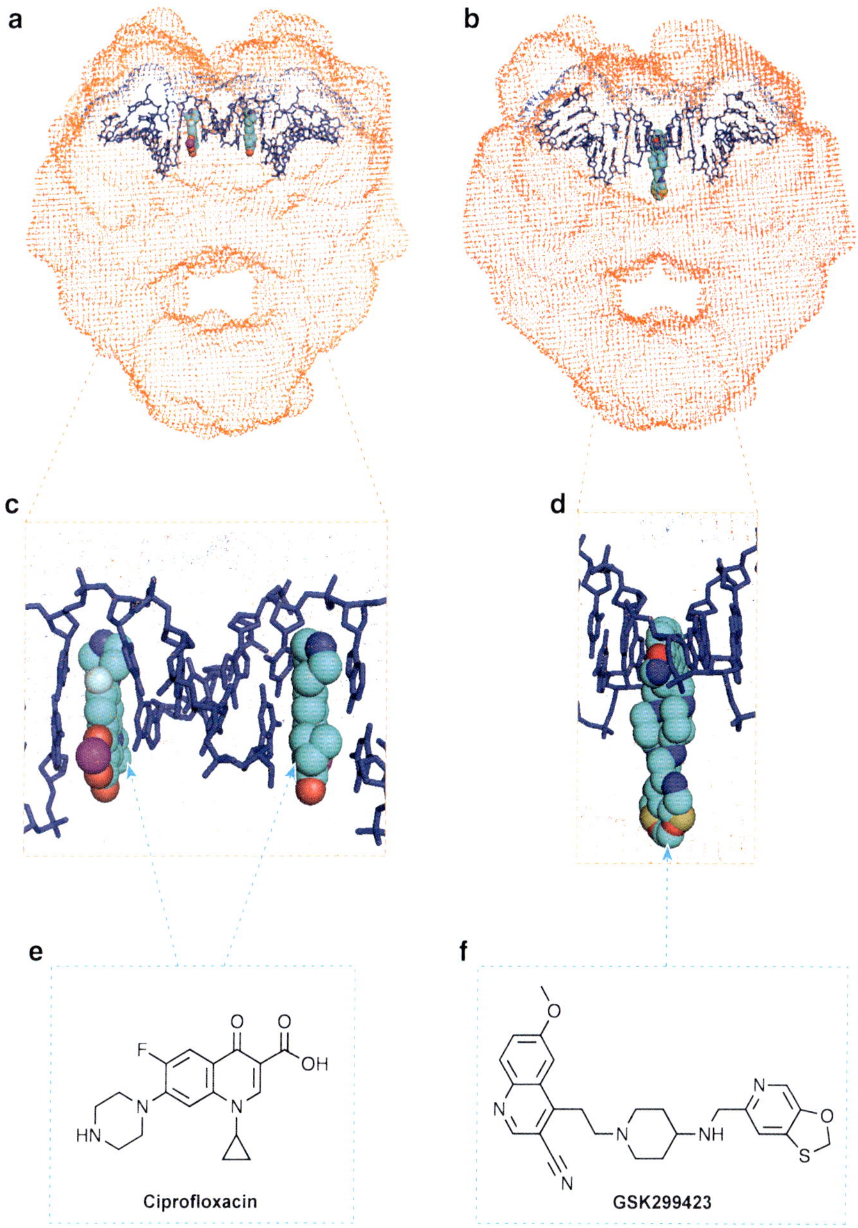

Fig. 9.4 Interfacial inhibition by Type II bacterial topoisomerase poisons. (**a**) Overview of the gyrase A cleavage complex trapped by ciprofloxacin (PDB ID code 2XCT (Bax et al. 2010)). (**b**) Overview of the gyrase A uncleaved complexed poisoned by GSK299423 [PDB ID code 2XCS (Bax et al. 2010)]. (**c**) Intercalation of ciprofloxacin (shown in *cyan* with nitrogen and oxygen atoms in *blue and red*, respectively) in the DNA breaks between the base pairs flanking each cleavage site of gyrase A. Catalytic manganese is represented in *magenta*. (**d**) Intercalation of GSK299423 (shown in *cyan* with nitrogen and oxygen and sulfur atoms in *blue, red and yellow*, respectively) in the uncleaved DNA at the interface of two gyrase A subunits. (**e**) Structure of ciprofloxacin. (**f**) Structure of GSK299423

(Pommier et al. 2010). Similarly to other topoisomerase poisons, fluoroquinolones trap bacterial Type II topoisomerases in a stabilized cleavage complex by stacking between the two base pairs flanking the cleavage site at the interface of a GyrA (gyrase, Fig. 9.4a and c) or a Par C (Topo IV) subunit dimer (Heddle et al. 2000; Laponogov et al. 2009). Recently, a novel class of bacterial Type II topoisomerases inhibitor that overcomes resistance to fluoroquinolone antibiotics has been reported by GlaxoSmithKline (Bax et al. 2010) (Fig. 9.4f). This novel inhibitor bridges the DNA and a transient non-hydrophobic pocket at the interface of a GyrA subunit dimer in the *Staphylococcus aureus* gyrase (Fig. 9.4b). The inhibitor binds in a site median from both cleavage sites and the resulting ternary complex is trapped in an uncleaved state (Bax et al. 2010) (Fig. 9.4d).

9.4 Generalization of the Interfacial Inhibition for Drug Discovery

The interfacial inhibition concept has implications for drug discovery since screening assays should also be designed to search for compounds that stabilize and not only inhibit the formation of macromolecular complexes. Such assays have the potential to lead to the discovery highly selective inhibitors of pharmacological targets.

References

Andoh T (1998) Bis(2,6-dioxopiperazines), catalytic inhibitors of DNA topoisomerase II, as molecular probes, cardioprotectors and antitumor drugs. *Biochimie* **80:** 235–246

Bax BD, Chan PF, Eggleston DS, Fosberry A, Gentry DR, Gorrec F, Giordano I, Hann MM, Hennessy A, Hibbs M, Huang J, Jones E, Jones J, Brown KK, Lewis CJ, May EW, Saunders MR, Singh O, Spitzfaden CE, Shen C, Shillings A, Theobald AJ, Wohlkonig A, Pearson ND, Gwynn MN (2010) Type IIA topoisomerase inhibition by a new class of antibacterial agents. *Nature* **466**(7309)**:** 935–940

Capranico G, Binaschi M (1998) DNA sequence selectivity of topoisomerases and topoisomerase poisons. *Biochim Biophys Acta* **1400**(1–3)**:** 185–194

Capranico G, De Isabella P, Tinelli S, Bigioni S, Zunino F (1993) Similar sequence specificity of mitoxantrone and VM-26 stimulation of in vitro DNA cleavage by mammalian DNA topoisomerase II. *Biochemistry* **32:** 3032–3048

Capranico G, Kohn KW, Pommier Y (1990a) Local sequence requirements for DNA cleavage by mammalian topoisomerase II in the presence of doxorubicin. *Nucleic Acids Res* **18**(22)**:** 6611–6619

Capranico G, Zunino F, Kohn KW, Pommier Y (1990b) Sequence-selective topoisomerase II inhibition by anthracycline derivatives in SV40 DNA: relationship with DNA binding affinity and cytotoxicity. *Biochemistry* **29**(2)**:** 562–569

Chrencik JE, Staker BL, Burgin AB, Pourquier P, Pommier Y, Stewart L, Redinbo MR (2004) Mechanisms of camptothecin resistance by human topoisomerase I mutations. *J Mol Biol* **339**(4)**:** 773–784

Christopoulos A (2002) Allosteric binding sites on cell-surface receptors: novel targets for drug discovery. *Nat Rev Drug Discov* **1**(3): 198–210

Classen S, Olland S, Berger JM (2003) Structure of the topoisomerase II ATPase region and its mechanism of inhibition by the chemotherapeutic agent ICRF-187. *Proc Natl Acad Sci USA* **100**(19): 10629–10634

Covey JM, Jaxel C, Kohn KW, Pommier Y (1989) Protein-linked DNA strand breaks induced in Mammalian cells by camptothecin, an inhibitor of topoisomerase I. *Cancer Res* **49:** 5016–5022

De Isabella P, Capranico G, Palumbo M, Sissi C, Krapcho AP, Zunino F (1993) Sequence selectivity of topoisomerase II DNA cleavage stimulated by mitoxantrone derivatives: relationship to drug DNA binding and cellular effects. *Molecular Pharmacol* **43:** 715–721

De Isabella P, Zunino F, Capranico G (1995) Base sequence determinants of amonafide stimulation of topoisomerase II DNA cleavage. *Nucleic Acids Res* **23**(2): 223–229

Fujimori A, Harker WG, Kohlhagen G, Hoki Y, Pommier Y (1995) Mutation at the catalytic site of topoisomerase I in CEM/C2, a human leukemia cell resistant to camptothecin. *Cancer Res* **55:** 1339–1346

Gentry AC, Juul S, Veigaard C, Knudsen BR, Osheroff N (2011) The geometry of DNA supercoils modulates the DNA cleavage activity of human topoisomerase I. *Nucleic Acids Res* **39**(3): 1014–1022

Heddle JG, Barnard FM, Wentzell LM, Maxwell A (2000) The interaction of drugs with DNA gyrase: a model for the molecular basis of quinolone action. *Nucleosides Nucleotides Nucleic Acids* **19**(8): 1249–1264

Hertzberg RP, Busby RW, Caranfa MJ, Holden KG, Johnson RK, Hecht SM, Kingsbury WD (1990) Irreversible trapping of the DNA-topoisomerase I covalent complex. *J Biol Chem* **265:** 19287–19295

Hertzberg RP, Caranfa MJ, Hecht SM (1989) On the mechanism of topoisomerase I inhibition by camptothecin: Evidence for binding to an enzyme-DNA complex. *Biochemistry* **28:** 4629–4638

Hsiang Y-H, Liu LF, Wall ME, Wani MC, Nicholas AW, Manikumar G, Kirschenbaum S, Silber R, Potmesil M (1989) DNA topoisomerase I-mediated DNA cleavage and cytotoxicity of camptothecin analogs. *Cancer Res* **49:** 4385–4389

Hsiang YH, Hertzberg R, Hecht S, Liu LF (1985) Camptothecin induces protein-linked DNA breaks via mammalian DNA topoisomerase I. *J Biol Chem* **260**(27): 14873–14878

Ioanoviciu A, Antony S, Pommier Y, Staker BL, Stewart L, Cushman M (2005) Synthesis and Mechanism of Action Studies of a Series of Norindenoisoquinoline Topoisomerase I Poisons Reveal an Inhibitor with a Flipped Orientation in the Ternary DNA-Enzyme-Inhibitor Complex As Determined by X-ray Crystallographic Analysis. *J Med Chem* **48**(15): 4803–4814

Ishida R, Sato M, Narita T, Utsumi KR, Nishimoto T, Morita T, Nagata H, Andoh T (1994) Inhibition of DNA topoisomerase II by ICRF-193 induces polyploidization by uncoupling chromosome dynamics from other cell cycle events. *J Cell Biol* **126**(6): 1341–1351

Jaxel C, Capranico G, Kerrigan D, Kohn KW, Pommier Y (1991) Effect of local DNA sequence on topoisomerase I cleavage in the presence or absence of camptothecin. *J Biol Chem* **266**(30): 20418–20423

Jaxel C, Kohn KW, Pommier Y (1988) Topoisomerase I interaction with SV40 DNA in the presence and absence of camptothecin. *Nucleic Acids Res* **16:** 11157–11170

Jaxel C, Kohn KW, Wani MC, Wall ME, Pommier Y (1989) Structure-activity study of the actions of camptothecin derivatives on mammalian topoisomerase I: evidence for a specific receptor site and a relation to antitumor activity. *Cancer Res* **49:** 1465–1469

Kepler JA, Wani MC, McNaull JN, Wall ME, Levine SG (1969) Plant antitumor agents. IV. An approach toward the synthesis of camptothecin. *J Org Chem* **34**(12): 3853–3858

Koster DA, Palle K, Bot ES, Bjornsti MA, Dekker NH (2007) Antitumour drugs impede DNA uncoiling by topoisomerase I. *Nature* **448**(7150): 213–217

Laponogov I, Sohi MK, Veselkov DA, Pan XS, Sawhney R, Thompson AW, McAuley KE, Fisher LM, Sanderson MR (2009) Structural insight into the quinolone-DNA cleavage complex of type IIA topoisomerases. *Nat Struct Mol Biol* **16**(6): 667–669

Leteurtre F, Fesen M, Kohlhagen G, Kohn KW, Pommier Y (1993) Specific interaction of camptothecin, a topoisomerase I inhibitor, with guanine residues of DNA detected by photoactivation at 365nm. *Biochemistry* **32:** 8955–8962

Leteurtre F, Kohlhagen G, Paull KD, Pommier Y (1994) Topoisomerase II inhibition by anthrapyrazoles, DuP 937 & DuP 941 (Losoxanthrone) and cytotoxicity in the NCI cell screen. *J Natl Cancer Inst* **86:** 1239–1244

Marchand C, Antony S, Kohn KW, Cushman M, Ioanoviciu A, Staker BL, Burgin AB, Stewart L, Pommier Y (2006) A novel norindenoisoquinoline structure reveals a common interfacial inhibitor paradigm for ternary trapping of the topoisomerase I-DNA covalent complex. *Mol Cancer Ther* **5**(2): 287–295

Monod J, Changeux JP, Jacob F (1963) Allosteric proteins and cellular control systems. *J Mol Biol* **6:** 306–329

Pommier Y, Capranico G, Orr A, Kohn KW (1991) Local base sequence preferences for DNA cleavage by mammalian topoisomerase II in the presence of amsacrine or teniposide. *Nucleic Acids Res* **19**(21): 5973–5980

Pommier Y, Cherfils J (2005) Interfacial inhibition of macromolecular interactions: nature's paradigm for drug discovery. *Trends Pharmacol Sci* **26**(3): 138–145

Pommier Y, Kohlhagen G, Kohn F, Leteurtre F, Wani MC, Wall ME (1995) Interaction of an alkylating camptothecin derivative with a DNA base at topoisomerase I-DNA cleavage sites. *Proc Natl Acad Sci USA* **92:** 8861–8865

Pommier Y, Leo E, Zhang H, Marchand C (2010) DNA topoisomerases and their poisoning by anticancer and antibacterial drugs. *Chem Biol* **17**(5): 421–433

Pommier Y, Marchand C (2005) Interfacial inhibitors of protein-nucleic acid interactions. *Curr Med Chem Anticancer Agents* **5**(4): 421–429

Pommier Y, Pourquier P, Urasaki Y, Wu J, Laco G (1999) Topoisomerase I inhibitors: selectivity and cellular resistance. *Drug Resist Updat* **2:** 307–318

Porter SE, Champoux JJ (1989) The basis for camptothecin enhancement of DNA breakage by eukaryotic topoisomerase I. *Nucleic Acids Res* **17**(21): 8521–8532

Redinbo MR, Stewart L, Kuhn P, Champoux JJ, Hol WG (1998) Crystal structures of human topoisomerase I in covalent and noncovalent complexes with DNA. *Science* **279**(5356): 1504–1513

Sirikantaramas S, Yamazaki M, Saito K (2008) Mutations in topoisomerase I as a self-resistance mechanism coevolved with the production of the anticancer alkaloid camptothecin in plants. *Proc Natl Acad Sci USA* **105**(18): 6782–6786

Sissi C, Bolgan L, Moro S, Zagotto G, Bailly C, Menta E, Capranico G, Palumbo M (1998) DNA-binding preferences of bisantrene analogues: relevance to the sequence specificity of drug-mediated topoisomerase II poisoning. *Mol Pharmacol* **54**(6): 1036–1045

Staker BL, Feese MD, Cushman M, Pommier Y, Zembower D, Stewart L, Burgin AB (2005) Structures of three classes of anticancer agents bound to the human topoisomerase I-DNA covalent complex. *J Med Chem* **48**(7): 2336–2345

Staker BL, Hjerrild K, Feese MD, Behnke CA, Burgin AB, Jr., Stewart L (2002) The mechanism of topoisomerase I poisoning by a camptothecin analog. *Proc Natl Acad Sci USA* **99**(24): 15387–15392

Tanizawa A, Fujimori A, Fujimori Y, Pommier Y (1994) Comparison of topoisomerase I inhibition, DNA damage, and cytotoxicity of camptothecin derivatives presently in clinical trials. *J Natl Cancer Inst* **86:** 836–842

Wall ME, Wani MC (1995) Camptothecin and taxol: discovery to clinic--thirteenth Bruce F. Cain Memorial Award Lecture. *Cancer Res* **55**(4): 753–760

Chapter 10
Topoisomerase I Inhibitors: Chemical Biology

Beverly A. Teicher

Topoisomerase I (Top1) is an essential enzyme in mammalian cells and Top1-knockout mice die very early in embryogenesis (Pommier 2006, 2009; Giles and Sharma 2005). The double-helical nature of DNA requires that there be a mechanism to resolve the tangles that arise from this structural feature. Topoisomerases are isomerase enzymes that act on the topology of DNA (Champoux 2001) (see Chaps. 1–5). Due to the size of the eukaryotic chromosome, removal of the supercoils can only be accomplished locally by introducing breaks into the DNA helix. Top1 releases the tension generated by winding/unwinding of DNA by wrapping around DNA and cleaving one strand permitting the helix to spin. Once DNA is relaxed, Top1 religates the broken strand. This process controls DNA replication, transcription, and protein synthesis. The first type I topoisomerase enzyme, originally called ω protein was discovered by James C. Wang (Wang 2009a, b). The DNA double-helical configuration makes the strands difficult to separate. In circular DNA in which double helical DNA is bent around and the two strands are topologically linked or knotted. Identical DNA loops with different numbers of twists are topoisomers, and cannot be interconverted by any process that does not involve the breaking of DNA strands. Topoisomerases I and II catalyze and guide the supercoiling, superlinking, and unknotting of DNA by creating transient breaks in the DNA using a conserved tyrosine as the catalytic residue (Champoux 2001). There are three main types of topology: Supercoiling, knotting, and catenation. When transcription or replication occurs, DNA needs to be free of these compact structures. In addition, during replication, the newly replicated duplex of DNA and the original duplex of DNA become intertwined and need to be completely separated to ensure genomic integrity as a cell divides (see Chaps. 1–5). As transcription proceeds, DNA ahead of the transcription fork becomes overwound or positively

B.A. Teicher (✉)
Developmental Therapeutics Program, National Cancer Institute,
6130 Executive Blvd., Rockville, MD 20852, USA
e-mail: teicherba@mail.nih.gov

Y. Pommier (ed.), *DNA Topoisomerases and Cancer*, Cancer Drug Discovery and Development, DOI 10.1007/978-1-4614-0323-4_10,

supercoiled, while DNA behind the transcription fork becomes underwound or negatively supercoiled. As replication occurs, DNA ahead of the replication fork becomes positively supercoiled, while DNA behind the replication fork becomes entangled forming precatenanes. An essential topological problem occurs at the end of replication, when daughter chromosomes must be fully disentangled before mitosis (Wang 1991).

Because DNA topoisomerase enzymes control the DNA topological state, they control cellular processes that involve DNA (Leppard and Champoux 2005). Topoisomerase activity is crucial for initiation and elongation during DNA synthesis, for the proper separation of sister chromatids during mitosis, for RNA transcription, and for nonhomologous or illegitimate recombination chromosomal rearrangements (Dean et al. 1987a, b; Brill et al. 1987; Goto and Wang 1985; Ishimi et al. 1992; Sundin and Varshavsky 1980, 1981; Pruss and Drlica 1989; Halligan et al. 1982; Bullock et al. 1985). Top1 associates preferentially with transcriptionally active genes and is thought to be involved in relaxing supercoils introduced by RNA polymerase during transcription (Garg et al. 1987; Stewart and Schutz 1987; Zhang et al. 1988).

10.1 Mechanism of Action

Chemical biology is the scientific discipline spanning the fields of chemistry and biology that involves application of chemical techniques and tools, often compounds, to study and manipulate biological systems. Chemical biology was instrumental in the discovery of Top1 since it was originally identified as the molecular target of the plant alkaloid camptothecin (Hsiang and Liu 1988; Hsiang et al. 1985; Wall et al. 1966; Wani and Wall 1969). Top1 is a validated target for cancer chemotherapy because of its identification as the sole target of camptothecin (Hsiang et al. 1985; Li and Liu 2001; Pommier et al. 1998, 1999). Camptothecin specifically inhibits the religation step of the Top1 catalyzed cleavage/relegation reaction, resulting in accumulation of a covalent reaction intermediate, referred to as the cleavable or cleavage complex or Top1cc (Hsiang et al. 1985; Porter and Champoux 1989; Nitiss and Wang 1996). The Top1cc is a reversible protein-DNA covalent complex and represents a unique type of cellular lesion. It has been extremely difficult to study the mechanism of camptothecin activity because the drug acts as an uncompetitive inhibitor and binds only to the transient enzyme substrate complex (Hertzberg et al. 1989; Horwitz et al. 1971). The 2.1 Å crystal structure of a camptothecin derivative, topotecan, bound to the Top1-DNA covalent complex resolved the structure of a camptothecin bound to the Top1-DNA complex (Staker et al. 2002). The crystal structure explains why the drug binds only to the enzyme – substrate complex and specifically blocks both DNA relegation and relaxation. The drug binds to the complex by intercalating between DNA bases of both strands at the enzyme-induced strand break and makes specific hydrogen bond contacts with both the DNA and the enzyme. The ternary structure demonstrates that topotecan is tightly wedged against the protein and phosphodiester backbone that could prevent DNA rotation (see Chap. 9).

The finding that Top1 requires no energy cofactor suggested that hydrolysis was not involved in the mechanism of the DNA cleavage; otherwise religation would require a coupled reaction to balance the unfavorable free energy of dehydration in an aqueous medium (Tse-Dinh et al. 1980). The proposed enzymatic mechanism involves two sequential trans-esterification reactions. In the cleavage reaction, the active site tyrosine (Tyr 732 in human Top1) acts as a nucleophile. The phenolic oxygen attacks a DNA phosphodiester bond, forming an intermediate in which the 3′ end of the broken strand is covalently attached by an O^4-phosphodiester bond to the Top1 tyrosine (Tse-Dinh et al. 1980; Wang 1994). The religation step consists of a transesterification involving nucleophilic attack by the hydroxyl oxygen at the 5′ end of the broken strand. Both the breakage and closure reactions generate phosphodiester bonds and the free energies of hydrolysis are similar. Therefore, the equilibrium constant is near unity and the reaction is freely reversible. However, the equilibrium has been shown to favor religation (Tse-Dinh et al. 1980). Top1 has been proposed to relax DNA via a mechanism of "controlled rotation" in which the DNA duplex located downstream of the cleavage site rotates around the phosphodiester bond between the +1 and −1 base pairs of the uncleaved strand, effectively passing the unbroken strand through the single-strand break with each complete rotation event (Stewart et al. 1998). Repair of topoI-mediated DNA damage has been reviewed (Pommier et al. 2006).

Top1 inhibitors exhibit S-phase cytotoxicity and G2-M cell cycle arrest. A replication fork collision between an advancing replication fork and the inhibitor-trapped Top1 cleavable complex, triggering replication fork arrest and breakage to generate a DNA double-strand break and a covalent Top1-DNA complex, has been proposed to explain the S-phase cytotoxicity (D'Arpa et al. 1990; Hsiang et al. 1989). This collision is responsible for the G2-M arrest and activation of DNA damage signals including nuclear factor kB activation, p53 up-regulation, replication protein A phosphorylation, Chk1 phosphorylation, and ATM/ATR activation (Li and Liu 2001; Tsao et al. 1992). Elevated Top1 levels in tumors are a factor in the antitumor activity of Top1 inhibitors (Coleman et al. 2002; Lynch et al. 1998). In the presence of inhibitors, Top1 is down regulated and targeted to the ubiquitin/proteasome pathway (Desai et al. 1997, 2003; Beidler and Cheng 1995). Camptothecin-Top1-DNA cleavable complexes are rapidly conjugated with SUMO, an ubiquitin-like protein, by UBC9, perhaps as a repair response (Table 10.1) (Desai et al. 2001; Mao et al. 2000) (see Chap. 17).

10.2 Camptothecins

Camptothecin was studied extensively in the Cancer Chemotherapy National Service Center of the National Cancer Institute during the 1960s. It was formulated in carboxymethylcellulose and administered by intraperitoneal injection to tumor-bearing rodents. Relative to other compounds evaluated, camptothecin had relatively poor activity (DeWys et al. 1968). However, the sodium salt of camptothecin

Table 10.1 Genes implicated in the cellular response of camptothecin induced DNA damage

Gene	Protein
ATM	Ataxia telangiectasia mutated; serine/threonine kinase; DNA binding checkpoint damage response; apoptosis induction
ATR/MEC1	Ataxia telangiectasia and Rad3 related; serine/threonine kinase; DNA replication negative regulation; DNA damage checkpoint
CHEK1, CHEK2	CHK1 checkpoint homolog; serine/threonine kinase; DNA damage checkpoint; response to DNA damage stimulus
RAD17/RAD24	DNA repair checkpoint protein
UBE2A	Ubiquitin-conjugating enzyme E2A; regulation of protein metabolism
TDP1	3′-tyrosyl-DNA phosphodiesterase 1; single strand DNA break repair; exonuclease
POLS/TRF4	DNA-directed polymerase sigma; nucleotidyltransferase; DNA double-strand break repair; DNA replication
MSH2/HNPCC	DNA mismatch repair protein mutS homolog; DNA double strand break repair
ERCC1/RAD26	Excision repair cross-complimenting gene 1 protein; response to X-ray; DNA damage response resulting in apoptosis
PNKP/PNK	Polynuclcotide kinase 3′-phosphatase; nucleotide-excision repair; DNA damage removal
CDC45L/CDC25	DNA replication initiation
WRN	Werner syndrome helicase; DNA replication fork processing; response to DNA damage stimulus
UBP1/LBP-1	Upstream binding protein 1 transcriptional repressor
MUS81	DNA endonuclease; response to DNA damage stimulus; DNA repair
RAD50	Single stranded DNA endodeoxyribonuclease; regulation of mitotic recombination; component of MRE11 complex
SUMO3	Ubiquitin protein binding
PARP-1	Poly(ADP-ribose)polymerase 1; response to DNA damage stimulus; DNA repair
EME1	Essential meiotic endonuclease 1 homolog; DNA endonuclease; response to DNA damage stimulus
MRE11	Single stranded DNA endodeoxyribonuclease; DNA-double-strand break repair via nonhomologous end joining
BRCA1/TP53BP1/MDC1	Mediator of DNA damage checkpoint 1; DNA repair complex

demonstrated significant activity and increased the survival time in mice bearing several lymphocytic leukemias (Gallo et al. 1971). Camptothecin sodium salt was found to be effective in patients with advanced disseminated melanoma or gastrointestinal malignancies (Gottlieb et al. 1970; Moertel et al. 1972). Severe toxicities included myelo-suppression, vomiting, diarrhea, and hemorrhagic cystitis and resulted in the discontinuation of the clinical trial of sodium camptothecin.

Although the sodium salt of camptothecin was found to be clinically active, its use was discontinued in the 1970s because of severe side effects and lack of understanding of the mechanism of action (Wall and Wani 1995). The Top1-targeted camptothecin derivatives, topotecan and irinotecan, and the Top2-targeted drugs doxorubicin, amsacrine, etoposide, and teniposide, stabilize the covalent topoisomerase-DNA complex, thereby preventing relegation (Giovanella et al. 1989; Kreuzer and Cozzarelli 1979; Drlica and Franco 1988; Liu 1989). Early experiments demonstrated that short exposure (<1 h) of cells in culture to camptothecin is relatively non-cytotoxic (Horwitz et al. 1971; Holm et al. 1989; O'Connor et al. 1991). This is consistent with a time-dependent conversion of Top1 cleavage complexes to DNA lesions by cellular metabolism. When cells expressing Top1 are exposed to the detergent sodium dodecyl sulfate (SDS), they undergo protein denaturation and quenching of the topoisomerization reaction (Wang 1985; Wang et al. 1990; Pommier et al. 1994). Any cleavable complexes present are trapped, because the enzymatic machinery necessary to catalyze relegation is no longer functional and covalently bound Top1-DNA complexes can be recovered intact and purified. This technique has been used to determine the preferred sites of Top1 enzymatic cleavage.

Today, many Top1-targeted agents currently in clinical investigation are based on the camptothecin structure. Camptothecin derivatives, topotecan and irinotecan, are the only FDA-approved Top1-targeted anticancer drugs. Despite clinical success, there are several problems with camptothecin-derived anticancer agents. A major limitation is the chemical equilibrium between camptothecin lactone form and the E ring-opened form. The E ring-opened carboxylate form has less than 10% the potency of the lactone form as a Top1 inhibitor and is inactive in cell culture, perhaps due to inability to cross the cell membrane (Hertzberg et al. 1989; Adams et al. 2000). Camptothecin analogs suffer from another drawback that further limits antitumor efficacy (Pommier et al. 2006; Chu et al. 1997; Schellens et al. 2000; Beretta et al. 2006; Maliepaard et al. 2001; Yang et al. 2000). Although these drugs can freely enter cells via passive diffusion across cell membranes, their intracellular concentration is reduced by efflux pumps in a wide variety of tissues. Multi-drug resistance (MDR) results from drug efflux by the well characterized P-glycoprotein (P-gp) (Chu et al. 1997). Both topotecan and irinotecan are substrates for the P-gp efflux pump. Additionally, all camptothecins are substrates for the efflux pump known as breast cancer resistant protein (BCRP) (Schellens et al. 2000; Beretta et al. 2006; Maliepaard et al. 2001; Yang et al. 2000). SN-38, the active species from irinotecan, is also conjugated and detoxified by UDP-glucuronosyl transferase (UGT) to yield an SN-38-glucuonide (Ciotti et al. 1999). SN-38 glucuronidation is specifically catalyzed by human liver UGT1A1, UGT1A3, UGT1A6, and UGT1A9 isoforms and is associated with increased efflux of the drug from colon cancer cells (Hanioka et al. 2001; Cummings et al. 2002). Cellular metabolism via carboxylesterases and UGTs plays an important role in the cytotoxicity of irinotecan in cell culture (Ahmed et al. 1999; Khanna et al. 2000). Genetic variability at the UGT1A1 promoter correlates with both the pharmacokinetics and toxicity of SN-38 (Ratain 2000, 2002).

10.3 Lactone Ring Modifications

10.3.1 Homocamptothecins

Modifying the metabolically liable camptothecin lactone ring from a six-membered α-hydroxylactone to a seven-membered β-hydroxylactone ring led to the development of the homocamptothecin family of compounds (Fig. 10.1) (Lesueur-Ginot et al. 1999; Demarquay et al. 2001, 2004; Troconiz et al. 2006; Morisaki et al. 2005; Bates et al. 2004; Solier et al. 2004; Lansiaux et al. 2001; Urasaki et al. 2000). Modification of the crucial E-ring, by insertion of a methylene group between the keto-group and the hydroxyl-substituent, preserved or enhanced Top1 enzyme inhibition. The homocamptothecins are potently cytotoxic and are active antitumor agents in human tumor xenografts (Lesueur-Ginot et al. 1999; Demarquay et al. 2001, 2004). The difluoro homocamptothecin derivative BN80915 (diflomotecan) is one of the most potent topoisomerase inhibitors as measured by the number of DNA-strand breaks and cytotoxicity in cell-based assays (Lansiaux et al. 2001). Diflomotecan was more effective than irinotecan in the human PC-3 prostate carcinoma xenograft producing tumor growth delays of 26–29 days when administered orally twice daily at a dose of 0.03 mg/kg for 14 days. In another study, diflomotecan produced about 28 days of tumor growth delay in the PC-3 human prostate carcinoma xenograft when administered orally once per day for 14 days at a dose of 0.06 mg/kg or weekly for 3 weeks at a dose of 1 mg/kg. In contrast to camptothecins, homocamptothecins undergo slow lactone ring opening in plasma. After 3 h in human plasma, the homocamptothecin BN80927 was more than 90% intact while 80% of SN38, the active species from irinotecan, was ring-opened. The half-life for ring opening of BN80927 was 21 h and for SN38 was less than 30 min (Demarquay et al. 2004). The homocamptothecins, like the camptothecins, are substrates for cellular efflux pumps such as ABCG2 (Table 10.2) (Morisaki et al. 2005; Bates et al. 2004). Cell lines which are resistant to camptothecins by overexpression of multidrug resistance efflux pumps or mutations in Top1 are also resistant to homocamptothecins (Urasaki et al. 2000).

In preclinical safety studies, the dose-limiting toxicity of diflomotecan was myelosuppression (Troconiz et al. 2006). A Phase I clinical study with diflomotecan was conducted to determine the maximum tolerated dose when diflomotecan was administered as a short intravenous infusion and to establish the appropriate pharmacokinetics and plasma concentration versus neutropenic effect relationships. The patients in the Phase I trial had a variety of solid tumors. Diflomotecan was administered as a 20 min intravenous infusion once every 3 weeks. The main toxicological side effects were hematological, especially severe neutropenia. The recommended dose was established to be 4 mg/m^2 for this route and schedule of administration. The time course of the neutropenia could be described by a PK/PD model using the neutrophil cell counts. Diflomotecan has high oral bioavailability (72–95%). The recommended Phase II clinical trial regimen is oral administration of 1–5 days every 3 weeks because it is relatively well tolerated, convenient, and mimics protracted exposure (Kroep and Gelderblom 2009).

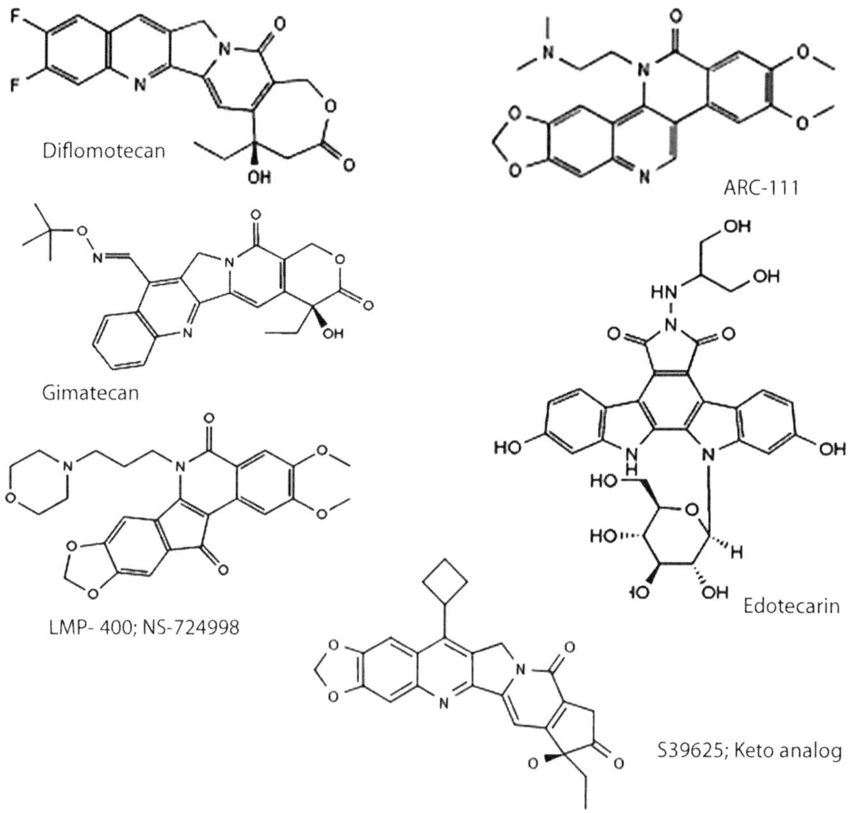

Fig. 10.1 Chemical structures of Top1 inhibitors

Recently, homocamptothecins with 9-benzylideneamino substituents in the nine position, trifluoromethyl groups in the seven position or phosphate esters were prepared to further increase metabolic stability aqueous solubility and antitumor efficacy (Guo et al. 2010; Zhu et al. 2010; Miao et al. 2010). These compounds are in early preclinical evaluation.

10.3.2 Hydroxy-Keto Analogs

As an alternate strategy to stabilize the camptothecin E-ring, keto analogs with a five-membered E-ring missing the lactone ring oxygen were synthesized (Fig. 10.1) (Hautefaye et al. 2003). The resulting five-membered ring should be much less labile under physiologic conditions. The compounds (S39625 and S38809) containing a five-membered keto ring were active against purified Top1 and selective against Top1 in yeast and human cancer cells. These compounds were more potent cytotoxic agents for humans toward colon, breast, and prostate cancer cells and leukemia

Table 10.2 Chemical and clinical characteristics of topoisomerase I inhibitors of varied structure are listed

Compound	Chemical class	Multidrug resistance substrate	Clinical trial status	Dose limiting toxicity
Topotecan	Camptothecin	Yes	Approved Ovarian ca Small cell lung ca	Neutropenia
Irinotecan	Camptothecin	Yes	Approved colorectal ca	Diarrhea neutropenia
Diflomotecan	Homocamptothecin	No	Phase II	Neutropenia
Gimatecan	Camptothecin	No	Phase II	Thrombocytopenia
Edotecarin	Indolocarbazole	Yes	Phase II	Neutropenia granulocytopenia
LMP776; LMP400	Indenoisoquinoline	No	Phase I	?
Genz644282	Dibenzonaphthyridinone	No	Phase I	?

cells than was camptothecin (Takagi et al. 2007; Dexheimer and Pommier 2008). The Top1-DNA cleavage complexes produced by the five-membered keto compounds were persistence both with purified Top1 and in cells following 1 h exposure to the compounds. These compounds were not substrates for either the ABCB1 (multidrug resistance-1/P-glycoprotein) or ABCG2 (mitoxantrone resistance/breast cancer resistance protein) efflux transporter. At nanomolar concentrations, the five-membered keto ring compounds induced intense and persistent histone γ-H2AX. To assess antitumor activity in vivo, HCT 116 human colon carcinoma cells were xenografted subcutaneously into nude mice and the five-membered keto compounds were administered by intravenous injection on days 10, 17, and 24. The compounds were active antitumor agents, and induced more than 88% inhibition of tumor growth at 12.5 mg/kg (Leonce et al. 2007).

10.3.3 Gimatecan

Gimatecan (ST1481) is a seven-position modified lipophilic camptothecin derivative that developed to provide rapid uptake and enhanced accumulation and to prolong and stabilize the Top1-DNA-drug ternary complex compared with conventional camptothecins (Fig. 10.1) (Perego et al. 2001, 2006; Di Francesco et al. 2005; De Cesare et al. 2001, 2004). Specifically, gimatecan is 7-t-butoxyiminomethyl-camptothecin. Gimatecan is very efficient in forming stable ternary complexes with DNA and Top1 resulting in a higher number of DNA strand breaks than topotecan and SN38 under the same conditions (Perego et al. 2006; Di Francesco et al. 2005). Unlike topotecan and SN38, gimatecan is not a substrate for the breast cancer resistance protein (BCRP), an efflux pump or for the multidrug resistance P-glycoprotein efflux pump (Table 10.2) (De Cesare et al. 2001; Perego et al. 2001).

Gimatecan has routinely been administered orally in preclinical in vivo studies; however, the formulation used in the in vivo studies contained 10% DMSO. Gimatecan administered daily orally at doses between 0.25 and 4 mg/kg was a highly effective antitumor agent in a wide variety of human tumor xenografts grown subcutaneously, intracranially, or intraperitoneally (De Cesare et al. 2001, 2004). Gimatecan is a highly effective antitumor agent toward the NCI-H460 human non-small lung carcinoma xenograft when treatment is initiated on day 3 post tumor cell implantation. Gimatecan administered orally daily 5 days per week for 5 weeks at doses of 0.25 or 0.5 mg/kg or every 8–10 days for 10 doses of 5 or 6 mg/kg produced tumor growth delays of 80–100 days. In mice bearing intracranial SW1787 human astrocytoma, gimatecan administered orally daily for 5 days per week for 4 weeks at a dose of 0.25 mg/kg increased median survival by 20 days. In a similar study in mice bearing intracranial LM human melanoma, median survival was increased 15 days by gimatecan treatment. Gimatecan antitumor activity was explored in subcutaneously implanted glioma xenografts alone and in combination with imatinib mesylate or everolimus. The combination regimen had more activity than any of the single agents (Vassal et al. 2008).

Gimatecan showed good tolerability in Phase I clinical trial. The absorption, metabolism, and excretion of [^{14}C] gimatecan were studied in patients after oral administration. Gimatecan had uncomplicated metabolism with rapid absorption (T_{max} was 1 h) and a long elimination phase with clearance half-life of 91 h (Woo et al. 2007). Fecal excretion was the main elimination pathway. The pharmacokinetics of gimatecan was further explored on two oral schedules, daily for 5 days of a 28-day cycle and Monday/Thursday continuously. The lower C_{max} and consistent drug exposure with the Monday/Thursday schedule may provide a wider therapeutic window for gimatecan (Woo et al. 2008). Gimatecan has undergone Phase II clinical study in advanced epithelial ovarian, fallopian tube, and peritoneal cancers, advanced breast cancer, malignant glioma, and metastatic colorectal cancer (Pecorelli et al. 2006; Mariani et al. 2006; Hochberg et al. 2006; Hu et al. 2009; Boni et al. 2004). These studies have found that gimatecan is active as a single agent with bone marrow suppression being the main toxicity.

10.3.4 Edotecarin

Among the novel non-camptothecin Top1 inhibitors, the indolocarbazoles are the most advanced (Long and Balasubramanian 2000; Long et al. 2002). The two most prominent of these compounds are NB-506 and edotecarin (PHA-782615; J-107088) (Fig. 10.1). Edotecarin is a derivative of NB-506 that as a Top1 inhibitor induces single-strand DNA cleavage more effectively than either NB-506 or camptothecin. Although Top1-mediated cleavage can be demonstrated with these compounds in vitro and in cell-based assays, other mechanisms contribute to the cytotoxicity of these compounds. Indolocarbazoles are also well known as kinase inhibitors.

Urasaki et al. (2001) used three cell lines with known mutants in three different Top1 domains, human prostate carcinoma cells DU-145/RC1 (mutation R364H), Chinese hamster fibroblasts DC3F/C10 (mutation G503S), and human leukemia CEM/C2 cells (mutation N722S). The Top1 enzymes in these cells are resistant to both camptothecin and NB-506. However, the three cell lines which were 2-logs or more resistant to camptothecin, only two to tenfold were resistant to NB-506 cytotoxicity, indicating that another mechanism contributes significantly to the cytotoxicity of this compound. Edotecarin (J-107088) emerged as an interesting novel indolocarbazole differing from camptothecin in selectivity in DNA cleavage at C/T-G compared with T-G/A for camptothecin and formation of very stable, persistent DNA-enzyme cleavage complexes. Like the camptothecins, edotecarin is subject to multi-drug resistance by efflux from cells via ATP-binding cassette transporters such as breast cancer resistance proteins (BCRP, MXR, ABCP) (Table 10.2) (Komatani et al. 2001). Edotecarin was tested extensively in human tumor xenografts including central nervous system tumors, colon cancer, and breast cancer alone and in combination with other anticancer agents (Cavazos et al. 2001; Ciomei et al. 2006, 2007). For administration to mice, edotecarin was dissolved in 20% polyethylene glycol 400 and water. The treatment schedule for edotecarin was once or twice weekly for two or more weeks. Edotecarin (30 mg/kg) produced 16–43 days of tumor growth delay in mice bearing HCT116 human colon carcinoma xenografts. In mice bearing human SKBR-3 breast carcinoma xenografts, edotecarin (30 or 150 mg/kg) once weekly for 4 weeks resulted in tumor growth delays of 24 and 60 days, respectively. In studies examining efficacy in CNS derived adult and pediatric tumors, edotecarin was administered by intraperitoneal injection in a vehicle containing 10% DMSO at a dose of 54 mg/kg on days 1–5 and 8–12. In the adult tumor xenografts, tumor growth delays ranged between 12 and 60 days while in the pediatric xenografts, the tumor growth delays ranged between 16 and more than 90 days. In preclinical safety studies, edotecarin was largely eliminated as unchanged parent molecule via biliary excretion.

Edotecarin has undergone several Phase I and Phase II clinical trials (Yamada et al. 2006; Hurwitz et al. 2007; Perez et al. 2002). Edotecarin has been administered to patients as a 2 h intravenous infusion once every 21 days. The recommended dose for Phase II for patients in Japan and in the United States was 13 mg/m^2 intravenously every 3 weeks. The dose limiting toxicity was hematologic toxicity especially neutropenia, leucopenia, and anemia. The pharmacokinetics of edotecarin was fully characterized (Yin et al. 2005). Steady-state plasma concentrations were rapidly achieved during infusion followed by a bi-exponential decline with a very steep initial phase and a relatively shallow terminal phase. Edotecarin has a moderate plasma clearance and a large volume of distribution. As in the preclinical studies, biliary excretion was the major route of elimination. Edotecarin has undergone Phase II clinical trials in irinotecan-naive metastatic colorectal cancer and breast cancer and Phase III clinical trial in glioblastoma multiforme (Nahum et al. 2003).

10.3.5 Indenoisoquinolines

The indenoquinoline NSC314622 was identified as a potential Top1 inhibitor by COMPARE analysis from 48-h cytotoxicity screening of the NCI 60-cell line panel (Fig. 10.1) (Long and Balasubramanian 2000). On further investigation, NSC314622 induces Top1-mediated DNA strand breaks at the same site as camptothecin and at additional sites. NSC314622 also inhibits Top1-mediated supercoiled DNA relaxation but not by intercalation into DNA. Exposure of MCF-7 breast cancer cells to NSC314622 for 1 h resulted in formation of protein-associated breaks in genomic DNA, reflecting formation of stabilized DNA-Top1 cleavable complexes. These findings initiated development of a series of more than 400 compounds to elucidate the structure activity relationship for indenoisoquinoline Top1 inhibitors (Pommier 2006, 2009; Marchand et al. 2006; Nagarajan et al. 2006a, b; Morrell et al. 2006, 2007a, b; Pommier and Cushman 2009). The indenoquinolines have several different characteristics from camptothecins (Table 10.2). They are chemically stable and do not contain the labile hydroxylactone E-ring characteristic of camptothecins. Indenoisoquinolines target different DNA sequences in formation of DNA-Top1 cleavable complexes than camptothecins and the complexes formed are much more stable than those formed by camptothecins. Co-crystal structures of camptothecin and two indenoisoquinolines in ternary complexes with Top1 and DNA show that the small molecules interact with the DNA by hydrophobic stacking interactions and with Top1 by a network of hydrogen bonds revealing a common interfacial inhibitory paradigm (Pommier 2006, 2009; Marchand et al. 2006). Various regions of the indenoisoquinoline molecule have been optimized for Top1 inhibitory activity including examination of nitrogen heterocycles on the lactam ring, nitration in the isoquinoline ring, length of the lactam side-chain, and substituents in the nine-position (Nagarajan et al. 2006b; Morrell et al. 2006, 2007a, b; Pommier and Cushman 2009). The potential of bisindenoisoquinolines has also been explored (Ciomei et al. 2007; Marchand et al. 2006). The in vivo efficacy of the bisindenoisoquinoline NSC 727357 was evaluated in the human melanoma xenograft LOX IMVI. Tumors were implanted subcutaneously in the axillary region and were allowed to reach approximately 88 mg before the start of the treatment. NSC 727357 was formulated as a solution in 10% DMSO in saline containing 0.05% Tween 80, and administered by intraperitoneal injection. Doses of 13.4, 20, and 30 mg/kg were administered once daily for 5 days, with the first treatment given on day 7 after tumor implantation. The compound was assessed in a preliminary study against LOX-IMVI, because it was one of the tumor cell lines that demonstrated growth inhibition in the hollow fiber assay. In this 14-day study, the bisindenoisoquinoline NSC 727357 appeared to be active against the melanoma xenografts with a reduction in median tumor weight on day 14 of 24% in the 13.4 mg/kg drug-treated group, 33% in the 20 mg/kg drug-treated group, and 56% in the 30 mg/kg drug-treated group. The tumor growth delay produced at the highest compound dose tested was 2.5 days.

Indenoisoquinoline derivatives, NSC-725776 and NSC-743400 (salt of 724998), have been selected for clinical development (Fig. 10.1) (Pommier 2006, 2009; Antony et al. 2006). Five-day safety studies were carried out in beagle dogs (Glaze et al. 2009). When administered as a 15-min intravenous infusion, the maximum tolerated dose for NSC-725776 was 3 mg/kg and for NSC-743400 was 7.5 mg/kg. Toxicity profiles for the indenoisoquinolines generally resemble that of topotecan, as the bone marrow and intestines are primary sites of normal tissue toxicity. An assay for γ-H2AX has been developed and validated as a pharmacodynamic biomarker for potential use in early clinical trials of the indenoisoquinoline derivatives (Pommier and Cushman 2009; Ji et al. 2007).

The indenoisoquinolines LMP400 (NSC 743400) and LMP776 (NSC 725776) have entered Phase 1 clinical trial. The treatment cycle is 28 days. On days 1–5 of each cycle, the study drug will be administered by intravenous infusion, followed by 23 days without drug. In addition to standard clinical determinations, the effect of LMP400 and LMP776 on the pharmacodynamic endpoint, γ-H2AX, is being determined in tumor biopsy and skin samples pre- and post-treatment. The pharmacodynamic response is defined as the mean percent nuclear area that is γ-H2AX positive.

10.3.6 Dibenzonaphthyridinones

Nitidine and fagaronine are benzo[*c*]phenanthridine alkaloids with good antitumor potency (Stermitz et al. 1975). Both compounds are active as Top1 inhibitors (Zee-Cheng and Cheng 1975; Janin et al. 1993). Synthetic compounds of this chemical class such as ARC-111 are as potent as camptothecin in stimulating Top1-mediated DNA cleavage using purified human Top1 and are more potent than irinotecan in many human tumor xenograft efficacy models (Fig. 10.1) (Ruchelman et al. 2002, 2003, 2004; Zhu et al. 2005, 2006; Feng et al. 2008a, b, c, 2009; Satyanarayana et al. 2008). An extensive structure-activity relationship was conducted around the dibenzo[c,h][1,6]naphthyridin-6-one family of compounds elucidated structural features associated with potent Top1-targeting activity and suitable pharmaceutical properties (Zhu et al. 2006; Feng et al. 2008a, b, c, 2009; Satyanarayana et al. 2008; Li et al. 2003). Enhanced Top1-targeting, cytotoxic potency, and robust antitumor activity were associated with: (Pommier 2006) Methoxy substituents at both the two- and three-positions of the A-ring (Pommier 2009), a 8,9-methylenedioxy moiety within the D-ring and (Giles and Sharma 2005) heteroatom substitution adjacent to the benzo ring that incorporates the methylenedioxy substituent. Aqueous solubility can be increased with polar substituents without loss of Top1 potency (Satyanarayana et al. 2008). These compounds are not substrates for MDR1 or BCRP efflux (Table 10.2). The compound 8,9-dimethoxy-5-(2-*N*,*N*-dimethylaminoethyl)-2,3-methylenedioxy-5H-dibenzo[c,h][1,6]naphthyridin-6-one (ARC-111, topovale) was selected for in-depth study in cell-based and efficacy models (Li et al. 2003; Ruchelman et al. 2005; Kurtzberg et al. 2007, 2008). The cytotoxicity of ARC-111 was assessed in seven human tumor cell

Table 10.3 Tumor growth delays and percent maximal body weight loss for human tumor xenograft bearing mice treated with ARC-111 and standard comparator drugs

Tumor line	Treatment	Tumor growth delay, days +/− SEM	% Body weight loss
HCT116 Colon Ca	ARC-111 (2 mg/kg iv[a], alt days for 2 weeks)	20.6 ± 4.4	10.2
	Irinotecan (60 mg/kg iv, each 4th day ×3)	17.0 ± 1.6	5.4
HT-29 Colon Ca	ARC-111 (2 mg/kg iv, alt days for 2 weeks)	9.1 ± 1.2	7.7
	Irinotecan (60 mg/kg iv, each 4th day ×3)	8.7 ± 2.4	6.8
NCI-H460 Non-Small Cell Lung Ca	ARC-111 (2 mg/kg iv, alt days for 2 weeks)	20.9 ± 2.7	10.1
	Docetaxel (20 mg/kg iv, alt days ×3)	20.9 ± 2.1	26.4
MiaPaCa2 Pancreatic Ca	ARC-111 (2 mg/kg iv, alt days for 2 weeks)	7.0 ± 1.1	5.3
	Gemcitabine (90 mg/kg iv, each 3rd day ×4)	7.0 ± 1.7	5.9

[a] Intravenous injection is abbreviated iv

lines of varied histology and resistance mechanisms by MTT assay or colony formation. Compared with topotecan and SN38, ARC-111 was a more potent cytotoxic agent and was highly effective in cells expressing the efflux pumps. ARC-111 is an active antitumor agent in SCID mice bearing human tumor xenografts. ARC-11 was as active as irinotecan in the HCT-8 colon carcinoma and as active as topotecan or irinotecan in the SKNEP anaplastic Wilm's xenograft (Li et al. 2003). ARC-111 and several congeners were also very effective antitumor agents in animals bearing the SJ-BT45 medulloblastoma (Ruchelman et al. 2005). The efficacy of ARC-111 was compared with irinotecan in human HCT116 colon cancer xenografts (Table 10.3). Irinotecan was administered at 60 mg/kg/day; iv; Q4D × 3, and ARC-111 was administered at 2 mg/kg/day; iv; QOD × 3 × 2 week. Tumor growth delays were 17 days for both irinotecan and ARC-111. A similar study was performed with the human HT29 colon cancer xenograft, and the tumor growth delays were 10 days for irinotecan and 9 days for ARC-111. ARC-111 was compared with docetaxel in human NCI-H460 non-small cell lung carcinoma xenografts. Docetaxel (20 mg/kg/day; iv; QOD × 3) and ARC-111 administration each resulted in a tumor growth delay of 21 days. ARC-111 was compared with gemcitabine in human MiaPaCa2 pancreatic cancer xenograft. Gemcitabine (90 mg/kg/day; iv; Q3D × 4) administration resulted a tumor growth delay of 7 days as did ARC-111 (Kurtzberg et al. 2007, 2008). A compound from this class-designated Genz644282 was selected for development and is currently in Phase I clinical trial.

In a recent study, to improve understanding of the forces that stabilize drug-Top1-DNA ternary complexes, the five-membered cyclopentadienone C-ring of the indenoisoquinoline system was replaced by six-membered nitrogen heterocyclic rings, resulting in dibenzo[c,h][1,6]naphthyridines that were synthesized by a novel route and tested for Top1 inhibition (Kiselev et al. 2010). Several of these compounds that had unique DNA cleavage site selectivities and were potent cytotoxic agents in cancer cell lines.

10.4 Predictive Markers and Biomarkers

10.4.1 Bone Marrow CFU-GM

Bone marrow is a normal tissue that is critically sensitive to many antineoplastic agents. Compounds including Top1 inhibitors kill rapidly dividing bone marrow progenitor cells resulting in acute reversible neutropenia and thrombocytopenia 4–20 days later (Table 10.2) (Pessina 2003). Repopulation of the marrow progenitor niche precedes recovery of peripheral cell counts by several days. A goal during preclinical development is to predict whether a new agent will be toxic to the bone marrow, whether the toxicity will be specific to one hematopoietic cell lineage and whether bone marrow progenitor cells will be much more sensitive to the agent than a variety of human malignant cells. Bone marrow granulocyte-macrophage-colony forming unit (CFU-GM) assays comparing the sensitivity of bone marrows across species have been useful in predicting the blood levels of agents that might be reached in patients compared with blood levels in preclinical efficacy and safety species. With many cytotoxic agents, the bone marrow of mice is less sensitive than human bone marrow, thus allowing blood levels to be achieved in preclinical efficacy testing that cannot be reached in patients. The bone marrow toxicity of several Top1 inhibitors has been studied (Table 10.4) (Kurtzberg et al. 2008; Pessina 2003; Masubuchi 2004; Erickson-Miller 1997). While human and canine bone marrow may have similar sensitivity to Top1 inhibitors, murine bone marrow is 4.5–27-fold less sensitive to these compounds. The differential sensitivity between murine and human bone marrow progenitor cells to Top1 inhibitors may explain, in part, why curative doses of topotecan and 9-aminocamptothecin in mice with human tumor xenografts are not achievable in patients (Erickson-Miller 1997). The corollary is that the compounds with the smallest or no differential in bone marrow progenitor sensitivity amongst species would likely have a better potential for reaching similar blood levels in patients as in mice, if bone marrow toxicity in dose-limiting in humans. From these data, camptothecin and ARC-111 would be predicted to be most promising; however, camptothecin suffers from metabolic instability.

Pessina et al. (2003) went further to suggest that through use of ratio of mouse/human IC_{90} values and the maximum tolerated dose of the compound in mice the maximum tolerated dose of the compound in patients could be predicted and thus the potential for achieving a therapeutic blood level in patients could be estimated.

Table 10.4 The concentrations of Top1 inhibitors (nM) inhibiting bone marrow CFU-GM from human canine and mouse are shown

Compound	Mouse CFU-GM IC_{50}, nM	Human CFU-GM IC_{50}, nM	Canine CFU-GM IC_{50}, nM	Canine CFU-GM IC_{90}, nM	Mouse CFU-GM IC_{90}, nM	Human CFU-GM IC_{90}, nM	Ratio mouse to human IC_{90}
Camptothecin	18	1.7	0.5	7.6	42	16	5.5
9-Amino-camptothecin	20	0.6	0.3	7.6	66	6.2	11
Topotecan	128/166	2.8/6.5	1.7	7.6	381/519	39/19	10/27
SN-38	108	10			331	26	13
ARC-111	8	1.9			28	6.2	4.5

The data are for continuous exposure (12–16 days) the cells to the compounds in a methylcellulose media over a broad concentration range of compound. The values represent 50% (IC_{50}) and 90% (IC_{90}) cell killing. Colonies of 30 cells or more were counted

10.4.2 Pharmacodynamic DNA Damage Markers

There is an increasing effort early in the clinical experience with investigational anticancer agents to confirm that the molecule is achieving the desired biological effect (Kummar et al. 2006, 2007). The driving forces are to discontinue molecules that for some reason are not "hitting" the desired therapeutic target (yet may be toxic), to efficiently select a dose of the investigational agent that achieved the desired biological effect and to facilitate the selection of patients who may best benefit from treatment with the new therapeutic. Thus, the identification of biomarkers, pharmacodynamic markers, and pharmacogenomic markers in the tumor and/or in the patient is often proceeding in parallel with preclinical development of potential new anticancer therapies. With greater frequency, the early clinical exploration of investigational anticancer agents is being integrated with pharmacodynamic assays (Pommier and Cushman 2009; Kummar et al. 2007). The anticipation is that the time required for anticancer drug development will be shortened through the application of pharmacokinetic and pharmacodynamic measurements and biomarker determinations in the earliest clinical trials.

Top1 inhibitors are highly targeted molecules that stabilize the DNA single-strand break-enzyme complex (Top1 cleavage complex). DNA single strand breaks result in replication fork collapse and the efficient formation of one-ended DNA double-strand breaks that have been described as replication-mediated double-strand breaks (Pommier 2009; Kurtzberg et al. 2007; Pommier et al. 2010). The Mre11·Rad50·Nbs1 (MRN) complex binds DNA double-strand breaks to repair DNA and activate checkpoints. Replication-mediated DNA double strand breaks induced by Top1 cleavage complexes interact with MRN, which activates the Chk2 checkpoint downstream from ATM (Fig. 10.2). In addition to activation of the ATM-Chk2 pathways, replication-mediated DNA double strand breaks also activate RPA2 phosphorylation, histone γ-H2AX, and BLM phosphorylation. Therefore, both ATM and Chk2 are recruited together with MRN and γ-H2AX and both Mre11 and Nbs1 are phosphorylated by ATM (Stracker et al. 2007). MRN is critically important for the functional activation of ATM-Chk2 and it is known that the NBS-, AT-, and Chk2-deficient cells are hypersensitive to camptothecin, thus suggesting that MRN and Chk2 may have prognostic value in selecting patients who could most benefit from treatment with a Top1 inhibitor (Takemura et al. 2006).

The phosphorylated histone H2AX (γ-H2AX) produced in response to DNA double-strand breaks can be detected by immunofluorescence and has been correlated directly with DNA damage severity and genomic repair (Fig. 10.2) (Pommier and Cushman 2009; Ji et al. 2007). A γ-H2AX immunocytochemical assay has been developed and validated to monitor response to DNA damage in human blood and tumor biopsies. Other markers of DNA damage studies were p53BP1, Chk2, and ATM. Formation of γ-H2AX foci were quantitative with DNA damage dosing with ionizing radiation and were detectable within 2 h of treatment. γ-H2AX formation appears to be a robust pharmacodynamic biomarker with potential for clinical monitoring of DNA damage in PBMC and tumor specimens from early clinical trial patients (Ji et al. 2007).

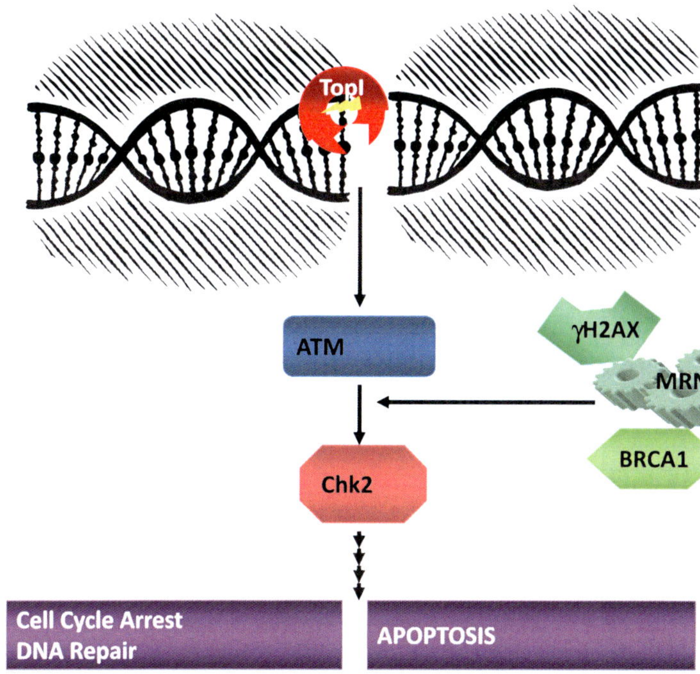

Fig. 10.2 Schematic showing pharmacodynamic markers in the molecular pathway involved in cellular responses to Top1 cleavage complexes. Top1 inhibition induced replication-mediated DNA double strand breaks activate ATM and Chk2. Phosphorylated histone H2AX (gamma-H2AX) occurs in response to the DNA double-strand breaks. Phosphorylation of Mre11 and Nbs1 two protein in the MRN complex (Mre11·Rad50·Nbs1) is also induced by replication-mediated DNA double strand breaks. Ultimately downstream of Chk2 either the cells are arrested in the cell cycle and DNA repair can occur or the cells proceed to apoptosis

10.4.3 Gene Signatures

The ready availability of genomic microarray technology for determination of RNA expression levels from varied biological samples has allowed the application of this technology to identification of biomarker gene signatures for diseases and drug response, drug sensitivity, and drug resistance (Weinstein and Pommier 2006; Potti et al. 2006; Potti and Nevins 2008; Riedel et al. 2008; Anguiano et al. 2008). A gene signature consists of a list of genes whose expression is correlated with the biological state of interest. Much of the early work in the application of this biomarker technology to oncology began with the NCI-60 cell line panel for which gene expression patterns have been profiled providing a baseline of cell line molecular characteristics. The NCI-60 gene expression profiles along with the vast database of compound response data for these cell lines facilitated the initial approaches to connecting gene expression patterns with sensitivity or resistance to particular compounds/drugs. Using cell-based drug sensitivity coupled with Affymetrix microarray data,

Potti et al. (2006) developed gene expression signatures that predict sensitivity to six chemotherapeutic agents including topotecan. The NCI-60 cell line data was used as a starting point and the gene signatures were then tested in an additional cell lines. The gene signature for topotecan sensitivity/resistance included about 150 genes. Data from the analysis of 13 ovarian cancer cell lines was used to link prediction of chemosensitivity to topotecan with expression of a deregulated oncogenic pathway. Ovarian cancer cell lines that were predicted to be topotecan resistant had a higher likelihood of Src pathway deregulation (Potti et al. 2006). The development of gene expression profiles that can predict response to investigational new agents should allow the selection of patients who can best benefit from these treatments in early clinical trials and shorten the time required for clinical trial (Potti and Nevins 2008; Riedel et al. 2008; Anguiano et al. 2008).

10.5 Conclusion

Top1 remains a target of active interest in the development of new anticancer agents because Top1 inhibitors are clearly active and effective anticancer drugs and because the current Top1-targeted drugs are molecules that can be improved upon (Pommier et al. 2010). There are currently camptothecin and non-camptothecin Top1 inhibitors in preclinical and clinical development. Each of these investigational molecules may have properties that lead to improved therapeutic benefits to patients. There are also very active preclinical efforts based upon protein phosphorylation levels and mRNA levels in tumor and blood samples to define biomarkers that can select patients most likely to benefit from treatment with investigational Top1 inhibitors and to guide clinical investigators toward definition of the lowest effective dose and optimal schedule for administration of these new agents. The convergence of these efforts should result in highly clinically effective second generation Top1 inhibitors for the treatment of malignant disease on patients.

References

Adams DJ, Dewhirst MW, Flowers JL, Gamcsik MP, Colvin OM, Manikumar G, Wani MC, Wall ME (2000) Camptothecin analogs with enhanced antitumor activity at acidic pH. Cancer Chemother Pharmacol 46:263–271

Ahmed F, Vyas V, Cornfield A et al (1999) In vitro activation of irinotecan to SN-38 by human liver and intestine. Anticancer Res 19:2067–2071

Anguiano A, Nevins JR, Potti A (2008) Towards the individualization of lung cancer therapy. Cancer 113:1760–1767

Antony S, Agama KK, Miao ZH, Hollingshead M, Holbeck SL, Wright MH, Varticovski L, Nagarajan M, Morrell A Cushman M, Pommier Y (2006) Bisindenoisoquinoline bis-1,3-{(5,6-dihydro-5,11-diketo-11H-indeno[1,2-c]isoquinoline)-6-propylamino}propane bis(trifluoroacetate) (NSC727357), a DNA intercalator and topoisomerase inhibitor with antitumor activity. Mol Pharmacol 70:1109–1120

Bates SE, Medina-Perez WY, Kohlhagen G, Antony S, Nadjem T, Robey RW, Pommier Y (2004) ABCG2 mediates differential resistance to SN-38 (7-ethyl-10-hydroxycamptothecin) and homocamptothecins. J Pharmacol Exp Therap 310:836–842

Beidler DR, Cheng YC (1995) Camptothecin induction of a time- and concentration-dependent decrease of topoisomerase I and its implication in camptothecin activity. Mol Pharmacol 47:907–914

Beretta GL, Perego P, Zunino F (2006) Mechanisms of cellular resistance to camptothecins. Curr Med Chem 13:3291–3305

Boni C, Gamucci T, Bonetti A, Bisagni G, Dallo E, Zanna C, Marsoni S, Sessa C, Ospedaliera A, Maria Nuova S, Emilia R (2004) A phase II study of the novel oral camptothecin SR1481 in pretreated metastatic colorectal cancer (CRC). J Clin Oncol 22 suppl:abstr 3684

Brill SJ, DiNardo S, Voelkel-Meiman K, Sternglanz R (1987) Need for DNA topoisomerase activity as a swivel for DNA replication for transcription of ribosomal RNA. Nature 326:414–416

Bullock P, Champoux JJ, Botchan M (1985) Association of crossover points with topoisomerase I cleavage sites: A model for non-homologous recombination. Science 230:954–958

Cavazos CM, Keir ST, Yoshinari T, Bigner DD, Friedman HS (2001) Therapeutic activity of the topoisomerase I inhibitor J-107088 [6-N-(1-hydroxymethyla-2-hydroxy)ethylamino-12,13-dihydro-13-(b-D-glucopyranosyl)-5H-indolo[2,3-a]-pyrrolo[3,4-c]carbazole-5,7(6H)-dione] against pediatric and adult central nervous system tumor xenografts. Cancer Chemother Pharmacol 48:250–254

Champoux JJ (2001) DNA topoisomerases: structure, function, and mechanism. Annu Rev Biochem 70:369–413

Chu X, Kato Y, Sugiyama Y (1997) Multiplicity of biliary excretion mechanisms for irinotecan, CPT-11, and its metabolites in rates. Cancer Res 57:1934–1938

Ciomei M, Croci V, Ciavolella A, Ballinari D, Pesenti E (2006) Antitumor efficacy of edotecarin as a single agent and in combination with chemotherapy agents in a xenograft model. Clin Cancer Res 12:2856–2861

Ciomei M, Croci V, Stellari F, Amboldi N, Giavarini R, Pesenti E (2007) Antitumor activity of edotecarin in breast carcinoma models. Cancer Chemother Pharmacol 60:229–235

Ciotti M, Basu N, Brangi M, Owens IS (1999) Glucuronidation of 7-ethyl-10-hydroxycamptothecin (SN-38) by human UDP-glucuronosyltransferases encoded at the UGT1 locus. Biochem Biophys Res Commun 260:199–202

Coleman LW, Rohr LR, Bronstein IB, Holden JA (2002) Human DNA topoisomerase I: an anticancer drug target present in human sarcomas. Hum Pathol 33:599–607

Cummings J, Boyd G, Ethell BT et al (2002) Enhanced clearance of topoisomerase I inhibitors from human colon cancer cells by glucuronidation. Biochem Pharmacol 63:607–613

D'Arpa P, Beardmore C, Liu LF (1990) Involvement of nucleic acid synthesis in cell killing mechanisms of topoisomerase poisons. Cancer Res 50:6919–6924

Dean FB, Bullock P, Murakami Y, Wobbe CR, Weissback L, Hurwitz J (1987) Simian virus 40 (SC40) DNA replication: SV40 large T antigen unwinds DNA containing the SV40 origin of replication. Proc Natl Acad Sci USA 84:16–20

Dean FB, Borowiec JA, Ishimi Y, Deb S, Tegtmyer P, Hurwitz J (1987) Simian virus 40 large tumor antigen requires three core replication origin domains for DNA unwinding and replication in vivo. Proc Natl Acad Sci USA 84:8267–8271

De Cesare M, Pratesi G, Veneroni S, Bergottini R, Zunino F (2004) Efficacy of the novel camptothecin gimatecan against orthotopic and metastatic human tumor xenograft models. Clin Cancer Res 10:7357–7364

De Cesare M, Pratesi G, Perego P, Carnini N, TTinelli S, Merlini L, Penco S, Pisano C, Bucci F, Vesci L, Pace S, Capocasa F, Carminati P, Zunino F (2001) Potent antitumor activity and improved pharmacological profile of ST1481, a novel 7-substituted camptothecin. Cancer Res 61:7189–7195

Di Francesco AM, Riccardi AS, Barone G, Rutella S, Meco D, Frapolli R, Zucchetti M, D'Incalci M, Pisano C, Carminati P, Riccardi R (2005) The novel lipophilic camptothecin analogue gimatecan is very active in vitro in human neuroblastoma: a comparative study with SN38 and topotecan. Biochem Pharm 70:1125–1136

Demarquay D, Huchet M, Coulomb H, Lesueur-Ginot L, Lavergne O, Kasprzyk PG, Bailly C, Camara J, Bigg DCH (2001) The homocamptothecin BN 80915 is a highly potent orally active topoisomerase I poison. Anti-Cancer Drugs 12:9–19

Demarquay D, Huchet M, Coulomb H, Lesueur-Ginot L, Lavergne O, Camara J, Kasprzyk PG, Prevost G, Bigg DCH (2004) BN80927: a novel homocamptothecin that inhibits proliferation of human cells in vitro and in vivo. Cancer Res 64:4942–4949

Desai SD, Zhang H, Rodriguez-Bauman A, Yang JM, Wu X, Gounder MK, Rubin EH, Liu LF (2003) Transcription-dependent degradation of topoisomerase I-DNA covalent complexes. Mol Cell Biol 23:2341–2350

Desai SD, Liu LF, Vazquez-Abad D, D'Arpa P (1997) Ubiquitin-dependent destruction of topoisomerase I is stimulated by the antitumor drug camptothecin. J Biol Chem 272:24159–24164

Desai SD, Li TK, Rodriguez-Bauman A, Rubin EH, Liu LF (2001) Ubiquitin-26S proteasome-mediated degradation of topoisomerase I as a resistance mechanism to camptothecin in tumor cells. Cancer Res 61:5926–5932

Drlica K, Franco RJ (1988) Inhibitors of DNA topoisomerases. Biochem 27:2252–2259

DeWys WD, Humphreys SR, Goldin A (1968) Studies on the therapeutic effectiveness of drugs with tumor weight and survival time indices of Walker 256 carcinosarcoma. Cancer Chemo Rep 52:229–242

Dexheimer TS, Pommier Y (2008) DNA cleavage assay for the identification of topoisomerase I inhibitors. Nature Protocols 3: 1736–1750

Erickson-MillerC(1997)DifferentialtoxicityofCamptothecin,Topotecanand9-Aminocamptothecin to Human, Canine, and Murine Myeloid Progenitors (CFU-GM) In Vitro. Cancer Chemother Pharmacol 1997; 39:467–472

Feng W, Satyanarayana M, Tsai YC, Liu AA, Liu LF, LaVoie EJ (2008) Facile formation of hydrophilic derivatives of 5H-8,9-dimethoxy-5-[2-(N,N-dimethylamino)ethyl]-2,3-methylenedioxydibenzo[c,h][1,6]naphthyridin-6-one (ARC-111) and its 12-aza analog via quaternary ammonium intermediates. Bioorg Med Chem Lett 18:3570–3572

Feng W, Satyanarayana M, Tsai YC, Liu AA, Liu LF, LaVoie EJ (2008) 11-Substituted 2,3-dimethoxy-8,9-methylenedioxybenzo[i]phenanthridine derivatives as novel topoisomerase I-targeting agents. Bioorg Med Chem 16:8598–8606

Feng W, Satyanarayana M, Cheng L, Liu AA, Tsai YC, Liu LF, LaVoie EJ (2008) Synthesis of N-substituted 5-[2-(N-alkylamino)ethyl]dibenzo[c,h][1,6]-naphthyridines as novel topoisomerase I-targeting antitumor agents. Bioorg Med Chem 16:9295–9301

Feng W, Satyanarayana M, Tsai YC, Liu AA, Liu LF, LaVoie EJ (2009) 12-Substituted 2,3-dimethoxy-8,9-methylenedioxybenzo[i]phenanthridines as novel topoisomerase I-targeting antitumor agents. Bioorg Med Chem 17:2877–2885

Gallo RC, Whang-Peng J, Adamson RH (1971) Studies on the antitumor activity, mechanism of action, and cell cycle effects of camptothecin. J Natl Cancer Inst 46:789–795

Garg LC, DiAngelo S, Jacob ST (1987) Role of DNA Topoisomerase I in the transcription of supercoiled rRNA gene. Proc Natl Acad Sci USA 84: 3185–3188

Giles I, Sharma RP (2005) Topoisomerase enzymes as therapeutic targets for cancer chemotherapy. Med Chem 1:383–394

Giovanella BC, Stehlin JS, Wall ME, Wani MC, Nicholas AW, Liu LF et al (1989) DNA topoisomerase I-targeted chemotherapy of human colon cancer xenografts. Science 246:1046–1048

Glaze E, Harder JB, McCormick D, Johnson W, Detrisac C, Pommier Y, Tomaszewski J (2009) Five-day intravenous toxicity study of indenoisoquinoline analogues in dogs. Proc Am Assoc Cancer Res 50: Abstr 2933

Goto T, Wang JC (1985) Cloning of yeast *TOP1*, the gene encoding DNA topoisomerase I, and construction of mutants defective in both DNA topoisomerase I and topoisomerase II. Proc Natl Acad Sci USA 82:7178–7182

Gottlieb JA, Guarino AM, Call JB, Oliverio VT, Block JB (1970) Preliminary pharmacologic and clinical evaluation of camptothecin sodium (NSC 100880). Cancer Chemo Rep 54:461–470

Guo W, Miao Z, Sheng C, Yao J, Feng H, Zhang W, Zhu L, Liu W, Cheng P, Zhang J, Che X, Wang W, Luo C, Xu Y (2010) Synthesis and evaluation of 9-benzylideneamino derivatives of homocamptothecin as potent inhibitors of DNA topoisomerase I. Europ J Med Chem 45: 2223–2228

Halligan BD, Davis JL, Edwards KA, Liu LF(1982) Intra-and inter-molecular strand transfer by HeLa DNA topoisomerase I. J Biol Chem 257:3995–4000

Hanioka N, Ozawa S, Jinno H, Ando M, Saito Y, Sawada J (2001) Human liver UDP-glucuronosyltransferase isoforms involved in the glucuronidation of 7-ethyl-10-hydroxycamptothecin. Xenobiotica 31:687–699

Hautefaye P, Cimetiere B, Pierre A, Leonce S, Hickman J, Laine W, Bailly C, Lavielle G (2003) Synthesis and pharmacological evaluation of novel non-lactone analogues of camptothecin. Bioorg Med Chem Lett 13: 2731– 2735

Hertzberg RP, Caranfa MJ, Holden KG, Jakas DR, Gallagher G, Mattern MR, Mong SM, Bartus JO, Johnson RK, Kingsbury WD (1989) Modification of the hydroxyl lactone ring of camptothecin: inhibition of mammalian topoisomerase I and biological activity. J Med Chem 32:715–720

Horwitz SB, Chang CK, Grollman AP (1971) On the mechanism of topoisomerase I inhibition by camptothecin: evidence for binding to an enzyme-DNA complex. Biochemistry 7:632–644

Hochberg FH, Supko J, Amato A, Salem N, Carminati P, Wen P (2006) Phase I trial and pharmacokinetic study or oral gimatecan in adults with malignant glioma. J Clin Oncol 24 suppl:abstr 1559

Holm C, Covey JM, Kerrigan D, Pommier Y (1989) Differeential requirement of DNA replication for the cytotoxicity of DNA topoiosmerase I and II inhibitors in Chinese hamster DC3F cells. Cancer Res 49:6365–6368

Hsiang YH, Hertzberg R, Hecht S, Liu LF (1985) Camptothecin induces protein-linked DNA breaks via mammalian DNA topoisomerse I. J Biol Chem 260:14873–14878

Hsiang YH, Liu LF (1988) Identification of mammalian DNA topoisomerase I as an intracellular target of the anticancer drug camptothecin. Cancer Res 48:1722–1726

Hsiang YH, Lihou MG, Liu LF (1989) Arrest of replication forks by drug-stabilized topoisomerase I-DNA cleavable complexes as a mechanism of cell killing by camptothecin. Cancer Res 49:5077–5082

Hu J, Wen LE, Abrey LE, Fadul C, Drappatz J, Salem N, Amato A, Carminati P, Supko J, Hochberg F (2009) Phase II trial of oral gimatecan in adults with recurrent glioblastoma. J Clin Oncol 27 suppl:abstr 2009.

Hurwitz HI, Cohen RB, McGovren JP, Hirawat S, Petros WP, Natsumeda Y, Yoshinari T (2007) A phase I study of the safety and pharmacokinetics of edotecarin (J-107088), a novel toposiosmerase I inhibitor, in patients with advanced solid tumors. Cancer Chemother Pharmacol 59:139–147

Ishimi Y, Sugasawa K, Hanaoka F, Eki T, Hurwitz J (1992) Topoisomerase II plays an essential role as a swivelase in the late stage of SV40 chromosome replication in vitro. J Biol Chem 267:462–466

Janin YL, Croisy A, Rious JL, Bisagni E (1993) Synthesis and evaluation of new 6-amino-substituted benzo[c]phenanthridine derivatives. J Med Chem 36:3686–3692

Ji JJ, Putvatana R, Zhang Y, Redon C, Sedelnikova O, Yang S, Pommier Y, Bonner W, Kinders R, Parchment R, Hollings head M, Low J, Murgo A, Tomaszewski JE, Doroshow J (2007) A validated assay for gamma-H2AX as a pharmacodynamic biomarker of response to DNA damage. Proc Am Assoc Cancer Res abstr 4027

Khanna R, Morton CL, danks MK, Potter PM (2000) Proficient metabolism of irinotecan by a human intestinal carboxylesterase. Cancer Res 60:4725–4738

Kreuzer KN, Cozzarelli NR (1979) *Escherechia coli* mutants thermosensitive for deoxyribonucleic acid gyrase subunit A: Effects on deoxyribonucleic acid replication, transcription, and bacterial growth. J Bacteriol 140:424–435

Kroep JR, Gelderblom H (2009) Diflomotecan, a promising homocamptothecin for cancer therapy. Exp Opin Invest Drugs 18:69–75

Komatani H, Kotani H, Hara Y, Nakagawa R, Matsumoto M, Arakawa H, Nishimura S (2001) Identification of breast cancer resistant protein/mitoxantrone resistance/placenta-specific, ATP-binding cassette transporter as a transporter of NB-506 and J-107088, topoisomerase I inhibitors with an indolocarbazole structure. Cancer Res 61:2827–2832

Kiselev E, Dexheimer TS, Pommier Y, Cushman MC (2010) Design, synthesis and evaluation of dibenzo[c,h][1,6]naphthyridines as topoisomerase I inhibitors and potential anticancer agents. J Med Chem 53:8716–8726

Kummar S, Gutierrez M, Doroshow JH, Murgo AJ (2006) Drug development in oncology: classical cytotoxics and molecularly targeted agents. Brit J Clin Pharmacol 62:15–26

Kummar S, Kinders R, Rubenstein L, Parchment RE, Murgo AJ, Collins J, Pickeral O, Low J, Steinberg SM, Gutierrez M, Yang S, Helman L, Wiltrout R, Tomaszewski JE, Doroshow JH (2007) Compressing drug development timelines in oncology using phase "0" trials. Nature Rev Cancer 7:131–139

Kurtzberg L, Battle T, Rouleau C, Bagley RG, Agata N, Yao M, Schmid S, Roth, S, Crawford J, Krumbholtz R, Yu X-J, Wang F, LaVoie E, Teicher BA (2007) Bone marrow and tumor line cytotoxicity and human tumor xenograft efficacy of non-camptothecin and camptothecin topoisomerase I inhibitors. Proc Am Assoc Cancer Res abstr 771

Kurtzberg L, Battle T, Rouleau C, Bagley RG, Agata N, Yao M, Schmid S, Roth, S, Crawford J, Krumbholtz R, Yu X-J, Wang F, LaVoie E, Teicher BA (2008) Bone marrow and tumor line cytotoxicity and human tumor xenograft efficacy of non-camptothecin and camptothecin topoisomerase I inhibitors. Molec Cancer Therap 7:3212–3222

Lansiaux A, Facompre M, Wattez N, Hildebrand M P, Bal C, Demarquay D, Lavergne O, Bigg DCH, Bailly C (2001) Apoptosis induced by the homocamptothecin anticancer drug BN80915 in HL-60 cells. Mol Pharmacol 60:450–461

Leonce S, Lansiaux A, Kraus-Berthier L, Giraudet S, David-Cordonnier MH, Hautefaye P, Lavielle G, Hickman J, Pierre A (2007) High stability of the cleavage complex induced by novel non-lactone camptothecin derivatives. Proc Amer Assoc Cancer Res 48: Abstr 787

Leppard JB, Champoux JJ (2005) Human DNA topoiosmerase I: relaxation, roles and damage control. Chromosoma 114:75–85

Lesueur-Ginot L, Demarquay D, Kiss R, Kasprzyk PG, Dassonneville L, Bailly C, Camara J, Lavergne O, Bigg DCH (1999) Homocamptothecin, an E-ring modified camptothecin with enhanced lactone stability, retains topoisomerase I-targeted activity and antitumor properties. Cancer Res 59:2939–2943

Li TK, Liu LF (2001) Tumor cell death induced by topoisomerase –targeting drugs. Ann Rev Pharmacol Toxicol 41:53–77

Li TK, Houghton PJ, Desai SD, Daroui P, Liu AA, Hars ES, Ruchelman AL, LaVoie EJ, Liu LF (2003) Characterization of ARC-111 as a novel topoisomerase I-targeting anticancer drug. Cancer Res 63:8400–8407

Liu LF (1989) DNA topoisomerase poisons as antitumor drugs. Ann Rev Biochem 58:351–375

Long BH, Balasubramanian BN (2000) Non-camptothecin topoisomerase I active compounds as potential anticancer agents. Exp Opin Ther Patents 10:655–686

Long BH, Rose WC, Vyas DM, Matson JA, Forenza S (2002) Discovery of antitumor indolocarbazoles: Rebeccamycin, NSC655649 and fluoroindolocabazoles. Curr Med Chem-Anticancer Agents 2:255–266

Lynch BJ, Komaromy-Hiller G, Bronstein IB, Holden JA (1998) Expression of DNA topoisomerase I, DNA topoisomerase II-α and p53 in metastatic malignant melanoma. Hum Pathol 29:1240–1245

Maliepaard M, van Gastelen MA, Tohgo A, Hausheer FH, van Waardenburg RC, de Jong LA, Pluim D, Beijnen JH, Schellens JH (2001) Circumvention of breast cancer resistance protein (BCRP)-mediated resistance to camptothecins in vitro using non-substrate drugs or the BCRP inhibitor GF120918. Clin Cancer Res 7:935–941

Mao Y, Sun M, Desai SD, Liu LF(2000) SUMO-1 conjugation to topoisomerase I: a possible repair response to topoisomerase-mediated DNA damage. Proc Natl Acad Sci USA 97:4046–4051

Mariani P, Moliterni A, DaPrada G, Hess D, Gamucci T, Zaniboni A, Malossi A, barbieri P, Marsoni S, Gianni L (2006) A phase II trial of the novel oral camptothecin grimatecan (G) in women with anthracycline (A) and taxane (T) pre-treated advanced breast cancer. J Clin Oncol 24 suppl:abstr 662

Marchand C, Antony S, Kohn KW, Cushman M, Ioanoviciu A, Staker BL, Burgin AB, Stewart L, Pommier Y (2006) A novel norindenoisoquinoline structure reveals a common interfacial inhibitor paradigm for ternary trapping of the topoisomerase I-DNA covalent complex. Mol Cancer Ther 5:287–295

Masubuchi N (2004) A predictive model of human myelotoxicity using five camptothecin derivatives and the in vitro colony-forming unit granulocyte/macrophage assay. Clin Cancer Res 10:6722–6731

Miao Z, Zhang J, You L, Wang J, Sheng C, Yao J, Zhang W, Feng H, Guo W, Zhou L, Liu W, Zhu L, Cheng P, Che X, Wang W, Luo C, Xu Y, Dong G (2010) Phosphate ester derivatives of homocamptothecin: synthesis, solution stabilities and antitumor activities. Bioorg Med Chem 18: 3140– 3146.

Moertel CG, Schutt AJ, Reitemeier RJ, Hahn RG (1972) Phase II study of camptothecin (NSC 100880) in the treatment of advanced gastrointestinal cancer. Cancer Chemo Rep 56:95–101

Morisaki K, Robey RW, Ozvegy-Laczka C, Honjo Y, Polgar O, Steadman K, Sarkadi B, Bates SE (2005) Single nucleotide polymorphisms modify the transporter activity of ABCG2. Cancer Chemother Pharmacol 56:161–172

Morrell A, Antony S, Kohlhagen G, Pommier Y, Cushman M (2006) A systematic study of nityrated indenoisoquinolines reveals a potent topoiosmerase I inhibitor. J Med Chem 49:7740–7753

Morrell A, Placzek MS, Steffen JD, Antony S, Agama K, Pommier Y, Cushman M (2007) Investigation of the lactam side chain length necessary for optimal indenoquinoline topoisomerase I inhibition and cytotoxicity in human cancer cell cultures. J Med Chem 50:2040–2048

Morrell A, Placzek M, Parmley S, Grella B, Antony S, Pommier Y, Cushman M (2007) Optimization of the indenone ring of indenoisoquinoline topoisomerase I inhibitors. J Med Chem 50:4388–4404

Nahum K, Shiba D, Padavanija P, Garcia M, Hurwitz HI, Mackintosh F, Natsumeda Y, Yatsuzuka N, Locker P, Gruia G (2003) Phase II efficacy and tolerability study of edotecarin (J107088) in patients with irinotecan-naïve metastatic colorectal cancer (MCRC). Proc Am Soc Oncol 22: abstr 1099

Nagarajan M, Morrell A, Antony S, Kohlhagen G, Agama K, Pommier Y, Ragazzon PA, Garbett NC, Chaires JB, Hollingshead M, Cushman M (2006) Synthesis and biological evaluation of bisindenoisoquinolines as topoisomerase I inhibitors. J Med Chem 49:5129–5140

Nagarajan M, Morrell A,Ioanoviciu A, Antony S, Kohlhagen G, Agama K, Hollingshead M, Pommier Y, Cushman M (2006) Synthesis and evaluation of indenoisoquinoline topoisomerase I inhibitors substituted with nitrogen heterocycles. J Med Chem 49:6283–6289

Nitiss JL, Wang JC (1996) Mechanisms of cell killing by drugs that trap covalent complexes between DNA topoisomerases and DNA. Mol Pharmaol 50:1095–1102

O'Connor PM, Nieves-Neira W, Kerrigan D et al (1991) S-Phase population analysis does not correlate with the cytotoxicity of camptothecin and 10,11-methylene-dooxycamptothecin in human colon carcinoma HT-29 cells. Cancer Commun 3:233–240

Pecorelli S, Ray-Coquard I, Colombo N, Katsaros D, Lhomme C, Lissoni A, Vermorken JB, DuBois A, Poveda A, Frigerio L (2006) A phase II study or oral gimatecan (ST1481) in women with progressing or recurring advanced epithelial ovarian, fallopian tube and peritoneal cancers. J Clin Oncol 24 suppl: abstr 5088

Perego P, Ciusani E, Gatti L, Carenini N, Corna E, Zunino F (2006) Sensitization to gimatecan-induced apoptosis by tumor necrosis factor-related apoptosis inducing ligand in prostate carcinoma cells. Biochem Pharm 71:791–798

Perego P, De Cesare M, De Isabella P, Carenini N, Beggiolin G, Pezzoni G, Palumbo M, Tartaglia L, Pratesi G, Pisano C, Carminati P, Scheffer GL, Zunino F (2001) A novel 7-modified camptothecin analog overcomes breast cancer resistance protein-associated resistance in a mitoxantrone-selected colon carcinoma cell line. Cancer Res 61:6034–6037

Perez RP, Hurwitz HI, Nahum K, Lee J, Shiba D, Garcia M et al (2002) Phase II trials of J-107088, a non-camptothecin topoisomerase I inhibitor, in irinotecan naïve/refractory metastatic colorectal cancer. Proc Am Soc Clin Oncol 21:abstr 632

Pessina A (2003) Application of the CFU-GM assay to predict acute drug-induced neutropenia: an international blind trial tovalidate a prediction model for the maximum tolerated dose (MTD) of myelosuppressive xenobiotics. Toxicological Sciences 75:355–367

Pommier Y, Tanizawa A, Kohn KW (1994) Mechanisms of topoisomerase I inhibition by anti-cancer drugs. In *Advances in Pharmacology*; Liu, L.F.; Academic Press: New York, *29B*, 73–92

Pommier Y, Barcelo JM, Rao VA, Sordet O, Jonson AG, Thibaut AG, Miao ZH, Séller JA, Zhang H, Marchand C, Agama K, Nitiss JL, Redon C (2006) Repair of topoisomerase I-mediated DNA damage. Prog Nuc Acid Res Molec Biol 81:179–229

Pommier Y (2009) DNA topoisomerase I inhibitors: chemistry, biology and interfacial inhibition. Chem Rev 109:2894–2902

Pommier Y (2006) Topoisomerase I inhibitors: camptothecins and beyond. Nat Rev Cancer 6:789–802

Pommier Y, Cushman M (2009) The indenoisoquinoline non-camptothecin topoisomerase I inhibitors: update and perspectives. Molec Cancer Therap 8: 1008–1014

Pommier Y, Pourquier P, Fan Y, Strumberg D (1998) Mechanism of action of eukaryotic DNA topoisomerase I and drugs targeted to the enzyme. Biochem Biophys Acta 1400:83–105

Pommier Y, Pourquier P, Urasaki Y, Wu J, Laco G (1999) Topoisomerase I inhibitors: selectivity and cellular resistance. Drug Resistance Update 2:307–318

Pommier Y, Leo E, Zhang HL, Marchand C (2010) DNA topoisomerases and their poisoning by anticancer and antibacterial drugs. Chem Biol 17:421–33

Potti A, Dressman HK, Bild A, Riedel RF, Chan G, Sayer R, Cragun J, Cottrill H, Kelley MJ, Petersen R, Harpole D, Marks J, Berchuck A, Ginsburg GS, Febbo P, Lancaster J, Nevins JR (2006) Genomic signatures to guide the use of chemotherapeutics. Nat Med 12:1294–1300

Potti A, Nevins JR (2008) Utilization of genomic signatures to direct use of primary chemotherapy. Curr Opin Genet Develop 18:62–67

Porter SE, Champoux JJ (1989) The basis for camptothecin enhancement of DNA breakage by eukaryotic topoisomerase I. Nuc Acids Res 17:8521–8532

Pruss GJ, Drlica K (1989) DNA supercoiling and prokaryotic transcription. Cell 56:521–523

Ratain MJ (2000) Insights into the pharmacokinetics and pharmacodynamics of irinotecan. Clin Cancer Res 6:3393–3394

Ratain MJ (2002) Irinotecan dosing: does the CPT in CPT-11 stand for "Can't predict toxicity"? J Clin Oncol 20:7–8

Riedel RF, Porrello A, Pontzer E, Chenette EJ, Hsu DS, Balakumaran B, Potti A, Nevins J, Febbo PG (2008) A genomic approach to identify molecular pathways associated with chemotherapy resistance. Mol Cancer Ther 7:3141–3149

Ruchelman AL, Houghton PJ, Zhou N, Liu AA, Liu LF, LaVoie EJ (2005) 5-(2-aminothyl) dibenzo[c,h]naphthyridin-6-ones: variation of N-alkyl substituents modulates sensitivity to efflux transporters associated with multidrug resistance. J Med Chem 48:792–804

Ruchelman AL, Singh SK, Wu XH, Ray A, Yang JM, Li TK, Liu AA, Liu LF, LaVoie EJ (2002) Diaza- and triazachrysenes: potent topoisomerase-targeting agents with exceptional antitumor activity against the human tumor xenograft MDA-MB-435. Bioog Med Chem Lett 12:3333–3336

Ruchelman AL, Singh SK, Wu X, Ray A, Yang JM, Li TK, Liu AA, Liu LF, LaVoie EJ (2003) 5H-dibenzo[c,h]naphthyridin-6-ones: novel topoisomerase I-targeting anticancer agents with potent cytotoxic activity. Bioorg Med Chem 11:2061–2073

Ruchelman AL, Zhu S, Zhou N, Liu AA, Liu LF, LaVoie EJ (2004) Dimethoxybenzo[i]phenanthridine-12-carboxylic acid derivatives and 6H-dibenzo[c,h][2,6]naphthyridin-5-ones with potent topoisomerase I-targeting activity and cytotoxicity. Biorg Med Chem Lett 14:5585–5589

Satyanarayana M, Feng W, Cheng L, Liu AA, Tsai YC, Liu LF, LaVoie EJ (2008) Syntheses and biological evaluation of topoisomerase I-targeting agents related to 11-[2-(N,N-dimethylamino) ethyl]-2,3-dimethoxy-8,9-methylenedioxy-11H-isoquino[4,3-c]cinnolin-12-one (ARC31). Bioorg Med Chem 16:7824–7831

Schellens JHM, Melirpaard M, Scheper RJ, Scheffer GL, Jonker JW, Smit JW, Beijnen JH, Schinkel AH (2000) Transport of topoisomerase I inhibitors by the breast cancer resistance protein. Ann NY Acad Sci 922:188–194

Solier S, Lansiaux A, Logette E, Wu J, Soret J, Tazi J, Bailly C, Desoche L, Solary E, Corcos L (2004) Topoisomerase I and II inhibitors control caspase-2 pre-messenger RNA splicing in human cells. Molec Cancer Res 2:53–61

Stermitz FR, Gillespie JP, Amoros LG, Romero R, Stermitz TA, Larson KA, Earl S, Ogg JE (1975) Synthesis and biological activity of some antitumor benzophenanthridinium salts. J Med Chem 18:708–713

Stracker TH, Morales M, Couto SS, Hussein H, Petrini JHJ (2007) The carboxy terminus of NBS1 is required for induction of apoptosis by the MRE11 complex. Nature 447:218–221

Staker BL, Hjerrild K, Feese MD, Behnke CA, Burgin AB, Stewart L (2002) The mechanism of topoisomerase I poisoning by a camptothecin analog. Proc Natl Acad Sci USA 99:15387–15392

Stewart AF, Schutz G (1987) Camptothecin-induced in vivo induced topoisomerase cleavages in the transcriptionally active tyrosine aminotransferase gene. Cell 50:1109–1117

Stewart L, Redinbo MR, Qiu X, Hol WGJ, Champoux JJ (1998) A model for the mechanism of human topoisomerase I. Science 279:1534–1541

Sundin O, Varshavsky A (1980) Terminal stages of SV40 DNA replication proceed via multiply intertwined catenated dimers. Cell 21:103–114

Sundin O, Varshavsky A (1981) Arrest of segregation leads to accumulation of highly intertwined catenated dimers. Cell 25:659–669

Takagi K, Dexheimer TS, Redon C, sordet O, Agama K, Lavielle G, Pierre A, Bates SE, Pommier Y (2007) Novel E-ring campotethecin keto analogues 9S38809 and S39625) are stable, potent, and selective topoisomerase I inhibitors without being substrates of drug efflux transporters. Mol Cancer Therap 6: 3229– 3238

Takemura H, Rao VA, Sordet O, Furuta T, Miao Z-H, Meng LH, Zhang H, Pommier Y (2006) Defective Mre-1-dependent activation of Chk2 by ataxia telangiectasia mutated in colorectal carcinoma cells in response to replication-dependent DNA double strand breaks. J Biol Chem 41:30814–30823

Troconiz IF, Garrido MJ, Segura C, Cendros J-M, Principe P, Peraire C, Obach R (2006) Phase I dose-finding study and a pharmacokinetic/pharmacodynamic analysis of the neutropenic response of intravenous diflomotecan in patients with advanced malignant tumors. Cancer Chemother Pharmacol 57:727–735

Tsao YP, D'Arpa P, Liu LF (1992) The involvement of active DNA synthesis in camptothecin-induced G2 arrest: altered regulation of p34cdc2/cyclin B. Cancer Res 52:1823–1829

Tse-Dinh Y-C, Kirkegaard K, Wang JC (1980) Covalent bonds between protein and DNA: Formation of phosphotyrosine linkage between certain DNA topoisomerases and DNA. J Biol Chem 255:5560–5565

Urasaki Y, Laco G, Takebayashi Y, Bailly C, Kohlhagen G, Pommier Y (2001) Use of campthecin-resistant mammalian cell lines to evaluate the role of topoisomerase I in the antiproliferative activity of the indolocarbazole, NB-506, and its topoisomerase I binding site. Cancer Res 61:504–508

Urasaki Y, Takebayashi Y, Pommier Y (2000) Activity of a novel camptothecin analogue, homo-camptothecin, in camptothecin-resistant cell lines with topoisomerase I alterations. Cancer Res 60:6577–6580

Vassal G, Hamelin N, Opolon P, Versace R, Geoerger B (2008) The topoisomerase I inhibitor gimatecan exhibits synergistic antitumor activity in combination with imatinib mesylate and everolimus against malignant glioma xenografts. J Clin Oncol 26 suppl:abstr 2073

Wang JC (1994) DNA Topoisomerases as targets of therapeutics: An overview. In Advances in Pharmacology, vol 29A; Liu, L.F.; Academic Press: New York, pp 1–19

Wang JC (2009) A journey in the world of DNA rings and beyond. Annu Rev Biochem 78:31–54

Wang JC (2009) Untangling the Double Helix. DNA Entanglement and the Action of the DNA Topoisomerases, Cold Spring Harbor Laboratory Press, Cold Spring Harbor, NY, 245 pp

Wang JC (1991) DNA topoisomerases: why so many? J Biol Chem 266:6659–6662

Wang JC (1985) DNA topoisomerases. Ann Rev Biochem 54:665–697

Wang JC, Caron PR, Kim RA (1990) The role of DNA topoisomerases in recombination and genome stability: A double-edged sword? Cell 62:403–406

Wall ME, Wani MC, Cook CE, Palmer KH, McPhail AT, Sim GM (1966) Plant antitumor agents. I. The isolation and structure of camptothecin, a novel alkaloidal leukemia and tumor inhibitor from Camptotheca acuminata. J Amer Chem Soc 88:3888–3890

Wall ME, Wani MC (1995) Camptothecin and taxol: discovery to clinic – thirteenth Bruce F. Cain Memorial Award lecture. Cancer Res 55:753–760

Wani MC, Wall ME (1969) Plant antitumor agents. II. The structure of two new alkaloids from Camptotheca acuminata. J Org Chem 34:1364–1367

Weinstein JN, Pommier Y (2006) Connecting genes, drugs and disease. Nature Biotech 24:1365–1366

Woo MM, Rodriguez L, Gu H, Crenshaw-Williams K, Rocha F, Freestone S, Dickson J, Jodrell D, Mangold JB (2007) Absorption, metabolism and excretion of 14C gimatecan (LBQ707) after oral administration in patients with advanced cancer. J Clin Oncol 25 suppl:abstr 2564

Woo MM, Zhang J, Rocha F, Fandi A, Schran HF (2008) Clinical pharmacokinetics (PK) of two oral dosing schedules of gimatecan in a phase I study: implications for safety and efficacy. J Clin Oncol 26 suppl:abstr 2512

Yang CH, Schneider E, Kuo ML, Volk EL, Rocchi E, Chen YC (2000) BCRP/MXR/ABCP expression in topotecan-resistant human breast carcinoma cells. Biochem Pharmacol 60:831–837

Yamada Y, Tamura T, Yamamoto N, Shimoyama T, Ueda Y, Murakami H, Kusaba H, Kamiya Y, Saka H, Tanigawara Y, McGovren JP, Natsumeda Y (2006) Phase I and pharmacokinetic study of edotecarin, a novel topoisomerase I inhibitor, administered once every 3 weeks in patients with solid tumors. Cancer Chemother Pharmacol 58:173–182

Yin D, Toler S, Guo F, Duncan B, Sharma A (2005) Pharmacokinetics (PK) of edotecarin (J-107088), a topoismerase I inhibitor, in patients with metastatic breast cancer (mBC) or glioblastoma (GBM). J Clin Soc 23 suppl:abstr 2073

Zee-Cheng KY, Cheng CC (1975) Preparation and antileukemic activity of some alkoxybenzo[c] phenanthridinium salts and corresponding dihydro derivatives. J Med Chem 18:66–71

Zhang H, Wang JC, Liu LF (1988) Involvement of DNA topoisomerase I in the transcription of human ribosomal RNA genes. Proc Natl Acad Sci USA 85:1060–1064

Zhu S, Ruchelman AL, Zhou N, Liu AA, Liu LF, LaVoie EJ (2005) Esters and amides of 2,3-dimethoxy-8,9-methylenedioxy-benzo[i]phenanthridine-12-carboxylic acid: potent cytotoxic and topoisomerase I-targeting agents. Bioorg Med Chem 13:6782–6794

Zhu S, Ruchelman AL, Zhou N, Liu AA, Liu LF, LaVoie EJ (2006) 6-Substituted 6H-dibenzo[c,h][2,6]naphthyridin-5-ones: Reversed lactam analogues of ARC-111 with potent topoisomerase I-targeting activity and cytotoxicity. Bioorg Med Chem 14:3131–3143

Zhu L, Miao Z, Sheng C, Guo W, Yao J, Liu W, Che X, Wang W, Cheng P, Zhang W (2010) Trifluoromethyl-promoted homocamptothecins: synthesis and bioloigcal activity. Europ J Med Chem 45: 2726–2732

Chapter 11
Topoisomerase II Inhibitors: Chemical Biology

Anna Rogojina, Stefan Gajewski, Karim Bahmed, Neil Osheroff, and John L. Nitiss

11.1 Introduction: Importance of Top2 as a Drug Target

DNA topoisomerases participate in a wide variety of DNA metabolic activities. Type II topoisomerases are critical during replication, transcription, and chromosome separation (Wang 2002). Topoisomerases are also the targets of several widely used active anticancer agents. The eukaryotic Top2 is the target of such widely used agents as doxorubicin, etoposide, and mitoxantrone (Deweese and Osheroff 2009; Nitiss 2009b; Pommier et al. 2010).

While it has been known for some time that many chemically diverse compounds target topoisomerase II (Top2), the molecular details of enzyme inhibition have remained obscure. The lack of detailed information concerning the enzyme-binding site for drugs has been a significant impediment to the development of a next generation of active and safer Top2 targeting agents.

There have been new developments in the molecular pharmacology of Top2 targeting agents that suggest that new agents might have useful properties. Some of the excitement has arisen from a more detailed understanding of the differential effects of targeting the two mammalian Top2 isoforms. Topoisomerase IIα (Top2α) is expressed preferentially in proliferating cells, and is essential for the completion of mitosis (Nitiss 2009a). By contrast, topoisomerase IIβ (Top2β) is expressed in all

N. Osheroff (✉)
Departments of Biochemistry and Medicine (Hematology/Oncology), School of Medicine, Vanderbilt University, 654 Robinson Research Building, 37232-0146, Nashville, TN, USA
e-mail: neil.osheroff@vanderbilt.edu

J.L. Nitiss (✉)
Department of Biopharmaceutical Sciences, University of Illinois at Chicago, 833 S. Wood Street, IL 60612-7231, Chicago, USA
e-mail: jlnitiss@uic.edu

Y. Pommier (ed.), *DNA Topoisomerases and Cancer*, Cancer Drug Discovery and Development, DOI 10.1007/978-1-4614-0323-4_11,

cells, and while it is required for normal development, it is not essential for cell proliferation (Austin and Marsh 1998). It has been suggested that some of the deleterious effects of Top2 targeting drugs are due to the action of these drugs against Top2β. For example, recent work by Liu and colleagues has suggested that targeting Top2β may be an important way that Top2 targeting drugs can lead to secondary malignancies (Azarova et al. 2007). If this hypothesis is partly correct, then drugs that are specific for Top2α may have therapeutic efficacy with a reduced probability of secondary malignancies.

As described below, FDA approved Top2 targeting drugs potentially suffer from additional issues. For example, most currently used Top2 targeting agents intercalate in DNA (the epipodophyllotoxins etoposide and teniposide are exceptions). Intercalation likely interferes with DNA metabolism by topoisomerase-independent mechanisms. In addition, anthracyclines and anthracenediones generate free radicals. While these topoisomerase-independent cytotoxic mechanisms may contribute to antitumor activity, they are also important for toxic effects against normal cells.

In this chapter, we provide an overview of the chemical biology of Top2 targeting agents. We emphasize agents that are currently approved or that have served as critical model compounds, and compounds that may act by different principles than currently approved agents. Wc introduce our current understanding of drug action, and highlight the limitations of our understanding of drug action.

11.2 Biochemical Mechanisms of Targeting Top2

Compounds that alter the catalytic activity of Top2 can be separated into two categories. Chemicals in the first category decrease the overall activity of the enzyme and are known as catalytic inhibitors. Chemicals in the second category increase levels of Top2-DNA cleaved DNA complexes. These latter compounds are said to "poison" the type II enzyme and convert it to a cellular toxin that initiate a number of mutagenic and potentially lethal consequence. Because of their actions, compounds that increase levels of cleavage complexes are referred to as "Top2 poisons" to distinguish them from catalytic inhibitors (Nitiss 2009b). Although many Top2 poisons also inhibit overall activity, the "gain of function" induced by these compounds in the cell (i.e., increased levels of cleavage complexes) is the dominant phenotype (Deweese and Osheroff 2009).

Top2 poisons increase the concentration of cleavage complexes by two non-mutually exclusive pathways: either they inhibit the ability of the enzyme to ligate cleaved DNA molecules or they increase the forward rate of enzyme-mediated DNA cleavage. Top2 poisons affect the DNA cleavage/ligation equilibrium by three distinct mechanisms. Interfacial Top2 poisons act primarily by inhibiting ligation, redox-dependent Top2 poisons also act primarily by inhibiting ligation, while DNA lesions act primarily by enhancing the forward rate of DNA cleavage.

11.2.1 Interfacial Top2 Poisons

Interfacial Top2 poisons are postulated to form non-covalent interactions with Top2 at the protein-DNA interface in the vicinity of the active site tyrosine (Binaschi et al. 2001; Deweese and Osheroff 2009; Pommier and Marchand 2005). It is notable that all Top2-targeted anticancer drugs that are currently used in the clinics fall into this category. In addition, a number of dietary bioflavonoids, such as the isoflavone genistein (which is prominent in soy) also function as interfacial Top2 poisons (Deweese and Osheroff 2009). Interfacial poisons ultimately inhibit DNA ligation by a conceptually straightforward mechanism; they slip between the cleaved bases and act as "molecular doorstops" that do not allow the DNA ends to be brought into register to allow rejoining. Because interfacial poisons interact with both the protein and DNA within the ternary enzyme-DNA-drug complex, they generally alter the DNA cleavage site specificity of the enzyme (Capranico et al. 1998). In addition, each of the two strand breaks generated by Top2 must be stabilized by a separate drug molecule.

Nonetheless, the precise mechanism of action of interfacial poisons remains unsolved. One of the first models for explaining the action of Top2 poisons postulated that intercalation into DNA occurs after DNA cleavage has occurred. Intercalation would unwind the DNA helix so that DNA ends are no longer precisely positioned for religation (D'Arpa and Liu 1989). The idea that intercalation is critical for the action of Top2 poisons is appealing, since it provides an explanation for agents that act primarily as inhibitors of enzyme-mediated religation. This hypothesis did not invoke a specific requirement for drug–protein interactions. While the hypothesis provided a way of thinking about the action of intercalating agents, it did not provide an explanation for the action of non-intercalating Top2 poisons such as epipodophyllotoxins, nor does it provide an explanation for the sequence selectivity seen with many intercalating agents.

A more detailed explanation has recently been elaborated for trapping of both Top1 and Top2 targeting agents. The model, termed interfacial inhibition, proposes that Top2 poisons bind at the DNA-protein interface (Pommier et al. 2010; Pommier and Marchand 2005). A demonstration of this model for Top1 poisons comes from the determined structures of several topoisomerase I-drug-DNA ternary complexes (Marchand et al. 2006; Staker et al. 2002, 2005). Camptothecins and other topoisomerase I poisons were found to intercalate between the −1 and +1 bases of DNA in the ternary complex, where the −1 base is the nucleotide that is covalently bound to Top1. In addition to the stacking interactions arising from intercalation of the drug, the structures also showed drug–protein interactions. This result is in agreement with previous findings that camptothecin did not form significant binary complexes with either DNA or Top1. The presence of the intercalated drug results in the displacement of the 5′-OH of the free DNA end relative to the 3′-phosphotyrosyl protein-DNA covalent complex, resulting in inhibition of ligation.

A similar type of interfacial inhibition has been observed in structures of bacterial type II topoisomerases in complex with fluoroquinolones and DNA (Laponogov et al. 2009; Wohlkonig et al. 2010). The fluoroquinolones in the structure stack between base pairs at the DNA cleavage site. While the interactions with DNA are mainly stabilized by π-π interactions, there are also contacts between the drug and conserved residues of the topoisomerase. Although the details of the ternary complexes require refinement, the presence of the fluoroquinolone likely displaces the 5′-phosphotyrosyl from the free 3′-OH and the displacement greatly reduces ligation rates. There are likely notable differences between these structures derived from prokaryotic enzymes and intercalating agents that target eukaryotic Top2. For example, the fluoroquinolones form a wedge- like structure, as opposed to the expected planar structure with the intercalating agents that target eukaryotic Top2. The interfacial inhibition model can readily accommodate the observation that not all intercalating agents are Top2 poisons. The model would suggest that some protein–drug interactions are needed for optimal stabilization of a drug: DNA: enzyme ternary complex. The protein–drug interactions distinguish the interfacial inhibition model from the simple intercalator model described above. In addition, in its simplest form, the simple intercalation model would suggest that intercalators interact with an enzyme-DNA cleaved complex. Since intercalative poisons display strong affinities for Top2, even in the absence of DNA (Froelich-Ammon et al. 1995a, b), it is reasonable that interactions with Top2 mediate the entry of these drugs into the ternary complex. Alternately, intercalation may precede DNA cleavage by Top2, with sites of cleavage mainly determined by intercalator: DNA interactions.

The most important non-intercalating interfacial Top2 poisons are etoposide and teniposide, both of which are epipodophyllotoxins. These compounds display little (if any) affinity for DNA in the absence of Top2 and several lines of evidence indicate that interactions with the enzyme are critical for drug function and mediate entry into the ternary complex (Burden et al. 1996; Kingma et al. 1999; Wilstermann et al. 2007). While no eukaryotic Top2 structures that include drugs have been determined (as of this date), NMR and binding studies of the binary enzyme-drug complex coupled with DNA functional (DNA cleavage) studies in the ternary complex have assigned functions to most parts of the etoposide molecule (Fig. 11.1) (Bender and Osheroff 2008; Wilstermann et al. 2007). The binding of etoposide to Top2 appears to be driven by interactions with the A–ring, B–ring, and potentially by stacking interactions with the E–ring (Bender and Osheroff 2008; Wilstermann et al. 2007). The E–ring methoxyl groups and the 4′-OH moiety are important for drug function, but do not contribute substantially to enzyme-drug binding or to DNA cleavage specificity (Bender and Osheroff 2008; Wilstermann et al. 2007). Neither the C4 gylcoside nor the D-ring of etoposide contacts the enzyme in the binary complex (Bender and Osheroff 2008; Wilstermann et al. 2007). However, both appear to interact with DNA in the ternary complex and influence the specificity of DNA cleavage (Bender and Osheroff 2008). Finally, while removal of the C4 glycoside has little effect on levels of etoposide-induced DNA cleavage by Top2, this group can be substituted with an aminoalkyl side chain (TOP-53), which increases the affinity of the drug for the enzyme (Wilstermann et al. 2007), or

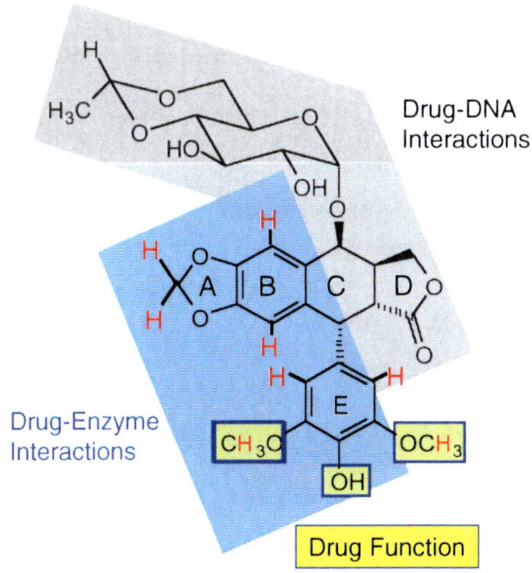

Fig. 11.1 Summary of etoposide substituents that interact with human Top2α. Protons that interact with the enzyme (as determined by saturation transfer difference ^{1}H NMR spectroscopy) are shown in red. Interactions between hydroxyl protons and the enzyme were obscured by the water peak and could not be visualized. The blue region on etoposide, including portions of the A–, B–, and E–rings is proposed to interact with Top2α in the binary drug-enzyme complex. E–ring substituents highlighted with *yellow boxes* are important for drug function and interact with the enzyme, but do not appear to contribute significantly to binding. We propose that interactions between etoposide and DNA in the ternary complex (are shaded in *gray*) are driven primarily by the D-ring, with additional contributions from the C4 sugar

a spermine moiety (F14512), which turns etoposide into a DNA-binding drug (Barret et al. 2008). Both modifications enhance the potency of the parent compound (Barret et al. 2008; Byl et al. 2001b; Gentry et al. 2011).

11.2.2 Redox-Dependent Top2 Poisons

A second class of Top2 poisons that inhibit DNA ligation functions by a very different and poorly understood mechanism. Compounds in this class require redox activity to facilitate their actions against Top2, and alter enzyme activity by covalently adducting to Top2 at amino acid residues outside of the active site (Bender et al. 2006; Deweese and Osheroff 2009; Lindsey et al. 2004; Wang et al. 2001). Several cysteine residues have been shown to be modified by "redox-dependent" Top2 poisons (Bender et al. 2007; Bender and Osheroff 2007), but the mechanism by which these modifications lead to modified enzyme function remains an enigma. Although (in some cases) there is a correlation between greater inhibition of ligation and enhanced stability of the closed N-terminal protein gate (Bender et al. 2006), the relationship between these two events is not understood.

Redox-dependent Top2 poisons are characterized by a number of dietary polyphenols such as EGGC (epigallocatechin gallate, which is found in green tea) as well as several environmental quinone-based toxins, including the benzene metabolite 1,4-benzoquinone, the acetaminophen metabolite N-acetyl *p*-benzoquinone imine (NAPQI), and polychlorinated biphenyls (PCB) quinone metabolites (Bandele et al. 2008; Bender et al. 2004, 2006; Lindsey et al. 2004). Since these compounds do not appear to function within the active site of Top2, they generally enhance DNA cleavage at sites that are intrinsically cut by the enzyme (Bandele et al. 2008). Moreover, because these agents require redox chemistry for activation, their ability to poison Top2 is abrogated by reducing agents (Bandele et al. 2008; Bender et al. 2004, 2006; Lindsey et al. 2004; Wang et al. 2001). Finally, while redox-dependent Top2 poisons enhance DNA cleavage when added to the protein-DNA complex, they display the distinguishing feature of inhibiting Top2 activity when incubated with the enzyme prior to the addition of DNA (Lindsey et al. 2004; Wang et al. 2001).

11.2.3 DNA Lesions as Top2 Poisons

Several forms of nucleic acid damage enhance Top2-mediated DNA cleavage (Kingma and Osheroff 1998; Sabourin and Osheroff 2000; Velez-Cruz et al. 2005). The type II enzymes are particularly sensitive to abasic sites, alkylated bases that contain exocyclic rings, and other lesions that distort the double helix.

DNA damage increases cleavage at naturally occurring sites of Top2 action (Kingma and Osheroff 1998; Sabourin and Osheroff 2000; Velez-Cruz et al. 2005). In order to enhance cleavage, lesions must be located within the four-base stagger that separates the two scissile bonds (Kingma and Osheroff 1998; Velez-Cruz et al. 2005). Unlike the interfacial and redox-dependent Top2 poisons discussed above, DNA lesions do not inhibit rates of Top2-mediated ligation (in fact, they generally are faster) and act primarily by enhancing the forward rate of DNA scission (Deweese and Osheroff 2009; Velez-Cruz et al. 2005).

The mechanistic basis for the effects of DNA lesions on Top2-mediated DNA cleavage is probably related to DNA structure. Structural and enzymological studies indicate that the DNA segment that is cleaved by Top2 contains a sharp (~150°) bend, which appears to play an important role in coordinating the two protomer subunits of the enzyme (Deweese et al. 2008; Deweese and Osheroff 2009; Dong and Berger 2007; Schmidt et al. 2010). Lesions that increase DNA flexibility or induce kinks or distortions in the double helix likely facilitate DNA bending and thus increase the forward rate of scission. This proposed mechanism accounts for the required positional specificity (i.e., between the scissile bonds) of lesions for DNA cleavage enhancement.

The physiological benefits of Top2 recognizing DNA lesions (if any) are unclear. However, both human type II topoisomerases appear to play roles in fragmenting genomic DNA and releasing chromosomal loops during apoptosis (Belyaev 2005; Solovyan et al. 2002). It has been suggested that the apoptotic activities of Top2 are enhanced (or perhaps triggered) by DNA lesions that are generated following the release of oxidative radicals from permeable mitochondria in apoptotic cells (Belyaev 2005; Solovyan et al. 2002).

11.3 Drugs That Target Top2: Approved Agents

The first drugs that target Top2 that were FDA approved were the anthracyclines doxorubicin (approved in 1974) and daunomycin (approved in 1979). The structures of several approved Top2 targeting agents are shown in Fig. 11.2. Much of the earlier clinical investigation with anthracyclines preceded the demonstration that anthracyclines target Top2. While some anthracyclines have substantial antitumor activity, they also have significant toxicities, including cardiotoxicity. Anthracyclines also generate free radicals that damage DNA and other cellular structures. The wide use of anthracyclines has prompted substantial investigation into the identification of safer and more active compounds. Current clinical use of anthracyclines and other approved Top2 targeting agents is discussed by Goldwasser and colleagues in Chap. 13. A more comprehensive picture of current advances in anthracyclines has been provided in a recent monograph (Krohn 2008).

Anthracyclines represent the largest group of approved Top2 targeting agents. In addition to doxorubicin, other approved anthracyclines include daunomycin,

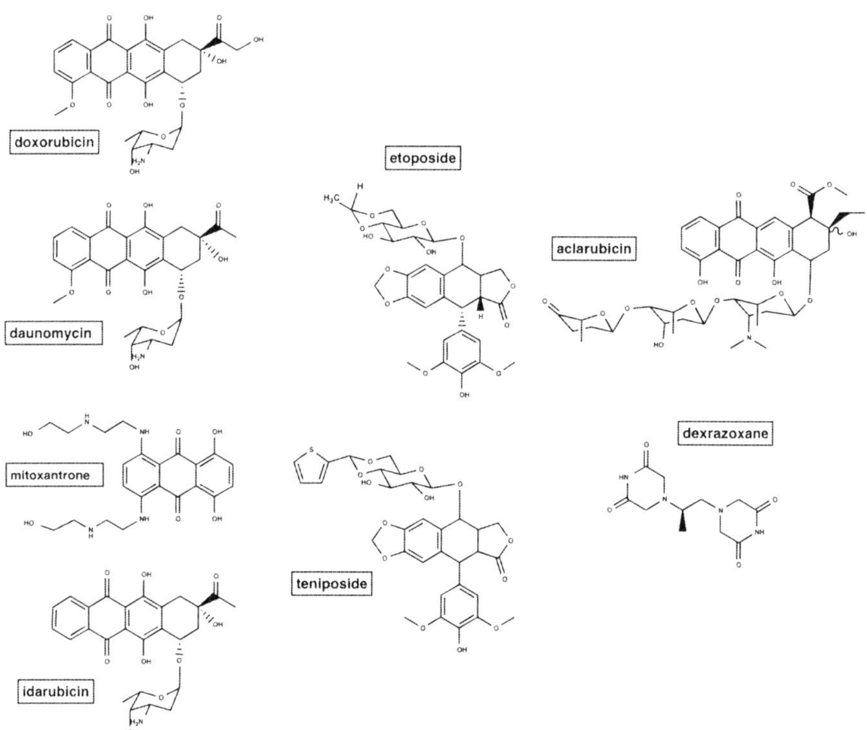

Fig. 11.2 Chemical structures of FDA-approved drugs targeting Top2. The structures of the anthracyclines, the epipodophyllotoxins etoposide and teniposide, the anthracenedione mitoxantrone, and the bisdioxopiperazine dexrazoxane are shown. FDA-approved agents that are not shown are the epipodophyllotoxin etoposide phosphate and the two approved liposomal doxorubicin formulations

idarubicin, and aclarubicin. Aclarubicin is unique among approved anthracyclines because it is not a Top2 poison, but is instead a Top2 catalytic inhibitor. Aclarubicin is discussed further in Sect. 5, along with other catalytic inhibitors of Top2. Since a major issue for anthracyclines has been safe and effective dosing, two liposomal formulations, Doxil® and Myocet® have been approved for use.

The quest for safer anthracyclines has led to an examination of other intercalating Top2 poisons. Mitoxantrone, an anthracenedione is a potent intercalating agent that has been approved for leukemias and advanced hormone refractory prostate cancer. Mitoxantrone is unique because it is the only Top2 poison that has been approved for a noncancer indication, multiple sclerosis (Giovannoni 2011). Like many anthracyclines, mitoxantrone can generate substantial cardiotoxicity (de Forni and Armand 1994; Hamzehloo and Etemadifar 2006).

Two non-intercalating Top2 poisons are currently approved for use, etoposide and teniposide (Baldwin and Osheroff 2005; Hande 1998). In addition, the water-soluble prodrug etoposide phosphate has also been approved for use. Etoposide phosphate is rapidly converted to etoposide in the plasma. Since epipodophyllotoxins are non-intercalating, drug action is very specific for targeting Top2 (Nitiss and Beck 1996). Mechanistic aspects of etoposide and other epipodophyllotoxins are discussed in Sect. 11.2.

Dexrazoxane (ICR-187), like aclarubicin, is a catalytic inhibitor of Top2. While dexrazoxane has limited anticancer activity, it is used to prevent anthracycline-induced cardiotoxicity. Dexrazoxane and other Top2 catalytic inhibitors are discussed further in Sect. 11.5.

11.4 Drugs That Target Top2: Significant Experimental Agents

A broad range of experimental agents has been identified that are Top2 poisons. While it is beyond the scope of the present chapter to provide a detailed discussion of the many experimental agents that can stimulate Top2-mediated cleavage, this section highlights some of the more unique compounds, the compounds that have been particularly important in the study of Top2 targeting agents, and compounds that may lead to new drugs. A selection of relevant structures is shown in Fig. 11.3.

11.4.1 Experimental Intercalating Agents

Probably no class of anticancer agents have been subjected to more detailed chemical analysis than anthracyclines (Krohn 2008). The demonstration that many intercalating agents are Top2 poisons has led to identification and study of many other classes of intercalating Top2 poisons. This section introduces a few compounds that have either been significant model compounds, or have been extensively examined clinically.

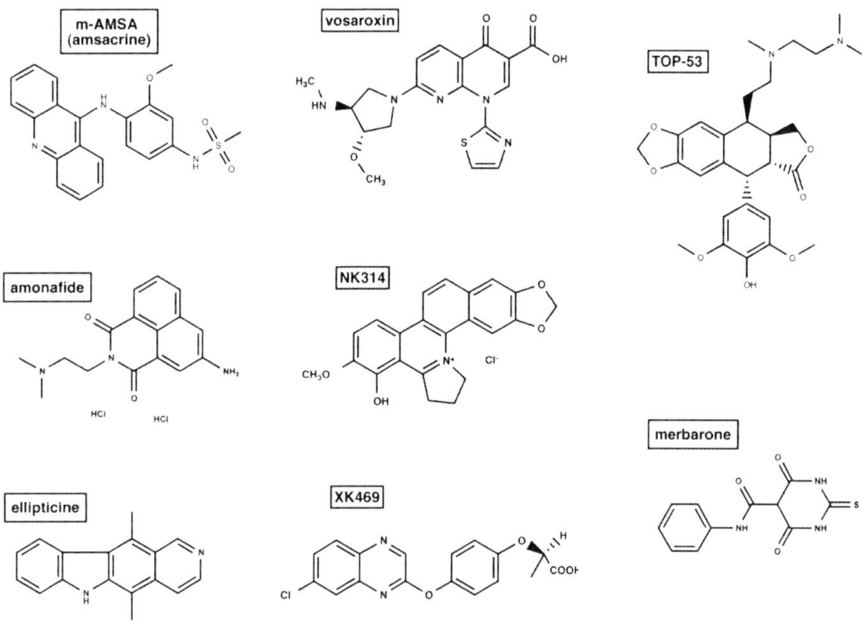

Fig. 11.3 Chemical structures of selected experimental agents targeting Top2. The structures of a variety of experimental Top2 targeting agents are illustrated. All of the compounds shown with the exception of merbarone are Top2 poisons; merbarone is a catalytic inhibitor. NK314 has been proposed to be a Top2α selective Top2 poison, while XK469 is a Top2β selective agent. The other Top2 poisons illustrated are not notably selective for either isoform

Amsacrine (*m*AMSA), an aminoacridine was the first agent shown to act as a Top2 poison (Minford et al. 1986; Pommier et al. 1985; Tewey et al. 1984). *m*AMSA has been widely used as an intercalating Top2 poison in laboratory studies, in part because it has very limited Top2-independent effects. *m*AMSA was extensively tested in a variety of tumor types, with limited activity except in leukemia. For many years *m*AMSA was available in the USA for treatment of relapsed acute myeloid leukemias (AML) (Arlin 1989), and it is still used in other countries. A large number of derivatives have been isolated, some with enhanced activity against nondividing cells (Baguley and Finlay 1988; Granzen et al. 1992; Turnbull et al. 1999). Some derivatives such as DACA have been reported to be dual Top1/Top2 inhibitors and are discussed in Sect. 11.5.

Amonafide is an example of a naphthalimide, and is a potent intercalating agent (Ingrassia et al. 2009). Amonafide has undergone extensive clinical testing, with limited activity except in leukemias (Asbury et al. 1997, 1998). In addition to the limited activity in solid tumors, amonafide showed unpredictable toxicity due to polymorphisms in genes involved in drug metabolism. Recently, amonafide derivatives have provoked renewed interest due the observation that amonafide is a poor substrate for p-glycoprotein-mediated drug efflux, and its activity in AML (Allen et al. 2010; Chau et al. 2008).

A variety of other intercalating agents have been frequently used as model compounds. These include ellipticine derivatives (Dereuddre et al. 1997; Multon et al. 1989; Riou et al. 1995), acridines (Adjei et al. 1998; Makhey et al. 2000), and many other chemical classes. In many cases, compounds were identified as Top2 poisons, but were not analyzed in great detail.

Vosaroxin (formerly voreloxin) is a first class quinolone derivative that is currently in phase II clinical trials for a variety of blood-borne and solid tumors (Krug et al. 2011; Scatena et al. 2010; Zhu et al. 2010). In contrast to antibacterial quinolones, vosaroxin is strongly intercalative and this interaction with DNA is essential for actions of the drug both as a Top2 poison and as a cellular toxin (Hawtin et al. 2010). Although vosaroxin enhances DNA cleavage mediated by Top2α and Top2β in vitro and in treated human cells, it does so at a very restricted selection of sites (Hawtin et al. 2010). In addition, the drug clearly has additional modes of action (which are undefined at the present time) that contribute to cytotoxicity (Hawtin et al. 2010; Walsby et al. 2011).

11.4.2 Other Epipodophyllotoxins

Epipodophyllotoxins have been the most significant non-intercalating Top2 poisons. Much synthetic chemistry has been devoted to the development of new epipodophyllotoxins (Huang et al. 1999; You 2005). Several epipodophyllotoxins derivatives have undergone significant preclinical and clinical development, including compounds such as GL331 (Huang et al. 1999), TOP-53 (Byl et al. 2001a), and F11782 (Kruczynski et al. 2004). F11782 has some properties of catalytic Top2 inhibitors (Jensen et al. 2003), suggesting that epipodophyllotoxins that target topoisomerases in unique ways may be possible.

11.4.3 Experimental Agents with Isoform Specificity

Human cells have two type II topoisomerase isoforms Top2α and Top2β (Nitiss 2009a). As noted in the introduction, it has been suggested that some of the deleterious effects of Top2 poisons may arise from targeting Top2β. One clear way that this could occur is because Top2α is normally not present in nonproliferating cells. Therefore, the Top2β can generate DNA damage, leading to oncogenic translocations or killing of nonproliferating cells (such as cardiac myocytes, as occurs with anthracyclines). However, the ability to target Top2β in nonproliferating cells could allow elimination of nonproliferating tumor cells. Drugs targeting both Top2α and Top2β could enhance the killing of proliferating tumor cells by causing higher levels of DNA damage than targeting a single isoform.

Toyoda and colleagues described a synthetic benzo[c]phenanthridine alkaloid that is highly specific for the Top2α isoform (Toyoda et al. 2008). While not completely specific for Top2α, it represents the first model compound that can be used to assess whether specific targeting of Top2α might be a safer anticancer strategy. However, recent results have suggested that NK314 is a dual inhibitor of Top2α and DNA-dependent protein kinase (DNA-PK) (Hisatomi et al. 2011), a protein involved in nonhomologous end joining (NHEJ). Critically, NHEJ is an important pathway for repairing Top2-mediated DNA damage, therefore the cytotoxicity of NK314 may arise from both targeting Top2α and inhibiting repair of the damage that is generated.

While recent results favor the hypothesis that specific targeting Top2α might be of therapeutic value, it remains plausible that specific targeting of Top2β may be clinically beneficial. Several agents that act against both t Top2α and β, such as mitoxantrone and *m*AMSA have been reported to preferentially target Top2β (Errington et al. 1999). Snapka and colleagues found that the XK469, a quinoxaline phenoxypropionic acid derivative, was selective for Top2β (Gao et al. 1999). They observed that Top2β−/− mouse cells were threefold resistant to XK469, whereas the same cells showed only minimal resistance to *m*AMSA (Snapka et al. 2001). While XK469 has minimal activity against Top2α, it has also been reported to result in increases in cyclinB1 levels (Lin et al. 2002; Subramanian et al. 2002). Nonetheless, XK469 or other derivatives are likely to be useful tools in assessing the cellular effects of specific targeting of Top2β. XK469 has been explored in phase 1 clinical trials, although antitumor activity has not yet been reported (Alousi et al. 2007; Undevia et al. 2008).

11.4.4 Combined Top1/Top2 Targeting Agents

Drugs targeting Top1 or Top2 act on different targets, with the anticipation that the mechanisms of resistance to the individual agents would be distinct. Early trials that sought to combine camptothecins with Top2 targeting drugs were complicated by toxicity, and partial antagonism depending on the details of scheduling (Bertrand et al. 1992). As an alternative to combining Top1 and Top2 targeting agents, several investigators have screened for compounds that could stimulate cleavage by both classes of topoisomerases. Somewhat surprisingly, several agents have been identified that are dual inhibitors of both Top1 and Top2 (Denny and Baguley 2003; Riou et al. 1993; Yamashita et al. 1991). The effects of dual Top1/Top2 inhibitors frequently parallel the biochemical effects of agents that act against only one topoisomerase. For example, the covalent complexes induced by the dual inhibitor saintopin occur at high levels, and with the same heat reversal seen with camptothecin or etoposide (Yamashita et al. 1991). One agent that has been characterized in detail was the benzopyridoindole intoplicine. Intoplicine was tested in phase 1 trials, and its utility was limited by hepatic toxicity (Newman et al. 1999; van Gijn et al. 1999). A quinoline derivative TAS-103 was also shown to stabilize cleavage by both Top1 and Top2 (Aoyagi et al. 1999). For TAS-103, results in yeast suggested that the major cytotoxic activity was directed against Top2 (Byl et al. 1999; Fortune et al. 1999). This result suggests that many dual inhibitors may preferentially target either Top1 or Top2, with more modest activity against the other enzyme. This is not necessarily a disadvantage, if potent targeting of both enzymes is difficult to achieve due to toxicity or schedule dependence. Several other compounds have been described as dual Top1/Top2 inhibitors including the phenazanine XR11576 (Lewis et al. 2007; Wang et al. 2002) and the acridine DACA (N-[2-(dimethylamino)ethyl]acridine-4-carboxamide) (Denny and Baguley 2003). While the notion of targeting both Top1 and Top2 with a single chemical entity remains an interesting concept, currently available agents have not led to high levels of clinical activity at safe dosage levels. Biochemical studies of dual topoisomerase inhibitors have been somewhat limited. However, the ability to target both Top1 and Top2, enzymes with very different active sites, suggests that topoisomerase targeting can be accomplished with minimal protein–drug interactions.

11.5 Catalytic Inhibitors of Top2

The Top2 targeting agents described in the preceding sections are topoisomerase poisons, generating enzyme-mediated DNA damage. Since Top2α is required for cell proliferation, catalytic inhibition may be partly involved in the action of Top2 poisons. Alternately, catalytic inhibitors might also be an effective anticancer drug strategy. The best characterized catalytic inhibitors of eukaryotic Top2 are the bisdioxopiperazines such as dexrazoxane (ICRF-187) and ICRF-193 (Ishida et al. 1991, 1995). Bisdioxopiperazines inhibit Top2 at a unique point in the enzyme catalytic cycle (Roca et al. 1994). After strand passage, Top2 hydrolyzes ATP and the N-terminal clamp opens, allowing release of the strand that had been cleaved by the enzyme. Bisdioxopiperazines block DNA dependent ATP hydrolysis by Top2 and prevent the opening of the N-terminal clamp (Jensen et al. 2000; Morris et al. 2000) (see Berger and Osheroff Chap. 3 for details of the Top2 catalytic cycle). While bisdioxopiperazines do not lead to greatly elevated levels of covalent complexes (but see (Huang et al. 2001) for an alternate perspective), the generation of a closed clamp might lead to interference with DNA metabolism (Germe and Hyrien 2005; Jensen et al. 2000; Park and Avraham 2006). Nonetheless, bisdioxopiperazines have been commonly used as model compounds for Top2 catalytic inhibitors. Bisdioxopiperazines have not been reported to have substantial antitumor activity, but dexrazoxane had been approved both as a cardioprotectant to prevent anthracyclines-induced cardiotoxicity (Cvetkovic and Scott 2005) and to minimize tissue damage following anthracyclines extravasation (Schulmeister 2008, 2011).

The mechanism of cardioprotection during anthracycline treatment by bisdioxopiperazines continues to be controversial. The generally accepted mechanism for cardioprotection had been prevention of free radical damage by iron chelation (Simunek et al. 2009). However, recently, Lyu and colleagues suggested that Top2β may play an important role in anthracycline-induced cardiotoxicity (Lyu et al. 2007). It had previously been shown that treatment of mammalian cells with bisdioxopiperazines leads to selective proteolytic degradation of Top2β (Xiao et al. 2003). Lyu and colleagues observed that dexrazoxane blocked DNA damage signaling cardiomyocytes treated with anthracyclines, but had no effect on DNA damage signaling induced by hydrogen peroxide. This observation suggests that doxorubicin induces DNA damage in cardiomyocytes, and elimination of Top2β, the only Top2 in cardiomyocytes that largely prevents anthracyclines-mediated damage. Further studies will be needed to resolve this critical issue. If Top2β plays an important role in cardiotoxicity of anthracyclines, then this will provide a major rationale for developing potent Top2α specific agents.

The above discussion fails to answer whether catalytic inhibition of Top2 might be a useful anticancer drug strategy. In addition to dexrazoxane, the anthracycline aclarubicin is also an FDA-approved agent. Aclarubicin does not enhance levels Top2-mediated cleavage. Instead, aclarubicin is a potent inhibitor both of Top2-mediated cleavage and Top2 catalytic activity (Jensen et al. 1990, 1991; Petersen et al. 1994). Aclarubicin likely inhibits Top2 by preventing the enzyme from binding to DNA. Like other anthracyclines, aclarubicin has multiple targets. For example, aclarubicin has been shown to stimulate DNA cleavage by eukaryotic Top1 (Nitiss et al. 1997). Therefore, it is unclear to what extent the antitumor activity of aclarubicin is due to its activity against Top2.

An additional agent that has been tested extensively in the clinic is merbarone (5-(*N*-phenylcarboxamido)-2-thiobarbituric acid). Merbarone is a potent Top2 inhibitor (Drake et al. 1989) that does not prevent association of the enzyme with DNA, but blocks Top2 DNA cleavage (Fortune and Osheroff 1998). Like aclarubicin, merbarone is not specific for Top2, and has been reported to generate DNA damage in a Top2-independent manner (Clifford et al. 2003). Merbarone has been tested in several clinical trials and did not exhibit any antitumor activity (e.g., (Look et al. 1995, 1996; Malik et al. 1997)).

More recently, there has been a renewed effort to develop new catalytic inhibitors of Top2. Since bacterial type II topoisomerases can be inhibited by agents that are competitive with ATP binding, one class of agents that are being developed are purine analogs (Chene et al. 2009; Furet et al. 2009). Chene and colleagues have described an ATP competitive inhibitor termed quinoline aminopurine compound 1 (QAP1). This compound is a sub-micromolar inhibitor that is active both in vivo and in vitro. While detailed mechanistic and antitumor results have not yet been reported, it would be expected that this class of compounds would block Top2 enzymatic activity and reduce (but perhaps not eliminate) enzyme-mediated cleavage. The testing of these and other compounds will be critical in finally establishing whether Top2 catalytic inhibition is a viable anticancer strategy.

11.6 Inferring Drug Action Through Topoisomerase Mutants

A central strategy for understanding biochemical mechanisms of anticancer drugs with defined targets has been the identification of mutants with altered sensitivity. In principle, mutants that confer drug resistance might identify sites on Top2 that are either involved in drug binding or in some other enzymatic step that is critical for drug action. Since Top2 poisons generate enzyme-mediated DNA damage, resistance could be mediated by mutations that reduce enzyme activity. In order to use mutations to understand the molecular details of drug action, the mutational screens that have been used to identify drug resistant mutations have tried to reduce the likelihood of identifying mutations that are drug resistant simply due to low enzyme activity or stability.

The major tool that has been used to identify drug resistant mutations in eukaryotic Top2 has been to use yeast strains that moderately overexpress Top2 (Nitiss et al. 1992). Since drug resistant mutation alleles of Top2 would be expected to be genetically recessive to drug sensitive alleles, screens have typically used yeast strains with a temperature sensitive allele of Top2 on the chromosome, thereby ensuring that the overexpressed allele is the only active Top2 in the cell. Since overexpression of Top2 by itself is not sufficient to ensure that mutants with relatively normal activity will be recovered, additional experimentation is needed to demonstrate that drug resistance is not due to gross alterations in enzyme activity. The test that has been applied most often has been to try to find mutants that are resistant to one class of agents (e.g., epipodophyllotoxins) but with normal sensitivity to other classes of agents (such as intercalating agents). In general, most mutants that have been obtained in yeast screens do not pass this test, and are resistant to all classes of Top2 poisons.

A full list of yeast Top2 mutants with altered sensitivity to Top2 targeting agents is shown in Tables 11.1 and 11.2. Table 11.1 shows drug resistant alleles obtained by many laboratories. One large-scale screen carried out by Jiang is not included, since none of the mutant alleles were characterized in detail (Jiang 2005). Overall, a relatively large number of mutants have been identified. In general, the drug resistant alleles identified in yeast Top2 frequently have reduced enzymatic activity (see Table 11.1 for exceptions) and typically confer resistance to multiple classes of Top2 poisons.

Since isolation of resistant mutants to Top2 targeting drugs has been a somewhat disappointing strategy for understanding the action of Top2 targeting agents, an alternate strategy that has shown some promise is the isolation of mutants in Top2, which specifically enhance sensitivity to specific Top2 targeting drugs (Dong et al. 2000; Rogojina and Nitiss 2008). The first indication that this might provide information about Top2 targeting agents was the observation that mutating yeast Ser740 led to hypersensitivity to etoposide (Hsiung et al. 1995). Interestingly, the biochemical properties of trapped Top2 complexes were also altered. Top2 cleavage induced by topoisomerase poisons can be readily reversed by heating, by increasing salt concentrations, or by the addition of EDTA (Tewey et al. 1984). The Ser740Trp mutant protein, treated with etoposide resulted in covalent complexes that were much more stable with respect to elevated temperature or exposure to high salt than complexes formed with wild-type protein (Hsiung et al. 1995). The generation of covalent complexes with enhanced stability suggests that the mutation of Ser740 to Trp enhances etoposide binding, although this hypothesis has not been directly

Table 11.1 Yeast mutants in Top2 with altered sensitivity to Top2 targeting agents

Mutation	Relevant agents	Biochemical alterations and notes	References
Yeast Top2 mutants conferring resistance to anti-topoisomerase drugs			
Lys438Gln	mAMSA, etoposide	Mutant constructed based on the human Top2α Arg450Gln mutation; yeast enzyme not characterized	Nitiss et al. (1994)
Pro473Ala/Leu474Val/Arg475Gly	mAMSA	Enzyme not characterized	Wasserman and Wang (1994a)
L474A/R475G	mAMSA	Reduced drug-dependent DNA cleavage, substantial reduction in enzyme activity	Wasserman and Wang (1994a)
L474A/L479P	mAMSA	Reduced drug-dependent DNA cleavage, substantial reduction in enzyme activity	Wasserman and Wang (1994b)
Lys477Ala	mAMSA	Enzyme not characterized	Wasserman and Wang (1994a)
Ala641Gly	mAMSA teniposide	Reduced drug-dependent DNA cleavage, wild-type enzyme activity	Wasserman and Wang (1994a)
Ala641Ser	Doxorubicin, mAMSA, etoposide	Reduced drug-dependent DNA cleavage, wild-type enzyme activity	Patel et al. (1997)
Gly737Asp	CP-115,953, etoposide	Enzyme not characterized	Liu et al. (1994)
Gly747Glu	Doxorubicin, mAMSA, etoposide	Reduced drug dependent DNA cleavage, substantial reduction in enzyme activity	Patel et al. (1997)
Top2-4/Pro820Gln	Etoposide	Temperature sensitive enzyme activity, reduced enzyme activity at the permissive temperature	Nitiss et al. (1992)
Pro823Ser	mAMSA, etoposide, CP-115,953	Enzyme not characterized	Liu et al. (1994)
Top2-5/Arg883Pro/Arg885Ile/Met886Ileu	mAMSA, etoposide	Temperature sensitive enzyme activity, wild-type enzyme activity at the permissive temperature, greatly reduced drug-induced DNA cleavage	Jannatipour et al. (1993)

(continued)

Table 11.1 (continued)

Yeast Top2 mutants showing hypersensitivity to anti-topoisomerase drugs			
Mutation	Relevant agents	Biochemical alterations and notes	References
Gly436Ser	CP-115,953, etoposide, ellipticine, mAMSA	Drug resistant in yeast cells due to reduced stability. Hypersensitive to multiple drugs in the absence of ATP. Wild-type cleavage in the presence of ATP	Sabourin et al. (1998)
Pro473Leu	mAMSA	Reduced enzyme activity. High levels of sensitivity to mAMSA. Preferential induction of single versus double strand breaks	Rogojina and Nitiss (2008)
Ala484Pro	mAMSA, CP-115,953, etoposide	Enzyme not characterized	Rogojina and Nitiss (2008)
Ph711Ileu	mAMSA, etoposide	Enzyme not characterized	Rogojina and Nitiss (2008)
His735Gln	mAMSA, CP-115,953, etoposide	Enzyme not characterized	Rogojina and Nitiss (2008)
Gly737Val	mAMSA	Wild-type enzyme activity. High levels of sensitivity to mAMSA	Rogojina and Nitiss (2008)
Gln739Trp	Etoposide, mAMSA	Protein was highly resistant to fluoroquinolones, TOP2-covalent complexes, formed in the presence of etoposide shown heat stability	Dong and Nitiss, unpublished
Ser740Trp	Etoposide	Enhanced levels of etoposide stabilized cleavage. Etoposide-induced covalent complexes showed enhanced stability. Reduced cleavage with fluoroquinclones	Hsiung et al. (1995)
Thr744Pro	mAMSA	Wild-type enzymatic activity. Enhanced DNA cleavage in the presence of mAMSA and fluoroquinolones. Hypersensitivity was not associated with heat-stable covalent complexes	Dong et al. (2000)
Leu787Ser	mAMSA, etoposide	Enzyme not characterized	Rogojina and Nitiss (2008)
His1011Tyr	Ellipticine	Wild-type enzyme activity, resistant to CP-115,953 and etoposide, hypersensitive to ellipticine, wild-type sensitivity to *m*AMSA	Elsea et al. (1995)
Leu1052Ileu	mAMSA, CP-115,953, etoposide	Enzyme not characterized	Rogojina and Nitiss (2008)

In some cases, the amino acid number listed differs from the published sequence due to a subsequently identified DNA sequencing error in the DNA of yeast Top2

Table 11.2 Human Top2 α mutants conferring resistance or hypersensitivity to anti-topoisomerase drugs

Human Top2 α mutants conferring resistance or hypersensitivity to anti-topoisomerase drugs			
Mutation	Relevant agents	Biochemical alterations and notes	References
Gly437Glu	mAMSA (H) Teniposide (H)	Mutant protein exhibits enhanced catalytic activity	Patel et al. (2000)
Arg450Gln	Etoposide (R) mAMSA (R)	Reduced drug-stabilized DNA cleavage. Greater effects on enzyme activity and in vitro drug sensitivity when combined with Pro803Ser	Bugg et al. (1991); Mao et al. (1999)
Arg487Lys	mAMSA (R)	Resistant to mAMSA in vitro, wild-type sensitivity to etoposide. Mutant has been independently isolated in mammalian cells at least three times	Hinds et al. (1991); Lee et al. (1992)
Glu571Lys	mAMSA (R)	Wild-type enzyme activity, reduced drug-stabilized cleavage	Patel et al. (2000)
His759Pro	Etoposide (R) Doxorubicin (R)	Reduced enzyme activity, reduced drug-stabilized cleavage	Suda et al. (2004)
His759Ala	Etoposide (R) Doxorubicin (R)	Reduced enzyme activity, reduced drug-stabilized cleavage	Suda et al. (2004)
Ser763Trp	Etoposide (H) mAMSA (R)	Etoposide hypersensitive, analog of yeast Ser740Trp	Strumberg et al. (1999a)
Ser763Ala	mAMSA (R)	Not hypersensitive to etoposide, resistant to mAMSA, reduced enzyme activity	Strumberg et al. (1999a)
Asn770Pro	Etoposide (R) Doxorubicin (R)	Reduced enzyme activity, reduced drug-stabilized cleavage	Suda et al. (2004)
Pro803Ser	Etoposide (R) mAMSA (R)	Weak biochemical effect as a single mutant. Greater effects on enzyme activity and in vitro drug sensitivity when combined with Arg450Gln	Kohno et al. (1995); Mao et al. (1999)

(continued)

Table 11.2 (continued)

Topoisomerase IIβ mutants conferring resistance or hypersensitivity to anti-topoisomerase drugs			
Mutation	Relevant agents	Biochemical alterations and notes	References
Gly465Gln	mAMSA (R) Etoposide (R) Ellipticine (R) DACA (R)	Reduced decatenation activity	Gilroy et al. (2006); Leontiou et al. (2004)
His514Tyr	mAMSA (H) Etoposide (H) AMCA (H) Ellipticine (R) DACA (R)	Enzyme not characterized	Leontiou et al. (2004); Leontiou et al. (2007)
Glu522Lys	Etoposide (H) Ellipticine (H) mAMSA (R)	Reduced cleavage in the presence of mAMSA	Leontiou et al. (2004); Leontiou et al. (2007)
Gly550Arg	mAMSA (R) Etoposide (R) Ellipticine (R) DACA (R)	Wild-type activity	Leontiou et al. (2007)
Ala596Thr	mAMSA (R) Etoposide (R) Ellipticine (R) DACA (R)	Enzyme not characterized	Leontiou et al. (2007)
Tyr606Cys	mAMSA (H) Etoposide (R) Ellipticine (R) DACA (R)	Wild-type activity	Leontiou et al. (2007)

Arg651Cys	mAMSA (H) Ellipticine (R) DACA (R)	Enzyme not characterized	Leontiou et al. (2007)
Asp661Asn	mAMSA (R) Etoposide (R) Ellipticine (R) DACA (R)	Reduced enzyme activity, reduced DNA cleavage in the presence of calcium	Leontiou et al. (2007)
Pro732Leu	mAMSA (R) Etoposide (R) Ellipticine (R)	Reduced enzyme activity, reduced DNA cleavage in the presence of calcium	Leontiou et al. (2007)

Drugs designated (*R*) are resistant to the agent listed, and drugs designated (*H*) are hypersensitive. In some cases, the amino acid number listed differs from the published sequence due to a subsequently identified DNA sequencing error in the cDNA of Top2α tested. Interestingly, the same effect is also seen with the homologous mutants in human Top2α (mutating Ser763 to Trp) (Strumberg et al. 1999a, b).

Other mutations near Ser740 also lead to hypersensitivity to other Top2 targeting agents. Changing Thr744 to Pro results in a protein with hypersensitivity to intercalating agents and fluoroquinolones, but does not change etoposide sensitivity (Dong et al. 2000). The observation that mutations within the same domain of Top2 can separately lead to sensitivity to Top2 targeting agents is consistent with the hypothesis that Top2 poisons since they lead to biochemically similar phenotypes act near each other, but target distinct protein determinants. More recently additional mutations have been identified that confer very high levels of sensitivity compared to wild-type Top2 (Rogojina and Nitiss 2008). A list of drug hypersensitive mutants from yeast Top2 is summarized in Table 11.1. While many of the newly identified mutants localize near the active site tyrosine, and may therefore enhance interfacial inhibitor binding, other amino acids that are mutated are far from domains that participate in DNA cleavage and religation.

The analysis of yeast Top2 mutants has been greatly aided by several of the structures of the yeast Top2 breakage reunion domain (Berger et al. 1996; Dong and Berger 2007; Fass et al. 1999; Schmidt et al. 2010). The structure of Dong and Berger reported in 2007 was particularly useful since it was the first structure of a eukaryotic Top2 breakage/reunion domain bound to DNA. In addition, the structure showed the Rossman fold residues much closer to the active site tyrosine than in previously solved structures (Schoeffler and Berger 2008). A reasonable inference is that the Dong and Berger structure represents the structure of the enzyme at point in the reaction cycle close to where cleavage and religation takes place. This structure is likely to be highly relevant to understanding the effects of Top2 poisons. Figure 11.4 shows the Dong and Berger structure highlighting amino acids conferring hypersensitivity to Top2 poisons. Interestingly, many (although not all) residues conferring hypersensitivity to Top2 poisons are likely to be close to the interface between the enzyme and DNA. These results are consistent with the interfacial inhibitor model discussed above.

Analysis of mutants of Top2 has also extended to an analysis of mutations in human Top2α or Top2β that alter sensitivity to Top2 poisons. Early studies led to the detection of mutations in Top2α in cell lines that were specifically resistant to Top2 poisons but not to other cytotoxic agents (Bugg et al. 1991; Danks et al. 1988; Lee et al. 1992; Zwelling et al. 1989). This approach is necessarily limited in the number of mutants that can be identified. Mutations were not identified in Top2β, although cell lines resistant to Top2 poisons often display reduced or ablated expression of Top2β (Khelifa et al. 1994; Nitiss and Beck 1996). Since human topoisomerases can be functionally expressed in yeast, the yeast model system has been applied to study the details of drug resistance in human type II topoisomerases (Gilroy et al. 2006; Hsiung et al. 1996; Leontiou et al. 2006; Patel et al. 2000). A summary of many of the mutants identified in human Top2 isoforms is shown in Table 11.2, and the positions of mutations from intercalator-resistant Top2β alleles is shown in Fig. 11.5. An interpretation of drug-resistant alleles of human Top2 isoforms is complicated by the lack of any structures of the breakage/reunion

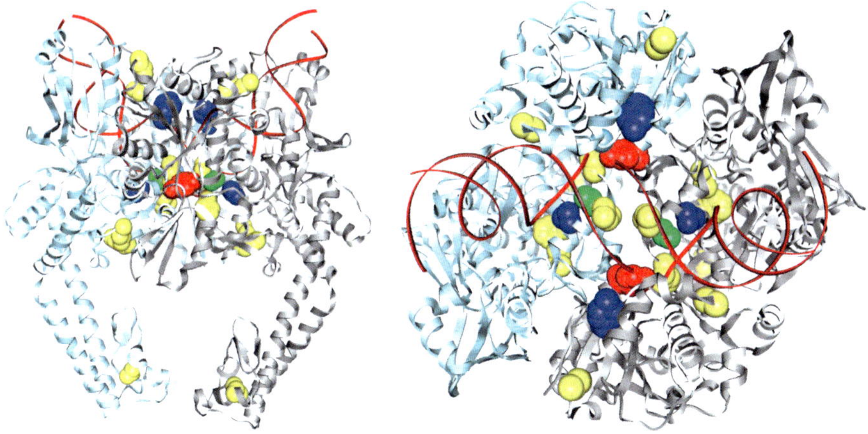

Fig. 11.4 Mutations in the breakage reunion domain of yeast Top2 that confer hypersensitivity to Top2 targeting agents. Amino acids that can be mutated to result in a Top2 enzyme with enhanced sensitivity to topoisomerase poisons. Two views of the Top2 protein are shown. The amino acids are illustrated on the Top2 (breakage/reunion domain) DNA complex determined by Dong and Berger (Dong and Berger 2007). Tyr 782, the residue that covalently binds to DNA is shown in *red*, Ser740 (etoposide hypersensitive) is shown in *green*, Pro473, Gly737, and Thr744 (mAMSA hypersensitive, with wild type sensitivity to etoposide) are shown in *blue*, and Gly436, Ala484, Ph711, His735, Gln739, Leu787, and Leu1052 (hypersensitive to etoposide and mAMSA) are shown in *yellow*

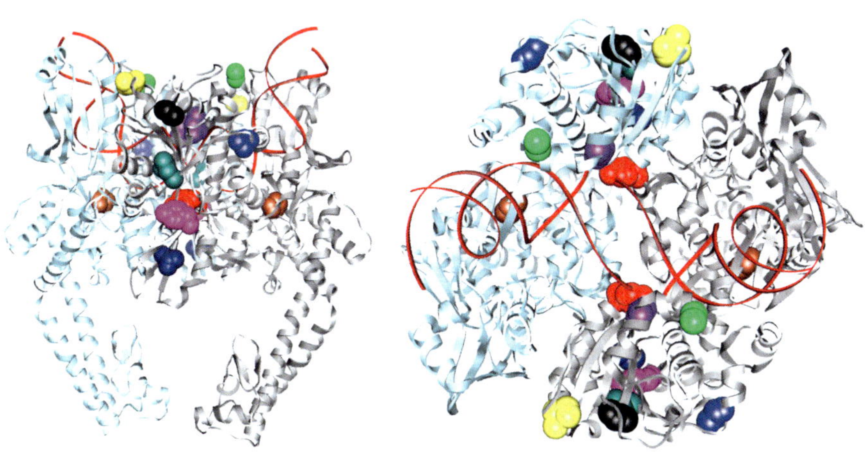

Fig. 11.5 Amino acids in Top2β that can be mutated to confer resistance to Top2 targeting agents. The mutations in Top2β listed in Table 11.2 were converted to yeast equivalents based on the homology between different eukaryotic topoisomerases. As in Fig. 11.4, two views of the Top2 protein are shown. The amino acids illustrated are βG465 = yT437 *yellow*, βH514 = yA486 *green*, βE522 = yE494_*purple*, βG550 = yG519 *black*, βA596 = yV566 *dark blue*, βY606 = yY579 *magenta*, βR651 = yL624 *teal*, βD661 = yD634 *blue*, and βP732 = yP693 *chocolate*. The active site tyrosine βY826 = Y782 *red*. Details of the individual mutations are in Table 11.2

domain of human type II topoisomerases. The alleles shown in Table 11.2 will prove valuable for interpreting structures once they are solved.

11.7 Top2 Poisons and Leukemia

Despite the importance of Top2α as a target for anticancer therapy, substantial evidence suggests that DNA cleavage mediated by the enzyme can trigger chromosomal translocations that lead to specific types of leukemia (Deweese and Osheroff 2009; Felix 1998, 2001; Felix et al. 1995, 2006; McClendon and Osheroff 2007). To this point, 2–3% of patients who receive regimens that include etoposide or other Top2-targeted drugs develop therapy-related AMLs. Most of these leukemias are characterized by translocations with breakpoints in the mixed lineage leukemia (*MLL*) gene at chromosomal band 11q23 (Felix 2001; Felix et al. 2006). The MLL protein is a histone methyltransferase that regulates the *Hox* genes, which control proliferation in hematopoietic cells (Felix 2001; Felix et al. 2006). Numerous breakpoints in *MLL* have been identified and are located in close proximity to Top2-DNA cleavage sites (Felix 2001; Felix et al. 2006; Mays et al. 2010). Although therapy-related malignancies are an unfortunate, but relatively common side effect of chemotherapy, *MLL*-involved leukemias are only observed in patients treated with Top2 poisons (Felix 1998, 2001; Felix et al. 1995).

Recently, development of acute promyelocytic leukemia (APL) has been observed in individuals treated with Top2-targeted drugs (Hasan et al. 2008; Mistry et al. 2005). Patients with these leukemias display translocations between the *PML* promyelocytic leukemia *(PML)* gene on chromosome 15 and the RARA (retinoic acid receptor a) gene on chromosome 17.

In addition to treatment-related leukemias, ~80% of infants with AML or acute lymphoblastic leukemia (ALL) display translocations that involve the *MLL* gene (Felix et al. 2006; Gilliland et al. 2004; Ross 2000; Ross et al. 1994, 1996; Strick et al. 2000). The chromosomal translocations associated with these cancers have been observed in utero, indicating that infant leukemias are initiated during pregnancy. Epidemiological studies indicate that the risk of developing these infant leukemias is increased >3-fold by the maternal consumption of foods that are high in naturally dietary Top2 poisons such as genistein or other bioflavonoids (Gilliland et al. 2004; Ross 2000; Ross et al. 1994).

The ability of Top2 poisons to *cause* rather than *cure* cancer may be related to cellular levels of cleavage complexes. If the concentration of enzyme-associated DNA strand breaks is sufficient, DNA recombination/repair pathways can be overwhelmed and drug treatment can result in cell death (Bender and Osheroff 2008; McClendon and Osheroff 2007). However, if the levels of breaks are not adequate to induce death, pathways that promote cell survival can lead to the formation of stable chromosomal translocations that ultimately lead to cancerous growth. Clearly, considerably more research in this area is necessary. Hopefully, it will be possible to develop novel Top2-targeted drugs with a decreased propensity to generate leukemias.

11.8 Looking Forward: Paths New and More Active Agents

Top2-targeted drugs have been used in the clinic for over 35 years. Like nearly all anticancer drug targets, efforts to develop Top2 targeting agents have met with some success, and many failures. In the following sections, we pose a series of challenges that need to be met to fully unlock the potential of Top2 as an anticancer drug target.

Challenge 1: Understanding the molecular details of how Top2 drugs work. Berger and Osheroff (Chap. 3) described our understanding of how the structure of Top2 allows the completion of a coordinated set of biochemical reactions. While biochemical studies of Top2 targeting agents have taught us a great deal of how drugs act on the enzyme, they have not provided the molecular details that allow us to design new Top2 targeting drugs. Novel Top2 inhibitors with design characteristic such as isoform specificity, increased potency, or sequence selectivity will likely be identified and optimized in part using structural approaches. If the interfacial inhibitor model is an important way of understanding Top2 drug action, we will need detailed structural information concerning multiple inhibitors with both Top2α and Top2β.

Challenge 2: What properties make a Top2 poison an active and safe drug? A very large number of drugs that target topoisomerases have been described. As discussed above, agents such as *m*AMSA are effective Top2 poisons, but disappointing in their clinical activity. While issues such as drug disposition and metabolism are clearly relevant, we still do not fully appreciate what the most relevant properties are that would merit extensive preclinical development. For example, are the current Top2 inhibitors sufficiently potent? Doxorubicin and mitoxantrone can trap covalent complexes in cells exposed to sub-micromolar concentrations. Would very potent non-intercalating Top2 targeting drugs be more active, or would they have narrow therapeutic windows?

Are mechanistic details of drug action important? Is the relative ATP independence of amonafide a useful characteristic, a detriment, or an irrelevant detail? Most of the clinically approved Top2 poisons inhibit enzyme-mediated religation. Would agents that primarily stimulate cleavage without blocking ligation have a different clinical spectrum of activity? Would it be useful to develop new Top2 targeting drugs with enhanced DNA sequence preference? A Top2 drug with a high sequence preference might lead to high levels of DNA cleavage at a limited number of sites, and may be an alternate way to minimize drug-stimulated oncogenic translocations.

Challenge 3: Are isoform-specific drugs a viable strategy for safer effective agents? As described in Sect. 11.4, there are several new small molecules that preferentially target either the Top2α or Top2β isoform. It will be exciting to learn whether this preserves antitumor activity while decreasing the risk of cardiotoxicity and secondary malignancies. For this challenge to be fully met, the molecular differences between Top2α and Top2β will need to be identified. At the time of writing this book, there was no three-dimensional structure of the breakage/reunion domain of either human Top2 isoform.

Challenge 4: Would catalytic inhibitors of Top2 have significant anticancer effects? The clinical experience with Top2 catalytic inhibitors as anticancer agents has been rather disappointing. As described above, merbarone has undergone extensive phase II trials with no evidence of clinical activity. Bisdioxopiperazines (especially razoxane, ICRF-154, a close relative of dexrazoxane) also underwent extensive clinical testing with little evidence of antitumor activity. Certainly, dexrazoxane has established itself as a useful adjunct to minimize cardiotoxicity of anthracyclines. Nonetheless, it remains quite possible that other catalytic inhibitors might have substantial activity in some clinical settings.

Challenge 5: Are we willing to commit effort to develop new agents against an "old" target? This final challenge may be the most difficult to overcome. Most clinicians, pharmacologists, and biochemists consulting this volume likely believe that further development of Top2 as a drug target is warranted, based on the clinical activity already exhibited, and the potential for new agents. We are currently seeing a renaissance of old agents, a renaissance brought on in part by the concept of synthetic lethality. The observation that PARP inhibitors are highly toxic to tumors, with deficiencies in Brca1 or Brca2, has opened up new ways of using agents that generate DNA damage (Fong et al. 2009; Lord and Ashworth 2008). Interestingly, Brca1 and Brca2 cells are hypersensitive to etoposide, suggesting that synthetic lethality approaches will be relevant to the use of Top2 targeting agents (Treszezamsky et al. 2007). While new approaches to the use of current Top2 inhibitors will certainly be of clinical value, there is outstanding promise in the next generation of Top2 targeting drugs.

Acknowledgments We thank Yves Pommier, the epitome of a gracious and helpful book editor, and Karin Nitiss for help with figures. Work in the authors' laboratories was supported by grants from the National Institute of Health and the American Lebanese Syrian Associated Charities (JLN).

References

Adjei AA, Charron M, Rowinsky EK, Svingen PA, Miller J, Reid JM, Sebolt-Leopold J, Ames MM, Kaufmann SH (1998) Effect of pyrazoloacridine (NSC 366140) on DNA topoisomerases I and II. *Clin Cancer Res* **4**(3)**:** 683–691

Allen SL, Kolitz JE, Lundberg AS, Bennett JM, Capizzi RL, Budman DR (2010) Phase I trials of amonafide as monotherapy and in combination with cytarabine in patients with poor-risk acute myeloid leukemia. *Leuk Res* **34**(4)**:** 487–491

Alousi AM, Boinpally R, Wiegand R, Parchment R, Gadgeel S, Heilbrun LK, Wozniak AJ, DeLuca P, LoRusso PM (2007) A phase 1 trial of XK469: toxicity profile of a selective topoisomerase IIbeta inhibitor. *Invest New Drugs* **25**(2)**:** 147–154

Aoyagi Y, Kobunai T, Utsugi T, Oh-hara T, Yamada Y (1999) In vitro antitumor activity of TAS-103, a novel quinoline derivative that targets topoisomerases I and II. *Jpn J Cancer Res* **90**(5)**:** 578–587

Arlin ZA (1989) Mitoxantrone and amsacrine: two important agents for the treatment of acute myelogenous leukemia (AML) and acute lymphoblastic leukemia (ALL). *Bone Marrow Transplant* **4 Suppl 1:** 57–59

Asbury R, Blessing JA, Look KY, Buller R, Lucci JA, 3 rd (1997) A phase II trial of amonafide in patients with nonsquamous cell carcinoma of the cervix. A Gynecologic Oncology Group study. *Am J Clin Oncol* **20**(6)**:** 626–627

Asbury R, Blessing JA, Podczaski E, Ball H (1998) A phase II trial of amonafide in patients with mixed mesodermal tumors of the uterus: a Gynecologic Oncology Group study. *Am J Clin Oncol* **21**(3): 306–307

Aubert B, et al. (BaBaR Collaboration) (2009) Measurement of D{0}-D[−over]{0} mixing from a time-dependent amplitude analysis of D{0}-->K+pi{−}pi{0} decays. *Phys Rev Lett* **103**(21): 211801

Austin CA, Marsh KL (1998) Eukaryotic DNA topoisomerase II beta. *Bioessays* **20**(3): 215–226

Azarova AM, Lyu YL, Lin CP, Tsai YC, Lau JY, Wang JC, Liu LF (2007) Roles of DNA topoisomerase II isozymes in chemotherapy and secondary malignancies. *Proc Natl Acad Sci USA* **104**(26): 11014–11019

Baguley BC, Finlay GJ (1988) Derivatives of amsacrine: determinants required for high activity against Lewis lung carcinoma. *J Natl Cancer Inst* **80**(3): 195–199

Baldwin EL, Osheroff N (2005) Etoposide, Topoisomerase II, and Cancer. *Curr Med Chem-Anticancer Agents* **5**: 363–372

Bandele OJ, Clawson SJ, Osheroff N (2008) Dietary polyphenols as topoisomerase II poisons: B ring and C ring substituents determine the mechanism of enzyme-mediated DNA cleavage enhancement. *Chem Res Toxicol* **21**: 1253–1260

Barret JM, Kruczynski A, Vispe S, Annereau JP, Brel V, Guminski Y, Delcros JG, Lansiaux A, Guilbaud N, Imbert T, Bailly C (2008) F14512, a potent antitumor agent targeting topoisomerase II vectored into cancer cells via the polyamine transport system. *Cancer Research* **68**(23): 9845–9853

Belyaev IY (2005) DNA loop organization and DNA fragmentation during radiation-induced apoptosis in human lymphocytes. *Radiats Biol Radioecol* **45**(5): 541–548

Bender RP, Ham AJ, Osheroff N (2007) Quinone-induced enhancement of DNA cleavage by human topoisomerase IIalpha: adduction of cysteine residues 392 and 405. *Biochemistry* **46**(10): 2856–2864

Bender RP, Lehmler HJ, Robertson LW, Ludewig G, Osheroff N (2006) Polychlorinated biphenyl quinone metabolites poison human topoisomerase IIα: altering enzyme function by blocking the N-terminal protein gate. *Biochemistry* **45**(33): 10140–10152

Bender RP, Lindsey RH, Jr., Burden DA, Osheroff N (2004) N-acetyl-p-benzoquinone imine, the toxic metabolite of acetaminophen, is a topoisomerase II poison. *Biochemistry* **43**(12): 3731–3739

Bender RP, Osheroff N (2007) Mutation of cysteine residue 455 to alanine in human topoisomerase IIalpha confers hypersensitivity to quinones: enhancing DNA scission by closing the N-terminal protein gate. *Chem Res Toxicol* **20**(6): 975–981

Bender RP, Osheroff N (2008) DNA topoisomerases as targets for the chemotherapeutic treatment of cancer. In *Checkpoint Responses in Cancer Therapy*, Dai W (ed), pp 57–91. Totowa, New Jersey: Humana Press

Berger JM, Gamblin SJ, Harrison SC, Wang JC (1996) Structure and mechanism of DNA topoisomerase II [published erratum appears in Nature 1996 Mar 14;380(6570):179]. *Nature* **379**(6562): 225–232

Bertrand R, O'Connor PM, Kerrigan D, Pommier Y (1992) Sequential administration of camptothecin and etoposide circumvents the antagonistic cytotoxicity of simultaneous drug administration in slowly growing human colon carcinoma HT-29 cells. *Eur J Cancer* **28A**(4–5): 743–748

Binaschi M, Bigioni M, Cipollone A, Rossi C, Goso C, Maggi CA, Capranico G, Animati F (2001) Anthracyclines: selected new developments. *Curr Med Chem Anticancer Agents* **1**(2): 113–130

Bugg BY, Danks MK, Beck WT, Suttle DP (1991) Expression of a mutant DNA topoisomerase II in CCRF-CEM human leukemic cells selected for resistance to teniposide. *Proc Natl Acad Sci USA* **88**(17): 7654–7658

Burden DA, Kingma PS, Froelich-Ammon SJ, Bjornsti MA, Patchan MW, Thompson RB, Osheroff N (1996) Topoisomerase II.etoposide interactions direct the formation of drug-induced enzyme-DNA cleavage complexes. *J Biol Chem* **271**(46): 29238–29244

Byl JA, Cline SD, Utsugi T, Kobunai T, Yamada Y, Osheroff N (2001a) DNA topoisomerase II as the target for the anticancer drug TOP-53: mechanistic basis for drug action. *Biochemistry* **40**(3): 712–718

Byl JA, Fortune JM, Burden DA, Nitiss JL, Utsugi T, Yamada Y, Osheroff N (1999) DNA topoisomerases as targets for the anticancer drug TAS-103: primary cellular target and DNA cleavage enhancement. *Biochemistry* **38**(47): 15573–15579

Capranico G, Guano F, Moro S, Zagotto G, Sissi C, Gatto B, Zunino F, Menta E, Palumbo M (1998) Mapping drug interactions at the covalent topoisomerase II-DNA complex by bisantrene/amsacrine congeners. *J Biol Chem* **273**(21): 12732–12739

Chau M, Christensen JL, Ajami AM, Capizzi RL (2008) Amonafide, a topoisomerase II inhibitor, is unaffected by P-glycoprotein-mediated efflux. *Leuk Res* **32**(3): 465–473

Chene P, Rudloff J, Schoepfer J, Furet P, Meier P, Qian Z, Schlaeppi JM, Schmitz R, Radimerski T (2009) Catalytic inhibition of topoisomerase II by a novel rationally designed ATP-competitive purine analogue. *BMC Chem Biol* **9**: 1

Clifford B, Beljin M, Stark GR, Taylor WR (2003) G2 arrest in response to topoisomerase II inhibitors: the role of p53. *Cancer Res* **63**(14): 4074–4081

Cvetkovic RS, Scott LJ (2005) Dexrazoxane : a review of its use for cardioprotection during anthracycline chemotherapy. *Drugs* **65**(7): 1005–1024

D'Arpa P, Liu LF (1989) Topoisomerase-targeting antitumor drugs. *Biochim Biophys Acta* **989**(2): 163–177

Danks MK, Schmidt CA, Cirtain MC, Suttle DP, Beck WT (1988) Altered catalytic activity of and DNA cleavage by DNA topoisomerase II from human leukemic cells selected for resistance to VM-26. *Biochemistry* **27**(24): 8861–8869

de Forni M, Armand JP (1994) Cardiotoxicity of chemotherapy. *Curr Opin Oncol* **6**(4): 340–344

Denny WA, Baguley BC (2003) Dual topoisomerase I/II inhibitors in cancer therapy. *Curr Top Med Chem* **3**(3): 339–353

Dereuddre S, Delaporte C, Jacquemin-Sablon A (1997) Role of topoisomerase II beta in the resistance of 9-OH-ellipticine- resistant Chinese hamster fibroblasts to topoisomerase II inhibitors. *Cancer Res* **57**(19): 4301–4308

Deweese JE, Burgin AB, Osheroff N (2008) Using 3′-bridging phosphorothiolates to isolate the forward DNA cleavage reaction of human topoisomerase IIalpha. *Biochemistry* **47**(13): 4129–4140

Deweese JE, Osheroff N (2009) The DNA cleavage reaction of topoisomerase II: wolf in sheep's clothing. *Nucleic Acids Res* **37**(3): 738–748

Dong J, Walker J, Nitiss JL (2000) A mutation in yeast topoisomerase II that confers hypersensitivity to multiple classes of topoisomerase II poisons. *J Biol Chem* **275**(11): 7980–7987

Dong KC, Berger JM (2007) Structural basis for gate-DNA recognition and bending by type IIA topoisomerases. *Nature* **450**(7173): 1201–1205

Drake FH, Hofmann GA, Mong SM, Bartus JO, Hertzberg RP, Johnson RK, Mattern MR, Mirabelli CK (1989) In vitro and intracellular inhibition of topoisomerase II by the antitumor agent merbarone. *Cancer Res* **49**(10): 2578–2583

Elsea SH, Hsiung Y, Nitiss JL, Osheroff N (1995) A yeast type II topoisomerase selected for resistance to quinolones. Mutation of histidine 1012 to tyrosine confers resistance to nonintercalative drugs but hypersensitivity to ellipticine. *J Biol Chem* **270**(4): 1913–1920

Errington F, Willmore E, Tilby MJ, Li L, Li G, Li W, Baguley BC, Austin CA (1999) Murine transgenic cells lacking DNA topoisomerase IIbeta are resistant to acridines and mitoxantrone: analysis of cytotoxicity and cleavable complex formation. *Mol Pharmacol* **56**(6): 1309–1316

Fass D, Bogden CE, Berger JM (1999) Quaternary changes in topoisomerase II may direct orthogonal movement of two DNA strands. *Nat Struct Biol* **6**(4): 322–326

Felix CA (1998) Secondary leukemias induced by topoisomerase-targeted drugs. *Biochim Biophys Acta* **1400**(1–3): 233–255

Felix CA (2001) Leukemias related to treatment with DNA topoisomerase II inhibitors. *Med Pediatr Oncol* **36**(5): 525–535

Felix CA, Hosler MR, Winick NJ, Masterson M, Wilson AE, Lange BJ (1995) ALL-1 gene rearrangements in DNA topoisomerase II inhibitor-related leukemia in children. *Blood* **85**(11): 3250–3256

Felix CA, Kolaris CP, Osheroff N (2006) Topoisomerase II and the etiology of chromosomal translocations. *DNA Repair (Amst)* **5**(9–10): 1093–1108

Fong PC, Boss DS, Yap TA, Tutt A, Wu P, Mergui-Roelvink M, Mortimer P, Swaisland H, Lau A, O'Connor MJ, Ashworth A, Carmichael J, Kaye SB, Schellens JH, de Bono JS (2009) Inhibition of poly(ADP-ribose) polymerase in tumors from BRCA mutation carriers. *N Engl J Med* **361**(2): 123–134

Fortune JM, Osheroff N (1998) Merbarone inhibits the catalytic activity of human topoisomerase IIalpha by blocking DNA cleavage. *J Biol Chem* **273**(28): 17643–17650

Fortune JM, Velea L, Graves DE, Utsugi T, Yamada Y, Osheroff N (1999) DNA topoisomerases as targets for the anticancer drug TAS-103: DNA interactions and topoisomerase catalytic inhibition. *Biochemistry* **38**(47): 15580–15586

Froelich-Ammon SJ, Burden DA, Patchan MW, Elsea SH, Thompson RB, Osheroff N (1995a) Increased drug affinity as the mechanistic basis for drug hypersensitivity of a mutant type II topoisomerase. *J Biol Chem* **270**: 28018–28021

Froelich-Ammon SJ, Patchan MW, Osheroff N, Thompson RB (1995b) Topoisomerase II binds to ellipticine in the absence or presence of DNA: characterization of enzyme-drug interactions by fluorescence spectroscopy. *J Biol Chem* **270**: 14998–15005

Furet P, Schoepfer J, Radimerski T, Chene P (2009) Discovery of a new class of catalytic topoisomerase II inhibitors targeting the ATP-binding site by structure based design. Part I. *Bioorg Med Chem Lett* **19**(15): 4014–4017

Gao H, Huang KC, Yamasaki EF, Chan KK, Chohan L, Snapka RM (1999) XK469, a selective topoisomerase IIbeta poison. *Proc Natl Acad Sci USA* **96**(21): 12168–12173

Gentry AC, Pitts SL, Jablonsky MJ, Bailly C, Graves DE, Osheroff N (2011) Interactions between the etoposide derivative F14512 and human type II topoisomerases: implications for the C4 spermine moiety in promoting enzyme-mediated DNA cleavage. *Biochemistry* **50**: 3240–3249

Germe T, Hyrien O (2005) Topoisomerase II-DNA complexes trapped by ICRF-193 perturb chromatin structure. *Embo Reports* **6**(8): 729–735

Gilliland DG, Jordan CT, Felix CA (2004) The molecular basis of leukemia. *Hematology Am Soc Hematol Educ Program*: 80–97

Gilroy KL, Leontiou C, Padget K, Lakey JH, Austin CA (2006) mAMSA resistant human topoisomerase IIbeta mutation G465D has reduced ATP hydrolysis activity. *Nucleic Acids Res* **34**(5): 1597–1607

Giovannoni G (2011) Promising emerging therapies for multiple sclerosis. *Neurol Clin* **29**(2): 435–448

Granzen B, Graves DE, Baguley BC, Danks MK, Beck WT (1992) Structure-activity studies of amsacrine analogs in drug resistant human leukemia cell lines expressing either altered DNA topoisomerase II or P-glycoprotein. *Oncol Res* **4**(11–12): 489–496

Hamzehloo A, Etemadifar M (2006) Mitoxantrone-induced cardiotoxicity in patients with multiple sclerosis. *Arch Iran Med* **9**(2): 111–114

Hande KR (1998) Clinical applications of anticancer drugs targeted to topoisomerase II. *Biochimica Et Biophysica Acta* **1400**(1–3): 173–184

Hasan SK, Mays AN, Ottone T, Ledda A, La Nasa G, Cattaneo C, Borlenghi E, Melillo L, Montefusco E, Cervera J, Stephen C, Satchi G, Lennard A, Libura M, Byl JA, Osheroff N, Amadori S, Felix CA, Voso MT, Sperr WR, Esteve J, Sanz MA, Grimwade D, Lo-Coco F (2008) Molecular analysis of t(15;17) genomic breakpoints in secondary acute promyelocytic leukemia arising after treatment of multiple sclerosis. *Blood* **112**(8): 3383–3390

Hawtin RE, Stockett DE, Byl JA, McDowell RS, Nguyen T, Arkin MR, Conroy A, Yang W, Osheroff N, Fox JA (2010) Voreloxin is an anticancer quinolone derivative that intercalates DNA and poisons topoisomerase II. *PLoS One* **5**(4): e10186

Hinds M, Deisseroth K, Mayes J, Altschuler E, Jansen R, Ledley FD, Zwelling LA (1991) Identification of a point mutation in the topoisomerase II gene from a human leukemia cell line containing an amsacrine-resistant form of topoisomerase II. *Cancer Res* **51**(17): 4729–4731

Hisatomi T, Sueoka-Aragane N, Sato A, Tomimasu R, Ide M, Kurimasa A, Okamoto K, Kimura S, Sueoka E (2011) NK314 potentiates anti-tumor activity with adult T-cell leukemia-lymphoma cells by inhibition of dual targets on topoisomerase II{alpha} and DNA-dependent protein kinase. *Blood*

Hsiung Y, Elsea SH, Osheroff N, Nitiss JL (1995) A mutation in yeast TOP2 homologous to a quinolone-resistant mutation in bacteria. Mutation of the amino acid homologous to Ser83 of Escherichia coli gyrA alters sensitivity to eukaryotic topoisomerase inhibitors. *J Biol Chem* **270**(35): 20359–20364

Hsiung Y, Jannatipour M, Rose A, McMahon J, Duncan D, Nitiss JL (1996) Functional expression of human topoisomerase II alpha in yeast: mutations at amino acids 450 or 803 of topoisomerase II alpha result in enzymes that can confer resistance to anti-topoisomerase II agents. *Cancer Res* **56**(1): 91–99

Huang KC, Gao H, Yamasaki EF, Grabowski DR, Liu S, Shen LL, Chan KK, Ganapathi R, Snapka RM (2001) Topoisomerase II poisoning by ICRF-193. *J Biol Chem* **276**(48): 44488–44494

Huang TS, Lee CC, Chao Y, Shu CH, Chen LT, Chen LL, Chen MH, Yuan CC, Whang-Peng J (1999) A novel podophyllotoxin-derived compound GL331 is more potent than its congener VP-16 in killing refractory cancer cells. *Pharm Res* **16**(7): 997–1002

Ingrassia L, Lefranc F, Kiss R, Mijatovic T (2009) Naphthalimides and azonafides as promising anti-cancer agents. *Curr Med Chem* **16**(10): 1192–1213

Ishida R, Hamatake M, Wasserman RA, Nitiss JL, Wang JC, Andoh T (1995) DNA topoisomerase II is the molecular target of bisdioxopiperazine derivatives ICRF-159 and ICRF-193 in Saccharomyces cerevisiae. *Cancer Res* **55**(11): 2299–2303

Ishida R, Miki T, Narita T, Yui R, Sato M, Utsumi KR, Tanabe K, Andoh T (1991) Inhibition of intracellular topoisomerase II by antitumor bis(2,6- dioxopiperazine) derivatives: mode of cell growth inhibition distinct from that of cleavable complex-forming type inhibitors. *Cancer Res* **51**(18): 4909–4916

Jannatipour M, Liu YX, Nitiss JL (1993) The top2-5 mutant of yeast topoisomerase II encodes an enzyme resistant to etoposide and amsacrine. *J Biol Chem* **268**(25): 18586–18592

Jensen LH, Nitiss KC, Rose A, Dong J, Zhou J, Hu T, Osheroff N, Jensen PB, Sehested M, Nitiss JL (2000) A novel mechanism of cell killing by anti-topoisomerase II bisdioxopiperazines. *J Biol Chem* **275**(3): 2137–2146

Jensen LH, Renodon-Corniere A, Nitiss KC, Hill BT, Nitiss JL, Jensen PB, Sehested M (2003) A dual mechanism of action of the anticancer agent F 11782 on human topoisomerase II alpha. *Biochem Pharmacol* **66**(4): 623–631

Jensen PB, Jensen PS, Demant EJ, Friche E, Sorensen BS, Sehested M, Wassermann K, Vindelov L, Westergaard O, Hansen HH, Srensen BS, Vindelv L (1991) Antagonistic effect of aclarubicin on daunorubicin-induced cytotoxicity in human small cell lung cancer cells: relationship to DNA integrity and topoisomerase II. *Cancer Res* **51**(19): 5093–5099

Jensen PB, Sorensen BS, Demant EJ, Sehested M, Jensen PS, Vindelov L, Hansen HH, Srensen BS, Vindelv L (1990) Antagonistic effect of aclarubicin on the cytotoxicity of etoposide and 4'-(9-acridinylamino)methanesulfon-m-anisidide in human small cell lung cancer cell lines and on topoisomerase II-mediated DNA cleavage. *Cancer Res* **50**(11): 3311–3316

Jiang X (2005) Random mutagenesis of the B'A' core domain of yeast DNA topoisomerase II and large-scale screens of mutants resistant to the anticancer drug etoposide. *Biochem Biophys Res Commun* **327**(2): 597–603

Khelifa T, Casabianca-Pignede MR, Rene B, Jacquemin-Sablon A (1994) Expression of topoisomerases II alpha and beta in Chinese hamster lung cells resistant to topoisomerase II inhibitors. *Mol Pharmacol* **46**(2): 323–328

Kingma PS, Burden DA, Osheroff N (1999) Binding of etoposide to topoisomerase II in the absence of DNA: decreased affinity as a mechanism of drug resistance. *Biochemistry* **38**(12): 3457–3461

Kingma PS, Osheroff N (1998) The response of eukaryotic topoisomerases to DNA damage. *Biochim Biophys Acta* **1400**(1–3): 223–232

Kohno K, Danks MK, Matsuda T, Nitiss JL, Beck WT (1995) A novel mutation of DNA topoisomerase IIalpha in an etoposide-resistant human cancer cell line. *Cellular Pharmacology* **2:** 97–90

Krohn K (ed) (2008) *Anthracycline Chemistry and Biology II: Mode of Action, Clinical Aspects and New Drugs*. Heidelberg: Springer, 224 pp

Kruczynski A, Barret JM, Van Hille B, Chansard N, Astruc J, Menon Y, Duchier C, Creancier L, Hill BT (2004) Decreased nucleotide excision repair activity and alterations of topoisomerase IIalpha are associated with the in vivo resistance of a P388 leukemia subline to F11782, a novel catalytic inhibitor of topoisomerases I and II. *Clin Cancer Res* **10**(9): 3156–3168

Krug LM, Crawford J, Ettinger DS, Shapiro GI, Spigel D, Reiman T, Temel JS, Michelson GC, Young DY, Hoch U, Adelman DC (2011) Phase II multicenter trial of voreloxin as second-line therapy in chemotherapy-sensitive or refractory small cell lung cancer. *J Thorac Oncol* **6**(2): 384–386

Laponogov I, Sohi MK, Veselkov DA, Pan XS, Sawhney R, Thompson AW, McAuley KE, Fisher LM, Sanderson MR (2009) Structural insight into the quinolone-DNA cleavage complex of type IIA topoisomerases. *Nat Struct Mol Biol* **16**(6): 667–669

Lee MS, Wang JC, Beran M (1992) Two independent amsacrine-resistant human myeloid leukemia cell lines share an identical point mutation in the 170 kDa form of human topoisomerase II. *J Mol Biol* **223**(4): 837–843

Leontiou C, Lakey JH, Austin CA (2004) Mutation E522K in human DNA topoisomerase IIbeta confers resistance to methyl N-(4′-(9-acridinylamino)-phenyl)carbamate hydrochloride and methyl N-(4′-(9-acridinylamino)-3-methoxy-phenyl) methane sulfonamide but hypersensitivity to etoposide. *Mol Pharmacol* **66**(3): 430–439

Leontiou C, Lakey JH, Lightowlers R, Turnbull RM, Austin CA (2006) Mutation P732L in human DNA topoisomerase IIbeta abolishes DNA cleavage in the presence of calcium and confers drug resistance. *Mol Pharmacol* **69**(1): 130–139

Leontiou C, Watters GP, Gilroy KL, Heslop P, Cowell IG, Craig K, Lightowlers RN, Lakey JH, Austin CA (2007) Differential selection of acridine resistance mutations in human DNA topoisomerase IIbeta is dependent on the acridine structure. *Mol Pharmacol* **71**(4): 1006–1014

Lewis LJ, Mistry P, Charlton PA, Thomas H, Coley HM (2007) Mode of action of the novel phenazine anticancer agents XR11576 and XR5944. *Anticancer Drugs* **18**(2): 139–148

Lin H, Liu XY, Subramanian B, Nakeff A, Valeriote F, Chen BD (2002) Mitotic arrest induced by XK469, a novel antitumor agent, is correlated with the inhibition of cyclin B1 ubiquitination. *Int J Cancer* **97**(1): 121–128

Lindsey RH, Jr., Bromberg KD, Felix CA, Osheroff N (2004) 1,4-Benzoquinone is a topoisomerase II poison. *Biochemistry* **43**(23): 7563–7574

Liu YX, Hsiung Y, Jannatipour M, Yeh Y, Nitiss JL (1994) Yeast topoisomerase II mutants resistant to anti-topoisomerase agents: identification and characterization of new yeast topoisomerase II mutants selected for resistance to etoposide. *Cancer Res* **54**(11): 2943–2951

Look KY, Blessing JA, Adelson MD, Morris M, Bookman MA (1996) A phase II trial of merbarone (NSC 336628) in the treatment of recurrent epithelial ovarian carcinoma. A Gynecologic Oncology Group Study. *Am J Clin Oncol* **19**(1): 7–9

Look KY, Blessing JA, Williams L, Morris M (1995) A phase II trial of merbarone (NSC 336628) as salvage therapy for squamous cell carcinoma of the cervix. A Gynecologic Oncology Group Study. *Am J Clin Oncol* **18**(5): 441–443

Lord CJ, Ashworth A (2008) Targeted therapy for cancer using PARP inhibitors. *Curr Opin Pharmacol* **8**(4): 363–369

Lyu YL, Kerrigan JE, Lin CP, Azarova AM, Tsai YC, Ban Y, Liu LF (2007) Topoisomerase II beta-Mediated DNA double-strand breaks: Implications in doxorubicin cardiotoxicity and prevention by dexrazoxane. *Cancer Research* **67**: 8839–8846

Makhey D, Yu C, Liu A, Liu LF, LaVoie EJ (2000) Substituted benz[a]acridines and benz[c]acridines as mammalian topoisomerase poisons. *Bioorg Med Chem* **8**(5): 1171–1182

Malik UR, Dutcher JP, Caliendo G, Lasala P, Mitnick R, Wiernik PH (1997) Phase II trial of merbarone in patients with malignant brain tumors. *Med Oncol* **14**(3–4): 159–162

Mao Y, Yu C, Hsieh TS, Nitiss JL, Liu AA, Wang H, Liu LF (1999) Mutations of human topoisomerase II alpha affecting multidrug resistance and sensitivity. *Biochemistry* **38**(33): 10793–10800

Marchand C, Antony S, Kohn KW, Cushman M, Ioanoviciu A, Staker BL, Burgin AB, Stewart L, Pommier Y (2006) A novel norindenoisoquinoline structure reveals a common interfacial inhibitor paradigm for ternary trapping of the topoisomerase I-DNA covalent complex. *Mol Cancer Ther* **5**(2)**:** 287–295

Mays AN, Osheroff N, Xiao Y, Wiemels JL, Felix CA, Byl JA, Saravanamuttu K, Peniket A, Corser R, Chang C, Hoyle C, Parker AN, Hasan SK, Lo-Coco F, Solomon E, Grimwade D (2010) Evidence for direct involvement of epirubicin in the formation of chromosomal translocations in t(15;17) therapy-related acute promyelocytic leukemia. *Blood* **115**(2)**:** 326–330

McClendon AK, Osheroff N (2007) DNA topoisomerase II, genotoxicity, and cancer. *Mutation Research* **623**(1–2)**:** 83–97

Minford J, Pommier Y, Filipski J, Kohn KW, Kerrigan D, Mattern M, Michaels S, Schwartz R, Zwelling LA (1986) Isolation of intercalator-dependent protein-linked DNA strand cleavage activity from cell nuclei and identification as topoisomerase II. *Biochemistry* **25**(1)**:** 9–16

Mistry AR, Felix CA, Whitmarsh RJ, Mason A, Reiter A, Cassinat B, Parry A, Walz C, Wiemels JL, Segal MR, Ades L, Blair IA, Osheroff N, Peniket AJ, Lafage-Pochitaloff M, Cross NC, Chomienne C, Solomon E, Fenaux P, Grimwade D (2005) DNA topoisomerase II in therapy-related acute promyelocytic leukemia. *New Engl J Med* **352**(15)**:** 1529–1538

Morris SK, Baird CL, Lindsley JE (2000) Steady-state and rapid kinetic analysis of topoisomerase II trapped as the closed-clamp intermediate by ICRF-193. *J Biol Chem* **275**(4)**:** 2613–2618

Multon E, Riou JF, LeFevre D, Ahomadegbe JC, Riou G (1989) Topoisomerase II-mediated DNA cleavage activity induced by ellipticines on the human tumor cell line N417. *Biochem Pharmacol* **38**(13)**:** 2077–2086

Newman RA, Kim J, Newman BM, Bruno R, Bayssas M, Klink-Alaki M, Pazdur R (1999) Phase I trial of intoplicine (RP 60475) administered as a 72 h infusion every 3 weeks in patients with solid tumors. *Anticancer Drugs* **10**(10)**:** 889–894

Nitiss JL (2009a) DNA topoisomerase II and its growing repertoire of biological functions. *Nature Reviews Cancer* **9**(5)**:** 327–337

Nitiss JL (2009b) Targeting DNA topoisomerase II in cancer chemotherapy. *Nature Reviews Cancer* **9**(5)**:** 338–350

Nitiss JL, Beck WT (1996) Antitopoisomerase drug action and resistance. *Eur J Cancer* **32A**(6)**:** 958–966

Nitiss JL, Liu YX, Harbury P, Jannatipour M, Wasserman R, Wang JC (1992) Amsacrine and etoposide hypersensitivity of yeast cells overexpressing DNA topoisomerase II. *Cancer Res* **52**(16)**:** 4467–4472

Nitiss JL, Pourquier P, Pommier Y (1997) Aclacinomycin A stabilizes topoisomerase I covalent complexes. *Cancer Res* **57**(20)**:** 4564–4569

Nitiss JL, Vilalta PM, Wu H, McMahon J (1994) Mutations in the gyrB domain of eukaryotic topoisomerase II can lead to partially dominant resistance to etoposide and amsacrine. *Mol Pharmacol* **46**(4)**:** 773–777

Park I, Avraham HK (2006) Cell cycle-dependent DNA damage signaling induced by ICRF-193 involves ATM, ATR, CHK2, and BRCA1. *Exp Cell Res* **312**(11)**:** 1996–2008

Patel S, Keller BA, Fisher LM (2000) Mutations at arg486 and glu571 in human topoisomerase IIalpha confer resistance to amsacrine: relevance for antitumor drug resistance in human cells. *Mol Pharmacol* **57**(4)**:** 784–791

Patel S, Sprung AU, Keller BA, Heaton VJ, Fisher LM (1997) Identification of yeast DNA topoisomerase II mutants resistant to the antitumor drug doxorubicin: implications for the mechanisms of doxorubicin action and cytotoxicity. *Mol Pharmacol* **52**(4)**:** 658–666

Petersen LN, Jensen PB, Sorensen BS, Engelholm SA, Spang-Thomsen M, Srensen BS (1994) Postincubation with aclarubicin reverses topoisomerase II mediated DNA cleavage, strand breaks, and cytotoxicity induced by VP-16. *Invest New Drugs* **12**(4)**:** 289–297

Pommier Y, Leo E, Zhang H, Marchand C (2010) DNA topoisomerases and their poisoning by anticancer and antibacterial drugs. *Chem Biol* **17**(5)**:** 421–433

Pommier Y, Marchand C (2005) Interfacial inhibitors of protein-nucleic acid interactions. *Curr Med Chem Anticancer Agents* **5**(4)**:** 421–429

Pommier Y, Minford JK, Schwartz RE, Zwelling LA, Kohn KW (1985) Effects of the DNA intercalators 4′-(9-acridinylamino)methanesulfon-m- anisidide and 2-methyl-9-hydroxyellipticinium on topoisomerase II mediated DNA strand cleavage and strand passage. *Biochemistry* **24**(23): 6410–6416

Riou JF, Fosse P, Nguyen CH, Larsen AK, Bissery MC, Grondard L, Saucier JM, Bisagni E, Lavelle F (1993) Intoplicine (RP 60475) and its derivatives, a new class of antitumor agents inhibiting both topoisomerase I and II activities. *Cancer Res* **53**(24): 5987–5993

Riou JF, Grondard L, Naudin A, Bailly C (1995) Effects of two distamycin-ellipticine hybrid molecules on topoisomerase I and II mediated DNA cleavage: relation to cytotoxicity. *Biochem Pharmacol* **50**(3): 424–428

Roca J, Ishida R, Berger JM, Andoh T, Wang JC (1994) Antitumor bisdioxopiperazines inhibit yeast DNA topoisomerase II by trapping the enzyme in the form of a closed protein clamp. *Proc Natl Acad Sci USA* **91**(5): 1781–1785

Rogojina AT, Nitiss JL (2008) Isolation and characterization of *m*AMSA-hypersensitive mutants cytotoxicity of Top2 covalent complexes containing DNA single strand breaks. *J Biol Chem* **283**(43): 29239–29250

Ross JA (2000) Dietary flavonoids and the MLL gene: A pathway to infant leukemia? *Proc Nat Acad Sci USA* **97**(9): 4411–4413

Ross JA, Potter JD, Reaman GH, Pendergrass TW, Robison LL (1996) Maternal exposure to potential inhibitors of DNA topoisomerase II and infant leukemia (United States): a report from the Children's Cancer Group. *Cancer Causes Control* **7**(6): 581–590

Ross JA, Potter JD, Robison LL (1994) Infant leukemia, topoisomerase II inhibitors, and the MLL gene. *J Nat Cancer Inst* **86**(22): 1678–1680

Sabourin M, Byl JAW, Hannah SE, Nitiss JL, Osheroff N (1998) A mutant yeast topoisomerase II (top2G437S) with differential sensitivity to anticancer drugs in the presence and absence of ATP. *J Biol Chem* **273**(44): 29086–29092

Sabourin M, Osheroff N (2000) Sensitivity of human type II topoisomerases to DNA damage: stimulation of enzyme-mediated DNA cleavage by abasic, oxidized and alkylated lesions. *Nucleic Acids Res* **28**(9): 1947–1954

Scatena CD, Kumer JL, Arbitrario JP, Howlett AR, Hawtin RE, Fox JA, Silverman JA (2010) Voreloxin, a first-in-class anticancer quinolone derivative, acts synergistically with cytarabine in vitro and induces bone marrow aplasia in vivo. *Cancer Chemother Pharmacol* **66**(5): 881–888

Schmidt BH, Burgin AB, Deweese JE, Osheroff N, Berger JM (2010) A novel and unified two-metal mechanism for DNA cleavage by type II and IA topoisomerases. *Nature* **465**(7298): 641–644

Schoeffler AJ, Berger JM (2008) DNA topoisomerases: harnessing and constraining energy to govern chromosome topology. *Q Rev Biophys* **41**(1): 41–101

Schulmeister L (2008) Dexrazoxane treatment for intrathoracic anthracycline extravasation. *Onkologie* **31**(11): 634

Schulmeister L (2011) Extravasation management: clinical update. *Semin Oncol Nurs* **27**(1): 82–90

Simunek T, Sterba M, Popelova O, Adamcova M, Hrdina R, Gersl V (2009) Anthracycline-induced cardiotoxicity: overview of studies examining the roles of oxidative stress and free cellular iron. *Pharmacol Rep* **61**(1): 154–171

Snapka RM, Gao H, Grabowski DR, Brill D, Chan KK, Li L, Li GC, Ganapathi R (2001) Cytotoxic mechanism of XK469: resistance of topoisomerase IIbeta knockout cells and inhibition of topoisomerase I. *Biochem Biophys Res Commun* **280**(4): 1155–1160

Solovyan VT, Bezvenyuk ZA, Salminen A, Austin CA, Courtney MJ (2002) The role of topoisomerase II in the excision of DNA loop domains during apoptosis. *J Biol Chem* **277**(24): 21458–21467

Staker BL, Feese MD, Cushman M, Pommier Y, Zembower D, Stewart L, Burgin AB (2005) Structures of three classes of anticancer agents bound to the human topoisomerase I-DNA covalent complex. *J Med Chem* **48**(7): 2336–2345

Staker BL, Hjerrild K, Feese MD, Behnke CA, Burgin AB, Jr., Stewart L (2002) The mechanism of topoisomerase I poisoning by a camptothecin analog. *Proc Natl Acad Sci USA* **99**(24): 15387–15392

Strick R, Strissel PL, Borgers S, Smith SL, Rowley JD (2000) Dietary bioflavonoids induce cleavage in the MLL gene and may contribute to infant leukemia. *Proc Natl Acad Sci USA* **97**: 4790–4795

Strumberg D, Nitiss JL, Dong J, Kohn KW, Pommier Y (1999a) Molecular analysis of yeast and human Type II topoisomerases. *J Biol Chem* **274**(40): 28246–28255

Strumberg D, Nitiss JL, Rose A, Nicklaus MC, Pommier Y (1999b) Mutation of a conserved serine residue in a quinolone-resistant type II topoisomerase alters the enzyme-DNA and drug interactions. *J Biol Chem* **274**(11): 7292–7301

Subramanian B, Nakeff A, Media J, Wentland M, Valeriote F (2002) Cellular drug action profile paradigm applied to XK469. *J Exp Ther Oncol* **2**(5): 253–263

Suda N, Ito Y, Imai T, Kikumori T, Kikuchi A, Nishiyama Y, Yoshida S, Suzuki M (2004) The alpha4 residues of human DNA topoisomerase IIalpha function in enzymatic activity and anticancer drug sensitivity. *Nucleic Acids Res* **32**(5): 1767–1773

Tewey KM, Chen GL, Nelson EM, Liu LF (1984) Intercalative antitumor drugs interfere with the breakage-reunion reaction of mammalian DNA topoisomerase II. *J Biol Chem* **259**(14): 9182–9187

Toyoda E, Kagaya S, Cowell IG, Kurosawa A, Kamoshita K, Nishikawa K, Iiizumi S, Koyama H, Austin CA, Adachi N (2008) NK314, a topoisomerase II inhibitor that specifically targets the alpha isoform. *J Biol Chem* **283**(35): 23711–23720

Treszezamsky AD, Kachnic LA, Feng Z, Zhang J, Tokadjian C, Powell SN (2007) BRCA1- and BRCA2-deficient cells are sensitive to etoposide-induced DNA double-strand breaks via topoisomerase II. *Cancer Res* **67**(15): 7078–7081

Turnbull RM, Meczes EL, Perenna Rogers M, Lock RB, Sullivan DM, Finlay GJ, Baguley BC, Austin CA (1999) Carbamate analogues of amsacrine active against non-cycling cells: relative activity against topoisomerases IIalpha and beta. *Cancer Chemother Pharmacol* **44**(4): 275–282

Undevia SD, Innocenti F, Ramirez J, House L, Desai AA, Skoog LA, Singh DA, Karrison T, Kindler HL, Ratain MJ (2008) A phase I and pharmacokinetic study of the quinoxaline antitumour Agent R(+)XK469 in patients with advanced solid tumours. *Eur J Cancer* **44**(12): 1684–1692

van Gijn R, ten Bokkel Huinink WW, Rodenhuis S, Vermorken JB, van Tellingen O, Rosing H, van Warmerdam LJ, Beijnen JH (1999) Topoisomerase I/II inhibitor intoplicine administered as a 24 h infusion: phase I and pharmacologic study. *Anticancer Drugs* **10**(1): 17–23

Velez-Cruz R, Riggins JN, Daniels JS, Cai H, Guengerich FP, Marnett LJ, Osheroff N (2005) Exocyclic DNA lesions stimulate DNA cleavage mediated by human topoisomerase II alpha in vitro and in cultured cells. *Biochemistry* **44**(10): 3972–3981

Walsby EJ, Coles SJ, Knapper S, Burnett AK (2011) The topoisomerase II inhibitor voreloxin causes cell cycle arrest and apoptosis in myeloid leukemia cells and acts in synergy with cytarabine. *Haematologica* **96**(3): 393–399

Wang H, Mao Y, Chen AY, Zhou N, LaVoie EJ, Liu LF (2001) Stimulation of topoisomerase II-mediated DNA damage via a mechanism involving protein thiolation. *Biochemistry* **40**(11): 3316–3323

Wang JC (2002) Cellular roles of DNA topoisomerases: a molecular perspective. *Nat Rev Mol Cell Biol* **3**(6): 430–440

Wang S, Miller W, Milton J, Vicker N, Stewart A, Charlton P, Mistry P, Hardick D, Denny WA (2002) Structure-activity relationships for analogues of the phenazine-based dual topoisomerase I/II inhibitor XR11576. *Bioorg Med Chem Lett* **12**(3): 415–418

Wasserman RA, Wang JC (1994a) Analysis of yeast DNA topoisomerase II mutants resistant to the antitumor drug amsacrine. *Cancer Res* **54**(7): 1795–1800

Wasserman RA, Wang JC (1994b) Mechanistic studies of amsacrine-resistant derivatives of DNA topoisomerase II. Implications in resistance to multiple antitumor drugs targeting the enzyme. *J Biol Chem* **269**(33): 20943–20951

Wilstermann AM, Bender RP, Godfrey M, Choi S, Anklin C, Berkowitz DB, Osheroff N, Graves DE (2007) Topoisomerase II - drug interaction domains: identification of substituents on etoposide that interact with the enzyme. *Biochemistry* **46**(28): 8217–8225

Wohlkonig A, Chan PF, Fosberry AP, Homes P, Huang J, Kranz M, Leydon VR, Miles TJ, Pearson ND, Perera RL, Shillings AJ, Gwynn MN, Bax BD (2010) Structural basis of quinolone inhibition of type IIA topoisomerases and target-mediated resistance. *Nat Struct Mol Biol* **17**(9): 1152–1153

Xiao H, Mao Y, Desai SD, Zhou N, Ting CY, Hwang JL, Liu LF (2003) The topoisomerase II beta circular clamp arrests transcription and signals a 26 S proteasome pathway. *Proc Natl Acad Sci USA* **100**(6): 3239–3244

Yamashita Y, Kawada S, Fujii N, Nakano H (1991) Induction of mammalian DNA topoisomerase I and II mediated DNA cleavage by saintopin, a new antitumor agent from fungus. *Biochemistry* **30**(24): 5838–5845

You Y (2005) Podophyllotoxin derivatives: current synthetic approaches for new anticancer agents. *Curr Pharm Des* **11**(13): 1695–1717

Zhu X, Ma Y, Liu D (2010) Novel agents and regimens for acute myeloid leukemia: 2009 ASH annual meeting highlights. *J Hematol Oncol* **3**: 17

Zwelling LA, Hinds M, Chan D, Mayes J, Sie KL, Parker E, Silberman L, Radcliffe A, Beran M, Blick M (1989) Characterization of an amsacrine-resistant line of human leukemia cells. Evidence for a drug-resistant form of topoisomerase II. *J Biol Chem* **264**(28): 16411–16420

Chapter 12
Topoisomerase I Inhibitors: Current Use and Prospects

Yan Makeyev, Franco Muggia, Arun Rajan, Giuseppe Giaccone, Takahisa Furuta, and Philippe Rougier

12.1 Historical Background

The two leading Top1 interacting drugs topotecan (Hycamptin) and irinotecan (Camptosar®, Campto®) were introduced into clinical studies in the 1980s and gained regulatory agency approvals by several countries for the treatment of various cancers in the 1990s. The history of the development of these camptothecin derivatives since sodium camptothecin's original studies from 1968 to 1972 was reviewed by O'Leary and Muggia (O'Leary and Muggia 1998), and has also been covered by books emanating from international symposia (Pantazis et al. 1996; Potmesil and Kohn 1991). The key chemical equilibrium in plasma and in tissues between the active lactone (closed) form of the E ring versus the inactive carboxylate was identified even before the discovery of topoisomerases. Other camptothecin derivatives have been developed, and new classes of Top1 interacting drugs are recently undergoing clinical study. However, this chapter will confine its review to the clinical underpinnings that support the use of the topotecan and irinotecan, principally because the role of new compounds and new formulations, while promising, has not been defined.

12.2 Irinotecan and Topotecan: Structure, Pharmacokinetics, and Pharmacogenomics

Although both irinotecan and topotecan are Top1 inhibitors, there are interesting differences in the pharmacokinetic and pharmacogenetic characteristics between them. *Irinotecan* is a prodrug metabolized by carboxylesterase to the potent active metabolite SN-38 and its stable lactone form (Fig. 12.1) (Kuhn 1998) that, in turn,

F. Muggia (✉)
New York University Langone Medical Center, New York University, New York, USA
e-mail: franco.muggia@nyumc.org

Y. Pommier (ed.), *DNA Topoisomerases and Cancer*, Cancer Drug Discovery and Development, DOI 10.1007/978-1-4614-0323-4_12,

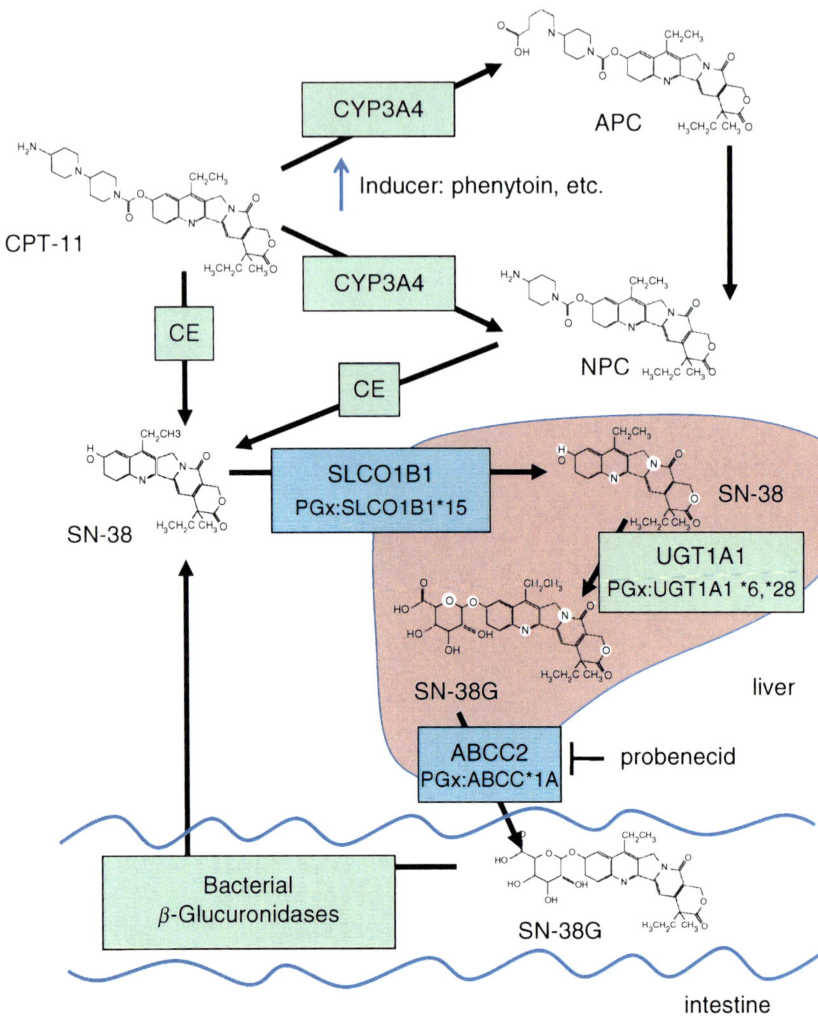

Fig. 12.1 Metabolism and elimination of irinotecan (CPT-11). Irinotecan is metabolized by carboxyesterase (CE) to the active metabolite, SN-38. A portion of irinotecan is metabolized by CYP3A4 to inactive metabolite, aminopentanecarboxylic acid (APC). SN-38 is taken to hepatocytes mainly by SLCO1B1 and then converted to SN-38 glucuronide (SN-38G) by UGT1A1. SN-38G is excreted to bile juice by ABCC2 and eliminated to small intestine. Some part of SN-38G by ß-glucuronidase of bacterial flow in the intestine. There are genetic differences in activity of SLCO1B1, UGT1A1 and ABCC2, which influence the kinetics of SN-38. *ABC* ATP-binding cassette transporters, *SLC*O solute carrier organic anion transporter, *UG*T uridine-diphosphoglucuronosyltransferase

inhibits Top1 and induces DNA double-strand breaks in cells in a replication-dependent manner, resulting in induction of apoptosis in cells mainly in the S phase. The DNA double-strand breaks are mainly repaired by homologous recombination (HR) and nonhomologous end joining (NHEJ) (Hoeijmakers 2001).

SN-38 is conjugated with glucuronic acid by uridine-diphosphoglucuronosyltransferase (UGT) to form an inactive metabolite, SN-38G (Mathijssen et al. 2003).

Of UGT proteins, UGT1A1 is the major protein that catalyzes the glucuronidation of SN-38 (Ando et al. 1998; Mackenzie et al. 1997). There are genetic differences in the activity of UGT1A1 that are associated with irinotecan toxicity via the alternation of bioavailability of SN-38. Ando (Ando et al. 2000) first investigated whether patients with variant UGT1A1 genotypes would be at higher risk for severe toxicity by irinotecan and found that genotypes either heterozygous or homozygous for *UGT1A1**28 would be significant risk factors for severe toxicity by irinotecan. Following this report, the relationship between UGT1A1 polymorphism and irinotecan toxicity has been studied intensively throughout the world. Onoue (Onoue and Inui 2008) reported that not only *UGT1A1**28 but also *UGT1A1**6 were associated with the occurrence of adverse events in irinotecan chemotherapy in Asians. Case reports of severe neutropenia due to these polymorphisms are often reported (Yokoyama et al. 2009). It is therefore recommended that the UGT1A1 genotype be measured in advance in patients scheduled for treatment with irinotecan-based regimens, especially in Asian populations.

Before conjugation of SN-38 with glucuronic acid in the liver, SN-38 needs to be incorporated into hepatocytes. Uptake of SN-38 to hepatocytes is mainly mediated by OATP1B1 (SLCO1B1) (Nozawa et al. 2005), which shows a genetic difference in activity. Xiang (Xiang et al. 2006) investigated the influence of SLCO1B1 *1a, *1b, *5, and *15 polymorphisms on the disposition of irinotecan and its metabolites and found that the *SLCO1B*1*15 haplotype might be associated with increased SN-38 levels, leading to an increased risk of toxicity. Takane (Takane et al. 2007) reported that a patient homozygous for the *SLCO1B1**15 allele developed severe toxicities after the first cycle of irinotecan-based regimen, including grade 3 diarrhea, grade 4 leukopenia, and grade 4 neutropenia. In addition to *UGT1A1* *6 and *28, screening of *SLCO1B1**15 is also suggested in order to avoid unpredictable severe toxicity when beginning irinotecan chemotherapy.

Irinotecan is metabolized by carboxylesterase to the active metabolite, SN-38, as noted above. However, irinotecan is also metabolized by CYP3A4 to an inactive metabolite, 7-ethyl-10-[4-*N*-(5-aminopentanoic acid)-1-piperidino]- carbonyloxy-camptothecin (APC) (Kuhn 1998). The elucidation of this metabolic pathway suggests the potential for drug-drug interactions on coadministration of irinotecan with other inducers or substrates of CYP3A4. Phenytoin is an anticonvulsant, which is not only metabolized by CYP3A4 but is also an inducer of it. Murry (Murry et al. 2002) studied the pharmacokinetic profile of irinotecan and its major metabolites with and without concomitant phenytoin administration in an individual patient and found that concomitant phenytoin resulted in a marked decrease in systemic exposure to irinotecan and SN-38 and an increase in exposure to APC. Similarly, Kuhn (Kuhn 2002) reported that enzyme-inducing antiepileptic drugs (EIAEDs) such as phenytoin and carbamazepine altered both the pharmacokinetics and pharmacodynamics of irinotecan and that peak concentrations and the area under the plasma-time curves for both irinotecan and SN-38 were significantly decreased in patients receiving EIAEDs. They recommended that irinotecan dosage should be increased in patients receiving stable doses of EIAEDs.

SN-38G is excreted from hepatocytes to bile ducts. This transport is mediated by ABCC2, which is polymorphic. ABCC2 -1774delG (*1A) is associated with grade 3/4 neutropenia in patients treated with irinotecan (Sai et al. 2010). Probenecid is known to inhibit the activity of ABCC2. Therefore, concomitant use of probenecid with irinotecan would decrease the biliary excretion of SN-38G, which might increase the risk of adverse events of irinotecan (Horikawa et al. 2002).

Topotecan 9-dimethylaminomethyl-10-hydroxycamptothecin, introduced by the National Cancer Institute (NCI) a decade after camptothecin sodium, and extensively developed by Glaxo SmithKline, has as its main advantages water solubility and predictable pharmacokinetics. In contrast to irinotecan, it has limited biliary excretion, and therefore, little gastrointestinal toxicity. On the other hand, because of the short half-life of its lactone form in plasma, the drug must be administered in repeated daily doses, and in contradistinction with irinotecan, is highly schedule dependent. The daily × 5 days schedule is the US Food & Drug Administration (FDA) approved schedule. Topotecan is cleared through renal excretion with urinary recovery ranging from 60% to 70% (Pratt et al. 1994; Stewart et al. 1994). Urinary secretion of topotecan is mediated by organic anion transporter 3 (OAT3) (Fig. 12.2). It is reported that single nucleotide polymorphisms (SNPs) of OAT3 are unlikely to influence mRNA expression and promote activity. Less than 40% of topotecan is eliminated through nonrenal routes, such as hepatic and biliary, so that plasma kinetics of topotecan could be influenced somewhat by the activity of CYPs. In fact, phenytoin is known as the inducer of CYPs and increases the clearance of topotecan (Zamboni et al. 1998). The human multidrug resistance gene MDR1 encodes P-glycoprotein (P-gp), which is an integral membrane protein and mediates ATP-dependent substrate efflux. MDR1 is polymorphic and is known to affect the absorption of substrates of MDR1, such as digoxin (Hoffmeyer et al. 2000). Topotecan is also a substrate of MDR1 (Crouthamel et al. 2006), but is an even greater substrate of ABCG2 that is commonly present in the gut and accounts for its erratic oral absorption (see next paragraph). Schaiquevich (Schaiquevich et al. 2007) studied the factors affecting the kinetics of topotecan in pediatric cancer patients and found that the most significant covariate was body surface area, which explained 54% of the interindividual variability for topotecan systemic clearance. They found that concomitant phenytoin, calculated glomerular filtration rate, and age (<0.5 years) were also related to clearance of topotecan. They reported the predictive formula of clearance of topotecan, which could potentially be useful for the optimization of topotecan dose.

Alternative dose schedules to the impractical daily × 5, every 3 weeks administration have been explored, but shorter or intermittent regimens may be less effective. Studies by Hochster and Liebes at New York University (Hochster et al. 1994, 1999), evaluated the pharmacology and clinical use of continuous infusion schedules alone and in combination, particularly in patients with gynecologic cancer (see Sect. 12.5). Also, the oral route was extensively studied by Schellens (Schellens et al. 1996) with limited bioavailability eventually being explained by ABCG2 expression in the gut; inhibitors of the ATP binding site of this transporter overcomes this erratic absorption (Muggia and Hudes 2003), and such observation including a clinical pharmacologic study has yet to be pursued. While oral topote-

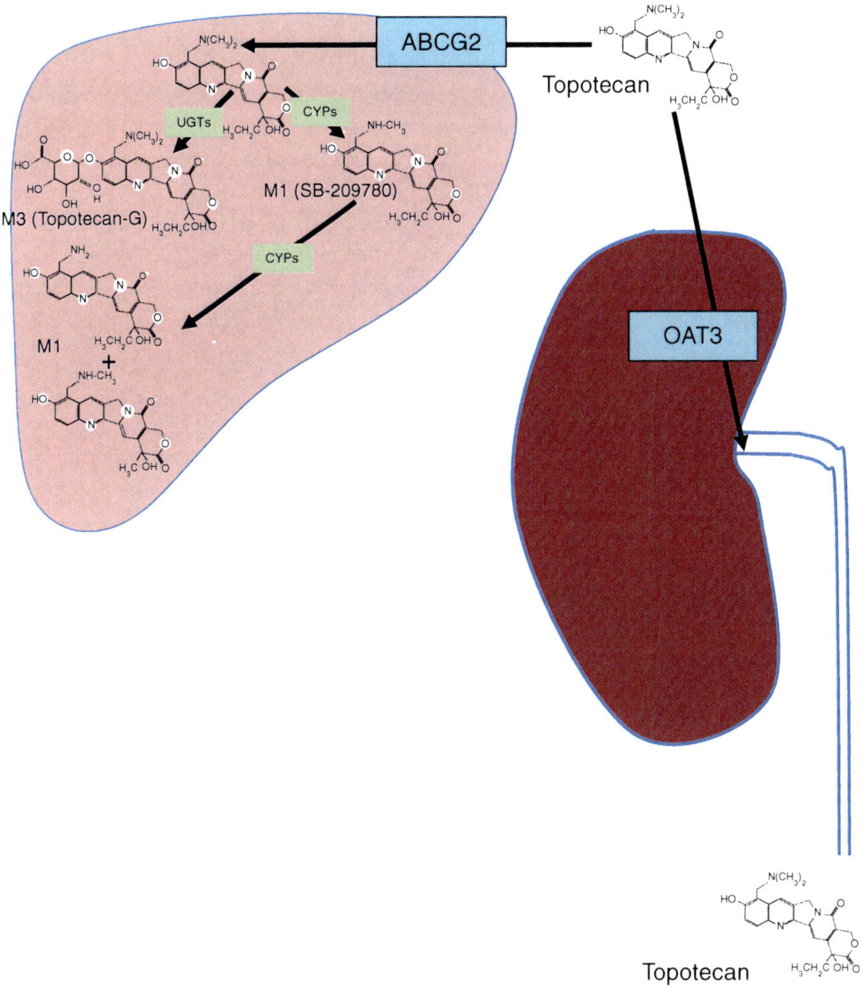

Fig. 12.2 Metabolism and elimination of topotecan. Topotecan is eliminated by the organic anion transporter (*OAT3*) in the kidneys and metabolized in the liver by UGTs and cytochromes P450

can eventually was approved for use in the USA in recurrent small cell lung cancer (SCLC), gastrointestinal toxicities as well as issues common to myelosuppressive cytotoxics in the face of unreliable pharmacology limited its wide adoption. A background to pharmacologic issues relating to topotecan and other inhibitors is contained within *The Camptothecins: Unfolding Their Anticancer Potential* (Liehr and Giovanella 2000).

As described above, the kinetics of irinotecan and topotecan are affected by genetics and drug–drug interaction as well as unknown factors. Clinicians must take these problems into consideration when treating patients with irinotecan- or topotecan-based therapy, which could contribute to more effective and safer Top1 inhibitor-based regimens (Furuta 2009).

12.3 Other Top1 Inhibitors

A number of camptothecin derivatives have been in clinical trial but have not been incorporated into clinical practice: *exatecan mesylate* (DX-8951f) was introduced by Daiichi Pharmaceutical Co., Ltd., Japan because of potency compared to irinotecan; *belotecan* (Camtobell, CKD602) is in use principally in Korea; *lurtotecan* was developed in a liposomal formulation before being dropped; the insoluble derivatives *9-aminocamptothecin* and *9-nitrocamptothecin* (rubitecan) underwent phase I and II development, including various solubilizer, oral administration, and intraperitoneally [summarized in *The Camptothecins –from discovery to the patient*(2000)].

Gimatecan (ST 1481) is the prototype of an orally administered lipophilic camptothecin analog in further development. In preclinical studies, it has shown greater activity and a wider therapeutic index compared to topotecan (De Cesare et al. 2004). Recently, interest has shifted to slow release forms of camptothecin itself or SN-38 with several preparations under development, particularly for colorectal cancer (CRC).
Karenitecin is a semisynthetic, 7-Silyl lipophilic camptothecin derivative with a more stable E-ring and consequently greater lactone stability than topotecan or irinotecan. In preclinical studies, karenitecin demonstrated greater antitumor activity compared to other camptothecins.

Edotecarin (J-107088) is a novel non-camptothecin Top1 inhibitor belonging to the family of indolocarbazoles. It causes DNA cleavage at a different site and forms more stable ternary complexes with DNA and Top1 when compared to camptothecin and its analogs.

Indenoisoquinolines are non-camptothecin inhibitors of Top1. They exhibit a unique set of properties when compared to camptothecins. These include greater chemical stability, trapping of Top1 cleavage sites at different locations of the cancer genome, and decreased propensity to act as substrates for multidrug resistance efflux pumps (ABCG2 and MDR-1) (Pommier and Cushman 2009). A phase I study of two novel compounds, LMP400 (NSC743400) and LMP776 (NSC725776), is ongoing in adults with relapsed solid tumors and lymphomas (NCT01051635). The primary endpoint of the study is to define the MTD and DLTs of these compounds. Being interested in these last four drugs in lung cancer, their initial clinical experience is summarized in the next section.

12.4 Role in Lung Cancer

Topotecan was approved for treatment of recurrent SCLC based on the results of a large phase III trial: patients who had relapsed at least 60 days after completion of first-line therapy received either topotecan at a dose of 1.5 mg/m^2/day × 5 every 21 days or CAV (cyclophosphamide 1,000 mg/m^2, doxorubicin 45 mg/m^2, and vincristine 2 mg) on day 1 of a 21 day cycle. Of the 211 patients treated, 107 received topotecan and 104 received CAV. The response rate (RR) to the two regimens was 24% and 18%, respectively ($p=0.285$). Median time to progression (TTP) and median survival for patients receiving topotecan versus CAV was 13.3 weeks versus 12.3 weeks ($p=0.552$) and 25 weeks versus 24.7 weeks ($p=0.795$), respectively. Significant adverse events included grade 4 neutropenia (with 38% of topotecan courses vs. 51% of CAV courses; $p<0.001$), grade 4 thrombocytopenia (10% and 1.4%; $p<0.001$), and grade 3/4 anemia (18% and 7%; $p<0.001$). This trial demonstrated that topotecan was at least as effective as CAV in patients with recurrent SCLC (von Pawel et al. 1999).

Oral topotecan at a dose of 2.3 mg/m^2/day × 5 given every 21 days was compared to best supportive care in a phase III study in relapsed SCLC. Seventy-one patients received topotecan and 70 best supportive care. Median survival improved in the topotecan group (26–13 weeks, $p=0.0104$) (O'Brien et al. 2006). Further, oral topotecan was compared to intravenous topotecan in a phase III study and demonstrated comparable activity and tolerability in patients with chemotherapy-sensitive SCLC (Eckardt et al. 2007). It has also been evaluated for the treatment of recurrent non-small cell lung cancer (NSCLC) after one prior regimen compared to intravenous docetaxel: 414 patients were randomized to oral topotecan at a dose of 2.3 mg/m^2/day × 5 repeated every 3 weeks and 415 to docetaxel at a dose of 75 mg/m^2 × 1 every 3 weeks. Survival at 1 year was 25% with topotecan and 29% with docetaxel. These results met predetermined criteria for non-inferiority of topotecan relative to docetaxel. Median survival was 28 weeks with topotecan compared to 31 weeks with docetaxel ($p=0.057$); median TTP was 11 weeks and 13 weeks, respectively ($p=0.02$). Common grade 3/4 adverse events were related to myelosuppression (Ramlau et al. 2006). Other ongoing studies evaluating topotecan in lung cancer are listed in Table 12.1.

Irinotecan has also been the subject of several phase III studies for patients with SCLC. In 2002, Noda et al. published results of a study in Japanese patients with extensive stage SCLC comparing irinotecan plus cisplatin versus etoposide plus cisplatin. An interim analysis after enrolling 154 patients (77 patients out of 115 to be accrued in each arm) resulted in early termination since a statistically significant

Table 12.1 Ongoing studies evaluating topotecan in lung cancer

Disease	Intervention	Primary outcome measures	Phase	Study ID
SCLC	Topotecan ± Aflibercept	PFS at 3 months	II	NCT00828139
SCLC or advanced solid tumors	Topotecan + Obatoclax Mesylate	Determination of MTD, RP2D, and toxicity profile (phase I) Overall response rate (phase II)	I/II	NCT00521144
SCLC	Topotecan + Doxorubicin	Determination of DLT Safety and efficacy	I	NCT00856037
NSCLC	Topotecan + Bevacizumab	PFS at 6 months	II	NCT00365547

PFS progression-free survival, *MTD* maximum tolerated dose, *RP2D* recommended phase 2 dose, *DLT* dose-limiting toxicity improvement in survival was shown in the experimental arm: the median survival in the irinotecan arm was 12.8 months compared to 9.4 months in the etoposide arm ($p=0.002$), and overall RR was 84% in patients receiving irinotecan plus cisplatin and 68% in the control arm ($p=0.02$) (Noda et al. 2002). To confirm these results in the North American population Hanna et al. conducted a phase III trial using a modified schedule in which treatment was repeated every 3 weeks in both arms. This study did not show any benefit of irinotecan plus cisplatin over etoposide plus cisplatin (331 patients; 221 patients in the experimental arm; response rates: 48% vs. 44%, median TTP: 4.1 months vs. 4.6 months, median overall survival (OS): 9.3 months vs. 10.2 months; $p=0.74$) (Hanna et al. 2006). Further, another phase III trial conducted in the North American population by the Southwest Oncology Group (S0124) using a treatment regimen identical to the Japanese trial also failed to confirm the survival benefit noted therein (651 eligible patients, 324 patients in the experimental arm; response rates: 60% vs. 57% ($p=0.56$), median progression free survival (PFS): 5.8 months vs. 5.2 months ($p=0.07$), median OS: 9.9 months vs. 9.1 months ($p=0.71$))(Lara et al. 2009). Therefore, although irinotecan + cisplatin is an active regimen, it has generally not replaced the etoposide + cisplatin regimen in SCLC.

Irinotecan has extensively been studied in advanced NSCLC, particularly in Japan, where this agent is currently marketed. Irinotecan has single agent activity similar to other cytotoxic agents and it has often been combined with platinum compounds.

Belotecan has been studied in patients with treatment-naïve extensive stage SCLC: 62 patients (49 males; median age: 66 years) received belotecan administered intravenously at a dose of 0.5 mg/m^2/day for 5 consecutive days every 3 weeks. Among 53 evaluable patients, 1 complete response (CR), 32 partial responses (PRs), and 10 stable disease (SD) were noted. The overall RR on an intent-to-treat basis was 53%, median TTP was 4.6 months, median OS was 10.4 months, and the 1-year survival rate was 50%. Toxicities resembled those of topotecan (Kim et al. 2010). Jeong reported results from a phase II study of belotecan in Asian patients with SCLC who had relapsed at least 3 months after achieving an objective response to first-line irinotecan-containing chemotherapy. Belotecan was initially administered at a dose of 0.5 mg/m^2/day × 5 every 3 weeks and subsequently the dose was modified 0.4, 0.5, or 0.6 mg/m^2/day × 5 based on toxicity: with 25 patients evaluable for response. 6 PRs (22%) and 13 SD (48%) were noted. The median TTP was 4.7 months (95% CI, 3.6–5.8) and median OS was 13.1 months (95% CI, 10.4–15.8). The most frequent grade 3/4 adverse events included neutropenia in 93% of patients and thrombocytopenia in 48% of patients (Jeong et al. 2010). Belotecan 0.5 mg/m^2/day from day 1 through day 4 with cisplatin at a dose of 60 mg/m^2 on day 1 every 3 weeks was a very active combination in 17 patients with previously untreated extensive stage SCLC: 14 PRs (83%, 95%CI: 63–100%) were seen in this study; the dose-limiting toxicity was grade 4 febrile neutropenia (Lee et al. 2007).

A phase III study is evaluating this combination versus etoposide plus cisplatin in patients with previously untreated extensive stage SCLC (COMBAT;

NCT00826644): the primary endpoint is assessment of RR and secondary endpoints including assessment of duration of response, TTP, and OS.

Karenitecin at a dose of 1 mg/m^2 intravenously for 5 consecutive days every 21 days was evaluated in a phase II trial conducted by the Cancer and Leukemia Group B (CALGB) in patients with relapsed or refractory NSCLC: of 52 patients who were eligible (27 males; median age: 63 years; 50% adenocarcinoma, 21% squamous cell carcinoma), 28 patients had relapsed disease and 24 patients had refractory disease. Of 50 patients evaluable, 2 PRs (3.8%) and 24 SD (46%) were seen, while 23 patients (44%) progressed. The median survival in patients with relapsed and refractory NSCLC was 10.4 months (95% CI, 8.5–17.0) and 6 months (95% CI, 3.7–9.7), respectively. One-year survival in the two groups was 36% (95% CI, 14–58%) and 21% (95% CI, 5–37%), respectively. The most frequent grade 3/4 toxicities were neutropenia (31%) and thrombocytopenia (25%). Improvement in survival after treatment with karenitecin in patients with relapsed or refractory NSCLC was comparable to the outcomes seen with other agents used in the second-line setting in these patients (Miller et al. 2005).

Gimatecan administered orally once a week at escalating doses starting at 0.27 mg/m^2/week for 3 weeks of a 4-week cycle has been evaluated in a phase I study in 33 advanced solid tumor patients that included 4 with NSCLC. The MTD using this schedule of administration was 2.4 mg/m^2/week. No objective responses were seen in this study. Major adverse events were anemia, neutropenia, leukopenia, fatigue, nausea, and vomiting (Zhu et al. 2009). By contrast, in another phase I study gimatecan administered daily at doses ranging from 0.8–7.2 mg/m^2/cycle demonstrated antitumor activity: 108 patients were treated including 21 patients with NSCLC and 6 PRs (2 with NSCLC) were seen. The dose limiting toxicity was thrombocytopenia (Sessa et al. 2007).

Edotecarin has been evaluated in several phase I and phase II trials. Yamada et al. conducted a phase I study of edotecarin in 24 Japanese patients, 7 of whom had lung cancer but no confirmed objective responses were seen. The most common grade 3/4 adverse events (AE) were neutropenia and leukopenia (Yamada et al. 2006). In another phase I study conducted by Hurwitz et al. 29 patients with advanced solid tumors, including 3 patients with NSCLC received edotecarin at escalating doses starting at 6 mg/m^2 administered intravenously every 21 days. The most common grade 3/4 AEs were neutropenia, leukopenia, and anemia. No objective responses were seen in three patients with NSCLC (Hurwitz et al. 2007). Two indenoisoquinolines are undergoing clinical studies, LMP400 (NSC743400) and LMP776 (NSC725776); their activity in lung cancer has not been established.

In summary, there is an established role for Top1 inhibitors in the treatment of previously treated lung cancers. Unfortunately, RRs and survival remain poor, and their potential in combination with other drugs and radiation as primary therapy are largely unexplored in phase III trials. New Top1 inhibitors exhibit chemical and pharmacogenomic properties that are different from topotecan and irinotecan warranting further evaluation.

12.5 Role in Gastrointestinal Malignancies

12.5.1 Colorectal

12.5.1.1 Topotecan

Topotecan has minimal activity in the patients with metastatic CRC, with a RR under 10% (Creemers et al. 1995). In a small phase I/II study, combination of topotecan with oxaliplatin did not show significant activity in 5-FU pretreated patients (Hutter et al. 2004).

12.5.1.2 Irinotecan

Antitumor Activity, Proof of Concept Studies

Single-agent irinotecan produced objective RR in the range of 14–27% in patients that developed disease progression during treatment with fluorouracil (Rougier et al. 1997; Shimada et al. 1996). In a randomized trial, 267 patients with advanced CRC were treated with either irinotecan or fluorouracil by continuous infusion, after failure of first-line fluorouracil-based therapy. Median survival was 10.8 month in irinotecan arm, and 8.5 month in fluorouracil arm. Quality of life was similar in both groups (Rougier et al. 1998). The most common grade 3–4 adverse events in irinotecan arm were diarrhea, neutropenia, vomiting, pain, and asthenia.

Irinotecan Efficacy in First-Line Treatment

In the first-line treatment, many schedules of combination of irinotecan and 5-FU/leucovorin or oral fluoropyrimidine have been developed, and demonstrated their efficacy (Table 12.2). The first was the IFL regimen combining weekly bolus 5-FU and leucovorin to irinotecan (125 mg/m² weekly for 4 weeks every 6 weeks), which was superior to bolus 5-FU and leucovorin alone in term of PFS, OS and (Saltz et al. 2000). In a subsequent phase III study, the IFL regimen was toxic and less effective than the FOLFOX regimen and fell out of routine use (Delaunoit et al. 2004; Goldberg et al. 2004). The second regimen, a combination of a weekly regimen using a 24 h 5-FU infusion (AIO regimen) and irinotecan (80 mg/m²) for 6 weeks every 8 weeks; was superior to the AIO regimen alone in terms of PFS and RR (Kohne et al. 2005), but the dose of 24 h 5-FU infusion had to be reduced from 2,300–2,000 mg/m². A third regimen, the base for most regimens used in 2010, was a combination of the LV5FU2 (bolus and infusion 5-FU over 48 h preceded by leucovorin) administered every 2 weeks with irinotecan administered as a 90 min infusion at the dose of 180 mg/m² before 5-FU was shown superior to LV5FU2

Table 12.2 Trials comparing a 5-FU-leucovorin combination to the same combination + irinotecan in first-line treatment in metastatic colorectal cancer

Study	A- control arm	B- experimental arm	PFS	OS	RR
Saltz et al. (2000)	Bolus FU/LV	IFL: Same + CPT	A: 4.3 mos.	A: 12.6 mos.	A: 21%
	4/6 week	125 mg/m² q week	B: 7.0 mos.	B: 14.8 mos.	B: 39%
	$n=226$	$n=231$	$P=0.004$	$P=0.04$	$P=0.001$
Köhne et.al. (2005)	AIO: 24 h FU infusion	Same + CPT	A: 6.4 mos.	A: 16.9 mos.	A: 34.4%
	6/8week	80 mg/m²/week	B: 8.5 mos.	B: 20.01 mos.	B: 62.2%
	$n=216$	$n=214$	$P<0.0001$	$P=0.278$	$P<0.0001$
Douillard et.al. (2000)	LV5FU2	Same + CPT:	A: 4.4 mos.	A: 14.1 mos.	A: 31%
	q2 weeks	180 mg/m² q2 week	B: 6.7 mos.	B: 17.4 mos.	B: 49%
	$n=188$	$n=199$	$P<0.001$	$P=0.031$	$P<0.001$

OS overall survival, *OR* overall response, *PFS* progression free survival, *CPT* irinotecan, *LV* leucovorin, FU 5-fluorouracil

alone in terms of OS, PFS, and RR; it was well tolerated (Douillard et al. 2000). A modification of this every 2 weeks regimen eliminating bolus 5-FU on day 2 became the FOLFIRI regimen, which was simpler to administer through portable pumps and had a similar activity and a better safety profile (Tournigand et al. 2004); it has also been combined with oral 5-FU with a good tolerance (Delord et al. 2007).

Irinotecan Efficacy in Second-Line Treatment

In second line, after failure on 5-FU, irinotecan has a demonstrated efficacy, alone compared to infusional 5-FU with a significant benefit in terms of OS and RR and without quality of life (QOL) reduction (Rougier et al. 1998); it has also been reported with a combination of LV5FU2 and irinotecan or oxaliplatin with interesting results in terms of PFS and RR (Rougier et al. 2002).

Irinotecan in the Strategy of Treatment of Patients with Metastatic Colorectal Cancer

Whether to use irinotecan in first-, second-, or even third-line therapy varies according to the context; for instance when PFS or response rates are not the main goals of the chemotherapy, the sequential use of the anticancer drugs may be as efficient as their combined use –except for a small advantage in OS when irinotecan is included (Seymour et al. 2007); when the RR and the PFS may be important for the QOL or the possibility of secondary resection irinotecan combinations are more suitable than 5-FU monotherapy. However, FOLFOX regimens are usually considered in this situation because it was superior to an IFL combination in the US trial (Goldberg et al. 2004) (but IFL is not the optimal comparator since the therapeutic index of FOLFIRI is better and in a randomized trial (Tournigand et al. 2004) FOLFOX was not superior to a FOLFIRI regimen). Thus, the choice between FOLFOX and FOLFIRI depends on the type of adjuvant treatment that the patient may have received and/or on the choice of the patient and physician based upon the respective side effects of these regimens. Clinical trials comparing oxaliplatin and irinotecan based combinations in first-line treatment of metastatic CRC are summarized in Table 12.2.

Results from a randomized phase II comparing XELOX and XELRI was also unable to show any superiority of one regimen over the other (Grothey et al. 2004); in this trial RR and PFS were in the same range but median OS was not reached (Table 12.3). Thus, contrary to IFL, in first-line treatment, irinotecan combinations with infusional 5-FU or oral 5-FU have the same antitumor effects as FOLFOX.

Irinotecan and Elderly Patients

In elderly patients suffering from metastatic CRC, the use of irinotecan seems to have the same efficacy as that of younger patients with a comparable safety profile (Folprecht et al. 2008). A randomized trial conducted to compare FOLFIRI with LV5FU2 has reported no concerns concerning tolerance (Mitry et al. 2008).

Irinotecan and Secondary Resections of Initially Unresectable Metastases

In case of unresectable metastases, irinotecan may contribute to render them more often resectable because of increased response rates (Barone et al. 2007); this important positive effect may be improved by combining irinotecan with 5-FU and oxaliplatin in a triplet regimen (FOLFOXIRI): a higher response rate and higher likelihood of resection has been reported compared to FOLFIRI (RR: 66% vs. 41%, $p=0.0002$ and R0 resections: 15% vs. 6%, $p=0.033$) (Falcone et al. 2007). Other triplet regimens have demonstrated high response rates and PFS with a similar schedule (named FOFIRINOX)(Ychou et al. 2008) and with a combination with tomudex (TOMOXIRI) (Maroun et al. 2006).

Irinotecan and Targeted Therapies

Results from many trials suggest that irinotecan is an excellent partner for antiangiogenic or anti-EGFR targeted drugs. In combination with bevacizumab, the efficacy of the IFL regimen was significantly superior to the one of the IFL regimen alone (Hurwitz et al. 2004). However, the IFL protocol is suboptimal – the FOLFIRI regimen was a better partner for bevacizumab in a randomized phase III trial reporting a higher overall survival and PFS with the combination of FOLFIRI + bevacizumab compared to IFL + bevacizumab (Fuchs et al. 2007); in the same study the combination of capecitabine + irinotecan + bevacizumab was not superior and resulted in a much higher toxicity.

Table 12.3 Trials comparing oxaliplatin and irinotecan-based combinations in first-line treatment of metastatic colorectal cancer

Study	A-control arm	B-experimental arm	C-experimental arm	TTP (median)	OS (median)	RR
Goldberg et al. (2004)	FOLFOX: $n=267$	IFL: $n=264$ CPT 125 mg/m²/week	IROX: $n=264$	A: 9.3mos.* B: 7 mos.* C: 6.5 mos. $P^*=0.002$	A: 19.5mos.* B: 15 mos.* C: 17.4 mos. $P=0.001$	A: 45%* B: 31%* C: 35% $P^*<0.001$
Tournigand et al. (2004)	FOLFOX Followed by FOLFIRI; $n=111$	FOLFIRI Followed by FOLFOX; $n=109$		A: 8.0 mos. B: 8.5 mos. $P=0.3$	A: 20.6 mos. B: 21.5 mos. $P=0.99$	A: 54% B: 56% NS
Grothey et al. (2003)	XELOX $n=82$	XELIRI CPT: 180 mg/m² every 2 week $n=79$		A: 7.9 mos. B: 7.9 mos. $P=0.3$	A: >16 mos. B: > 16 mos. NS	A: 51% B: 43% $P=0.3$

OS overall survival, *OR* overall response, *PFS* progression free survival, *CPT* irinotecan, *LV* leucovorin, FU 5-fluorouracil
*Statistically significant difference between the arms

In combination with anti-EGFR, and especially the antibodies cetuximab and panitumumab, irinotecan is also an excellent partner especially in *kras* wild-type tumors (Lievre et al. 2008). In the CRYSTAL trial FOLIRI combined to cetuximab results in significantly better response rate and PFS but not in OS when the global population was considered (Van Cutsem et al. 2009a), however the OS was significantly better in the *kras* wild-type population justifying the use of the combination of FOLFIRI + cetuximab in the *kras* wild type as first-line treatment.

Irinotecan as Part of Adjuvant Treatments

In the adjuvant setting, irinotecan after resection of high-risk colon cancer(Van Cutsem et al. 2009b) or very high-risk colon cancer (Ychou et al. 2009b), FOLFIRI regimen did not demonstrate any efficacy over LV5FU2. After resection of liver metastases from colorectal cancer, FOLFIRI was also not superior to LV5FU2 (Ychou et al. 2009a). Thus, there is no indication for irinotecan in adjuvant in high-risk patient following resection.

Predictive and Prognostic Factors When Irinotecan Is Used

Predictive factors for response and tolerance have not been used routinely but many predictive factors have been reported with the use of irinotecan alone or in combination with 5-FU, particularly by Lenz and coworkers (Lenz 2006; Vallbohmer et al. 2006).

In summary, irinotecan is an active and useful drug in colorectal cancer in all the situations except in adjuvant. It can be combined in promising regimens with other active drugs, with targeted therapies, and with radiation in colorectal cancers. Characterizing tumors by *kras* status and by microsatellite instability, coupled with further pharmacogenetic and pharmacodynamic information will undoubtedly enhance its usefulness in this common cancer.

12.5.2 Gastroesophageal Malignancies

Current frontline therapy of metastatic gastric (including gastroesophageal junction, GEJ) and esophageal cancers is based on cisplatin and/or 5-fluorouracil combinations. However, a search for alternative chemotherapy regimens continues due to toxicity considerations or identification of cisplatin resistance. Topotecan did not demonstrate clinically significant anti-neoplastic activity in gastroesophageal malignancies (Asbury et al. 2000; Benedetti et al. 1997; Macdonald et al. 2000; Saltz et al. 1997). Single agent irinotecan has modest activity against squamous carcinoma (Muhr-Wilkenshoff et al. 2003) and adenocarcinoma of the esophagus (Enzinger et al. 2005), or in chemotherapy naïve patients with gastric malignancies(Futatsuki et al. 1994; Kohne et al. 2003). Combinations of the irinotecan with 5-FU, cisplatin, or docetaxel were evaluated in phase II studies yielding response rates of 13–58% (Table 12.4).

Table 12.4 Trails of irinotecan in combination with cytotoxic agents in gastroesophageal malignancies

Authors	*N*	Clinical setting	Dose and schedule	Efficacy
Ilson et al. (1999)	35	Chemo naïve patients with advanced adenocarcinoma (23) or squamous cell carcinoma (12) of esophagus	CPT65 mg/m^2 Cis 30 mg/m^2 4/6 week	CR 2, PR 18 MDR 4.2 mo
Blanke et al. (2001)	38	Chemo naïve patients with recurrent adenocarcinoma of the GEJ or stomach	CPT 125 mg/m^2 + LV20 mg/m^2+ FU 500 mg/m^2, 4/6 week	CR 1, PR 7 OR 22% MS 7.6 mo. TTP 4.3 mo.
Ajani et al. (2002)	36	Chemo naïve patients with recurrent adenocarcinoma of the GEJ or stomach	CPT 65 mg/m^2 Cis 30 mg/m^2, 4/6 week	CR 4, PR 17 OR 58% TTP 24 week MS 9 mo.
Assersohn et al. (2004)	38	Second-line CT, primary refractory and resistant esophageal and gastric carcinoma, 37 patients received platinum-based CT	CPT 180 mg/m^2 FU 400 mg/m^2 bolus LV 125 mg/m^2 FU 1,200 mg/m^2 CIVI over 48 h, q2week	CR 2, PR 9 OR 29% SD 34% FFS 3.7 mo. OS 6.4 mo.
Bouche et al. (2004)	136	Chemo naïve patients with metastatic gastric cancer	Arm A "LV5FU2": LV 200 mg/m^2 FU 400 mg/m^2 bolus, FU 600 mg/m^2 22-h CIV × 2 days q2week	A: OR 13% MPFS 3.2 mo. OS 6.8 mo.
			Arm B:LV5FU2+ Cis 50 mg/m^2 × 2 days, q2week	B: OR 27% MPFS 4.9 mo. OS 9.5 mo.
			Arm C: LV5FU2+ CPT 180 mg/m^2 q2week	C: OR 40% MPFS 6.9 mo. OS 11.3 mo.

(continued)

Table 12.4 (continued)

Authors	*N*	Clinical setting	Dose and schedule	Efficacy
Pozzo et al. (2004)	115	Patients with metastatic adenocarcinoma of the GEJ or stomach. Randomized phase II trial.	Arm A: CPT 80 mg/m^2 LV 500 mg/m^2 FU 2,000 mg/m^2 CIV, 6/7 week Arm B: CPT 200 mg/m^2 Cis 60 mg/m^2, q3week	CR 5.1% PR 37.3% TTP 6.5 mo. OS 10.7 mo. CR 1.8% PR 30.4% TTP 4.2 mo. OS 6.9 mo.
Beretta et al. (2006)	30	Patient with metastatic gastric cancer, poor clinical performance, and/or ≥65 year old	FOLFIRI: CPT 180 mg/m^2, FU 400 mg/m^2 bolus, LV 100 mg/m^2 day 1,2 FU 600 mg/m^2 22-h CIV × 2 days, q2week	CR 2, PR 10 OR 40% TTP 5.5 mo.
Park et al. (2006)	46	Chemo naïve patients with metastatic gastric cancer	CPT 70 mg/m^2 Docetaxel 30 mg/m^2 on days 1 and 8, q3weeks	PR 21 OR = 45.7% TTP 4.5 mo OS 8.2 mo.
Di Lauro et al. (2007)	40	Chemo naïve patients with metastatic gastric or GEJ adenocarcinoma.	CPT 150 mg/m^2 Docetaxel 60 mg/m^2 on day 1 Oxaliplatin 85 mg/m^2 on day 2, q3weeks	CR 2, PR 18 ORR 50% TTP 6.5 mo. OS 11.5 mo.

CR complete response, *PR* partial response, *SD* stable disease, *PD* progressive disease, *OS* overall survival, *OR* overall response, *MDR* median duration of response, *PFS* progression free survival, *FFS* median failure-free survival, *TTP* median time to progression, *CPT* irinotecan, *Cis* cisplatin, *LV* leucovorin, *FU* 5-fluorouracil, *GEJ* gastroesophageal junction

Table 12.5 Selected studies of irinotecan containing regimens in combination with targeted agents in gastroesophageal malignancies

Authors	*N*	Clinical setting	Combination therapy	Efficacy
Pinto et al. (2007)	38	Chemo naïve patients with advanced adenocarcinoma of the GEJ or stomach	FOLFIRI + Cetuximab	ORR 44% TTP 8 mo. OS 16 mo.
Kanzler et al. (2009)	48	Chemo naïve patients with advanced adenocarcinoma of the GEJ or stomach	CPT + FU + LV + Cetuximab	ORR 42% TTP 8.5 mo. OS 16.6 mo.
Woell et al. (2009)	51	Chemo naïve patients with advanced gastric adenocarcinoma	CPT + Oxaliplatin + Cetuximab	ORR 63% TTP 6.2 mo. OS 9.5 mo.
Shah et al. (2006)	47	Chemo naïve patients with advanced adenocarcinoma of the GEJ or stomach	CPT + Cis + Bevacizumab	ORR 65% TTP 8.3 mo. OS 12.3 mo

CR complete response, *PR* partial response, *SD* stable disease, *PD* progressive disease, *OS* overall survival, *OR* overall response, *MDR* median duration of response, *PFS* progression free survival, *FFS* median failure-free survival, *TTP* median time to progression, *CPT* irinotecan, *Cis* cisplatin, *LV* leucovorin, *FU* 5-fluorouracil, *GEJ* gastroesophageal junction

Bi-weekly irinotecan 180 mg/m^2 IV with leucovorin and 5-FU 1,200 mg/m^2 by continuous infusion over 48 h were studied in 38 patients with 5-FU or platinum resistant disease. Overall response rate was 29% and median OS was 6.4 months (Assersohn et al. 2004). In a phase III trial of 333 chemotherapy naïve patients with adenocarcinoma of the stomach or gastroesophageal junction were randomly assigned to receive either IF (irinotecan 80 mg/m^2, leucovorin 500 mg/m^2, 5-FU 2,000 mg/m^2 over 22 h, for 6 out 7 weeks) or CF (cisplatin 100 mg/m^2, with 5-FU 1,000 mg/m^2 a day, one day 1–5, every 4 weeks): OS was 9.0 versus 8.7 months, respectively – showing non-inferiority for the IF arm. Irinotecan/5-FU is a potential alternative for patients who cannot tolerate cisplatin due to coexisting medical conditions (Dank et al. 2008), poor performance status, or advanced age (Beretta et al. 2006).

Several phase II trial demonstrated feasibility of combining of irinotecan-containing regimens with anti-EGFR, anti-VEGF monocolonal antibodies (Table 12.5). In the FOLCETUX study, the cetuximab/FOLFIRI combination for a maximum of 24 weeks (with an option to continue cetuximab alone) in 38 previously untreated patients with advanced gastroesophageal adenocarcinoma had an overall RR of 44% with a CR in four patients and a PR in 11 patients, and the median OS was 16 months. Bevacizumab added to irinotecan and cisplatin was evaluated in 47 patients with metastatic gastric or GEJ adenocarcinoma. Median TTP was 8.3 months and median OS was 12.3 months (Shah et al. 2006). Molecular markers of irinotecan efficacy may enhance its use in irinotecan-containing regimens as a cytotoxic backbone to improve the treatment of advanced or potentially resectable gastroesophageal cancers (Vallbohmer et al. 2006).

12.6 Gynecologic Malignancies

12.6.1 Ovarian Cancer

Topotecan gained approval by the US FDA in 1999 following completion of two randomized studies in recurrent epithelial ovarian cancer (EOC) that compared topotecan with paclitaxel (ten Bokkel Huinink et al. 1997). The studies showed similar survival, while PFS in one favored topotecan. Subsequently, the drug became widely used for the treatment of EOC utilizing modifications of the FDA approved dose-schedule of 1.5 mg/m^2/day × 5 days every 21 days: (1) most often in this same schedule the doses were reduced to 1.25 and to 1.0 mg/m^2/day; (2) a daily × 3 dose that was studied and deemed more practical; (3) a continuous infusion schedule spanning 10–21 days; and (4) a weekly schedule. Data comparing the various schedules are confined to a handful of studies, but mechanistic considerations favor the more protracted schedules. On the other hand, topotecan on a daily × 5 schedule has been compared to other drugs utilized in recurrent EOC: versus paclitaxel in the initial registration studies, versus pegylated liposomal doxorubicin (PLD) in PLD registration study (Gordon et al. 2001), and versus canfosfamide in the latter's failed registration study. Topotecan's eventual role in EOC has been relegated to the recurrent setting for the treatment of platinum-resistant disease –even if its activity is less in patients relapsing within 6 months of first-line platinum-based therapy, than in patients considered "platinum-sensitive."

Because of its myelosuppression, even if predictable, it has been challenging to integrate topotecan in the first-line treatment of EOC. A pilot study led by New York University for the New York Cancer Consortium used IV by continuous 14-day infusion (and eventually a brief attempt at substituting by oral topotecan stopped because of erratic toxicities) preceded by cisplatin (Hochster et al. 2006). The regimen was very active with RR 80% in patients with postsurgical residual disease, but the extent of myelosuppression far exceeded what is obtained with platinum-taxane-based doublets. The Gynecologic Oncology Group (GOG) and its international collaborators tested four cycles of several doublets in sequence with carboplatin and paclitaxel versus eight cycles of the latter as the reference first-line standard doublet in the largest phase III study conducted in ovarian cancer. The topotecan containing doublet used 3 days of topotecan 0.75 mg/m^2/day combined with carboplatin at an AUC of 5 on day 3 (a less myelosuppressive sequence). No differences in outcome emerged among any of the four arms in comparison to the reference standard doublet (Bookman et al. 2009). Consolidation trials of topotecan following platinum-taxane remissions have also proven negative in phase III trials versus just observation (Pfisterer et al. 2006). The New York Cancer Consortium has explored combinations of topotecan by continuous 14-day infusion preceded and followed by 80 mg/m^2 of oxaliplatin in 28-day cycles, and a phase II study in second- or third-line (LaNatra et al. 2009). Unlike the cisplatin-containing doublet, it is associated with less myelosuppression. The 14-day topotecan schedule by infusion or orally has also been combined with the pegylated liposomal doxorubicin in a phase I study conducted mostly in EOC; activity was seen in patients receiving the infusion topotecan combination (Mirchandani et al. 2005).

Irinotecan has definite activity in EOC, and in particular, against the more platinum-resistant clear cell histology (Adachi et al. 1999; Shimizu et al. 1998; Sugiyama et al. 1996). Both topotecan and irinotecan have been studied for use in intraperitoneal (IP) administration, because of favorable pharmacodynamics of the lactone form in the relatively acidic pH of the peritoneal fluid (Alberts et al. 2006). Preclinical studies suggest that topotecan's activity by the IP route could be enhanced by intravenous bevacizumab (Shah et al. 2009). Reversal of resistance by adding erlotinib has also been tried in refractory EOC (Muggia et al. 2006).

12.6.2 Cancer of the Uterine Cervix

A phase III study by the GOG provided the first evidence of a survival advantage of a chemotherapy combination (topotecan + cisplatin) over cisplatin by itself in patients with metastatic or recurrent cervical cancer (Long et al. 2005). Many of the patients entered in this study had received cisplatin as a radiosensitizer prior to developing metastatic disease and may have accounted for the modest performance of the single agent arm. However, the result stimulated further use of topotecan in this disease. In GOG 204, a study of four platinum-based doublets for the initial therapy of metastatic or residual disease, the topotecan and cisplatin doublet did not fare any better than paclitaxel, vinorelbine, or gemcitabine as part of the doublet (Monk et al. 2009). A cisplatin + paclitaxel regimen is being compared by the GOG against the non-platinum combination of paclitaxel + topotecan. Irinotecan has also demonstrated activity in this setting; in combination with cisplatin, the activity was insufficient to be incorporated into GOG 204 (Muggia et al. 2004). Both topotecan and irinotecan deserve some consideration as radiosensitizers as part of chemoradiation in locally advanced disease, backed by pilot studies exploring such use.

12.7 Primary Brain Neoplasms

Glioblastoma multiforme (GBM) and anaplastic astrocytoma (AA) are the most common histological subtypes of primary brain neoplasms. The median survival of a patient with GBM after a complete resection is 13 month compared with 8.8 months for patients with incomplete resection (Lacroix et al. 2001). Addition of temozolomide (TMZ) to surgery and radiation can improve survival (Stewart 2002), but its benefit maybe confined to the tumors with epigenetic silenced MGMT (O^6-methylguanine–DNA methyltransferase), a DNA-repair gene (Hegi et al. 2005). Irinotecan and its metabolites have limited penetration into cerebrospinal fluid in nonhuman primate model, and there is lack of data on the pharmacokinetics of irinotecan in cerebrospinal fluid (CSF) in humans (Chabner and Longo 2005; Blaney et al. 1998).

However, Friedman et al. demonstrated activity of irinotecan in patients with progressive or recurrent malignant gliomas (Friedman et al. 1999b). Irinotecan was administered at 125 mg/m^2, weekly for 4 weeks, followed by 2-weeks of rest. Nine of sixty (15%) patients enrolled in the trial had PR, defined as ≥50% reduction in tumor size, maintained for 4 weeks, with an additional 36 (55%) stable for at least 12 weeks. Grade 3 toxicities were infrequent and were limited to diarrhea, nausea, and neutropenia – perhaps related to increased clearance of irinotecan and decreased plasma concentrations of its active metabolites, SN-38 and SN-38G relative to pharmacokinetics observed in the patients treated for colorectal carcinomas. The increased clearance of irinotecan as well as low incidence of side effects were attributed to concurrent use of enzyme-inducing antiepileptic drugs (EIAED) (phenytoin, carbamazepine, phenobarbital) and dexamethasone. Several phase II studies, summarized in Table 12.6, demonstrate tolerable toxicity and limited activity of single agent irinotecan in adult patients with malignant gliomas.

Irinotecan 125 mg/m^2 on days 6, 13, and 20 with temozolomide 200 mg/m^2 for 5 days, later changed to temozolomide 200 mg/m^2 daily for 5 days and irinotecan 350 mg/m^2 on day 6, both repeated every 28 days were given to 18 patients with GBM, and 14 patients with WHO grade III anaplastic gliomas. Grade 3 and 4 myelosuppression occurred in seven patients, whereas non-hematological toxicity, mostly gastrointestinal, was not severe. Fifteen patients in GBM group responded to treatment (2CR, 3PR, 10 SD) while all 14 with anaplastic gliomas responded to treatment (CR 3, PR 2, SD 9) and PFS6 was 71% (Gruber and Buster 2004).

Overexpression of vascular endothelial growth factor (VEGF) is hallmark of malignant gliomas (Plate et al. 1992), and it correlates with higher tumor grade and worse outcome (Salmaggi et al. 2003). Several phase II trials, summarized in Table 12.7, combined bevacizumab 10 mg/kg and irinotecan every 2 weeks in the treatment of patients with malignant gliomas. Vredenburgh enrolled 32 patients with recurrent grade 3 and 4 gliomas. Patients with intracranial hemorrhage on initial brain MRI or on anticoagulation were excluded. One patient each died from pulmonary embolism and arterial ischemic stroke, and four others were removed from study due to thromboembolic complications; CNS hemorrhages or grade 3/4 hematological toxicities were not observed and PFS at 6 months was 38%. Friedman evaluated single agent bevacizumab, and combination of irinotecan and bevacizumab, in a phase II, noncomparative, multicenter study enrolling 167 patients with recurrent GBM randomly assigned to bevacizumab 10 mg/kg every 2 weeks with or without irinotecan, dosed with respect to EIAED use. Grade 3 or greater toxicities were reported in 46.4% of patients in bevacizumab, arm and 65.8% in combination arm. The most common serious side effects in bevacizumab-alone arm were hypertension and convulsion, while convulsion, neutropenia, venous thromboembolism, and fatigue were common in the bevacizumab and irinotecan group. This study demonstrated an improvement in response rate and PFS at 6 months relative to results observed in single agent irinotecan studies; therefore, the role of irinotecan given in combination with bevacizumab is unclear.

Topotecan has substantially higher penetration into CSF in nonhuman primate model (Blaney et al. 1998), and significant CSF penetration in humans (Baker et al.

Table 12.6 Selected phase II studies of a single agent irinotecan in malignant glioma patients

Authors	*N*	Clinical setting	Dose and schedule	Efficacy
Friedman et al. (1999b)	60	GBM, AA, AO Prior therapy, N: S-50, RT-53, CT-41, other-8	125 mg/m^2 qwk, 4/6 week	PR 9 (15%) SD 33 (55%) for ≥12 week
Chamberlain et al. (2002)	40	GBM, all patients had prior S, RT, CT	400 mg/m^2 and 500 mg/m^2 in 3 week	Progressive disease Median OS, 4 mo
Raymond et al. (2003)	52	GBM, Group A (*n*=25) inoperable or incomplete resection, no prior CT or RT Group B (*n*=27) relapsed after RT, S-22	Group A: 350 mg/m^2 q3week, ≤3 cycles, then RT Group B: 350 mg/m^2 q3week, ≤6 cycles	Group A: PFS6 26% Group B: PFS6, 43% ORR 2.2%
Prados et al. (2006)	51	GBM, AA, AOA, AOD Prior therapy: CT ≤1 regimen Concurrent EIAED (*n*=29)	Not on EIAED 350 mg/m^2 q3week On EIAED 750 mg/m^2 q3week	PR 3 (5.8%) SD 17 (33.3%) PFS6, 17.6%
Chamberlain and Glantz (2008)	22	TMZ-refractory AO, 1p19q co-deleted Prior S, RT, CT	On non-EIAED 350 mg/m^2 q3week On EIAED 600 mg/m^2 q3week	PR 5 (22%) SD 8 (36%) PFS6 33%
Chamberlain et al. (2008)	40	TMZ-refractory AA Prior S, RT, CT	On non-EIAED 350 mg/m^2 q3week On EIAED 600 mg/m^2 q3week	CR 1 PR 4 (10%) SD 23 (85%) PFS6 40%
Santisteban et al. (2009)	64	Recurrent gliomas (astrocytoma, oligodendroglioma, oligoastrocytoma)	Schedule A: 125 mg/m^2 qwk, 4/6 week Schedule B: 300 mg/m^2 q3week (If prior nitrosourea CT-20% dose reduction)	A: PFS6 6.25% B: PFS6 18.75%

AA anaplastic astrocytoma, *AO* anaplastic oligodendroglioma, *AOA* anaplastic oligoastrocytoma, *CR* complete response, *GBM* glioblastoma multiforme, *PD* progressive disease, *PR* partial response, *SD* stable disease, *OS* overall survival, *PFS6* progression-free survival at 6 months, *TTP* time to progression, *S* surgery, *RT* radiotherapy, *CT* chemotherapy, *TMZ* temozolomide, *CPT* irinotecan, *EIAED* enzyme inducing antiepileptic drugs

Table 12.7 Summary of phase II studies of irinotecan and bevacizumab in malignant glioma patients

Authors	*N*	Clinical setting	Dose and schedule	Efficacy
Vredenburgh et al. (2007a)	32	GBM 23, AA 9 Prior therapy: S, RT, TMZ	CPT and BV 10 mg/kg q2week × 3, q6 week CPT 340 mg/m^2 (EIAID+) CPT 125 mg/m^2 (EIAED-)	CR1 PR 19 SD 11 Median PFS 24 week PFS6, 38%
Vredenburgh et al. (2007b)	35	GBM Prior therapy RT, TMZ (S-not reported)	Cohort 1 ($n=23$) same as above Cohort 2 ($n=12$) CPT on days 1, 8, 22, 29, q6week; BV 15 mg/kg q3week CPT 350 mg/m^2 (EIAID+) CPT 125 mg/m^2 (EIAED-)	CR (by PET CT) 6 PR 20 13 PD mPFS 24 week PFS6, 46%
Desjardins et al. (2008)	33	Recurrent WHO grade III gliomas 25 AA, 8 AO	Cohort 1 BV 10 mg/m^2+ CPT q 2 week; ($n=9$) Cohort 2 CPT on days 1, 8, 22, 29, q6week; BV 15 mg/kg q3week ($n=24$) CPT 350 mg/m^2 (EIAID+) CPT 125 mg/m^2 (EIAED–)	CR3 PR17 SD11 mPFS 30 week PFS6, 55%
Kreisl et al. (2009)	48	Recurrent GBM Heavily pretreated	BV 10 mg/m^2+ CPT q 2 week CPT q2 week added at progression CPT 340 mg/m^2 (EIAID+) CPT 125 mg/m^2 (EIAED–)	CR 1 PR16 PFS6, 29% No OR After addition of CPT
Friedman et al. (2009)	167	Recurrent GBM	BV 10 mg/m^2 q 2 week ($n=85$) BV 10 mg/m^2+ CPT q 2 week ($n=82$) CPT 340 mg/m^2 (EIAID+) CPT 125 mg/m^2 (EIAED–)	BV alone Median OS 8.7 mo PFS6, 42.6% BV + CPT mOS 9.2 mo PFS6, 50.3%

AA anaplastic astrocytoma, *AO* anaplastic oligodendroglioma, *AOA* anaplastic oligoastrocytoma, *CR* complete response, *GBM* glioblastoma multiforme, *PD* progressive disease, *PR* partial response, *SD* stable disease, *OS* overall survival, *PFS6* progression free survival at 6 months, *TTP* time to progression, *BV* bevacizumab, *CPT* irinotecan, *TMZ* temozolomide

1996). Topotecan monotherapy was evaluated in adult and pediatric patients with recurrent primary brain neoplasms in multiple phase II trials, but it did not show significant clinical activity (Blaney et al. 1996; Friedman et al. 1999a; Macdonald et al. 1996). Stewart evaluated pharmacokinetically guided topotecan dosing in children with medulloblastoma and supratentorial primitive neuroectodermal tumors after maximal surgical resection (Stewart et al. 2004). Topotecan dosing was individualized to attain the target plasma concentration AUC of 120–160 ng/mL × h, as described by Santana (Santana et al. 2003). Out of 36 evaluable patients, 4 had complete response, 6 had partial response, and stable disease was observed in 17 patients. Most commonly observed toxicity was hematological, and there were no treatment-related deaths.

Topotecan was shown to have activity as a salvage regimen in primary CNS lymphomas. Fischer reported a study of 27 patients with relapsed or refractory disease after up to four previous chemotherapy regimens (in 26) and whole brain irradiation (in 12). Patients received 5 daily doses of topotecan every 3 weeks and 9 (5 CR and 4 PR) of 27 patients responded to therapy (Fischer et al. 2004). A smaller study of 15 patients demonstrated 3 CR and 3 PR, with acceptable toxicity and no treatment-related deaths (Voloschin et al. 2008).

Grabenbauer et al. reported an exploratory, randomized phase II study in 140 patients with GBM with an experimental arm consisting of topotecan 0.5 mg/m^2 daily CIVI for 21 days during whole brain radiation. This was followed by three 5-day courses of standard intravenous bolus topotecan (1.25 mg/m^2 a day). Progression-free survival at 6 months was 56% for chemoradiation arm and 40% for patients treated with radiation alone; however, this benefit disappeared in the subsequent 2 months of follow-up with median survivals of 14.6 and 15.9 months, respectively (Grabenbauer et al. 2009).

In summary, currently available data demonstrate limited single agent activity of either irinotecan or topotecan in the treatment of primary brain neoplasms. However, the addition of irinotecan to bevacizumab requires further study. Both, topotecan and irinotecan need to be explored in combination with targeted agents, especially, in the setting of intrinsic or acquired chemoresistance to alkylating agents such as BCNU and temozolomide.

12.8 Myelodysplastic Syndromes and Miscellaneous Uses

Topotecan has had some encouraging results in treatment of myelodysplasia and chronic myelomonocytic leukemias (Beran et al. 1996); however, its intrinsic myelosuppression has inhibited further development as other drugs with activity in this challenging area have appeared. In addition, combinations with cytarabine and etoposide have been investigated in various hematologic malignancies (Vey et al. 1999).

12.9 Conclusion

We have provided highlights of nearly two decades of clinical use of the Top1 inhibitors, irinotecan and topotecan. These drugs have broad activity and a predictable toxicity spectrum resulting in an established role for these drugs particularly in pulmonary, gastrointestinal, and gynecologic cancers. Their full potential has not been reached: only rudimentary studies have been done in oral administration (coupled with measures to improve bioavailability), radiosensitization, intraperitoneal delivery, and methods to reverse drug resistance. Perhaps the science in this volume will have an impact in their subsequent development, resulting in further improvement in therapeutic use of these agents. Research with new formulations (providing sustained exposure) and new drug families targeting topoisomerase will hopefully stimulate further study on sensitivity and resistance markers associated with this class of drug.

References

The Camptothecins: Unfolding Their Anticancer Potential. (2000) Proceedings of a conference. March 17–20, 2000, Arlington, Virginia, USA. *Ann N Y Acad Sci* **922:** xi-xii, 1–363

Adachi S, Ogasawara T, Yamasaki N, Shibahara H, Kanazawa R, Tsuji Y, Takemura T, Koyama K (1999) A pilot study of CPT-11 and cisplatin for ovarian clear cell adenocarcinoma. *Jpn J Clin Oncol* **29**(9)**:** 434–437

Ajani JA, Baker J, Pisters PWT, Ho L, Mansfield PF, Feig BW, Charnsangavej C (2002) CPT-11 plus cisplatin in patients with advanced, untreated gastric or gastroesophageal junction carcinoma: results of a phase II study. *Cancer* **94**(3)**:** 641–646

Alberts DS, Markman M, Muggia F, Ozols RF, Eldermire E, Bookman MA, Chen T, Curtin J, Hess LM, Liebes L, Young RC, Trimble E (2006) Proceedings of a GOG workshop on intraperitoneal therapy for ovarian cancer. *Gynecologic Oncology* **103**(3)**:** 783–792

Ando Y, Saka H, Ando M, Sawa T, Muro K, Ueoka H, Yokoyama A, Saitoh S, Shimokata K, Hasegawa Y (2000) Polymorphisms of UDP-glucuronosyltransferase gene and irinotecan toxicity: a pharmacogenetic analysis. *Cancer Res* **60**(24)**:** 6921–6926

Ando Y, Saka H, Asai G, Sugiura S, Shimokata K, Kamataki T (1998) UGT1A1 genotypes and glucuronidation of SN-38, the active metabolite of irinotecan. *Ann Oncol* **9**(8)**:** 845–847

Asbury RF, Lipsitz S, Graham D, Falkson CI, Baez L, Benson AB, 3 rd (2000) Treatment of squamous cell esophageal cancer with topotecan: an Eastern Cooperative Oncology Group Study (E2293). *Am J Clin Oncol* **23**(1)**:** 45–46

Assersohn L, Brown G, Cunningham D, Ward C, Oates J, Waters JS, Hill ME, Norman AR (2004) Phase II study of irinotecan and 5-fluorouracil/leucovorin in patients with primary refractory or relapsed advanced oesophageal and gastric carcinoma. *Ann Oncol* **15**(1)**:** 64–69

Baker SD, Heideman RL, Crom WR, Kuttesch JF, Gajjar A, Stewart CF (1996) Cerebrospinal fluid pharmacokinetics and penetration of continuous infusion topotecan in children with central nervous system tumors. *Cancer Chemotherapy and Pharmacology* **37**(3)**:** 195–202

Barone C, Nuzzo G, Cassano A, Basso M, Schinzari G, Giuliante F, D'Argento E, Trigila N, Astone A, Pozzo C (2007) Final analysis of colorectal cancer patients treated with irinotecan and 5-fluorouracil plus folinic acid neoadjuvant chemotherapy for unresectable liver metastases. *Br J Cancer* **97**(8)**:** 1035–1039

Benedetti JK, Burris HA, 3 rd, Balcerzak SP, Macdonald JS (1997) Phase II trial of topotecan in advanced gastric cancer: a Southwest Oncology Group study. *Invest New Drugs* **15**(3)**:** 261–264

Beran M, Kantarjian H, O'Brien S, Koller C, al-Bitar M, Arbuck S, Pierce S, Moore M, Abbruzzese J, Andreeff M, Keating M, Estey E (1996) Topotecan, a topoisomerase I inhibitor, is active in the treatment of myelodysplastic syndrome and chronic myelomonocytic leukemia. *Blood* **88**(7): 2473–2479

Beretta E, Di Bartolomeo M, Buzzoni R, Ferrario E, Mariani L, Gevorgyan A, Bajetta E (2006) Irinotecan, fluorouracil and folinic acid (FOLFIRI) as effective treatment combination for patients with advanced gastric cancer in poor clinical condition. *Tumori* **92**(5): 379–383

Blaney SM, Phillips PC, Packer RJ, Heideman RL, Berg SL, Adamson PC, Allen JC, Sallan SE, Jakacki RI, Lange BJ, Reaman GH, Horowitz ME, Poplack DG, Balis FM (1996) Phase II evaluation of topotecan for pediatric central nervous system tumors. *Cancer* **78**(3): 527–531

Blaney SM, Takimoto C, Murry DJ, Kuttesch N, McCully C, Cole DE, Godwin K, Balis FM (1998) Plasma and cerebrospinal fluid pharmacokinetics of 9-aminocamptothecin (9-AC), irinotecan (CPT-11), and SN-38 in nonhuman primates. *Cancer Chemother Pharmacol* **41**(6): 464–468

Blanke CD, Haller DG, Benson AB, Rothenberg ML, Berlin J, Mori M, Hsieh YC, Miller LL (2001) A phase II study of irinotecan with 5-fluorouracil and leucovorin in patients with previously untreated gastric adenocarcinoma. *Ann Oncol* **12**(11): 1575–1580

Bookman MA, Brady MF, McGuire WP, Harper PG, Alberts DS, Friedlander M, Colombo N, Fowler JM, Argenta PA, De Geest K, Mutch DG, Burger RA, Swart AM, Trimble EL, Accario-Winslow C, Roth LM (2009) Evaluation of New Platinum-Based Treatment Regimens in Advanced-Stage Ovarian Cancer: A Phase III Trial of the Gynecologic Cancer InterGroup. *J Clin Oncol* **27**(9): 1419–1425

Bouche O, Raoul JL, Bonnetain F, Giovannini M, Etienne PL, Lledo G, Arsene D, Paitel JF, Guerin-Meyer V, Mitry E, Buecher B, Kaminsky MC, Seitz JF, Rougier P, Bedenne L, Milan C, Federation Francophone de Cancerologie Digestive G (2004) Randomized multicenter phase II trial of a biweekly regimen of fluorouracil and leucovorin (LV5FU2), LV5FU2 plus cisplatin, or LV5FU2 plus irinotecan in patients with previously untreated metastatic gastric cancer: a Federation Francophone de Cancerologie Digestive Group Study-FFCD 9803. *J Clin Oncol* **22**(21): 4319–4328

Chabner BA, Longo DL (2005) Cancer chemotherapy and biotherapy. 17, p 387

Chamberlain MC (2002) Salvage chemotherapy with CPT-11 for recurrent glioblastoma multiforme. *Journal of Neuro-Oncology* **56**(2): 183–188

Chamberlain MC, Glantz MJ (2008) CPT-11 for recurrent temozolomide-refractory 1p19q co-deleted anaplastic oligodendroglioma. *Journal of Neuro-Oncology* **89**(2): 231–238

Chamberlain MC, Wei-Tsao DD, Blumenthal DT, Glantz MJ (2008) Salvage chemotherapy with CPT-11 for recurrent temozolomide-refractory anaplastic astrocytoma. *Cancer* **112**(9): 2038–2045

Creemers GJ, Wanders J, Gamucci T, Vallentin S, Dirix LY, Schoffski P, Hudson I, Verweij J (1995) Topotecan in colorectal cancer: a phase II study of the EORTC early clinical trials group. *Ann Oncol* **6**(8): 844–846

Crouthamel MH, Wu D, Yang Z, Ho RJ (2006) A novel MDR1 G1199T variant alters drug resistance and efflux transport activity of P-glycoprotein in recombinant Hek cells. *J Pharm Sci* **95**(12): 2767–2777

Dank M, Zaluski J, Barone C, Valvere V, Yalcin S, Peschel C, Wenczl M, Goker E, Cisar L, Wang K, Bugat R (2008) Randomized phase III study comparing irinotecan combined with 5-fluorouracil and folinic acid to cisplatin combined with 5-fluorouracil in chemotherapy naive patients with advanced adenocarcinoma of the stomach or esophagogastric junction. *Ann Oncol* **19**(8): 1450–1457

De Cesare M, Pratesi G, Veneroni S, Bergottini R, Zunino F (2004) Efficacy of the novel camptothecin gimatecan against orthotopic and metastatic human tumor xenograft models. *Clin Cancer Res* **10**(21): 7357–7364

Delaunoit T, Goldberg RM, Sargent DJ, Morton RF, Fuchs CS, Findlay BP, Thomas SP, Salim M, Schaefer PL, Stella PJ, Green E, Mailliard JA (2004) Mortality associated with daily bolus

5-fluorouracil/leucovorin administered in combination with either irinotecan or oxaliplatin. *Cancer* **101**(10): 2170–2176

Delord JP, Bennouna J, Artru P, Perrier H, Husseini F, Desseigne F, Francois E, Faroux R, Smith D, Piedbois P, Naman H, Douillard JY, Bugat R (2007) Phase II study of UFT with leucovorin and irinotecan (TEGAFIRI): first-line therapy for metastatic colorectal cancer. *Br J Cancer* **97**(3): 297–301

Desjardins A, Reardon DA, Herndon JE, 2nd, Marcello J, Quinn JA, Rich JN, Sathornsumetee S, Gururangan S, Sampson J, Bailey L, Bigner DD, Friedman AH, Friedman HS, Vredenburgh JJ (2008) Bevacizumab plus irinotecan in recurrent WHO grade 3 malignant gliomas. *Clin Cancer Res* **14**(21): 7068–7073

Di Lauro L, Nunziata C, Arena MG, Foggi P, Sperduti I, Lopez M (2007) Irinotecan, docetaxel and oxaliplatin combination in metastatic gastric or gastroesophageal junction adenocarcinoma. *British Journal of Cancer* **97**(5): 593–597

Douillard JY, Cunningham D, Roth AD, Navarro M, James RD, Karasek P, Jandik P, Iveson T, Carmichael J, Alakl M, Gruia G, Awad L, Rougier P (2000) Irinotecan combined with fluorouracil compared with fluorouracil alone as first-line treatment for metastatic colorectal cancer: a multicentre randomised trial. *Lancet* **355**(9209): 1041–1047

Eckardt JR, von Pawel J, Pujol JL, Papai Z, Quoix E, Ardizzoni A, Poulin R, Preston AJ, Dane G, Ross G (2007) Phase III study of oral compared with intravenous topotecan as second line therapy in small-cell lung cancer. *J Clin Oncol* **25**(15): 2086–2092

Enzinger PC, Kulke MH, Clark JW, Ryan DP, Kim H, Earle CC, Vincitore MM, Michelini AL, Mayer RJ, Fuchs CS (2005) A phase II trial of irinotecan in patients with previously untreated advanced esophageal and gastric adenocarcinoma. *Dig Dis Sci* **50**(12): 2218–2223

Falcone A, Ricci S, Brunetti I, Pfanner E, Allegrini G, Barbara C, Crino L, Benedetti G, Evangelista W, Fanchini L, Cortesi E, Picone V, Vitello S, Chiara S, Granetto C, Porcile G, Fioretto L, Orlandini C, Andreuccetti M, Masi G (2007) Phase III trial of infusional fluorouracil, leucovorin, oxaliplatin, and irinotecan (FOLFOXIRI) compared with infusional fluorouracil, leucovorin, and irinotecan (FOLFIRI) as first-line treatment for metastatic colorectal cancer: the Gruppo Oncologico Nord Ovest. *J Clin Oncol* **25**(13): 1670–1676

Fischer L, Thiel E, Klasen HA, Kirchen H, Jahnke K, Korfel A (2004) Response of relapsed or refractory primary central nervous system lymphoma (PCNSL) to topotecan. *Neurology* **62**(10): 1885–1887

Folprecht G, Seymour MT, Saltz L, Douillard JY, Hecker H, Stephens RJ, Maughan TS, Van Cutsem E, Rougier P, Mitry E, Schubert U, Kohne CH (2008) Irinotecan/fluorouracil combination in first-line therapy of older and younger patients with metastatic colorectal cancer: combined analysis of 2,691 patients in randomized controlled trials. *J Clin Oncol* **26**(9): 1443–1451

Friedman HS, Kerby T, Fields S, Zilisch JE, Graden D, McLendon RE, Houghton PJ, Arbuck S, Cokgor I, Friedman AH (1999a) Topotecan treatment of adults with primary malignant glioma. The Brain Tumor Center at Duke. *Cancer* **85**(5): 1160–1165

Friedman HS, Petros WP, Friedman AH, Schaaf LJ, Kerby T, Lawyer J, Parry M, Houghton PJ, Lovell S, Rasheed K, Cloughsey T, Stewart ES, Colvin OM, Provenzale JM, McLendon RE, Bigner DD, Cokgor I, Haglund M, Rich J, Ashley D, Malczyn J, Elfring GL, Miller LL (1999b) Irinotecan therapy in adults with recurrent or progressive malignant glioma. *Journal of Clinical Oncology* **17**(5): 1516–1525

Friedman HS, Prados MD, Wen PY, Mikkelsen T, Schiff D, Abrey LE, Yung WKA, Paleologos N, Nicholas MK, Jensen R, Vredenburgh J, Huang J, Zheng M, Cloughesy T (2009) Bevacizumab alone and in combination with irinotecan in recurrent glioblastoma. *J Clin Oncol* **27**(28): 4733–4740

Fuchs CS, Marshall J, Mitchell E, Wierzbicki R, Ganju V, Jeffery M, Schulz J, Richards D, Soufi-Mahjoubi R, Wang B, Barrueco J (2007) Randomized, controlled trial of irinotecan plus infusional, bolus, or oral fluoropyrimidines in first-line treatment of metastatic colorectal cancer: results from the BICC-C Study. *J Clin Oncol* **25**(30): 4779–4786

Furuta T (2009) Pharmacogenomics in chemotherapy for GI tract cancer. *J Gastroenterol* **44**(10): 1016–1025

Futatsuki K, Wakui A, Nakao I, Sakata Y, Kambe M, Shimada Y, Yoshino M, Taguchi T, Ogawa N (1994) Late phase II study of irinotecan hydrochloride (CPT-11) in advanced gastric cancer. CPT-11 Gastrointestinal Cancer Study Group. *Gan To Kagaku Ryoho* **21**(7): 1033–1038

Goldberg RM, Sargent DJ, Morton RF, Fuchs CS, Ramanathan RK, Williamson SK, Findlay BP, Pitot HC, Alberts SR (2004) A randomized controlled trial of fluorouracil plus leucovorin, irinotecan, and oxaliplatin combinations in patients with previously untreated metastatic colorectal cancer. *J Clin Oncol* **22**(1): 23–30

Gordon AN, Fleagle JT, Guthrie D, Parkin DE, Gore ME, Lacave AJ (2001) Recurrent epithelial ovarian carcinoma: a randomized phase III study of pegylated liposomal doxorubicin versus topotecan. *J Clin Oncol* **19**(14): 3312–3322

Grabenbauer GG, Gerber K-D, Ganslandt O, Richter A, Klautke G, Birkmann J, Meyer M (2009) Effects of concurrent topotecan and radiation on 6-month progression-free survival in the primary treatment of glioblastoma multiforme. *Int J Radiat Oncol Biol Phys* **75**(1): 164–169

Grothey A, Jordan K, O K (2003) Randomized Phase II trial of capecitabine plus irinotecan (CapIri) vs capecitabine plus oxaliplatin (CapOx) as first-line therapy of advanced colorectal cancer (ACRC). *Proc Am Soc Clin Oncol* **1022**(Abstract 1022)

Grothey A, Jordan K, Kellner O, Constantin C, Dietrich G, Kroening H, Mantovani L, Schlichting C, Forstbauer H, Schmoll H-J (2004) Capecitabine/ irinotecan (CapIri) and capecitabine/oxaliplatin (CapOx) are active second-line protocols in patients with advanced colorectal cancer (ACRC) after failure of first-line combination therapy: Results of a randomized phase II study. *J Clin Oncol (Meeting Abstracts)* **22**

Gruber ML, Buster WP (2004) Temozolomide in combination with irinotecan for treatment of recurrent malignant glioma. *American Journal of Clinical Oncology* **27**(1): 33–38

Hanna N, Bunn PA, Jr., Langer C, Einhorn L, Guthrie T, Jr., Beck T, Ansari R, Ellis P, Byrne M, Morrison M, Hariharan S, Wang B, Sandler A (2006) Randomized phase III trial comparing irinotecan/cisplatin with etoposide/cisplatin in patients with previously untreated extensive-stage disease small-cell lung cancer. *J Clin Oncol* **24**(13): 2038–2043

Hegi ME, Diserens A-C, Gorlia T, Hamou M-F, de Tribolet N, Weller M, Kros JM, Hainfellner JA, Mason W, Mariani L, Bromberg JEC, Hau P, Mirimanoff RO, Cairncross JG, Janzer RC, Stupp R (2005) MGMT Gene Silencing and Benefit from Temozolomide in Glioblastoma. *N Engl J Med* **352**(10): 997–1003

Hochster H, Liebes L, Speyer J, Sorich J, Taubes B, Oratz R, Wernz J, Chachoua A, Raphael B, Vinci R (1994) Phase I trial of low-dose continuous topotecan infusion in patients with cancer: an active and well-tolerated regimen. *J Clin Oncol* **12**(3): 553–559

Hochster H, Wadler S, Runowicz C, Liebes L, Cohen H, Wallach R, Sorich J, Taubes B, Speyer J (1999) Activity and Pharmacodynamics of 21-Day Topotecan Infusion in Patients With Ovarian Cancer Previously Treated With Platinum-Based Chemotherapy. *J Clin Oncol* **17**(8): 2553-

Hochster HS, Plimack ER, Mandeli J, Wadler S, Runowicz C, Goldberg G, Speyer J, Wallach R, Muggia F (2006) Prolonged topotecan infusion with cisplatin in the first-line treatment of ovarian cancer: An NYGOG and ECOG study. *Gynecologic Oncology* **100**(2): 324–329

Hoeijmakers JH (2001) Genome maintenance mechanisms for preventing cancer. *Nature* **411**(6835): 366–374

Hoffmeyer S, Burk O, von Richter O, Arnold HP, Brockmoller J, Johne A, Cascorbi I, Gerloff T, Roots I, Eichelbaum M, Brinkmann U (2000) Functional polymorphisms of the human multidrug-resistance gene: multiple sequence variations and correlation of one allele with P-glycoprotein expression and activity in vivo. *Proc Natl Acad Sci USA* **97**(7): 3473–3478

Horikawa M, Kato Y, Tyson CA, Sugiyama Y (2002) The potential for an interaction between MRP2 (ABCC2) and various therapeutic agents: probenecid as a candidate inhibitor of the biliary excretion of irinotecan metabolites. *Drug Metab Pharmacokinet* **17**(1): 23–33

Hurwitz H, Fehrenbacher L, Novotny W, Cartwright T, Hainsworth J, Heim W, Berlin J, Baron A, Griffing S, Holmgren E, Ferrara N, Fyfe G, Rogers B, Ross R, Kabbinavar F (2004) Bevacizumab plus irinotecan, fluorouracil, and leucovorin for metastatic colorectal cancer. *N Engl J Med* **350**(23): 2335–2342

Hurwitz HI, Cohen RB, McGovren JP, Hirawat S, Petros WP, Natsumeda Y, Yoshinari T (2007) A phase I study of the safety and pharmacokinetics of edotecarin (J-107088), a novel topoisomerase I inhibitor, in patients with advanced solid tumors. *Cancer Chemother Pharmacol* **59**(1): 139–147

Hutter G, Szelenyi H, Deckert PM, Keilholz U, Thiel E (2004) Phase I/II trial of topotecan given as continuous infusion in combination with oxaliplatin in 5-FU-pretreated patients with colorectal cancer. *Cancer Chemotherapy & Pharmacology* **54**(2): 178–184

Ilson DH, Saltz L, Enzinger P, Huang Y, Kornblith A, Gollub M, O'Reilly E, Schwartz G, DeGroff J, Gonzalez G, Kelsen DP (1999) Phase II trial of weekly irinotecan plus cisplatin in advanced esophageal cancer. *Journal of Clinical Oncology* **17**(10): 3270–3275

Jeong J, Cho BC, Sohn JH, Choi HJ, Kim SH, Lee YJ, Jung MK, Shin SJ, Park MS, Kim SK, Chang J, Kim JH (2010) Belotecan for relapsing small-cell lung cancer patients initially treated with an irinotecan-containing chemotherapy: A phase II trial. *Lung Cancer* **70**(1): 77–81

Kanzler S, Trarbach T, Seufferlein T, Kubicka S, Lordick F, Geissler M, Daum S, Galle PR, Moehler M, German Arbeitsgemeinschaft Internistische Onkologie (2009) Cetuximab with irinotecan/folinic acid/5-FU as first-line treatment in advanced gastric cancer: A nonrandomized multicenter AIO phase II study. *J Clin Oncol (Meeting Abstracts)* **27**(15 S): 4534-

Kim SJ, Kim JS, Kim SC, Kim YK, Kang JY, Yoon HK, Song JS, Lee SH, Moon HS, Kim JW, Kim KH, Kim CH, Shim BY, Kim HK (2010) A multicenter phase II study of belotecan, new camptothecin analogue, in patients with previously untreated extensive stage disease small cell lung cancer. *Lung Cancer* **68**(3): 446–449

Kohne CH, Catane R, Klein B, Ducreux M, Thuss-Patience P, Niederle N, Gips M, Preusser P, Knuth A, Clemens M, Bugat R, Figer I, Shani A, Fages B, Di Betta D, Jacques C, Wilke HJ (2003) Irinotecan is active in chemonaive patients with metastatic gastric cancer: a phase II multicentric trial. *British Journal of Cancer* **89**(6): 997–1001

Kohne CH, van Cutsem E, Wils J, Bokemeyer C, El-Serafi M, Lutz MP, Lorenz M, Reichardt P, Ruckle-Lanz H, Frickhofen N, Fuchs R, Mergenthaler HG, Langenbuch T, Vanhoefer U, Rougier P, Voigtmann R, Muller L, Genicot B, Anak O, Nordlinger B (2005) Phase III study of weekly high-dose infusional fluorouracil plus folinic acid with or without irinotecan in patients with metastatic colorectal cancer: European Organisation for Research and Treatment of Cancer Gastrointestinal Group Study 40986. *J Clin Oncol* **23**(22): 4856–4865

Kreisl TN, Kim L, Moore K, Duic P, Royce C, Stroud I, Garren N, Mackey M, Butman JA, Camphausen K, Park J, Albert PS, Fine HA (2009) Phase II trial of single-agent bevacizumab followed by bevacizumab plus irinotecan at tumor progression in recurrent glioblastoma. *J Clin Oncol* **27**(5): 740–745

Kuhn JG (1998) Pharmacology of irinotecan. *Oncology (Williston Park)* **12**(8 Suppl 6): 39–42

Kuhn JG (2002) Influence of anticonvulsants on the metabolism and elimination of irinotecan. A North American Brain Tumor Consortium preliminary report. *Oncology (Williston Park)* **16**(8 Suppl 7): 33–40

Lacroix M, Abi-Said D, Fourney DR, Gokaslan ZL, Shi W, DeMonte F, Lang FF, McCutcheon IE, Hassenbusch SJ, Holland E, Hess K, Michael C, Miller D, Sawaya R (2001) A multivariate analysis of 416 patients with glioblastoma multiforme: prognosis, extent of resection, and survival. *Journal of Neurosurgery* **95**(2): 190–198

LaNatra N, Hochster H, Muggia F, Blank SV, Curtin J, Fishman D, Shapira IE, Goldberg GL, Parise S, Tiersten A (2009) Oxaliplatin plus continuous infusion topotecan: First stage of an ongoing phase II study for recurrent ovarian cancer: A New York Cancer Consortium study (#N01-CM62204). *J Clin Oncol (Meeting Abstracts)* **27**(15 S): 5556-

Lara PN, Jr., Natale R, Crowley J, Lenz HJ, Redman MW, Carleton JE, Jett J, Langer CJ, Kuebler JP, Dakhil SR, Chansky K, Gandara DR (2009) Phase III trial of irinotecan/cisplatin compared with etoposide/cisplatin in extensive-stage small-cell lung cancer: clinical and pharmacogenomic results from SWOG S0124. *J Clin Oncol* **27**(15): 2530–2535

Lee DH, Kim SW, Bae KS, Hong JS, Suh C, Kang YK, Lee JS (2007) A phase I and pharmacologic study of belotecan in combination with cisplatin in patients with previously untreated extensive-stage disease small cell lung cancer. *Clin Cancer Res* **13**(20): 6182–6186

Lenz HJ (2006) Pharmacogenomics and colorectal cancer. *Adv Exp Med Biol* **587**: 211–231

Liehr JG and Giovanella B (2000) Introduction Annals of the New York Academy of Sciences, 922

Lievre A, Bachet JB, Boige V, Cayre A, Le Corre D, Buc E, Ychou M, Bouche O, Landi B, Louvet C, Andre T, Bibeau F, Diebold MD, Rougier P, Ducreux M, Tomasic G, Emile JF, Penault-Llorca F, Laurent-Puig P (2008) KRAS mutations as an independent prognostic factor in patients with advanced colorectal cancer treated with cetuximab. *J Clin Oncol* **26**(3): 374–379

Long HJ, 3 rd, Bundy BN, Grendys EC, Jr., Benda JA, McMeekin DS, Sorosky J, Miller DS, Eaton LA, Fiorica JV (2005) Randomized phase III trial of cisplatin with or without topotecan in carcinoma of the uterine cervix: a Gynecologic Oncology Group Study. *J Clin Oncol* **23**(21): 4626–4633

Macdonald D, Cairncross G, Stewart D, Forsyth P, Sawka C, Wainman N, Eisenhauer E (1996) Phase II study of topotecan in patients with recurrent malignant glioma. National Clinical Institute of Canada Clinical Trials Group. *Ann Oncol* **7**(2): 205–207

Macdonald JS, Jacobson JL, Ketchel SJ, Weiss G, Taylor S, Mills G, Kuebler JP, Rivkin S, Conrad M (2000) A phase II trial of topotecan in esophageal carcinoma: a Southwest Oncology Group study (SWOG 9339). *Invest New Drugs* **18**(2): 199–202

Mackenzie PI, Owens IS, Burchell B, Bock KW, Bairoch A, Belanger A, Fournel-Gigleux S, Green M, Hum DW, Iyanagi T, Lancet D, Louisot P, Magdalou J, Chowdhury JR, Ritter JK, Schachter H, Tephly TR, Tipton KF, Nebert DW (1997) The UDP glycosyltransferase gene superfamily: recommended nomenclature update based on evolutionary divergence. *Pharmacogenetics* **7**(4): 255–269

Maroun JA, Jonker D, Seymour L, Goel R, Vincent M, Kocha W, Cripps C, Fisher B, Lister D, Malpage A, Chiritescu G (2006) A National Cancer Institute of Canada Clinical Trials Group Study-IND.135: Phase I/II study of irinotecan (camptosar), oxaliplatin and raltitrexed (tomudex) (COT) in patients with advanced colorectal cancer. *Eur J Cancer* **42**(2): 193–199

Mathijssen RH, Marsh S, Karlsson MO, Xie R, Baker SD, Verweij J, Sparreboom A, McLeod HL (2003) Irinotecan pathway genotype analysis to predict pharmacokinetics. *Clin Cancer Res* **9**(9): 3246–3253

Miller AA, Herndon JE, 2nd, Gu L, Green MR (2005) Phase II trial of karenitecin in patients with relapsed or refractory non-small cell lung cancer (CALGB 30004). *Lung Cancer* **48**(3): 399–407

Mirchandani D, Hochster H, Hamilton A, Liebes L, Yee H, Curtin JP, Lee S, Sorich J, Dellenbaugh C, Muggia FM (2005) Phase I study of combined pegylated liposomal doxorubicin with protracted daily topotecan for ovarian cancer. *Clin Cancer Res* **11**(16): 5912–5919

Mitry E, Phelip JM, Bonnetain F, Lavau Denes S, Adhoute X (2008) Phase III trial of chemotherapy with or without irinotecan in the front-line treatment of metastatic colorectal cancer in elderly patients (FFCD 2001–02 trial): Results of a planned interim analysis. Gastrointestinal Cancers Symposium Orlando, FL

Monk BJ, Sill MW, McMeekin DS, Cohn DE, Ramondetta LM, Boardman CH, Benda J, Cella D (2009) Phase III Trial of Four Cisplatin-Containing Doublet Combinations in Stage IVB, Recurrent, or Persistent Cervical Carcinoma: A Gynecologic Oncology Group Study. *J Clin Oncol* **27**(28): 4649–4655

Muggia F, Kosloff R, Liebes L, Hochster H (2006) Topotecan Continuous Infusion: CA-125 Responses Including Patients Pretreated with Other Schedules of Topotecan. *Oncologist* **11**(5): 529–531

Muggia FM, Blessing JA, McGehee R, Monk BJ (2004) Cisplatin and irinotecan in squamous cell carcinoma of the cervix: a phase II study of the Gynecologic Oncology Group. *Gynecologic Oncology* **94**(2): 483–487

Muggia FM, Hudes GR (2003) Boosting Bioavailability to Topotecan: What Do We Gain? *J Clin Oncol* **21**(1): 177-

Muhr-Wilkenshoff F, Hinkelbein W, Ohnesorge I, Wolf KJ, Riecken EO, Zeitz M, Scherubl H (2003) A pilot study of irinotecan (CPT-11) as single-agent therapy in patients with locally advanced or metastatic esophageal carcinoma. *Int J Colorectal Dis* **18**(4): 330–334

Murry DJ, Cherrick I, Salama V, Berg S, Bernstein M, Kuttesch N, Blaney SM (2002) Influence of phenytoin on the disposition of irinotecan: a case report. *J Pediatr Hematol Oncol* **24**(2): 130–133

Noda K, Nishiwaki Y, Kawahara M, Negoro S, Sugiura T, Yokoyama A, Fukuoka M, Mori K, Watanabe K, Tamura T, Yamamoto S, Saijo N (2002) Irinotecan plus cisplatin compared with etoposide plus cisplatin for extensive small-cell lung cancer. *N Engl J Med* **346**(2): 85–91

Nozawa T, Minami H, Sugiura S, Tsuji A, Tamai I (2005) Role of organic anion transporter OATP1B1 (OATP-C) in hepatic uptake of irinotecan and its active metabolite, 7-ethyl-10-hydroxycamptothecin: in vitro evidence and effect of single nucleotide polymorphisms. *Drug Metab Dispos* **33**(3): 434–439

O'Brien ME, Ciuleanu TE, Tsekov H, Shparyk Y, Cucevia B, Juhasz G, Thatcher N, Ross GA, Dane GC, Crofts T (2006) Phase III trial comparing supportive care alone with supportive care with oral topotecan in patients with relapsed small-cell lung cancer. *J Clin Oncol* **24**(34): 5441–5447

O'Leary J, Muggia FM (1998) Camptothecins: a review of their development and schedules of administration. *Eur J Cancer* **34**(10): 1500–1508

Onoue M, Inui K (2008) [Role of UGT1A1*28 and UGT1A1*6 for irinotecan-induced adverse drug reaction]. *Gan To Kagaku Ryoho* **35**(7): 1080–1085

Pantazis P, Giovanella BC, Rothenberg ML (eds) (1996) The camptothecins: from discovery to the patient. New York, N.Y. :: New York Academy of Sciences

Park SR, Chun JH, Yu MS, Lee JH, Ryu KW, Choi IJ, Kim CG, Lee JS, Kim YW, Bae JM, Kim HK (2006) Phase II study of docetaxel and irinotecan combination chemotherapy in metastatic gastric carcinoma. *British Journal of Cancer* **94**(10): 1402–1406

Pfisterer J, Weber B, Reuss A, Kimmig R, du Bois A, Wagner U, Bourgeois H, Meier W, Costa S, Blohmer J-U, Lortholary A, Olbricht S, Stahle A, Jackisch C, Hardy-Bessard A-C, Mobus V, Quaas J, Richter B, Schroder W, Geay J-F, Luck H-J, Kuhn W, Meden H, Nitz U, Pujade-Lauraine E (2006) Randomized Phase III Trial of Topotecan Following Carboplatin and Paclitaxel in First-line Treatment of Advanced Ovarian Cancer: A Gynecologic Cancer Intergroup Trial of the AGO-OVAR and GINECO. *J Natl Cancer Inst* **98**(15): 1036–1045

Pinto C, Di Fabio F, Siena S, Cascinu S, Rojas Llimpe FL, Ceccarelli C, Mutri V, Giannetta L, Giaquinta S, Funaioli C, Berardi R, Longobardi C, Piana E, Martoni AA (2007) Phase II study of cetuximab in combination with FOLFIRI in patients with untreated advanced gastric or gastroesophageal junction adenocarcinoma (FOLCETUX study). *Annals of Oncology* **18**(3): 510–517

Plate KH, Breier G, Weich HA, Risau W (1992) Vascular endothelial growth factor is a potential tumour angiogenesis factor in human gliomas in vivo. *Nature* **359**(6398): 845–848

Pommier Y, Cushman M (2009) The indenoisoquinoline noncamptothecin topoisomerase I inhibitors: update and perspectives. *Mol Cancer Ther*

Potmesil M, W.Kohn K (eds) (1991) *DNA Topoisomerases in Cancer*: Oxford University Press, New York, 331 pp

Pozzo C, Barone C, Szanto J, Padi E, Peschel C, Bukki J, Gorbunova V, Valvere V, Zaluski J, Biakhov M, Zuber E, Jacques C, Bugat R (2004) Irinotecan in combination with 5-fluorouracil and folinic acid or with cisplatin in patients with advanced gastric or esophageal-gastric junction adenocarcinoma: results of a randomized phase II study. *Annals of Oncology* **15**(12): 1773–1781

Prados MD, Lamborn K, Yung WKA, Jaeckle K, Robins HI, Mehta M, Fine HA, Wen PY, Cloughesy T, Chang S, Nicholas MK, Schiff D, Greenberg H, Junck L, Fink K, Hess K, Kuhn J, North American Brain Tumor C (2006) A phase 2 trial of irinotecan (CPT-11) in patients with recurrent malignant glioma: a North American Brain Tumor Consortium study. *Neuro-Oncology* **8**(2): 189–193

Pratt CB, Stewart C, Santana VM, Bowman L, Furman W, Ochs J, Marina N, Kuttesch JF, Heideman R, Sandlund JT, et al. (1994) Phase I study of topotecan for pediatric patients with malignant solid tumors. *J Clin Oncol* **12**(3): 539–543

Ramlau R, Gervais R, Krzakowski M, von Pawel J, Kaukel E, Abratt RP, Dharan B, Grotzinger KM, Ross G, Dane G, Shepherd FA (2006) Phase III study comparing oral topotecan to intravenous docetaxel in patients with pretreated advanced non-small-cell lung cancer. *J Clin Oncol* **24**(18): 2800–2807

Raymond E, Fabbro M, Boige V, Rixe O, Frenay M, Vassal G, Faivre S, Sicard E, Germa C, Rodier JM, Vernillet L, Armand JP (2003) Multicentre phase II study and pharmacokinetic analysis of irinotecan in chemotherapy-naive patients with glioblastoma. *Annals of Oncology* **14**(4): 603–614

Rougier P, Bugat R, Douillard JY, Culine S, Suc E, Brunet P, Becouarn Y, Ychou M, Marty M, Extra JM, Bonneterre J, Adenis A, Seitz JF, Ganem G, Namer M, Conroy T, Negrier S, Merrouche Y, Burki F, Mousseau M, Herait P, Mahjoubi M (1997) Phase II study of irinotecan in the treatment of advanced colorectal cancer in chemotherapy-naive patients and patients pretreated with fluorouracil-based chemotherapy. *J Clin Oncol* **15**(1): 251–260

Rougier P, Lepille D, Bennouna J, Marre A, Ducreux M, Mignot L, Hua A, Mery-Mignard D (2002) Antitumour activity of three second-line treatment combinations in patients with metastatic colorectal cancer after optimal 5-FU regimen failure: a randomised, multicentre phase II study. *Ann Oncol* **13**(10): 1558–1567

Rougier P, Van Cutsem E, Bajetta E, Niederle N, Possinger K, Labianca R, Navarro M, Morant R, Bleiberg H, Wils J, Awad L, Herait P, Jacques C (1998) Randomised trial of irinotecan versus fluorouracil by continuous infusion after fluorouracil failure in patients with metastatic colorectal cancer. *Lancet* **352**(9138): 1407–1412

Sai K, Saito Y, Maekawa K, Kim SR, Kaniwa N, Nishimaki-Mogami T, Sawada J, Shirao K, Hamaguchi T, Yamamoto N, Kunitoh H, Ohe Y, Yamada Y, Tamura T, Yoshida T, Matsumura Y, Ohtsu A, Saijo N, Minami H (2010) Additive effects of drug transporter genetic polymorphisms on irinotecan pharmacokinetics/pharmacodynamics in Japanese cancer patients. *Cancer Chemother Pharmacol* **66**(1): 95–105

Salmaggi A, Eoli M, Frigerio S, Silvani A, Gelati M, Corsini E, Broggi G, Boiardi A (2003) Intracavitary VEGF, bFGF, IL-8, IL-12 levels in primary and recurrent malignant glioma. *J Neurooncol* **62**(3): 297–303

Saltz LB, Cox JV, Blanke C, Rosen LS, Fehrenbacher L, Moore MJ, Maroun JA, Ackland SP, Locker PK, Pirotta N, Elfring GL, Miller LL (2000) Irinotecan plus fluorouracil and leucovorin for metastatic colorectal cancer. Irinotecan Study Group. *N Engl J Med* **343**(13): 905–914

Saltz LB, Schwartz GK, Ilson DH, Quan V, Kelsen DP (1997) A phase II study of topotecan administered five times daily in patients with advanced gastric cancer. *Am J Clin Oncol* **20**(6): 621–625

Santana VM, Zamboni WC, Kirstein MN, Tan M, Liu T, Gajjar A, Houghton PJ, Stewart CF (2003) A Pilot Study of Protracted Topotecan Dosing Using a Pharmacokinetically Guided Dosing Approach in Children with Solid Tumors. *Clin Cancer Res* **9**(2): 633–640

Santisteban M, Buckner JC, Reid JM, Wu W, Scheithauer BW, Ames MM, Felten SJ, Nikcevich DA, Wiesenfeld M, Jaeckle KA, Galanis E (2009) Phase II trial of two different irinotecan schedules with pharmacokinetic analysis in patients with recurrent glioma: North Central Cancer Treatment Group results. *Journal of Neuro-Oncology* **92**(2): 165–175

Schaiquevich P, Panetta JC, Iacono LC, Freeman BB, 3 rd, Santana VM, Gajjar A, Stewart CF (2007) Population pharmacokinetic analysis of topotecan in pediatric cancer patients. *Clin Cancer Res* **13**(22 Pt 1): 6703–6711

Schellens JH, Creemers GJ, Beijnen JH, Rosing H, de Boer-Dennert M, McDonald M, Davies B, Verweij J (1996) Bioavailability and pharmacokinetics of oral topotecan: a new topoisomerase I inhibitor. *Br J Cancer* **73**(10): 1268–1271

Sessa C, Cresta S, Cerny T, Baselga J, Rota Caremoli E, Malossi A, Hess D, Trigo J, Zucchetti M, D'Incalci M, Zaniboni A, Capri G, Gatti B, Carminati P, Zanna C, Marsoni S, Gianni L (2007) Concerted escalation of dose and dosing duration in a phase I study of the oral camptothecin gimatecan (ST1481) in patients with advanced solid tumors. *Ann Oncol* **18**(3): 561–568

Seymour MT, Maughan TS, Ledermann JA, Topham C, James R, Gwyther SJ, Smith DB, Shepherd S, Maraveyas A, Ferry DR, Meade AM, Thompson L, Griffiths GO, Parmar MK, Stephens RJ (2007) Different strategies of sequential and combination chemotherapy for patients with poor prognosis advanced colorectal cancer (MRC FOCUS): a randomised controlled trial. *Lancet* **370**(9582): 143–152

Shah DK, Shin BS, Veith J, Toth K, Bernacki RJ, Balthasar JP (2009) Use of an anti-vascular endothelial growth factor antibody in a pharmacokinetic strategy to increase the efficacy of intraperitoneal chemotherapy. *J Pharmacol Exp Ther* **329**(2): 580–591

Shah MA, Ramanathan RK, Ilson DH, Levnor A, D'Adamo D, O'Reilly E, Tse A, Trocola R, Schwartz L, Capanu M, Schwartz GK, Kelsen DP (2006) Multicenter Phase II Study of

Irinotecan, Cisplatin, and Bevacizumab in Patients With Metastatic Gastric or Gastroesophageal Junction Adenocarcinoma. *J Clin Oncol* **24**(33): 5201–5206

Shimada Y, Rougier P, Pitot H (1996) Efficacy of CPT-11 (irinotecan) as a single agent in metastatic colorectal cancer. *Eur J Cancer* **32A Suppl 3:** S13-17

Shimizu Y, Umezawa S, Hasumi K (1998) A phase II study of combined CPT-11 and mitomycin-C in platinum refractory clear cell and mucinous ovarian carcinoma. *Ann Acad Med Singapore* **27**(5): 650–656

Stewart CF, Baker SD, Heideman RL, Jones D, Crom WR, Pratt CB (1994) Clinical pharmacodynamics of continuous infusion topotecan in children: systemic exposure predicts hematologic toxicity. *J Clin Oncol* **12**(9): 1946–1954

Stewart CF, Iacono LC, Chintagumpala M, Kellie SJ, Ashley D, Zamboni WC, Kirstein MN, Fouladi M, Seele LG, Wallace D, Houghton PJ, Gajjar A (2004) Results of a phase II upfront window of pharmacokinetically guided topotecan in high-risk medulloblastoma and supratentorial primitive neuroectodermal tumor. *J Clin Oncol* **22**(16): 3357–3365

Stewart LA (2002) Chemotherapy in adult high-grade glioma: a systematic review and meta-analysis of individual patient data from 12 randomised trials. *Lancet* **359**(9311): 1011–1018

Sugiyama T, Nishida T, Kataoka A, Imaishi K, Komai K, Ushijima K, Hasuo Y, Ookura N, Yakushiji M (1996) [Combination of irinotecan hydrochloride (CPT-11) and cisplatin as a new regimen for patients with advanced ovarian cancer]. *Materials science research international* **48**(9): 827–834

Takane H, Miyata M, Burioka N, Kurai J, Fukuoka Y, Suyama H, Shigeoka Y, Otsubo K, Ieiri I, Shimizu E (2007) Severe toxicities after irinotecan-based chemotherapy in a patient with lung cancer: a homozygote for the SLCO1B1*15 allele. *Ther Drug Monit* **29**(5): 666–668

ten Bokkel Huinink W, Gore M, Carmichael J, Gordon A, Malfetano J, Hudson I, Broom C, Scarabelli C, Davidson N, Spanczynski M, Bolis G, Malmstrom H, Coleman R, Fields S, Heron J (1997) Topotecan versus paclitaxel for the treatment of recurrent epithelial ovarian cancer. *J Clin Oncol* **15**(6): 2183–2193

Tournigand C, Andre T, Achille E, Lledo G, Flesh M, Mery-Mignard D, Quinaux E, Couteau C, Buyse M, Ganem G, Landi B, Colin P, Louvet C, de Gramont A (2004) FOLFIRI followed by FOLFOX6 or the Reverse Sequence in Advanced Colorectal Cancer: A Randomized GERCOR Study. *J Clin Oncol* **22**(2): 229–237

Vallbohmer D, Iqbal S, Yang DY, Rhodes KE, Zhang W, Gordon M, Fazzone W, Schultheis AM, Sherrod AE, Danenberg KD, Lenz HJ (2006) Molecular determinants of irinotecan efficacy. *Int J Cancer* **119**(10): 2435–2442

Van Cutsem E, Kohne CH, Hitre E, Zaluski J, Chang Chien CR, Makhson A, D'Haens G, Pinter T, Lim R, Bodoky G, Roh JK, Folprecht G, Ruff P, Stroh C, Tejpar S, Schlichting M, Nippgen J, Rougier P (2009a) Cetuximab and chemotherapy as initial treatment for metastatic colorectal cancer. *N Engl J Med* **360**(14): 1408–1417

Van Cutsem E, Labianca R, Bodoky G, Barone C, Aranda E, Nordlinger B, Topham C, Tabernero J, Andre T, Sobrero AF, Mini E, Greil R, Di Costanzo F, Collette L, Cisar L, Zhang X, Khayat D, Bokemeyer C, Roth AD, Cunningham D (2009b) Randomized phase III trial comparing biweekly infusional fluorouracil/leucovorin alone or with irinotecan in the adjuvant treatment of stage III colon cancer: PETACC-3. *J Clin Oncol* **27**(19): 3117–3125

Vey N, Kantarjian H, Beran M, O'Brien S, Cortes J, Koller C, Estey E (1999) Combination of topotecan with cytarabine or etoposide in patients with refractory or relapsed acute myeloid leukemia: results of a randomized phase I/II study. *Invest New Drugs* **17**(1): 89–95

Voloschin AD, Betensky R, Wen PY, Hochberg F, Batchelor T (2008) Topotecan as salvage therapy for relapsed or refractory primary central nervous system lymphoma. *J Neurooncol* **86**(2): 211–215

von Pawel J, Schiller JH, Shepherd FA, Fields SZ, Kleisbauer JP, Chrysson NG, Stewart DJ, Clark PI, Palmer MC, Depierre A, Carmichael J, Krebs JB, Ross G, Lane SR, Gralla R (1999) Topotecan versus cyclophosphamide, doxorubicin, and vincristine for the treatment of recurrent small-cell lung cancer. *J Clin Oncol* **17**(2): 658–667

Vredenburgh J, Desjardins A, Herndon J, Dowell J, Reardon D, Quinn J, Rich J, Sathornsumetee S, Gururangan S, Wagner M, Bigner D, Friedman A, Friedman H (2007a) Phase II trial of bevacizumab and irinotecan in recurrent malignant glioma. *Clinical cancer research* **13**(4): 1253–1259

Vredenburgh JJ, Desjardins A, Herndon JE, II, Marcello J, Reardon DA, Quinn JA, Rich JN, Sathornsumetee S, Gururangan S, Sampson J, Wagner M, Bailey L, Bigner DD, Friedman AH, Friedman HS (2007b) Bevacizumab Plus Irinotecan in Recurrent Glioblastoma Multiforme. *J Clin Oncol* **25**(30): 4722–4729

Woell E, Greil R, Eisterer W, Fridrik M, Grunberger B, Zabernigg A, Mayrbaurl B, Russ G, Thaler J (2009) Oxaliplatin, irinotecan, and cetuximab in advanced gastric cancer. First efficacy results of a multicenter phase II trial (AGMT Gastric-2) of the Arbeitsgemeinschaft Medikamentoese Tumortherapie (AGMT). *J Clin Oncol (Meeting Abstracts)* **27**(15 S): 4538-

Xiang X, Jada SR, Li HH, Fan L, Tham LS, Wong CI, Lee SC, Lim R, Zhou QY, Goh BC, Tan EH, Chowbay B (2006) Pharmacogenetics of SLCO1B1 gene and the impact of *1b and *15 haplotypes on irinotecan disposition in Asian cancer patients. *Pharmacogenet Genomics* **16**(9): 683–691

Yamada Y, Tamura T, Yamamoto N, Shimoyama T, Ueda Y, Murakami H, Kusaba H, Kamiya Y, Saka H, Tanigawara Y, McGovren JP, Natsumeda Y (2006) Phase I and pharmacokinetic study of edotecarin, a novel topoisomerase I inhibitor, administered once every 3 weeks in patients with solid tumors. *Cancer Chemother Pharmacol* **58**(2): 173–182

Ychou M, Hohenberger W, Thezenas S, Navarro M, Maurel J, Bokemeyer C, Shacham-Shmueli E, Rivera F, Kwok-Keung Choi C, Santoro A (2009a) A randomized phase III study comparing adjuvant 5-fluorouracil/folinic acid with FOLFIRI in patients following complete resection of liver metastases from colorectal cancer. *Ann Oncol* **20**(12): 1964–1970

Ychou M, Raoul JL, Douillard JY, Gourgou-Bourgade S, Bugat R, Mineur L, Viret F, Becouarn Y, Bouche O, Gamelin E, Ducreux M, Conroy T, Seitz JF, Bedenne L, Kramar A (2009b) A phase III randomised trial of LV5FU2+irinotecan versus LV5FU2 alone in adjuvant high-risk colon cancer (FNCLCC Accord02/FFCD9802). *Ann Oncol* **20**(4): 674–680

Ychou M, Viret F, Kramar A, Desseigne F, Mitry E, Guimbaud R, Delpero JR, Rivoire M, Quenet F, Portier G, Nordlinger B (2008) Tritherapy with fluorouracil/leucovorin, irinotecan and oxaliplatin (FOLFIRINOX): a phase II study in colorectal cancer patients with non-resectable liver metastases. *Cancer Chemotherapy & Pharmacology* **62**(2): 195–201

Yokoyama S, Imamura Y, Hatano N, Fukuoka T, Usui H, Morita Y (2009) [Two cases of advanced colorectal cancer with UGT1A1*28 homozygosity treated by FOLFIRI]. *Gan To Kagaku Ryoho* **36**(7): 1159–1161

Zamboni WC, Gajjar AJ, Heideman RL, Beijnen JH, Rosing H, Houghton PJ, Stewart CF (1998) Phenytoin alters the disposition of topotecan and N-desmethyl topotecan in a patient with medulloblastoma. *Clin Cancer Res* **4**(3): 783–789

Zhu AX, Ready N, Clark JW, Safran H, Amato A, Salem N, Pace S, He X, Zvereva N, Lynch TJ, Ryan DP, Supko JG (2009) Phase I and pharmacokinetic study of gimatecan given orally once a week for 3 of 4 weeks in patients with advanced solid tumors. *Clin Cancer Res* **15**(1): 374–381

Chapter 13
Topoisomerase II Inhibitors: Current Use and Prospects

Olivier Mir, William Dahut, François Goldwasser, and Christopher Heery

13.1 Introduction

DNA topoisomerase II (Top2)-targeted drugs are amongst the oldest anticancer agents available in oncology and hematology. They remain largely used because of their dramatic clinical effect in highly proliferative malignancies. These diseases are frequently very rapidly life threatening and/or responsible for organ failures. As a result, Top2-targeted drugs have a particular role in cancer therapy because they are the cornerstone of emergency treatments for bulky diseases when the treatment priority is not to obtain disease stability and delay disease progression, but to induce rapid tumor regression. Top2-targeted drugs are typically prescribed to patients with progressive disease on Friday, for whom treatment cannot be delayed to Monday. All Top2-targeted drugs are responsible for bone marrow acute toxicity, usually resulting in marked asthenia. Epipodophyllotoxins given by IV route and anthracyclins also share side effects (complete alopecia and phanerian toxicity) feared by the patients because they affect physical presentation and social life. However, their clinical antitumoral effect as induction therapies is usually clinically beneficial to the patient within few days. Etoposide is frequently combined with cisplatin, in germ-cell tumors, small-cell lung cancers, poorly differentiated adenocarcinomas of unknown origin, osteosarcomas, while doxorubicin is commonly associated with an alkylating agent, such as cyclophosphamide (AC protocol in breast cancer) or ifosfamide (AL protocol in soft-tissue sarcomas). Considered in this chapter are the epipodophyllotoxins, anthracyclines, and anthrapyrazoles, and amsacrine. Table 13.1 summarizes the role of these agents in the treatment strategies of solid tumors and hematologic malignancies in 2011.

O. Mir (✉)
Department of Clinical Oncology, Hopital Cochin, Paris, France
e-mail: olivier.mir@cch.aphp.fr

Y. Pommier (ed.), *DNA Topoisomerases and Cancer*, Cancer Drug Discovery and Development, DOI 10.1007/978-1-4614-0323-4_13,

Table 13.1 Clinical role of topoisomerase II poisons in the therapeutic armamentarium

	Etoposide	Doxorubicin	4′epi-doxorubicin	Mitoxantrone	Amsacrine
1st Hand	▪ Small-cell lung cancers	▪ Bone and Soft tissue sarcomas	▪ Breast cancers	Adult lympho-blastic leukemia	Pediatric and adult acute leukemias
	▪ Merkel carcinomas	▪ Breast cancers	▪ Esophageal and gastric cancers		
	▪ Testicular and ovarian germ cell tumors	▪ Bladder cancer			
	▪ Poorly differentiated and undifferentiated carcinomas of unknown origin	▪ Multiple Myeloma			
	▪ Poorly differentiated endocrine tumors	▪ Hodgkin's and non-Hodgkin's lymphomas			
	▪ Osteosarcomas and Ewing's sarcomas.	▪ Anaplastic thyroid cancer			
	▪ Endocrine prostate cancer				
	▪ Aggressive thymomas				
	▪ Neuroblastomas				
	▪ Kaposi's sarcomas				
2nd line	▪ Relapsed adult acute lymphoblastic and nonlymphocytic leukemia	▪ Adrenal cortical carcinoma (op'ddd failure)		– Prostate cancer	
	▪ Refractory testicular cancers (VIP)	▪ Ovarian cancer		– Breast cancer	
	▪ Hodgkin's and non-Hodgkin's lymphomas			– Resistant adult acute myelogenous and lympho-blastic leukemia	
	▪ Gestational trophoblastic disease (methotrexate failure)			– Lymphomas	
	▪ Adrenal cortical carcinoma (op'ddd failure)				
	▪ Epithelial ovarian cancer (taxane- and platinum-resistant)				
	▪ [illegible]				

In presence of specific features	▪ Metastatic gastric cancers ▪ Adenocarcinomas with overexpression of hCG		
Other uses	▪ Intensification with autologous bone marrow transplantation ▪ Radiosensitizer (non-small-cell lung cancer,…)		▪ Intensification with autologous bone marrow transplantation

13.2 Epipodophyllotoxins

The epipodophyllotoxins etoposide (VP-16) and teniposide (VM-26) exert their antineoplastic effect by selectively targeting Top2 (Pommier et al. 2010) (see Chap. 11). In contrast to the parent compound podophyllotoxin, these two glycosidic, semisynthetic derivatives of podophyllotoxin are inactive against tubulin. Etoposide was introduced in clinical trials in 1971 and was approved by the Food and Drug Administration (FDA) for marketing by Bristol Laboratories under the trade name Vepesid in early 1984. Teniposide (VM-26) was approved by the US FDA in 1992 for refractory childhood leukemia.

13.2.1 Pharmacokinetics

The pharmacokinetics of intravenous etoposide follows a two-compartment pharmacokinetic model with a terminal half-life of 6–8 h. Inter- and intra-patient variability is around 35% (Hande et al. 1984; Rodman et al. 1994). The peak plasma concentration and the area under the curve *(AUC)* are proportional to the administered dose up to of 800 mg/m^2 (Allen and Creaven 1975), and the elimination half-life is independent of dose. Etoposide penetrates the CSF poorly, with CSF concentrations less than 5% of simultaneously measured plasma levels (D'Incalci et al. 1986; Hande et al. 1984). Pleural fluid and ascitic fluid penetration of etoposide are poor. Etoposide is extensively protein bound (96%) (Stewart et al. 1990), metabolized by the liver (Arbuck et al. 1986; D'Incalci et al. 1982; Hande et al. 1984, 1990) and eliminated in the bile (10–15% as unchanged drug) and urine (35% as unchanged drug) (D'Incalci et al. 1986). Etoposide is not hemodialyzable (Suzuki et al. 1997). Several metabolites of etoposide have been identified in humans. The main metabolite is etoposide-glucuronide, which is eliminated in the urine. A catechol metabolite with significant cytotoxic activity is formed following etoposide O-demethylation in the liver. Cytochrome P450 3A metabolizes etoposide to a catechol metabolite, which is further oxidized to a quinone. The etoposide-*o*-dihydroxy also can be converted to the *o*-quinone derivative (D'Incalci et al. 1982, 1986; Hande et al. 1984). Etoposide clearance is not correlated to body surface area, and some authors proposed to replace the iv dose of 150 mg/m^2 by a fixed dose of 260 mg (D'Incalci et al. 1986). Parameters necessary for prescription of etoposide include:

- Albumin serum levels because of increased unbound etoposide in patients with hypoalbuminemia.
- Bilirubin serum concentrations: elevated serum bilirubin concentrations, competes for albumin binding, and also increases the concentration of the free or biologically active drug, resulting in greater hematologic toxicity. Minor alterations in liver function, such as transaminase elevations do not require dose reduction. Therefore, etoposide dose should be reduced by 50% in patients with total bilirubin

levels of 1.5–3.0 mg/dL. No etoposide should be given in patients with more than 5.0 mg/dL bilirubin (Hande et al. 1990).
- Estimated creatinin clearance. Etoposide dosage should be reduced in proportion to reductions in creatinine clearance.

Oral absorption of etoposide varies from 25% to 75% (Toffoli et al. 2004). There is no evidence of first-pass metabolism after oral administration. Etoposide phosphate has a more predictable and better oral bioavailability, compared to etoposide (Budman et al. 1994). Etoposide phosphate (Etopophos) simplifies the formulation of etoposide by being water soluble and readily converted to etoposide in the patient plasma by host endogenous phosphatase. Etoposide phosphate appears to have equivalent antineoplastic activity to etoposide. Etoposide phosphate can be given rapidly, over 5 min without signs of hypotension or acute effects (Sessa et al. 1995). Since it is not formulated with polyethylene glycol, polysorbate 80, or ethanol, etoposide phosphate does not cause acidosis, even when given at high doses. When given as a continuous infusion, etoposide phosphate is stable in pumps for at least 7 days.

13.2.2 Pharmacodynamics

The acute toxicity of etoposide is schedule dependent (D'Incalci et al. 1986; Pommier and Goldwasser 2011). At standard dose, given 3 consecutive days, the dose-limiting acute toxicity is mainly granulocytopenia, with nadir between days 8 and 14 and recovery at day 20. Anemia and thrombocytopenia are also common. Hematologic toxicity correlates better to the AUC of unbound etoposide than to the AUC of total etoposide (Ratain et al. 1991). Alopecia is universal with the standard iv protocol (EP), but frequently avoided orally using the 25 mg 3 times a day schedule. Nausea, hypotension, especially in case of rapid infusion, and anaphylactoid reactions are possible.

At high dose, in intensification regimens with bone marrow support, the dose-limiting toxicities become mucositis and hepatotoxicity. The maximal tolerated dose of etoposide administered as a single agent is between 2.5 and 3.5 g/m^2 depending on the conditioning regimen (Einhorn et al. 2007; Hande et al. 1984).

Late toxicities have to be in mind in patients with curable disease. Efforts to reduce the cumulative dose of etoposide are necessary to minimize these risks.

13.2.2.1 Secondary Leukemia

Etoposide is mutagenic in patients. Acute myelogenous leukemia (AML) cases related to prior treatment with epipodophyllotoxins (etoposide and teniposide) have been characterized and are certainly favored by the increased frequency of illegitimate recombination events induced by topoisomerase II poisons (Pommier and Goldwasser 2011). In contrast to alkylating agent-associated secondary AML, epipodophyllotoxin-associated AML exhibits a shorter latency period with a median of 24–30 months (Armstrong et al. 2009; Le Deley et al. 2003; Smith et al. 1999). Their phenotype is most often monocytic (FAB M4 or M5). In many patients, leukemic cells have an 11q23 abnormality. The follow-up of patients treated with epipodophyllotoxins by the National Cancer Institute Cancer Therapy Evaluation Program (NCI-CTEP) did not show evidence of significant variations in the incidence of secondary leukemias in patients who had received low (less than 1.5 g/m^2), moderate (between 1.5 and 2.99 g/m^2), or high cumulative doses (more than 3 g/m^2). Most other studies found a correlation between the cumulative dose of etoposide and the risk of secondary leukemias. In another report of 212 patients treated with PEB for germ cell tumors, 5 patients developed acute nonlymphocytic leukemia (ANLL) for a mean cumulative risk of 4.7% (Pedersen-Bjergaard et al. 1991). All these patients had cumulative etoposide doses above 2,000 mg/m^2, whereas none of the 130 patients with cumulative dose below 2,000 mg/m^2 developed leukemia. In a series of 734 children treated with epipodophyllotoxins, 21 developed secondary AML. The overall risk of developing a secondary leukemia was 3.8%. In a case-control study of the French society of pediatric oncology, 61 patients with secondary leukemia were matched with 196 controls. In multivariate analysis, the risk of leukemia correlated with the type of primary tumor (excess risk in case of Hodgkin's disease and osteosarcoma) and with the cumulative dose of etoposide. The risk of leukemia in patients who received more than 6 g/m^2 was 200-fold higher. Not only etoposide but also its catechol and quinone metabolites can induce in vitro Top2 cleavage complexes near the translocation breakpoints and are likely to also play a role in the creation of Top2-mediated chromosomal breakage. These leukemias frequently involved the long arm of chromosome 11, with translocation of the *MLL* gene at chromosome band 11q23. The *MLL* (myeloid-lymphoid leukemia or mixed-lineage leukemia) gene resides at 11q23. Most of the breakpoints occur in a 9-kilobase region that includes exons 5–11 of the *MLL* gene. This genomic region includes DNA sequences, potentially involved for illegitimate recombinations, such as Alu sequences, VDJ recombinase recognition sites, and Top2 consensus-binding sequences. DNA topoisomerase II cleavage assays have shown a correspondence between Top2 cleavage sites and the translocation breakpoints. The mechanism of the translocation might be a chromosomal breakage by Top2 followed by the recombination of DNA free ends during DNA repair (Pommier and Goldwasser 2011).

13.2.2.2 Increased Cardiovascular Risks

Treatment with the BEP regimen increases the long-term risk of cardiovascular disease in survivors of testicular cancer. Treatment with cisplatin, bleomycin, and etoposide (BEP) has a 5.7-fold higher risk (95% CI, 1.9–17.1 fold) for coronary artery disease compared with surgery only and a 3.1-fold higher risk (95% CI, 1.2–7.7 fold) for myocardial infarction compared with age-matched male controls from the general population (Haugnes et al. 2010).

13.2.3 Combination Strategies et Drug Interactions

Etoposide is used in combination with other DNA damaging agents, especially radiotherapy (Baas et al. 2010), cisplatin, and alkylating agents. The EP protocol combines etoposide and cisplatin and is one of the gold standard in cancer chemotherapy for several diseases. This combination can be used as first-line therapy in testicular cancer, small cell lung cancer, poorly differentiated metastatic adenocarcinomas, poorly differentiated endocrine carcinomas (Fjallskog et al. 2001). The combination of cisplatin and etoposide can produce significant responses in patients with heavily pretreated and poorly differentiated/rapidly progressing neuroendocrine tumors. The toxicity is considerable, and nephrotoxicity is the dose-limiting factor. Therefore, in elderly patients, or patients with severe comorbidities, treatment adaptations and replacement of cisplatin by carboplatin and iv etoposide by oral etoposide are frequently necessary.

In combination with cisplatin, etoposide can be given as a 1 h infusion for 5 consecutive days at the dose of 100 mg/m^2, especially in germ-cell tumors. Otherwise, it is frequently given for 3 consecutive days at the dose of 120–150 mg/m^2/day. In metastatic small-cell lung cancer, the first cycle may be the worst tolerated because of frequent bone marrow involvement at the time of diagnosis. Etoposide is stable if given in the same infusion than cisplatin. Prolonged fractionated oral administration of etoposide may present a theoretical advantage over intravenous administration of the bolus. Pharmacokinetics highlighted no interaction between etoposide and carboplatin (Thiery-Vuillemin et al. 2010).

The combination of etoposide with alkylating agents is used through the iv route or orally.

13.2.4 Clinical Role in 2011

Etoposide is one of the most widely used antitumor agents in pediatric oncology as well as chemotherapeutic agents used in conditioning regimen prior to allo-HSCT for childhood ALL.

Etoposide is the cornerstone in adult oncology for the treatment of germ-cell tumors and small-cell lung cancers. In men with good-prognosis germ cell tumors, two standard chemotherapy regimens were compared that contained bleomycin, etoposide, and cisplatin but differed in the scheduling and total dose of cisplatin, the total dose of bleomycin, and the scheduling and dose intensity of etoposide: either 3B(90)E(500)P or 4B(30)E(360)P. The trial was stopped early at a median follow-up of 33 months after a planned interim analysis found a survival benefit for the more dose-intense regimen, and the survival benefit of 3B(90)E(500)P was maintained with long-term follow-up. The aim of this analysis was to determine if this survival benefit was maintained with long-term follow-up (Grimison et al. 2010).

In extensive-disease small-cell lung cancer, the first line may be either a platinum derivative combined with irinotecan or with etoposide (Jiang et al. 2010; Schmittel et al. 2011). Small-cell lung carcinomas (SCLC) represent less than 20% of all lung cancers. As it is an aggressive tumor, on account of its high and early risk of dissemination, only a third of patients have limited-stage disease at diagnosis. For these patients, the current state-of-the-art treatment involves cisplatin-etoposide chemotherapy combined with chest radiotherapy. In extensive disease, radiotherapy has also a place in the management of SCLC: PCI reduces the risk of brain metastases and significantly improves overall survival, so that cisplatin (or carboplatin)-etoposide followed by PCI in responding patients has become the standard treatment Etoposide is used in various second-line therapies, still potentially curative, in Hodgkin's lymphomas (Josting et al. 2010) and NHL (Kim et al. 2010). Etoposide is part of salvage combination therapies in patients with relapsed/chemoresistant gestational trophoblastic disease (Feng et al. 2011).

The role of etoposide has increased in pediatric osteosarcomas. By contrast, it has been replaced by other agents in ovarian, gastric, and non-small-cell lung cancer. An exception is the clinical presentation with specific features suggesting the efficacy of etoposide: dramatic tumor growth, bulky disease, high LDH levels (Germann et al. 2002). Oral etoposide is used for the treatment of patients with numerous cancers who cannot be treated with intensive chemotherapy for various reasons, such as age and comorbidities. Patients with Merkel-cell carcinoma are treated with etoposide-containing regimens if they have disease localized to the primary site and nodes, or at least one of the following high risk features: recurrence after initial therapy, involved nodes, primary tumor size greater than 1 cm, gross residual disease after surgery, or occult primary with nodes (Poon et al. 2004; Poulsen et al. 2003). Etoposide is combined with alkylating agents, for intensification with bone marrow support (Chrzanowska et al. 2010; Ibrahim et al. 1992).

Teniposide (VM-26) is used in pediatric tumors and in neuro-oncology. It is highly active in combination in pediatric hematologic malignancies including both acute myelocytic (AML) and lymphocytic leukemias (ALL). Teniposide is a highly effective salvage therapy for initial induction failures in childhood ALL and also has been incorporated in salvage therapy for both Hodgkin's and non-Hodgkin's lymphoma. Activity has also been shown in bladder cancer (by both intravenous and intravesical routes), neuroblastoma, and small-cell lung cancer, and responses have been noted in tumors of the central nervous system.

13.3 Anthracyclines

Several compounds are in the clinical armamentarium (see Chap. 11).

13.3.1 Doxorubicin

Doxorubicin (trade name Adriamycin; also known as hydroxyldaunorubicin) is an anthracycline antibiotic only used in cancer chemotherapy. A single hydroxyl group differentiates doxorubicin from the natural product daunorubicin. Both can be traced to their discovery in Italy in the 1950s (Arcamone et al. 1969) in a new strain of *Streptomyces* (Arcamone et al. 1972).

13.3.2 Daunorubicin

Daunorubicin (daunomycin) was isolated in 1963 from *Streptomyces peucetius* (Dimarco et al. 1964). It is an anthracycline composed of the amino sugar daunosamine, linked through a glycosidic bond to daunomycione, a red-pigmented naphthacenequinone nucleus (Young et al. 1981).

13.3.3 Idarubicin

Idarubicin, also known as 4-demethoxydaunorubicin or 4-DMDR, was also synthesized by Arcamone and coworkers (**Arcamone** et al. 1976). It was designed to investigate the influence of the methoxyl group at the C-4 position of the tetracyclic aglycone, which is not present in other anthracyclines. Arcamone synthesized the same compound without the C-4 methyoxyl group, creating 4-demethoxydaunorubicin. Testing of the new compound showed five to eight times higher potency than daunorubicin, with potent antitumor effects. It was hoped that idarubicin's increased potency would improve its cardiotoxicity profile relative to daunorubicin.

13.3.4 Epirubicin

Epirubicin (4′-epi-doxorubicin) was synthesized by Arcamone et al. and reported in 1975 (Arcamone et al. 1975). Like idarubicin, it was created to improve the effectiveness of anthracyclines while decreasing their side effects, particularly their cardiotoxicity. Epirubicin differs in structure from daunorubicin by exchange of the natural amino sugar duanosamine (3-amino-2,3,6-trideoxy-L-*lyxo*-hexose) for the 4′-epi analog, 3-amino-2,3,6-trideoxy-L-*arabino*-hexose (Arcamone et al. 1975).

13.3.5 Pharmacokinetics of Anthracyclines

13.3.5.1 Doxorubicin

Doxorubicin is commonly administered as a single intravenous infusion of 45–75 mg/m^2 every 21 days. However, because cardiotoxicity has been linked to peak plasma concentrations, while antitumor effect is closely related to AUC, a prolonged infusion over 96 h may be safer and more effective (Legha et al. 1982; Synold and Doroshow 1996). Weekly dosing at roughly one third of the 3-week dose level (20–30 mg/m^2) has been shown to have less cardiotoxicity with similar cytotoxic effects on tumor cells (Von Hoff et al. 1979).

Doxorubicin has a relative volume of distribution of 1,780 L/m^2 (S.D., 1,120 L/m^2) (Benjamin et al. 1973). Although Benjamin et al. initially described a biphasic clearance of doxorubicin from plasma, later analysis of their data indicated a triphasic decline in plasma concentration. The first, second, and third half-lives last 12 (± 8) minutes, 3.3 (± 2.2) hours, and 29.6 (± 13.5) hours, respectively (Benjamin et al. 1974). Urinary excretion of unchanged drug is 5–10% (Benjamin et al. 1974; Takanashi and Bachur 1976). Doxorubicin is heavily bound to protein in plasma, at 74 ± 1.7%, while its main metabolite, doxorubicinol, is bound at 76 ± 1.4% (Greene et al. 1983). Doxorubicin clearance is influenced most directly by hepatic function (Greene et al. 1983; Takanashi and Bachur 1976). Nearly 50% of each dose is secreted in bile, some of it metabolically altered. This finding has led to dose reduction in patients with elevated bilirubin (Benjamin et al. 1974; Harris and Gross 1975). The long terminal half-life of doxorubicin is a result of prolonged tissue binding, which also allows for effective tissue concentrations to persist for up to a week after each dose (Greene et al. 1983).

13.3.5.2 Daunorubicin

Daunorubicin is commonly administered in short infusions of 35–45 mg/m^2 daily for 3 days as induction for acute myelogenous leukemia. After infusion, daunorubicin is rapidly converted to its active metabolites of daunorubicinol and C^4-*O*-demethyl daunorubicin, along with their corresponding breakdown products, which include aglycones (Huffman and Bachur 1972). Their primary half-life is about 45 min, with a secondary half-life of about 55 h (Alberts et al. 1971). Daunorubicinol then becomes the predominant circulating form of the drug, with a half-life of 37.2 h (Bachur 1971; Robert et al. 1992). Daunorubicin is also heavily protein-bound and will quickly become more concentrated in tissue than in plasma. Volume of distribution for daunorubicin has been reported as 942 L/m^2 (S.D., 549 L/m^2) (Alberts et al. 1971).

As with doxorubicin, clearance of daunorubicin is mainly mediated through hepatic function; however, daunorubicin converts to its active metabolites more rapidly than doxorubicin.

13.3.5.3 Idarubicin

Idarubicin is typically administered in doses of 10–15 mg/m^2 for multiple days, depending on the regimen in which it is being used (Wiernik et al. 1992). However, it is also given as one high dose/cycle for leukemia induction (Weiss et al. 2002). Idarubicin has a triphasic elimination, with half-lives of 9.6 min, 3.2, and 34.7 h, respectively (Smith et al. 1987). Its terminal half-life is 27 h (±5.5 h), with a volume of distribution of 63.9 ± 12.6 L/kg and a total clearance of 1.9 L/kg/h. Urinary excretion is 5% of the dose/24 h (Lu et al. 1986).

Clearance is mediated largely by hepatic metabolism; patients with liver dysfunction may have prolonged elevation of plasma concentrations (Lu et al. 1986). The dose should be decreased by 25% if bilirubin 1.5–3 mg/dL, and by 50% if bilirubin 3.1–5 mg/dL. Although renal clearance is a minor elimination route (Lu et al. 1986), it is recommended that the dose be reduced by 25% if creatinine clearance is less than 10 mL/min.

13.3.5.4 Epirubicin

Epirubicin is commonly given as 50–120 mg/m^2 every 3 weeks (Bedano et al. 2006; Poole et al. 2006; Roth et al. 2007; Taamma et al. 1999). It was developed to maximize the antitumor effect of anthracyclines, while decreasing their cardiotoxicity. Preclinical studies showed decreased concentrations of epirubicin in the heart and spleen at similar time points, while tumor concentrations were comparable to other anthracyclines (Ganzina 1983). Like other anthracyclines, epirubicin has a triphasic elimination, with half-lives of 4.8 min, 2.6, and 38 h respectively. Again, this is related to strong protein binding causing slow terminal elimination. Volume of distribution is 1,430 L/m^2 (±500 L/m^2) (Weenen et al. 1983).

13.3.6 Pharmacodynamics of Anthracylines

13.3.6.1 Doxorubicin

Like all anthracyclines, doxorubicin carries risks of myelosuppression, mucositis, alopecia, severe extravasation injury to local tissue, and cardiotoxicity, with cardiotoxicity clearly a function of peak concentrations (Legha et al. 1982). Von Hoff et al. developed a table outlining the probability of cardiotoxicity based on cumulative dose and age, with weekly dosing compared to a triweekly dosing schedule (Von Hoff et al. 1979). Not surprisingly, the triweekly schedule had a higher likelihood of cardiotoxicity at the same cumulative doses by age group. It has become common practice to limit patients to a cumulative dose of no more than 450 mg/m^2. However, caution is advised. For instance, a 65-year-old patient receiving doxorubicin every 3 weeks would have a 6.1% chance of developing clinically significant cardiotoxicity at a cumulative dose of 450 mg/m^2. The same patient would have only a 1.6% chance of cardiotoxicity if the same cumulative dose were given as lower individual doses administered weekly.

It has been postulated that the peak concentration of doxorubicin correlates better than AUC with cardiotoxicity because of doxorubicin's rapid hepatic conversion to metabolites containing free radicals. This speculation is based on a study by Cummings et al. in which two patients who developed cardiotoxicity also developed high levels of 7-deoxyaglycones after doxorubicin infusion (Cummings et al. 1986).

13.3.6.2 Daunorubicin

Daunorubicin and doxorubicin have similar risks for myelosuppression, mucositis, extravasation injury, and cardiotoxicity. LeFrak et al. first described cardiomyopathy and electrocardiogram abnormalities in patients receiving doxorubicin (Lefrak et al. 1973), and similar toxicities are seen with daunorubicin. Incidence of cardiotoxicity is around 1–2% and can be life threatening (Halazun et al. 1974; Von Hoff et al. 1977). As with doxorubicin, the risk of cardiotoxicity is related to dose, but this risk is of greater concern when daunorubicin is administered to children (Von Hoff et al. 1977).

13.3.6.3 Idarubicin

The most common doses of idarubicin carry a high risk of prolonged cytopenias, which can require growth factor support and transfusions. Cardiotoxicity remains a concern, but there is controversy over the effect of idarubicin on myocardium. Multiple studies have found no cardiotoxicity with administration of idarubicin (Borchmann et al. 1997; Toffoli et al. 1997, 2000). However, Anderlini et al. showed worsening of left ventricular ejection fraction in patients without prior exposure to other anthracyclines, and symptoms of congestive heart failure in patients with previous exposure to anthracyclines or with known cardiovascular disease (Anderlini et al. 1995).

13.3.6.4 Epirubicin

Side effects of epirubicin are similar to those of idarubicin, and both have a better cardiotoxicity profile than doxorubicin. Epirubicin is safe, with a low risk of cardiotoxicity (Ryberg et al. 1998), at a cumulative dose of 900 mg/m^2, almost double the safe dose of doxorubicin (about 450 mg/m^2). As with any "safe" dose, this should be seen as a general guideline, with individual patient characteristics taken into consideration.

13.3.7 Current Clinical Role of Anthracyclines

13.3.7.1 Doxorubicin

Solid Tumors

Doxorubicin is used to treat numerous tumor types in combination with a variety of other agents. It has been shown to improve time to progression and overall survival in patients with advanced thymoma (Fornasiero et al. 1991; Loehrer et al. 1994).

Doxorubicin is part of a regimen that improves outcome from 61% to 72% for patients with nonmetastatic Ewing's sarcoma and PNET; it does not improve outcomes for metastatic disease (Grier et al. 2003). Kaposi's sarcoma is now treated primarily with pegylated liposomal doxorubicin due to an improved response rate (58.7% vs 23.3%) compared to bleomycin and vincristine (Stewart et al. 1998). Recurrent or metastatic ovarian cancer has been treated with pegylated liposomal doxorubicin, but with minimal clinical benefit (Ferrandina et al. 2008; Mutch et al. 2007; Pectasides et al. 2008). Adjuvant therapy including doxorubicin and cisplatin for advanced-stage endometrial cancer improved 5-year survival compared to whole-abdominal irradiation (Randall et al. 2006). Patients with metastatic endometrial cancer benefit from the use of doxorubicin, cisplatin, and paclitaxel, but are at high risk for peripheral neuropathy (Fleming et al. 2004). Carcinoid tumor responds to a combination of streptozocin and doxorubicin, with improvement in time to progression (20 months vs 6.9 months) and survival (2.2 years vs 1.4 years) compared to streptozocin plus fluorouracil (Moertel et al. 1992). Doxorubicin is most commonly used as an adjuvant in the treatment of breast cancer. Multiple studies have shown its ability to reduce the risk of recurrence in higher-risk populations (Burstein et al. 2005; Dang et al. 2008; Fisher et al. 2004; Hutchins et al. 2005; Jones et al. 2006; Mamounas et al. 2005; Martin et al. 2003, 2005; Romond et al. 2005; Sparano et al. 2008). Doxorubicin may be used in combination with methotrexate, vinblastine, and cisplatin for bladder cancer in the neoadjuvant and metastatic settings, with significantly improved disease-free survival in patients treated in the neoadjuvant setting for locally advanced disease (38% vs 15%) (Grossman et al. 2003; Han et al. 2008; Logothetis et al. 1990). Doxorubicin has also been tested in soft tissue sarcoma, with evidence of activity based on response rates, but no clear survival benefit (Le Cesne et al. 2000; Worden et al. 2005). Finally, doxorubicin as monotherapy has been shown to be ineffective in hepatocellular carcinoma (Lai et al. 1988).

Hematologic Malignancies

Doxorubicin has been a staple of induction therapy for multiple myeloma and is used in combination with vincristine and bortezomib, both with dexamethasone (Oakervee et al. 2005; Segeren et al. 1999). Hodgkin's lymphoma is most commonly treated with ABVD (doxorubicin, bleomycin, vincristine, and dacarbazine), but for high-risk patients, BEACOPP (bleomycin, etoposide, doxorubicin, cyclophosphamide, vincristine, procarbazine, and prednisone) is also considered (Bonadonna et al. 2004; Canellos et al. 1992; Dann et al. 2007; Diehl et al. 2003; Engert et al. 2007). When indicated, doxorubicin is part of the standard R-CHOP therapy for follicular non-Hodgkin's lymphoma (rituximab, cyclophosphamide, hydroxyldaunorubicin, oncovin, and prednisone) (Czuczman et al. 2004). R-CHOP is also the standard regimen for mantle cell lymphoma (Lenz et al. 2005) and more aggressive non-Hodgkin's lymphomas such as diffuse large B-cell lymphoma (Feugier et al. 2005; Habermann et al. 2006; Wilson et al. 1993, 2002). Burkitt's lymphoma, a very aggressive disease, is treated with CODOX-M (cyclophosphamide, doxorubicin, oncovin, methotrexate, leucovorin, and intrathecal methotrexate or cytarabine) or dose-adjusted R-EPOCH (rituximab, etoposide, prednisone, oncovin, cyclophosphamide, hydroxyldaunorubicin, and intrathecal methotrexate) (Magrath et al. 1996; Rizzieri et al. 2004). Pre-B-cell and T-cell lymphoblastic lymphoma or leukemia also respond to Hyper-CVAD (cyclophosphamide, mesna, vincristine, doxorubicin, dexamethasone, methotrexate, cytarabine, leucovorin, and intrathecal methotrexate and cytarabine) (Larson et al. 1998; Thomas et al. 2004).

13.3.7.2 Daunorubicin

Daunorubicin is used primarily as induction and consolidation therapy for leukemia. In acute myelogenous leukemia, it is used in the 7+3 regimen in combination with cytarabine, but is not as effective as idarubicin (Wiernik et al. 1992). It is also used for induction and consolidation in acute promyelocytic leukemia in combination with cytarabine and all-trans retinoic acid (Ades et al. 2006; Fenaux 1993). Daunorubicin is also used in the Linker regimen for induction and consolidation in acute lymphoblastic leukemia, in combination with vincristine, prednisone, L-asparaginase, and prednisone (Linker et al. 1987, 1991).

13.3.7.3 Idarubicin

As noted above, idarubicin has been shown to be more effective than daunorubicin in the standard 7+3 regimen for induction and consolidation therapy for acute myelogenous leukemia (Wiernik et al. 1992). It is also used in the FLAG regimen (with fludarabine and cytarabine) in relapsed acute myelogenous leukemia (Pastore et al. 2003). With all-trans retinoic acid, arsenic trioxide, and gemtuzumab, it is used for induction in acute promyelocytic leukemia (Estey et al. 2006). Idarubicin and cytarabine are used in combination as a salvage regimen for refractory or recurrent acute lymphocytic leukemia as well (Weiss et al. 2002).

13.3.7.4 Epirubicin

Epirubicin has been used as part of a salvage regimen for refractory germ cell tumors in combination with cisplatin. In a phase II study, 9 of 30 patients had a complete response, and 7 of those 9 were in long-term remission at the time of publication (Bedano et al. 2006). Epirubicin is also used in combination with 5-fluorouracil (5-FU), cisplatin, and bleomycin or mitomycin for metastatic head and neck cancer (Hasbini et al. 1999; Taamma et al. 1999). ECF (epirubicin, cisplatin, and 5-FU) is a second-line therapy for metastatic or locally advanced gastric cancer, with a slightly different side effect profile to ECX (epirubicin, cisplatin, and capecitibine), EOF (epirubicin, oxaliplatin, and 5-FU), and EOX (epirubicin, oxaliplatin, and capecitabine) (Cunningham et al. 2008; Roth et al. 2007). ECF is also used in the neoadjuvant and adjuvant settings to significantly improve surgical resection outcomes in selected patients with cancers of the lower esophagus and esophagogastric junction (Cunningham et al. 2006). This combination can also be used in metastatic esophageal cancer, with similar outcomes to those in advanced gastric cancer (Cunningham et al. 2008). Adding epirubicin to CMF in adjuvant breast cancer treatment has shown benefit over CMF alone (Poole et al. 2006). Other regimens involving epirubicin have been developed for the adjuvant setting, but they are rarely chosen over doxorubicin-containing regimens in this setting (Joensuu et al. 2006; Levine et al. 2005; Moebus et al. 2010; Roche et al. 2006). Epirubicin is also used in various combinations for metastatic breast cancer (Langley et al. 2005).

13.4 Anthrapyrazoles: Mitoxantrone

Mitoxantrone (1,4-dihydroxy-5,8-bis(((2-[(2-hydroxyethyl)amino]ethyl)amino))-9,10-anthracene-dione dihydrochloride) was synthesized by Murdock in 1979 (Murdock et al. 1979). Murdock et al. believed that anthracyclines could be altered to be less complex, allowing more efficient intercalation into DNA. As with the newer anthracyclines, the goal was to retain the antitumor activity of doxorubicin while reducing toxicity.

13.4.1 Pharmacokinetics of Mitoxantrone

Mitoxantrone can be given in intravenous doses of 8–12 mg/m^2 every 21–28 days (Forstpointner et al. 2004; Herold et al. 2007; Robak et al. 2006; Rodriguez et al. 1995; Zinzani et al. 2004). For leukemia, it can be given daily for 3–5 days at intravenous doses of 5–10 mg/m^2 (Ho et al. 1988; Sternberg et al. 2000; Wierzbowska et al. 2008). Clearance is triphasic, with short, middle, and terminal half-lives of 6–9 min, 1–3 h, and 20.8–21.5 h, respectively (Alberts et al. 1983; Ehninger et al. 1985; Mulder et al. 1989). Renal clearance accounts for only 4–5% of the dose over a 48 h period. Biliary excretion is the major route of elimination, accounting for around 30% of each dose (Alberts et al. 1983; Ehninger et al. 1985). Therefore, patients with bilirubin >3 should have a 25% dose reduction. No dose reduction is required for renal dysfunction. Volume of distribution has been reported from 1,875 to 2,248 L/m^2.

13.4.2 Pharmacodynamics of Mitoxantrone

Dose-limiting toxicities of mitoxantrone include leukopenia and thrombocytopenia, both of which are dose-related and reversible. Green discolorations of urine and serum have been noted at doses ≥10 mg/m^2. Above 12 mg/m^2, leukopenia and thrombocytopenia can be severe and prolonged (Alberts et al. 1980; Von Hoff et al. 1980). Nausea and vomiting are common, though easily controlled with antiemetics. Alopecia and increased risk of infection are also common with chronic use of mitoxantrone (Martinelli Boneschi et al. 2005).

Two phase I studies showed no cardiotoxicity. However, a later prospective study of mitoxantrone found that 6 of 20 patients had a decrease in left ventricular ejection fraction of at least 10% at total doses of 26–98 mg/m^2 (Vorobiof et al. 1985). Data from patients treated with mitoxantrone for multiple sclerosis indicate that cardiotoxicity risk increases with cumulative dose, but subclinical cardiac events can occur at doses below those considered safe. Overall, cardiotoxicity is seen in only 0.2–0.5% of patients, which represents a lower risk than with anthracyclines (Pattoneri et al. 2007).

13.4.3 Current Clinical Role of Mitoxantrone

Until docetaxel showed improved progression-free and overall survival, mitoxantrone was the standard of care for metastatic castration-resistant prostate cancer (Tannock et al. 1996, 2004). It is still approved for the use of metastatic prostate cancer for palliation. It was also approved for use in the treatment of refractory multiple sclerosis, based on preliminary data published in 2002 (Hartung et al. 2002).

Currently, the only other neoplastic indications for mitoxantrone are lymphoma and leukemia. For patients with indolent lymphomas requiring treatment, mitoxantrone can be combined with fludarabine as an alternative to R-CHOP for initial therapy (Zinzani et al. 2004). It can also be combined with rituximab and either fludarabine and cyclophosphamide or chlorambucil and prednisone in the same patient population (Forstpointner et al. 2004; Herold et al. 2007). In mantle cell lymphoma, the combination of rituximab, fludarabine, cyclophosphamide, and mitoxantrone is also effective (Forstpointner et al. 2004). For more aggressive, refractory lymphomas, mitoxantrone, mesna, ifosfamide, and etoposide constitute a possible salvage regimen (Rodriguez et al. 1995).

Mitoxantrone is also used in patients with recurrent or refractory acute myelogenous leukemia, and can be combined with etoposide and cytarabine (Ho et al. 1988), cladrabine and cytarabine (Wierzbowska et al. 2008), or cytarabine alone (Sternberg et al. 2000). For refractory and recurrent acute lymphocytic leukemia, mitoxantrone is combined with cladrabine and cyclophosphamide, a toxic regimen that requires close monitoring (Robak et al. 2006).

13.5 Amsacrine

Amsacrine, or 4'(9-acridinylamino)-methancsulfon-m-aniside (m-AMSA) is the unique aminoacridine anticancer agent to undergo full clinical development. Since it was initially described in 1974 by Cain and coworkers (Cain and Atwell 1974), m-AMSA first entered clinical evaluation under National Cancer Institute (NCI) sponsorship in 1976 (Cassileth and Gale 1986; Louie and Issell 1985).

13.5.1 Pharmacokinetics of Amsacrine

The volume of distribution of amsacrine exceeds the total water content, indicating amsacrine sequestration of the drug at some site, mostly the liver and/or protein binding. Amsacrine has a biphasic plasma disappearance curve with a $t_{1/2}\alpha$ of 10–30 min and a $t_{1/2}\beta$ of 7–9 h (Hall et al. 1983). Amsacrine is bound to plasma proteins and is eliminated primarily by metabolism in the liver and both parent and metabolites are excreted in the bile. In the liver, the major metabolite is the amsacrine-glutathion-5′-conjugate. Amsacrine and, to a greater degree, its metabolites are also excreted in urine. Patients with liver disease have a reduced ability to clear amsacrine from the plasma. Patients with moderate renal dysfunction but normal liver function clear amsacrine adequately (Arlin et al. 1980; Cassileth and Gale 1986; Louie and Issell 1985). However, in patients with severe renal impairment, amsacrine plasma clearance is markedly reduced, underlying that urinary excretion also must be an important route for the elimination of unchanged amsacrine. The optimal schedule of administration for amsacrine appears to be a single daily dose. It seems that little advantage is gained by continuous infusion schedules. Patients with normal hepatic function or mild liver dysfunction should tolerate full drug doses. Patients with significant liver dysfunction manifested by serum bilirubin greater than 2 mg/dL should have an initial 30% dose reduction. Subsequent dose escalation may be possible based on clinical tolerance. Patients with moderate renal dysfunction (serum creatinine in the range of 1.2–2 mg/dL) should receive full-dose therapy; however, oliguric patients or those with more serious renal disease (serum creatinine greater than 2 mg/dL) should have an initial 30% dose reduction (Arlin et al. 1980; Cassileth and Gale 1986; Louie and Issell 1985).

13.5.2 Pharmacodynamics of Amsacrine

The oral route is not used because of large and unpredictable inter-individual variability in absorption. Subsequent trials have used the intravenous route exclusively. Although a number of schedules of administration have been tested, the optimal schedules appear to be 150 mg/m^2/day for 5 days for adult patients with leukemia (Cassileth and Gale 1986; Louie and Issell 1985). In all phase I trials, the dose-limiting toxicity was myelosuppression (Cassileth and Gale 1986; Louie and Issell 1985). Antitumor activity was seen in a variety of tumor types, especially leukemias and lymphomas (Cassileth and Gale 1986; Louie and Issell 1985).

Myelosuppression is the most important and dose-limiting toxicity. The degree of myelosuppression is dose dependent and at standard doses, is reversible. Leukopenia, thrombocytopenia, and to a lesser extent anemia occur in virtually all patients. The WBC nadir occurs around the tenth day after administration, with hematologic recovery by the 25th day. Amsacrine causes phlebitis. Consequently, it is recommended to dilute amsacrine in 500 mL of 5% dextrose and to use a central line for continuous infusion or repeated treatments to avoid reactions at the injection site. Hearing loss and allergic reactions (anaphylaxis, urticaria and rashes, allergic edema) are relatively rare (Weiss 1992). Nausea and vomiting are common with amsacrine. Stomatitis becomes dose limiting for treatments with very high doses in association with bone marrow rescue (Meloni et al. 1990). The incidence of hepatotoxicity may reach 35%. Elevation of bilirubin, the most frequent abnormality, is usually dose related and reversible (Appelbaum and Shulman 1982). Since amsacrine is conjugated in the liver and is excreted in large part via the biliary system, at least 30% dose reduction is generally recommended in patients with impaired hepatic function (elevated bilirubin). Patients may develop arrhythmia, conducting disturbances, congestive heart failure during and after amsacrine administration (Weiss et al. 1983, 1986). More commonly, the heart rate is decreased by about 10%. Because hypokalemia may exacerbate arrhythmias, it has been recommended that serum potassium levels be maintained at or above 4 mEq/l at the time of drug administration. In most patients, amsacrine produces a significant prolongation (0,05–0,064 s) of the corrected QT (QT_c) interval. The amsacrine-associated QT_c prolongation may persist for up to 90 min. Tachyarrhythmias in the setting of QT_c prolongation usually arise by triggered automaticity and may be precipitated by adrenergic hyperactivity (Louie and Issell 1985; Weiss et al. 1983, 1986). Amsacrine also may reduce significantly the serum sodium and magnesium concentrations 20 min after the start of the infusion. The decrease in magnesium levels may contribute to the amsacrine-induced cardiac arrhythmias (Seymour 1993). Nevertheless, amsacrine has been administered safely to patients with myocardial dysfunction.

13.5.3 Clinical Role in 2011

Amsacrine is used primarily in the treatment of hematologic malignancies, with emphasis on pediatric and adult acute leukemias, and some activity in lymphomas (Cassileth and Gale 1986; Louie and Issell 1985). A variety of phase II trials demonstrated no useful activity against human solid tumor. Amsacrine has substantial efficacy in acute myeloblastic leukemia (AML) (Berman et al. 1989; Burnett et al. 2011) and acute lymphoblastic leukemia (ALL) (Zohren et al. 2009). In AML, m-AMSA has been demonstrated to be as effective as daunorubicin when combined with araC. It can provide high remission rates even in patients with previous exposure to anthracyclines and in both ALL and AML patients refractory to primary induction therapy. m-AMSA is also used in intensive consolidation therapy.

References

Ades L, Chevret S, Raffoux E, de Botton S, Guerci A, Pigneux A, Stoppa AM, Lamy T, Rigal-Huguet F, Vekhoff A, Meyer-Monard S, Maloisel F, Deconinck E, Ferrant A, Thomas X, Fegueux N, Chomienne C, Dombret H, Degos L, Fenaux P (2006) Is cytarabine useful in the treatment of acute promyelocytic leukemia? Results of a randomized trial from the European Acute Promyelocytic Leukemia Group. *J Clin Oncol* **24**(36): 5703–5710

Alberts DS, Bachur NR, Holtzman JL (1971) The pharmacokinetics of daunomycin in man. *Clin Pharmacol Ther* **12**(1): 96–104

Alberts DS, Griffith KS, Goodman GE, Herman TS, Murray E (1980) Phase I clinical trial of mitoxantrone: a new anthracenedione anticancer drug. *Cancer Chemother Pharmacol* **5**(1): 11–15

Alberts DS, Peng YM, Leigh S, Davis TP, Woodward DL (1983) Disposition of mitoxantrone in patients. *Cancer Treat Rev* **10 Suppl B**: 23–27

Allen LM, Creaven PJ (1975) Comparison of the human pharmacokinetics of VM-26 and VP-16, two antineoplastic epipodophyllotixin glucopyranoside derivatives. *Eur J Cancer* **11**(10): 697–707

Anderlini P, Benjamin RS, Wong FC, Kantarjian HM, Andreeff M, Kornblau SM, O'Brien S, Mackay B, Ewer MS, Pierce SA, et al. (1995) Idarubicin cardiotoxicity: a retrospective study in acute myeloid leukemia and myelodysplasia. *J Clin Oncol* **13**(11): 2827–2834

Appelbaum FR, Shulman HM (1982) Fatal hepatotoxicity associated with AMSA therapy. *Cancer Treat Rep* **66**(10): 1863–1865

Arbuck SG, Douglass HO, Crom WR, Goodwin P, Silk Y, Cooper C, Evans WE (1986) Etoposide pharmacokinetics in patients with normal and abnormal organ function. *J Clin Oncol* **4**(11): 1690–1695

Arcamone F, Bernardi L, Giardino P, Patelli B, Marco A, Casazza AM, Pratesi G, Reggiani P (1976) Synthesis and antitumor activity of 4-demethoxydaunorubicin, 4-demethoxy-7,9-diepidaunorubicin, and their beta anomers. *Cancer Treat Rep* **60**(7): 829–834

Arcamone F, Cassinelli G, Fantini G, Grein A, Orezzi P, Pol C, Spalla C (1969) Adriamycin, 14-hydroxydaunomycin, a new antitumor antibiotic from S. peucetius var. caesius. *Biotechnol Bioeng* **11**(6): 1101–1110

Arcamone F, Cassinelli G, Franceschi G, Penco S (1972) Structure and physicochemical properties of adriamycin (doxorubicin). In *International Symposium on Adriamycin*, Carter S, Di Marco A, Ghione M, Krakoff I, Mathe G (eds), pp 9–22. New York: Springer-Verlag

Arcamone F, Penco S, Vigevani A, Redaelli S, Franchi G, DiMarco A, Casazza AM, Dasdia T, Formelli F, Necco A, Soranzo C (1975) Synthesis and antitumor properties of new glycosides of daunomycinone and adriamycinone. *J Med Chem* **18**(7): 703–707

Arlin ZA, Sklaroff RB, Gee TS, Kempin SJ, Howard J, Clarkson BD, Young CW (1980) Phase I and II trial of 4'-(9-acridinylamino)methanesulfon-m-anisidide in patients with acute leukemia. *Cancer Res* **40**(9): 3304–3306

Armstrong GT, Liu Q, Yasui Y, Neglia JP, Leisenring W, Robison LL, Mertens AC (2009) Late mortality among 5-year survivors of childhood cancer: a summary from the Childhood Cancer Survivor Study. *J Clin Oncol* **27**(14): 2328–2338

Baas P, Belderbos JS, van den Heuvel M (2010) Chemoradiation therapy in nonsmall cell lung cancer. *Curr Opin Oncol* **23**(2): 140–149

Bachur NR (1971) Daunorubicinol, a major metabolite of daunorubicin: isolation from human urine and enzymatic reactions. *J Pharmacol Exp Ther* **177**(3): 573–578

Bedano PM, Brames MJ, Williams SD, Juliar BE, Einhorn LH (2006) Phase II study of cisplatin plus epirubicin salvage chemotherapy in refractory germ cell tumors. *J Clin Oncol* **24**(34): 5403–5407

Benjamin RS, Riggs CE, Jr., Bachur NR (1973) Pharmacokinetics and metabolism of adriamycin in man. *Clin Pharmacol Ther* **14**(4): 592–600

Benjamin RS, Wiernik PH, Bachur NR (1974) Adriamycin chemotherapy--efficacy, safety, and pharmacologic basis of an intermittent single high-dosage schedule. *Cancer* **33**(1): 19–27

Berman E, Arlin ZA, Gaynor J, Miller W, Gee T, Kempin SJ, Mertelsmann R, Andreeff M, Reich L, Nahmias N, et al. (1989) Comparative trial of cytarabine and thioguanine in combination with amsacrine or daunorubicin in patients with untreated acute nonlymphocytic leukemia: results of the L-16M protocol. *Leukemia* **3**(2): 115–121

Bonadonna G, Bonfante V, Viviani S, Di Russo A, Villani F, Valagussa P (2004) ABVD plus subtotal nodal versus involved-field radiotherapy in early-stage Hodgkin's disease: long-term results. *J Clin Oncol* **22**(14): 2835–2841

Borchmann P, Hubel K, Schnell R, Engert A (1997) Idarubicin: a brief overview on pharmacology and clinical use. *Int J Clin Pharmacol Ther* **35**(2): 80–83

Budman DR, Igwemezie LN, Kaul S, Behr J, Lichtman S, Schulman P, Vinciguerra V, Allen SL, Kolitz J, Hock K, et al. (1994) Phase I evaluation of a water-soluble etoposide prodrug, etoposide phosphate, given as a 5-minute infusion on days 1, 3, and 5 in patients with solid tumors. *J Clin Oncol* **12**(9): 1902–1909

Burnett A, Wetzler M, Lowenberg B (2011) Therapeutic advances in acute myeloid leukemia. *J Clin Oncol* **29**(5): 487–494

Burstein HJ, Parker LM, Keshaviah A, Doherty J, Partridge AH, Schapira L, Ryan PD, Younger J, Harris LN, Moy B, Come SE, Schumer ST, Bunnell CA, Haldoupis M, Gelman R, Winer EP (2005) Efficacy of pegfilgrastim and darbepoetin alfa as hematopoietic support for dose-dense every-2-week adjuvant breast cancer chemotherapy. *J Clin Oncol* **23**(33): 8340–8347

Cain BF, Atwell GJ (1974) The experimental antitumour properties of three congeners of the acridylmethanesulphonanilide (AMSA) series. *Eur J Cancer* **10**(8): 539–549

Canellos GP, Anderson JR, Propert KJ, Nissen N, Cooper MR, Henderson ES, Green MR, Gottlieb A, Peterson BA (1992) Chemotherapy of advanced Hodgkin's disease with MOPP, ABVD, or MOPP alternating with ABVD. *N Engl J Med* **327**(21): 1478–1484

Cassileth PA, Gale RP (1986) Amsacrine: a review. *Leuk Res* **10**(11): 1257–1265

Chrzanowska M, Sobiak J, Grund G, Wachowiak J (2010) Pharmacokinetics of high-dose etoposide administered in combination with fractionated total-body irradiation as conditioning for allogeneic hematopoietic stem cell transplantation in children with acute lymphoblastic leukemia. *Pediatr Transplant* **15**(1): 96–102

Cummings J, Milstead R, Cunningham D, Kaye S (1986) Marked inter-patient variation in adriamycin biotransformation to 7-deoxyaglycones: evidence from metabolites identified in serum. *Eur J Cancer Clin Oncol* **22**(8): 991–1001

Cunningham D, Allum WH, Stenning SP, Thompson JN, Van de Velde CJ, Nicolson M, Scarffe JH, Lofts FJ, Falk SJ, Iveson TJ, Smith DB, Langley RE, Verma M, Weeden S, Chua YJ, Participants MT (2006) Perioperative chemotherapy versus surgery alone for resectable gastroesophageal cancer. *N Engl J Med* **355**(1): 11–20

Cunningham D, Starling N, Rao S, Iveson T, Nicolson M, Coxon F, Middleton G, Daniel F, Oates J, Norman AR (2008) Capecitabine and oxaliplatin for advanced esophagogastric cancer. *N Engl J Med* **358**(1): 36–46

Czuczman MS, Weaver R, Alkuzweny B, Berlfein J, Grillo-Lopez AJ (2004) Prolonged clinical and molecular remission in patients with low-grade or follicular non-Hodgkin's lymphoma treated with rituximab plus CHOP chemotherapy: 9-year follow-up. *J Clin Oncol* **22**(23): 4711–4716

D'Incalci M, Farina P, Sessa C, Mangioni C, Conter V, Masera G, Rocchetti M, Pisoni MB, Piazza E, Beer M, Cavalli F (1982) Pharmacokinetics of VP16-213 given by different administration methods. *Cancer Chemother Pharmacol* **7**(2–3): 141–145

D'Incalci M, Rossi C, Zucchetti M, Urso R, Cavalli F, Mangioni C, Willems Y, Sessa C (1986) Pharmacokinetics of etoposide in patients with abnormal renal and hepatic function. *Cancer Res* **46**(5): 2566–2571

Dang C, Fornier M, Sugarman S, Troso-Sandoval T, Lake D, D'Andrea G, Seidman A, Sklarin N, Dickler M, Currie V, Gilewski T, Moynahan ME, Drullinsky P, Robson M, Wasserheit-Leiblich C, Mills N, Steingart R, Panageas K, Norton L, Hudis C (2008) The safety of dose-dense doxorubicin and cyclophosphamide followed by paclitaxel with trastuzumab in HER-2/neu overexpressed/amplified breast cancer. *J Clin Oncol* **26**(8): 1216–1222

Dann EJ, Bar-Shalom R, Tamir A, Haim N, Ben-Shachar M, Avivi I, Zuckerman T, Kirschbaum M, Goor O, Libster D, Rowe JM, Epelbaum R (2007) Risk-adapted BEACOPP regimen can reduce the cumulative dose of chemotherapy for standard and high-risk Hodgkin lymphoma with no impairment of outcome. *Blood* **109**(3): 905–909

Diehl V, Franklin J, Pfreundschuh M, Lathan B, Paulus U, Hasenclever D, Tesch H, Herrmann R, Dorken B, Muller-Hermelink HK, Duhmke E, Loeffler M (2003) Standard and increased-dose BEACOPP chemotherapy compared with COPP-ABVD for advanced Hodgkin's disease. *N Engl J Med* **348**(24): 2386–2395

Dimarco A, Gaetani M, Orezzi P, Scarpinato BM, Silvestrini R, Soldati M, Dasdia T, Valentini L (1964) 'Daunomycin', a New Antibiotic of the Rhodomycin Group. *Nature* **201**: 706–707

Ehninger G, Proksch B, Heinzel G, Schiller E, Weible KH, Woodward DL (1985) The pharmacokinetics and metabolism of mitoxantrone in man. *Invest New Drugs* **3**(2): 109–116

Einhorn LH, Williams SD, Chamness A, Brames MJ, Perkins SM, Abonour R (2007) High-dose chemotherapy and stem-cell rescue for metastatic germ-cell tumors. *N Engl J Med* **357**(4): 340–348

Engert A, Franklin J, Eich HT, Brillant C, Sehlen S, Cartoni C, Herrmann R, Pfreundschuh M, Sieber M, Tesch H, Franke A, Koch P, de Wit M, Paulus U, Hasenclever D, Loeffler M, Muller RP, Muller-Hermelink HK, Duhmke E, Diehl V (2007) Two cycles of doxorubicin, bleomycin, vinblastine, and dacarbazine plus extended-field radiotherapy is superior to radiotherapy alone in early favorable Hodgkin's lymphoma: final results of the GHSG HD7 trial. *J Clin Oncol* **25**(23): 3495–3502

Estey E, Garcia-Manero G, Ferrajoli A, Faderl S, Verstovsek S, Jones D, Kantarjian H (2006) Use of all-trans retinoic acid plus arsenic trioxide as an alternative to chemotherapy in untreated acute promyelocytic leukemia. *Blood* **107**(9): 3469–3473

Fenaux P (1993) The role of all-trans-retinoic acid in the treatment of acute promyelocytic leukemia. *Acta Haematol* **89 Suppl 1**: 22–27

Feng F, Xiang Y, Wan X, Geng S, Wang T (2011) Salvage combination chemotherapy with floxuridine, dactinomycin, etoposide, and vincristine (FAEV) for patients with relapsed/chemoresistant gestational trophoblastic neoplasia. *Ann Oncol*

Ferrandina G, Ludovisi M, Lorusso D, Pignata S, Breda E, Savarese A, Del Medico P, Scaltriti L, Katsaros D, Priolo D, Scambia G (2008) Phase III trial of gemcitabine compared with pegylated liposomal doxorubicin in progressive or recurrent ovarian cancer. *J Clin Oncol* **26**(6): 890–896

Feugier P, Van Hoof A, Sebban C, Solal-Celigny P, Bouabdallah R, Ferme C, Christian B, Lepage E, Tilly H, Morschhauser F, Gaulard P, Salles G, Bosly A, Gisselbrecht C, Reyes F, Coiffier B (2005) Long-term results of the R-CHOP study in the treatment of elderly patients with diffuse large B-cell lymphoma: a study by the Groupe d'Etude des Lymphomes de l'Adulte. *J Clin Oncol* **23**(18): 4117–4126

Fisher B, Jeong JH, Anderson S, Wolmark N (2004) Treatment of axillary lymph node-negative, estrogen receptor-negative breast cancer: updated findings from National Surgical Adjuvant Breast and Bowel Project clinical trials. *J Natl Cancer Inst* **96**(24): 1823–1831

Fjallskog ML, Granberg DP, Welin SL, Eriksson C, Oberg KE, Janson ET, Eriksson BK (2001) Treatment with cisplatin and etoposide in patients with neuroendocrine tumors. *Cancer* **92**(5): 1101–1107

Fleming GF, Brunetto VL, Cella D, Look KY, Reid GC, Munkarah AR, Kline R, Burger RA, Goodman A, Burks RT (2004) Phase III trial of doxorubicin plus cisplatin with or without paclitaxel plus filgrastim in advanced endometrial carcinoma: a Gynecologic Oncology Group Study. *J Clin Oncol* **22**(11): 2159–2166

Fornasiero A, Daniele O, Ghiotto C, Piazza M, Fiore-Donati L, Calabro F, Rea F, Fiorentino MV (1991) Chemotherapy for invasive thymoma. A 13-year experience. *Cancer* **68**(1): 30–33

Forstpointner R, Dreyling M, Repp R, Hermann S, Hanel A, Metzner B, Pott C, Hartmann F, Rothmann F, Rohrberg R, Bock HP, Wandt H, Unterhalt M, Hiddemann W (2004) The addition of rituximab to a combination of fludarabine, cyclophosphamide, mitoxantrone (FCM) significantly increases the response rate and prolongs survival as compared with FCM alone in patients with relapsed and refractory follicular and mantle cell lymphomas: results of a prospective randomized study of the German Low-Grade Lymphoma Study Group. *Blood* **104**(10): 3064–3071

Ganzina F (1983) 4'-epi-doxorubicin, a new analogue of doxorubicin: a preliminary overview of preclinical and clinical data. *Cancer Treat Rev* **10**(1): 1–22

Germann N, Gross-Goupil M, Wasserman E, Emile JF, Misset JL, Reynes M, Goldwasser F (2002) The chemotherapy of metastatic gastric adenocarcinomas with hypersecretion of alpha-fetoprotein or beta-human chorionic gonadotrophin: report of two cases. *Ann Oncol* **13**(4): 632–636

Greene RF, Collins JM, Jenkins JF, Speyer JL, Myers CE (1983) Plasma pharmacokinetics of adriamycin and adriamycinol: implications for the design of in vitro experiments and treatment protocols. *Cancer Res* **43**(7): 3417–3421

Grier HE, Krailo MD, Tarbell NJ, Link MP, Fryer CJ, Pritchard DJ, Gebhardt MC, Dickman PS, Perlman EJ, Meyers PA, Donaldson SS, Moore S, Rausen AR, Vietti TJ, Miser JS (2003) Addition of ifosfamide and etoposide to standard chemotherapy for Ewing's sarcoma and primitive neuroectodermal tumor of bone. *N Engl J Med* **348**(8): 694–701

Grimison PS, Stockler MR, Thomson DB, Olver IN, Harvey VJ, Gebski VJ, Lewis CR, Levi JA, Boyer MJ, Gurney H, Craft P, Boland AL, Simes RJ, Toner GC (2010) Comparison of two standard chemotherapy regimens for good-prognosis germ cell tumors: updated analysis of a randomized trial. *J Natl Cancer Inst* **102**(16): 1253–1262

Grossman HB, Natale RB, Tangen CM, Speights VO, Vogelzang NJ, Trump DL, deVere White RW, Sarosdy MF, Wood DP, Jr., Raghavan D, Crawford ED (2003) Neoadjuvant chemotherapy plus cystectomy compared with cystectomy alone for locally advanced bladder cancer. *N Engl J Med* **349**(9): 859–866

Habermann TM, Weller EA, Morrison VA, Gascoyne RD, Cassileth PA, Cohn JB, Dakhil SR, Woda B, Fisher RI, Peterson BA, Horning SJ (2006) Rituximab-CHOP versus CHOP alone or with maintenance rituximab in older patients with diffuse large B-cell lymphoma. *J Clin Oncol* **24**(19): 3121–3127

Halazun JF, Wagner HR, Gaeta JF, Sinks LF (1974) Proceedings: Daunorubicin cardiac toxicity in children with acute lymphocytic leukemia. *Cancer* **33**(2): 545–554

Hall SW, Friedman J, Legha SS, Benjamin RS, Gutterman JU, Loo TL (1983) Human pharmacokinetics of a new acridine derivative, 4'-(9-acridinylamino)methanesulfon-m-anisidide (NSC 249992). *Cancer Res* **43**(7): 3422–3426

Han KS, Joung JY, Kim TS, Jeong IG, Seo HK, Chung J, Lee KH (2008) Methotrexate, vinblastine, doxorubicin and cisplatin combination regimen as salvage chemotherapy for patients with advanced or metastatic transitional cell carcinoma after failure of gemcitabine and cisplatin chemotherapy. *Br J Cancer* **98**(1): 86–90

Hande KR, Wedlund PJ, Noone RM, Wilkinson GR, Greco FA, Wolff SN (1984) Pharmacokinetics of high-dose etoposide (VP-16-213) administered to cancer patients. *Cancer Res* **44**(1): 379–382

Hande KR, Wolff SN, Greco FA, Hainsworth JD, Reed G, Johnson DH (1990) Etoposide kinetics in patients with obstructive jaundice. *J Clin Oncol* **8**(6): 1101–1107

Harris PA, Gross JF (1975) Preliminary pharmacokinetic model for adriamycin (NSC-123127). *Cancer Chemother Rep* **59**(4): 819–825

Hartung HP, Gonsette R, Konig N, Kwiecinski H, Guseo A, Morrissey SP, Krapf H, Zwingers T (2002) Mitoxantrone in progressive multiple sclerosis: a placebo-controlled, double-blind, randomised, multicentre trial. *Lancet* **360**(9350): 2018–2025

Hasbini A, Mahjoubi R, Fandi A, Chouaki N, Taamma A, Lianes P, Cortes-Funes H, Alonso S, Armand JP, Cvitkovic E, Raymond E (1999) Phase II trial combining mitomycin with 5-fluorouracil, epirubicin, and cisplatin in recurrent and metastatic undifferentiated carcinoma of nasopharyngeal type. *Ann Oncol* **10**(4): 421–425

Haugnes HS, Wethal T, Aass N, Dahl O, Klepp O, Langberg CW, Wilsgaard T, Bremnes RM, Fossa SD (2010) Cardiovascular risk factors and morbidity in long-term survivors of testicular cancer: a 20-year follow-up study. *J Clin Oncol* **28**(30): 4649–4657

Herold M, Haas A, Srock S, Neser S, Al-Ali KH, Neubauer A, Dolken G, Naumann R, Knauf W, Freund M, Rohrberg R, Hoffken K, Franke A, Ittel T, Kettner E, Haak U, Mey U, Klinkenstein C, Assmann M, von Grunhagen U (2007) Rituximab added to first-line mitoxantrone, chlorambucil, and prednisolone chemotherapy followed by interferon maintenance prolongs survival in patients with advanced follicular lymphoma: an East German Study Group Hematology and Oncology Study. *J Clin Oncol* **25**(15): 1986–1992

Ho AD, Lipp T, Ehninger G, Illiger HJ, Meyer P, Freund M, Hunstein W (1988) Combination of mitoxantrone and etoposide in refractory acute myelogenous leukemia--an active and well-tolerated regimen. *J Clin Oncol* **6**(2): 213–217

Huffman DH, Bachur NR (1972) Daunorubicin metabolism in acute myelocytic leukemia. *Blood* **39**(5): 637–643

Hutchins LF, Green SJ, Ravdin PM, Lew D, Martino S, Abeloff M, Lyss AP, Allred C, Rivkin SE, Osborne CK (2005) Randomized, controlled trial of cyclophosphamide, methotrexate, and fluorouracil versus cyclophosphamide, doxorubicin, and fluorouracil with and without tamoxifen for high-risk, node-negative breast cancer: treatment results of Intergroup Protocol INT-0102. *J Clin Oncol* **23**(33): 8313–8321

Ibrahim A, Goldwasser F, Pico JL. (1992) Autologous hematopoietic stem cells transplantation. In *Handbook of Chemotherapy in Clinical Oncology*, Droz JP, Cvitkovic E, Armand JP, Khoury S (ed). F.I.I.S

Jiang J, Liang X, Zhou X, Huang L, Huang R, Chu Z, Zhan Q (2010) A meta-analysis of randomized controlled trials comparing irinotecan/platinum with etoposide/platinum in patients with previously untreated extensive-stage small cell lung cancer. *J Thorac Oncol* **5**(6): 867–873

Joensuu H, Kellokumpu-Lehtinen PL, Bono P, Alanko T, Kataja V, Asola R, Utriainen T, Kokko R, Hemminki A, Tarkkanen M, Turpeenniemi-Hujanen T, Jyrkkio S, Flander M, Helle L, Ingalsuo S, Johansson K, Jaaskelainen AS, Pajunen M, Rauhala M, Kaleva-Kerola J, Salminen T, Leinonen M, Elomaa I, Isola J (2006) Adjuvant docetaxel or vinorelbine with or without trastuzumab for breast cancer. *N Engl J Med* **354**(8): 809–820

Jones SE, Savin MA, Holmes FA, O'Shaughnessy JA, Blum JL, Vukelja S, McIntyre KJ, Pippen JE, Bordelon JH, Kirby R, Sandbach J, Hyman WJ, Khandelwal P, Negron AG, Richards DA, Anthony SP, Mennel RG, Boehm KA, Meyer WG, Asmar L (2006) Phase III trial comparing doxorubicin plus cyclophosphamide with docetaxel plus cyclophosphamide as adjuvant therapy for operable breast cancer. *J Clin Oncol* **24**(34): 5381–5387

Josting A, Muller H, Borchmann P, Baars JW, Metzner B, Dohner H, Aurer I, Smardova L, Fischer T, Niederwieser D, Schafer-Eckart K, Schmitz N, Sureda A, Glossmann J, Diehl V, DeJong D, Hansmann ML, Raemaekers J, Engert A (2010) Dose intensity of chemotherapy in patients with relapsed Hodgkin's lymphoma. *J Clin Oncol* **28**(34): 5074–5080

Kim JE, Lee DH, Yoo C, Kim S, Kim SW, Lee JS, Park CJ, Huh J, Suh C (2010) BEAM or BuCyE high-dose chemotherapy followed by autologous stem cell transplantation in non-Hodgkin's lymphoma patients: a single center comparative analysis of efficacy and toxicity. *Leuk Res* **35**(2): 183–187

Lai CL, Wu PC, Chan GC, Lok AS, Lin HJ (1988) Doxorubicin versus no antitumor therapy in inoperable hepatocellular carcinoma. A prospective randomized trial. *Cancer* **62**(3): 479–483

Langley RE, Carmichael J, Jones AL, Cameron DA, Qian W, Uscinska B, Howell A, Parmar M (2005) Phase III trial of epirubicin plus paclitaxel compared with epirubicin plus cyclophosphamide as first-line chemotherapy for metastatic breast cancer: United Kingdom National Cancer Research Institute trial AB01. *J Clin Oncol* **23**(33): 8322–8330

Larson RA, Dodge RK, Linker CA, Stone RM, Powell BL, Lee EJ, Schulman P, Davey FR, Frankel SR, Bloomfield CD, George SL, Schiffer CA (1998) A randomized controlled trial of filgrastim during remission induction and consolidation chemotherapy for adults with acute lymphoblastic leukemia: CALGB study 9111. *Blood* **92**(5): 1556–1564

Le Cesne A, Judson I, Crowther D, Rodenhuis S, Keizer HJ, Van Hoesel Q, Blay JY, Frisch J, Van Glabbeke M, Hermans C, Van Oosterom A, Tursz T, Verweij J (2000) Randomized phase III study comparing conventional-dose doxorubicin plus ifosfamide versus high-dose doxorubicin plus ifosfamide plus recombinant human granulocyte-macrophage colony-stimulating factor in advanced soft tissue sarcomas: A trial of the European Organization for Research and Treatment of Cancer/Soft Tissue and Bone Sarcoma Group. *J Clin Oncol* **18**(14): 2676–2684

Le Deley MC, Leblanc T, Shamsaldin A, Raquin MA, Lacour B, Sommelet D, Chompret A, Cayuela JM, Bayle C, Bernheim A, de Vathaire F, Vassal G, Hill C (2003) Risk of secondary leukemia after a solid tumor in childhood according to the dose of epipodophyllotoxins and anthracyclines: a case-control study by the Societe Francaise d'Oncologie Pediatrique. *J Clin Oncol* **21**(6): 1074–1081

Lefrak EA, Pitha J, Rosenheim S, Gottlieb JA (1973) A clinicopathologic analysis of adriamycin cardiotoxicity. *Cancer* **32**(2): 302–314

Legha SS, Benjamin RS, Mackay B, Ewer M, Wallace S, Valdivieso M, Rasmussen SL, Blumenschein GR, Freireich EJ (1982) Reduction of doxorubicin cardiotoxicity by prolonged continuous intravenous infusion. *Ann Intern Med* **96**(2): 133–139

Lenz G, Dreyling M, Hoster E, Wormann B, Duhrsen U, Metzner B, Eimermacher H, Neubauer A, Wandt H, Steinhauer H, Martin S, Heidemann E, Aldaoud A, Parwaresch R, Hasford J, Unterhalt M, Hiddemann W (2005) Immunochemotherapy with rituximab and cyclophosphamide, doxorubicin, vincristine, and prednisone significantly improves response and time to treatment failure, but not long-term outcome in patients with previously untreated mantle cell lymphoma: results of a prospective randomized trial of the German Low Grade Lymphoma Study Group (GLSG). *J Clin Oncol* **23**(9): 1984–1992

Levine MN, Pritchard KI, Bramwell VH, Shepherd LE, Tu D, Paul N (2005) Randomized trial comparing cyclophosphamide, epirubicin, and fluorouracil with cyclophosphamide, methotrexate, and fluorouracil in premenopausal women with node-positive breast cancer: update of National Cancer Institute of Canada Clinical Trials Group Trial MA5. *J Clin Oncol* **23**(22): 5166–5170

Linker CA, Levitt LJ, O'Donnell M, Forman SJ, Ries CA (1991) Treatment of adult acute lymphoblastic leukemia with intensive cyclical chemotherapy: a follow-up report. *Blood* **78**(11): 2814–2822

Linker CA, Levitt LJ, O'Donnell M, Ries CA, Link MP, Forman SJ, Farbstein MJ (1987) Improved results of treatment of adult acute lymphoblastic leukemia. *Blood* **69**(4): 1242–1248

Loehrer PJ, Sr., Kim K, Aisner SC, Livingston R, Einhorn LH, Johnson D, Blum R (1994) Cisplatin plus doxorubicin plus cyclophosphamide in metastatic or recurrent thymoma: final results of an intergroup trial. The Eastern Cooperative Oncology Group, Southwest Oncology Group, and Southeastern Cancer Study Group. *J Clin Oncol* **12**(6): 1164–1168

Logothetis CJ, Dexeus FH, Finn L, Sella A, Amato RJ, Ayala AG, Kilbourn RG (1990) A prospective randomized trial comparing MVAC and CISCA chemotherapy for patients with metastatic urothelial tumors. *J Clin Oncol* **8**(6): 1050–1055

Louie AC, Issell BF (1985) Amsacrine (AMSA)–a clinical review. *J Clin Oncol* **3**(4): 562–592

Lu K, Savaraj N, Kavanagh J, Feun LG, Burgess M, Bodey GP, Loo TL (1986) Clinical pharmacology of 4-demethoxydaunorubicin (DMDR). *Cancer Chemother Pharmacol* **17**(2): 143–148

Magrath I, Adde M, Shad A, Venzon D, Seibel N, Gootenberg J, Neely J, Arndt C, Nieder M, Jaffe E, Wittes RA, Horak ID (1996) Adults and children with small non-cleaved-cell lymphoma have a similar excellent outcome when treated with the same chemotherapy regimen. *J Clin Oncol* **14**(3): 925–934

Mamounas EP, Bryant J, Lembersky B, Fehrenbacher L, Sedlacek SM, Fisher B, Wickerham DL, Yothers G, Soran A, Wolmark N (2005) Paclitaxel after doxorubicin plus cyclophosphamide as adjuvant chemotherapy for node-positive breast cancer: results from NSABP B-28. *J Clin Oncol* **23**(16): 3686–3696

Martin M, Pienkowski T, Mackey J, Pawlicki M, Guastalla JP, Weaver C, Tomiak E, Al-Tweigeri T, Chap L, Juhos E, Guevin R, Howell A, Fornander T, Hainsworth J, Coleman R, Vinholes J, Modiano M, Pinter T, Tang SC, Colwell B, Prady C, Provencher L, Walde D, Rodriguez-Lescure A, Hugh J, Loret C, Rupin M, Blitz S, Jacobs P, Murawsky M, Riva A, Vogel C (2005) Adjuvant docetaxel for node-positive breast cancer. *N Engl J Med* **352**(22): 2302–2313

Martin M, Villar A, Sole-Calvo A, Gonzalez R, Massuti B, Lizon J, Camps C, Carrato A, Casado A, Candel MT, Albanell J, Aranda J, Munarriz B, Campbell J, Diaz-Rubio E (2003) Doxorubicin in combination with fluorouracil and cyclophosphamide (i.v. FAC regimen, day 1, 21) versus methotrexate in combination with fluorouracil and cyclophosphamide (i.v. CMF regimen, day 1, 21) as adjuvant chemotherapy for operable breast cancer: a study by the GEICAM group. *Ann Oncol* **14**(6): 833–842

Martinelli Boneschi F, Rovaris M, Capra R, Comi G (2005) Mitoxantrone for multiple sclerosis. *Cochrane Database Syst Rev* (4): CD002127

Meloni G, De Fabritiis P, Petti MC, Mandelli F (1990) BAVC regimen and autologous bone marrow transplantation in patients with acute myelogenous leukemia in second remission. *Blood* **75**(12): 2282–2285

Moebus V, Jackisch C, Lueck HJ, du Bois A, Thomssen C, Kurbacher C, Kuhn W, Nitz U, Schneeweiss A, Huober J, Harbeck N, von Minckwitz G, Runnebaum IB, Hinke A, Kreienberg R, Konecny GE, Untch M (2010) Intense dose-dense sequential chemotherapy with epirubicin, paclitaxel, and cyclophosphamide compared with conventionally scheduled chemotherapy in high-risk primary breast cancer: mature results of an AGO phase III study. *J Clin Oncol* **28**(17): 2874–2880

Moertel CG, Lefkopoulo M, Lipsitz S, Hahn RG, Klaassen D (1992) Streptozocin-doxorubicin, streptozocin-fluorouracil or chlorozotocin in the treatment of advanced islet-cell carcinoma. *N Engl J Med* **326**(8): 519–523

Mulder PO, Sleijfer DT, Willemse PH, de Vries EG, Uges DR, Mulder NH (1989) High-dose cyclophosphamide or melphalan with escalating doses of mitoxantrone and autologous bone marrow transplantation for refractory solid tumors. *Cancer Res* **49**(16): 4654–4658

Murdock KC, Child RG, Fabio PF, Angier RB, Wallace RE, Durr FE, Citarella RV (1979) Antitumor agents. 1. 1,4-Bis[(aminoalkyl)amino]-9,10-anthracenediones. *J Med Chem* **22**(9): 1024–1030

Mutch DG, Orlando M, Goss T, Teneriello MG, Gordon AN, McMeekin SD, Wang Y, Scribner DR, Jr., Marciniack M, Naumann RW, Secord AA (2007) Randomized phase III trial of gemcitabine compared with pegylated liposomal doxorubicin in patients with platinum-resistant ovarian cancer. *J Clin Oncol* **25**(19): 2811–2818

Oakervee HE, Popat R, Curry N, Smith P, Morris C, Drake M, Agrawal S, Stec J, Schenkein D, Esseltine DL, Cavenagh JD (2005) PAD combination therapy (PS-341/bortezomib, doxorubicin and dexamethasone) for previously untreated patients with multiple myeloma. *Br J Haematol* **129**(6): 755–762

Pastore D, Specchia G, Carluccio P, Liso A, Mestice A, Rizzi R, Greco G, Buquicchio C, Liso V (2003) FLAG-IDA in the treatment of refractory/relapsed acute myeloid leukemia: single-center experience. *Ann Hematol* **82**(4): 231–235

Pattoneri P, Pela G, Montanari E, Pesci I, Moruzzi P, Borghetti A (2007) Evaluation of the myocardial performance index for early detection of mitoxantrone-induced cardiotoxicity in patients with multiple sclerosis. *Eur J Echocardiogr* **8**(2): 144–150

Pectasides D, Xiros N, Papaxoinis G, Aravantinos G, Sykiotis C, Pectasides E, Psyrri A, Koumarianou A, Gaglia A, Gouveris P, Economopoulos T (2008) Gemcitabine and pegylated liposomal doxorubicin alternating with cisplatin plus cyclophosphamide in platinum refractory/resistant, paclitaxel-pretreated, ovarian carcinoma. *Gynecol Oncol* **108**(1): 47–52

Pedersen-Bjergaard J, Daugaard G, Hansen SW, Philip P, Larsen SO, Rorth M (1991) Increased risk of myelodysplasia and leukaemia after etoposide, cisplatin, and bleomycin for germ-cell tumours. *Lancet* **338**(8763): 359–363

Pommier Y, Goldwasser F (2011) Topoisomerase II Inhibitors: The Epipodophyllotoxins. In *Cancer Chemotherapy and Biotherapy: Principles and Practice*, Chabner BA, Longo DL (ed), Fifth Edition edn, 19, pp 392–410. Philadelphia: Lippincott Williams & Wilkins

Pommier Y, Leo E, Zhang H, Marchand C (2010) DNA topoisomerases and their poisoning by anticancer and antibacterial drugs. *Chem Biol* **17**(5): 421–433

Poole CJ, Earl HM, Hiller L, Dunn JA, Bathers S, Grieve RJ, Spooner DA, Agrawal RK, Fernando IN, Brunt AM, O'Reilly SM, Crawford SM, Rea DW, Simmonds P, Mansi JL, Stanley A, Harvey P, McAdam K, Foster L, Leonard RC, Twelves CJ (2006) Epirubicin and cyclophosphamide, methotrexate, and fluorouracil as adjuvant therapy for early breast cancer. *N Engl J Med* **355**(18): 1851–1862

Poon D, Yap SP, Mancer K, Quek ST, Soh LT (2004) Induction chemotherapy followed by radiotherapy in Merkel-cell carcinoma. *Lancet Oncol* **5**(8): 509–510

Poulsen M, Rischin D, Walpole E, Harvey J, Mackintosh J, Ainslie J, Hamilton C, Keller J, Tripcony L (2003) High-risk Merkel cell carcinoma of the skin treated with synchronous carboplatin/etoposide and radiation: a Trans-Tasman Radiation Oncology Group Study--TROG 96:07. *J Clin Oncol* **21**(23): 4371–4376

Randall ME, Filiaci VL, Muss H, Spirtos NM, Mannel RS, Fowler J, Thigpen JT, Benda JA (2006) Randomized phase III trial of whole-abdominal irradiation versus doxorubicin and cisplatin chemotherapy in advanced endometrial carcinoma: a Gynecologic Oncology Group Study. *J Clin Oncol* **24**(1): 36–44

Ratain MJ, Mick R, Schilsky RL, Vogelzang NJ, Berezin F (1991) Pharmacologically based dosing of etoposide: a means of safely increasing dose intensity. *J Clin Oncol* **9**(8): 1480–1486

Rizzieri DA, Johnson JL, Niedzwiecki D, Lee EJ, Vardiman JW, Powell BL, Barcos M, Bloomfield CD, Schiffer CA, Peterson BA, Canellos GP, Larson RA (2004) Intensive chemotherapy with and without cranial radiation for Burkitt leukemia and lymphoma: final results of Cancer and Leukemia Group B Study 9251. *Cancer* **100**(7): 1438–1448

Robak T, Blonski JZ, Gora-Tybor J, Jamroziak K, Dwilewicz-Trojaczek J, Tomaszewska A, Konopka L, Ceglarek B, Dmoszynska A, Kowal M, Kloczko J, Stella-Holowiecka B, Sulek K, Calbecka M, Zawilska K, Kuliczkowski K, Skotnicki AB, Warzocha K, Kasznicki M (2006) Cladribine alone and in combination with cyclophosphamide or cyclophosphamide plus mitoxantrone in the treatment of progressive chronic lymphocytic leukemia: report of a prospective, multicenter, randomized trial of the Polish Adult Leukemia Group (PALG CLL2). *Blood* **108**(2): 473–479

Robert J, Rigal-Huguet F, Hurteloup P (1992) Comparative pharmacokinetic study of idarubicin and daunorubicin in leukemia patients. *Hematol Oncol* **10**(2): 111–116

Roche H, Fumoleau P, Spielmann M, Canon JL, Delozier T, Serin D, Symann M, Kerbrat P, Soulie P, Eichler F, Viens P, Monnier A, Vindevoghel A, Campone M, Goudier MJ, Bonneterre J, Ferrero JM, Martin AL, Geneve J, Asselain B (2006) Sequential adjuvant epirubicin-based and docetaxel chemotherapy for node-positive breast cancer patients: the FNCLCC PACS 01 Trial. *J Clin Oncol* **24**(36): 5664–5671

Rodman JH, Murry DJ, Madden T, Santana VM (1994) Altered etoposide pharmacokinetics and time to engraftment in pediatric patients undergoing autologous bone marrow transplantation. *J Clin Oncol* **12**(11): 2390–2397

Rodriguez MA, Cabanillas FC, Hagemeister FB, McLaughlin P, Romaguera JE, Swan F, Velasquez W (1995) A phase II trial of mesna/ifosfamide, mitoxantrone and etoposide for refractory lymphomas. *Ann Oncol* **6**(6): 609–611

Romond EH, Perez EA, Bryant J, Suman VJ, Geyer CE, Jr., Davidson NE, Tan-Chiu E, Martino S, Paik S, Kaufman PA, Swain SM, Pisansky TM, Fehrenbacher L, Kutteh LA, Vogel VG, Visscher DW, Yothers G, Jenkins RB, Brown AM, Dakhil SR, Mamounas EP, Lingle WL, Klein PM, Ingle JN, Wolmark N (2005) Trastuzumab plus adjuvant chemotherapy for operable HER2-positive breast cancer. *N Engl J Med* **353**(16): 1673–1684

Roth AD, Fazio N, Stupp R, Falk S, Bernhard J, Saletti P, Koberle D, Borner MM, Rufibach K, Maibach R, Wernli M, Leslie M, Glynne-Jones R, Widmer L, Seymour M, de Braud F (2007) Docetaxel, cisplatin, and fluorouracil; docetaxel and cisplatin; and epirubicin, cisplatin, and fluorouracil as systemic treatment for advanced gastric carcinoma: a randomized phase II trial of the Swiss Group for Clinical Cancer Research. *J Clin Oncol* **25**(22): 3217–3223

Ryberg M, Nielsen D, Skovsgaard T, Hansen J, Jensen BV, Dombernowsky P (1998) Epirubicin cardiotoxicity: an analysis of 469 patients with metastatic breast cancer. *J Clin Oncol* **16**(11): 3502–3508

Schmittel A, Sebastian M, Fischer von Weikersthal L, Martus P, Gauler TC, Kaufmann C, Hortig P, Fischer JR, Link H, Binder D, Fischer B, Caca K, Eberhardt WE, Keilholz U (2011) A German multicenter, randomized phase III trial comparing irinotecan-carboplatin with etoposide-carboplatin as first-line therapy for extensive-disease small-cell lung cancer. *Ann Oncol*

Segeren CM, Sonneveld P, van der Holt B, Baars JW, Biesma DH, Cornellissen JJ, Croockewit AJ, Dekker AW, Fibbe WE, Lowenberg B, van Marwijk Kooy M, van Oers MH, Richel DJ, Schouten HC, Vellenga E, Verhoef GE, Wijermans PW, Wittebol S, Lokhorst HM (1999) Vincristine, doxorubicin and dexamethasone (VAD) administered as rapid intravenous infusion for first-line treatment in untreated multiple myeloma. *Br J Haematol* **105**(1): 127–130

Sessa C, Zucchetti M, Cerny T, Pagani O, Cavalli F, De Fusco M, De Jong J, Gentili D, McDaniel C, Prins C, et al. (1995) Phase I clinical and pharmacokinetic study of oral etoposide phosphate. *J Clin Oncol* **13**(1): 200–209

Seymour JF (1993) Induction of hypomagnesemia during Amsacrine treatment. *Am J Hematol* **42**(3): 262–267

Smith DB, Margison JM, Lucas SB, Wilkinson PM, Howell A (1987) Clinical pharmacology of oral and intravenous 4-demethoxydaunorubicin. *Cancer Chemother Pharmacol* **19**(2): 138–142

Smith MA, Rubinstein L, Anderson JR, Arthur D, Catalano PJ, Freidlin B, Heyn R, Khayat A, Krailo M, Land VJ, Miser J, Shuster J, Vena D (1999) Secondary leukemia or myelodysplastic syndrome after treatment with epipodophyllotoxins. *J Clin Oncol* **17**(2): 569–577

Sparano JA, Wang M, Martino S, Jones V, Perez EA, Saphner T, Wolff AC, Sledge GW, Jr., Wood WC, Davidson NE (2008) Weekly paclitaxel in the adjuvant treatment of breast cancer. *N Engl J Med* **358**(16): 1663–1671

Sternberg DW, Aird W, Neuberg D, Thompson L, MacNeill K, Amrein P, Shulman LN (2000) Treatment of patients with recurrent and primary refractory acute myelogenous leukemia using mitoxantrone and intermediate-dose cytarabine: a pharmacologically based regimen. *Cancer* **88**(9): 2037–2041

Stewart CF, Arbuck SG, Fleming RA, Evans WE (1990) Changes in the clearance of total and unbound etoposide in patients with liver dysfunction. *J Clin Oncol* **8**(11): 1874–1879

Stewart S, Jablonowski H, Goebel FD, Arasteh K, Spittle M, Rios A, Aboulafia D, Galleshaw J, Dezube BJ (1998) Randomized comparative trial of pegylated liposomal doxorubicin versus bleomycin and vincristine in the treatment of AIDS-related Kaposi's sarcoma. International Pegylated Liposomal Doxorubicin Study Group. *J Clin Oncol* **16**(2): 683–691

Suzuki S, Koide M, Sakamoto S, Matsuo T (1997) Pharmacokinetics of carboplatin and etoposide in a haemodialysis patient with Merkel-cell carcinoma. *Nephrol Dial Transplant* **12**(1): 137–140

Synold TW, Doroshow JH (1996) Anthracycline dose intensity: clinical pharmacology and pharmacokinetics of high-dose doxorubicin administered as a 96-hour continuous intravenous infusion. *J Infus Chemother* **6**(2): 69–73

Taamma A, Fandi A, Azli N, Wibault P, Chouaki N, Hasbini A, Couteau C, Armand JP, Cvitkovic E (1999) Phase II trial of chemotherapy with 5-fluorouracil, bleomycin, epirubicin, and cisplatin for patients with locally advanced, metastatic, or recurrent undifferentiated carcinoma of the nasopharyngeal type. *Cancer* **86**(7): 1101–1108

Takanashi S, Bachur NR (1976) Adriamycin metabolism in man. Evidence from urinary metabolites. *Drug Metab Dispos* **4**(1): 79–87

Tannock IF, de Wit R, Berry WR, Horti J, Pluzanska A, Chi KN, Oudard S, Theodore C, James ND, Turesson I, Rosenthal MA, Eisenberger MA (2004) Docetaxel plus prednisone or mitoxantrone plus prednisone for advanced prostate cancer. *N Engl J Med* **351**(15): 1502–1512

Tannock IF, Osoba D, Stockler MR, Ernst DS, Neville AJ, Moore MJ, Armitage GR, Wilson JJ, Venner PM, Coppin CM, Murphy KC (1996) Chemotherapy with mitoxantrone plus prednisone or prednisone alone for symptomatic hormone-resistant prostate cancer: a Canadian randomized trial with palliative end points. *J Clin Oncol* **14**(6): 1756–1764

Thiery-Vuillemin A, Dobi E, Nguyen T, Royer B, Montange D, Maurina T, Kalbacher E, Bazan F, Villanueva C, Demarchi M, Chaigneau L, Ivanaj A, Pivot X (2010) Duration: escalation study of oral etoposide with carboplatin in patients with varied solid tumors. *Anticancer Drugs* **21**(10): 958–962

Thomas DA, O'Brien S, Cortes J, Giles FJ, Faderl S, Verstovsek S, Ferrajoli A, Koller C, Beran M, Pierce S, Ha CS, Cabanillas F, Keating MJ, Kantarjian H (2004) Outcome with the hyper-CVAD regimens in lymphoblastic lymphoma. *Blood* **104**(6)**:** 1624–1630

Toffoli G, Corona G, Basso B, Boiocchi M (2004) Pharmacokinetic optimisation of treatment with oral etoposide. *Clin Pharmacokinet* **43**(7)**:** 441–466

Toffoli G, Sorio R, Aita P, Crivellari D, Corona G, Bearz A, Robieux I, Colussi AM, Stocco F, Boiocchi M (2000) Dose-finding and pharmacologic study of chronic oral idarubicin therapy in metastatic breast cancer patients. *Clin Cancer Res* **6**(6)**:** 2279–2287

Toffoli G, Sorio R, Aita P, Crivellari D, Corona G, Rimondi G, Bearz A, Stocco F, Robieux I, Boiocchi M (1997) Pharmacology of chronic oral daily administration of idarubicin. *Haematologica* **82**(5 Suppl)**:** 1–3

Von Hoff DD, Layard MW, Basa P, Davis HL, Jr., Von Hoff AL, Rozencweig M, Muggia FM (1979) Risk factors for doxorubicin-induced congestive heart failure. *Ann Intern Med* **91**(5)**:** 710–717

Von Hoff DD, Pollard E, Kuhn J, Murray E, Coltman CA, Jr. (1980) Phase I clinical investigation of 1,4-dihydroxy-5,8-bis (((2-[(2-hydroxyethyl)amino]ethyl) amino))-9,10-anthracenedione dihydrochloride (NSC 301739), a new anthracenedione. *Cancer Res* **40**(5)**:** 1516–1518

Von Hoff DD, Rozencweig M, Layard M, Slavik M, Muggia FM (1977) Daunomycin-induced cardiotoxicity in children and adults. A review of 110 cases. *Am J Med* **62**(2)**:** 200–208

Vorobiof DA, Iturralde M, Falkson G (1985) Assessment of ventricular function by radionuclide angiography in patients receiving 4'-epidoxorubicin and mitoxantrone. *Cancer Chemother Pharmacol* **15**(3)**:** 253–257

Weenen H, Lankelma J, Penders PG, McVie JG, ten Bokkel Huinink WW, de Planque MM, Pinedo HM (1983) Pharmacokinetics of 4'-epi-doxorubicin in man. *Invest New Drugs* **1**(1)**:** 59–64

Weiss MA, Aliff TB, Tallman MS, Frankel SR, Kalaycio ME, Maslak PG, Jurcic JG, Scheinberg DA, Roma TE (2002) A single, high dose of idarubicin combined with cytarabine as induction therapy for adult patients with recurrent or refractory acute lymphoblastic leukemia. *Cancer* **95**(3)**:** 581–587

Weiss RB (1992) The anthracyclines: will we ever find a better doxorubicin? *Semin Oncol* **19**(6)**:** 670–686

Weiss RB, Grillo-Lopez AJ, Marsoni S, Posada JG, Jr., Hess F, Ross BJ (1986) Amsacrine-associated cardiotoxicity: an analysis of 82 cases. *J Clin Oncol* **4**(6)**:** 918–928

Weiss RB, Moquin D, Adams JD, Griffin JD, Zimbler H (1983) Electrocardiogram abnormalities induced by amsacrine. *Cancer Chemother Pharmacol* **10**(2)**:** 133–134

Wiernik PH, Banks PL, Case DC, Jr., Arlin ZA, Periman PO, Todd MB, Ritch PS, Enck RE, Weitberg AB (1992) Cytarabine plus idarubicin or daunorubicin as induction and consolidation therapy for previously untreated adult patients with acute myeloid leukemia. *Blood* **79**(2)**:** 313–319

Wierzbowska A, Robak T, Pluta A, Wawrzyniak E, Cebula B, Holowiecki J, Kyrcz-Krzemien S, Grosicki S, Giebel S, Skotnicki AB, Piatkowska-Jakubas B, Kuliczkowski K, Kielbinski M, Zawilska K, Kloczko J, Wrzesien-Kus A (2008) Cladribine combined with high doses of arabinoside cytosine, mitoxantrone, and G-CSF (CLAG-M) is a highly effective salvage regimen in patients with refractory and relapsed acute myeloid leukemia of the poor risk: a final report of the Polish Adult Leukemia Group. *Eur J Haematol* **80**(2)**:** 115–126

Wilson WH, Bryant G, Bates S, Fojo A, Wittes RE, Steinberg SM, Kohler DR, Jaffe ES, Herdt J, Cheson BD, et al. (1993) EPOCH chemotherapy: toxicity and efficacy in relapsed and refractory non-Hodgkin's lymphoma. *J Clin Oncol* **11**(8)**:** 1573–1582

Wilson WH, Grossbard ML, Pittaluga S, Cole D, Pearson D, Drbohlav N, Steinberg SM, Little RF, Janik J, Gutierrez M, Raffeld M, Staudt L, Cheson BD, Longo DL, Harris N, Jaffe ES, Chabner BA, Wittes R, Balis F (2002) Dose-adjusted EPOCH chemotherapy for untreated large B-cell lymphomas: a pharmacodynamic approach with high efficacy. *Blood* **99**(8)**:** 2685–2693

Worden FP, Taylor JM, Biermann JS, Sondak VK, Leu KM, Chugh R, McGinn CJ, Zalupski MM, Baker LH (2005) Randomized phase II evaluation of 6 g/m2 of ifosfamide plus doxorubicin and granulocyte colony-stimulating factor (G-CSF) compared with 12 g/m2 of ifosfamide plus doxorubicin and G-CSF in the treatment of poor-prognosis soft tissue sarcoma. *J Clin Oncol* **23**(1): 105–112

Young RC, Ozols RF, Myers CE (1981) The anthracycline antineoplastic drugs. *N Engl J Med* **305**(3): 139–153

Zinzani PL, Pulsoni A, Perrotti A, Soverini S, Zaja F, De Renzo A, Storti S, Lauta VM, Guardigni L, Gentilini P, Tucci A, Molinari AL, Gobbi M, Falini B, Fattori PP, Ciccone F, Alinari L, Martelli M, Pileri S, Tura S, Baccarani M (2004) Fludarabine plus mitoxantrone with and without rituximab versus CHOP with and without rituximab as front-line treatment for patients with follicular lymphoma. *J Clin Oncol* **22**(13): 2654–2661

Zohren F, Czibere A, Bruns I, Fenk R, Schroeder T, Graf T, Haas R, Kobbe G (2009) Fludarabine, amsacrine, high-dose cytarabine and 12 Gy total body irradiation followed by allogeneic hematopoietic stem cell transplantation is effective in patients with relapsed or high-risk acute lymphoblastic leukemia. *Bone Marrow Transplant* **44**(12): 785–792

Chapter 14
Transcriptional Stress by Camptothecin: Mechanisms and Implications for the Drug Antitumor Activity

Giovanni Capranico, Laura Baranello, Davide Bertozzi, and Jessica Marinello

14.1 Introduction

Poisoning of DNA topoisomerases by small molecules is widespread in nature from bacteria to animals, and has been a conserved mechanism of cell killing during evolution. Nevertheless, we still lack a complete understanding of the molecular basis of the high antitumor activity of several DNA topoisomerase poisons in animal models and human patients. Mammalian DNA topoisomerase I (Top1) is the sole target of the plant alkaloid camptothecin (CPT). Because of their activity against human solid tumors, the water-soluble camptothecin derivatives topotecan and irinotecan have obtained US Food and Drug Administration approval for ovarian and small-cell lung cancers, and colorectal cancers, respectively. Camptothecin is a noncompetitive inhibitor of Top1, and the poisoning activity is highly reversible *in vitro* and *in vivo* (Covey et al. 1989; Tanizawa et al. 1994; Capranico et al. 1997; Pommier et al. 1998; Anderson and Osheroff 2001; Li and Liu 2001; Staker et al. 2002). Camptothecin interacts with active site amino acid residues and DNA base pairs at the cleavage site preventing strand religation and therefore increasing the half-life of the Top1-DNA cleavage complex (Top1cc). The camptothecin action becomes lethal when a collision occurs between a Top1cc and an advancing replication fork as it can lead to an irreversible DNA break, that is, a break that cannot be resealed by Top1 (Strumberg et al. 2000; Li and Liu 2001; Pommier 2006). The irreversible cuts can eventually activate multiple responses in proliferating cells including S-phase checkpoint, activation of specific transcription factors, G2 arrest and cell death. Moreover, it must be noted that the poison has an inhibitory effect on the enzymatic activity as the enzyme is unable to complete the reaction cycle when

G. Capranico (✉)
"G. Moruzzi" Department of Biochemistry, University of Bologna, via Irnerio 48, 40126 Bologna, Italy
e-mail: giovanni.capranico@unibo.it

Y. Pommier (ed.), *DNA Topoisomerases and Cancer*, Cancer Drug Discovery and Development, DOI 10.1007/978-1-4614-0323-4_14,

camptothecin freezes a Top1-DNA complex. Thus, the topological state of the domain encompassing the frozen Top1 likely remains fixed until the enzyme is liberated from camptothecin.

Although the established cellular effects of camptothecin are peculiar of DNA damage responses, Top1cc occurs primarily in actively transcribed regions, but the transcription-dependent effects of Top1cc are not yet fully known. To understand the mechanism of action of an effective drug, one needs to establish the cellular functions of its cellular target. In the case of camptothecins, different recent reports have revealed unexpected new roles for Top1 activity in living cells. Here, we discuss the hypothesis that Top1 poisoning can uncouple fundamental transcription regulation processes leading to unbalanced molecular pathways and cancer growth arrest. The new mechanism may contribute to the pharmacological activity of camptothecins together with the induction of replicative DNA damage and the activation of DNA-damage checkpoints pathways.

14.2 DNA Topoisomerase I and Transcription-Generated DNA Supercoils

Mammalian Top1 is enriched in transcribed genomic regions as established by Top1 DNA cleavage sites (Champoux 2001; Wang 2002; Pommier 2006) and chromatin immunoprecipitation (ChIP) (Khobta et al. 2006). Top1 has been shown to activate gene transcription, and to bind to general transcription factors at promoters (Kretzschmar et al. 1993; Merino et al. 1993; Shykind et al. 1997). Early studies in the yeast *Saccharomyces cerevisiae* indicated that neither Top1 nor Top2 are essential for transcription by RNA polymerase II (Champoux 2001; Wang 2002). However, plasmids carrying transcriptionally active genes are found to be extremely negatively supercoiled when isolated from mutants lacking both Top1 and Top2, and slightly negatively supercoiled in mutants lacking Top1 only (Brill and Sternglanz 1988; French et al. 2011).

Thus, a main molecular function of Top1 is generally considered to be the relaxation of transcription-dependent DNA supercoils (Champoux 2001; Wang 2002). It is well established that waves of positive and negative supercoils are generated ahead and behind the elongating RNA polymerase if the translocating transcriptional apparatus cannot turn around the DNA template (the twin supercoiled-domain model) (Wu et al. 1988; Champoux 2001; Wang 2002). The twin supercoiling model has been supported by several findings (Liu and Wang 1987; Wang and Giaever 1988; Wang 2002). A critical prediction of the model is that the localized degree of supercoiling may exceed the average supercoiling state of intracellular DNA (Liu and Wang 1987). Within a topological domain, that may have diverse consequences. First, a high degree of template positive supercoiling can inhibit further transcription by tightening the DNA helix, particularly when the transcription rate is high (Drolet 2006). As a consequence, the Top1 function may be the relaxation of torsional stress to allow a normal rate of RNA synthesis. Secondly, it is interesting to point out that localized changes of DNA supercoiling can be exploited to regulate other nuclear processes (Wang and Giaever 1988). For instance, it has been shown *in vitro* that DNA recombination may be coupled to transcription through topology changes of the DNA template (Wang 1996). Therefore, Top1 may act as a regulator of DNA recombinations by modulating the local superhelicity of the DNA template. This is supported by the observation that the lack of both TOP1 and TOP2 genes increases rDNA recombination in yeast cells (Christman et al. 1988).

14.3 Regulation of Nucleosome Remodeling and Chromatin Structure by DNA Topoisomerase I

Another source of torsional stress of the nuclear genome is the continuous remodeling of nucleosomes in active regions. Top1 has been implicated in chromatin regulation since early investigations. Genetic studies of Top1 and/or Top2 mutants in *Schizosaccharomyces pombe* suggested a major function of Top1, but not of Top2, in the regulation of chromatin structure during all cell-cycle phases (Uemura and Yanagida 1984). Subsequently, it has been suggested that a main Top1 function may be the regulation of nucleosome remodeling by modulating the torsional tension generated by the assembly and/or disassembly of nucleosomes (Felsenfeld et al. 2000; Wang 2002).

This role of Top1 can have a main impact on the regulation of transcription and related processes. Nucleosomes can strongly suppress transcription, and a number of transcription factors act to permit efficient transcription elongation by modulating nucleosome position and assembly (Sims et al. 2004). In principle, positive supercoiling ahead of RNA polymerases could uncoil the negative supercoils associated with nucleosomes, thereby decondensing chromatin fibers and enabling polymerase passage. By investigating the effects of positive supercoiling on yeast 2-μ minichromosomes, Lee et al. (Lee and Garrard 1991) showed that minichromosomes having positive supercoils are preferentially sensitive to DNase I digestion and more accessible to internal nuclease cleavage. Relaxation *in vitro* of minichromosomes does not reverse the increased sensitivity to nuclease digestion, indicating that positive supercoils may drive the generation, but not the maintenance, of nucleosome conformations that favor elongation (Lee and Garrard 1991). Certainly, a chromatin template poses additional topological problems relative to a protein-free DNA template, and a topoisomerase could be involved in the translocation of a RNA polymerase through nucleosomes (Felsenfeld et al. 2000). Transcriptional studies showed that either Top1 or Top2 is required for efficient transcription of a chromatin template, but not for *in vitro* transcription with naked DNA (Mondal and Parvin 2001; Mondal et al. 2003). Interestingly, as repression was detected without topoisomerases only when RNA transcripts were above 200 bp, chromatin repression of transcription is dependent on the length of the transcript. The authors explained their findings by an accumulation of positive supercoils that inhibit further translocation of RNA polymerases along the template (Mondal et al. 2003).

In a recent publication, Bermejo and coworkers have investigated the contribution of Top2 in S phase transcription of *S. cervisiae* to understand how this enzyme might solve topological constraints arising when replication forks encounter transcription. Genome-wide analyses revealed that Top2 preferentially binds to promoter and transcription termination regions, but is not needed to license the transcriptional program as shown in Top2 mutants (Bermejo et al. 2009). This is probably due to the contribution of Top1. As Top2 has been implicated in DNA looping, it was hypothesized that it contributes to the formation of architectural domain containing one or more transcription units in which Top1 has a fundamental role in coordinating fork progression and ongoing transcription (Bermejo et al. 2009).

Other publications are somewhat in conflict with a role of Top1 in the relaxation of transcription-generated supercoils. In a kinetic study of DNA relaxation by Top1 or Top2, Top2 was found much more efficient than Top1 in changing the linking number of DNA when assembled into nucleosomes (Salceda et al. 2006). The catalytic assays were conducted *in vitro* with minichromosomes, isolated from yeast strains that had their DNA under either positive or negative supercoiling tension. Apparently, the DNA strand-rotation mechanism of Top1 does not efficiently relax chromatin that imposes barriers to DNA twist diffusion (Salceda et al. 2006). In that study, the relaxation efficiency of topoisomerases was assessed without ongoing transcription, and therefore it remains to be determined whether Top1 and Top2 are equally efficient in a transcription-coupled relaxation activity with a chromatin template.

An attractive hypothesis is that a main function of Top1 during transcription is to regulate nucleosome assembly/disassembly and conformational changes by relaxing twist alterations generated by the process (Lavelle 2007). Recently, we have determined the effects of stable depletion of Top1 activity on global gene expression and telomeric chromatin in *S. cerevisiae* (Lotito et al. 2008). In ΔTOP1 yeast strain, transcription of telomere-proximal genes was increased, and glucose utilization and energy production pathways were downregulated. Interestingly, the lack of Top1 activity increases histone H4 acetylation and H3K4 dimethylation at telomere-proximal regions. Those findings suggest that Top1 can affect gene expression at telomere-proximal regions through regulations of chromatin structure and histone modifications.

At a cellular level, it was interesting to note that ΔTOP1 did not activate telomere-proximal genes or repress genes of the glucose and energy production pathways when cells were grown under pH-stressed conditions (Lotito et al. 2008). As telomere-proximal regions are known to be enriched for stress-activated genes, the reported results provide strong evidence for a global role of Top1 in the regulation of the balance of cellular transcripts in highly proliferating yeast cells under optimal growth conditions. Thus, the Top1 activity may result in an increased efficiency of the transcriptional programs appropriate for the actual environmental conditions of yeast growth. In line with this conclusion, early findings showed that Top1 is required for an efficient repression of general transcription at the stationary phase in *S. cerevisiae* (Choder 1991) suggesting that Top1 can optimize the transcriptional program of the stationary phase.

14.4 Topological Stress Is an Immediate Effect of Camptothecin in Living Cells

Multiple studies are using camptothecins as molecular tools to dissect checkpoint pathways activated by DNA damage at replication forks. Moreover, camptothecin has been invaluable in experiments aimed at defining Top1 functions. We here intend to discuss the cellular and molecular effects of camptothecin that are not related to DNA replication and checkpoint activation. Thus, we will focus on: (1) early drug effects, which are independent from replicative DNA damage; and (2) effects that are detected at relatively low drug concentrations.

A first interesting observation was derived from a study focused on DNA topology and chromatin organization of a reporter plasmid in mammalian cells (Duann et al. 1999). In that study, cells were treated with 10 μM camptothecin at 37°C for 10 min. The drug effects were shown to be Top1-dependent with camptothecin treatments resulting in increased linking numbers of recovered plasmid DNA. The authors proposed that camptothecin-induced DNA breaks triggered immediate and general chromatin reorganization (Duann et al. 1999). As the drug effects were immediate (a marked change of the linking number of episomal DNA circles was detected within 3 min of treatments), the observations could also be explained by camptothecin inhibition of Top1 catalytic activity, suggesting an involvement of Top1 in chromatin structure and nucleosome organization (Duann et al. 1999). Notably, the studied mammalian cells contain other topoisomerases, including Top2, which therefore does not effectively resolve excess torsional tension due to Top1 inhibition.

Since camptothecin stabilizes the Top1 DNA cleavage complex, the DNA cleavage activity and the inhibition of the catalytic reaction by the drug are intrinsically linked together and cannot be split apart. However, recent findings support the view that inhibition of Top1 activity is a significant aspect of the drug action at enzyme and cellular levels. Camptothecins have been shown to markedly inhibit Top1 catalytic activity in single-molecule experiments (Koster et al. 2007). DNA uncoiling by Top1 was found to be slow but continuous in the presence of camptothecins, and the reported measurements showed that uncoiling occurs roughly 20-fold slower in the presence of topotecan than by Top1 alone (Koster et al. 2007). Moreover, topotecan, significantly hindered Top1-mediated DNA uncoiling with a more pronounced effect on the removal of positive versus negative supercoils (Koster et al. 2007), in agreement with previous molecular modeling calculations (Sari and Andricioaei 2005). As camptothecin treatments result in an immediate accumulation of positive supercoils in plasmid DNAs in yeast and mammalian cells (Duann et al. 1999; Koster et al. 2007), one may conclude that the drug affects specifically the enzyme activity in the nucleus of living cells. This may have an impact on chromatin structure as suggested previously (Duann et al. 1999).

Interestingly, camptothecin-induced chromatin reorganization did not involve nucleosome removal from the DNA template (Duann et al. 1999), suggesting an alteration by the drug of nucleosome conformation and/or positions along the studied DNA regions. To assess such hypothesis, we have investigated the *in vivo* camptothecin effects on histone modifications by ChIP. In one study, 10 μM camptothecin appeared to induce a more accessible chromatin conformation specifically at transcribed loci, since it caused a decrease of histone H1, and increases of core histone H3 and H4 acetylation along a human histone gene cluster on chromosome six but not at repressed α-satellite DNAs (Khobta et al. 2006). Because histone-modifying enzymes can be associated with RNA polymerases either at promoters or during elongation (Sims et al. 2004), the study shows that Top1 may be involved in a transcription-coupled regulation of chromatin structure in living cells.

14.5 Camptothecin Effects on Top1 Mobility, Nuclear Localization, and Protein Degradation

Camptothecin exerts early effects on Top1 protein mobility, nuclear localization, and degradation, which are likely dependent on transcription-related processes. Investigations by photobleaching of cells expressing biofluorescent Top1-GFP chimeras have shown that camptothecin rapidly affects Top1 mobility. During interphase, Top1 accumulates in the nucleolus and not in the nucleoplasm, although the enzyme interchanges constantly between the two compartments (Danks et al. 1996; Christensen et al. 2002; Cohen et al. 2008). A very likely candidate responsible for targeting Top1 to defined nuclear locations has been proposed to be the N-terminal domain, from amino acid residues 1–200 of the human enzyme. This domain distinguishes eukaryotic Top1 from the minimal Top1 variant of vaccinia virus (Shuman and Moss 1987) and other microbial enzymes (Grainge and Jayaram 1999; Pommier et al. 2010). The large part of the N-terminal domain minimally contributes to Top1 activity *in vitro* (Lisby et al. 2001), but it is believed to determine the biological properties of the enzyme. Most notably, it seems to be a docking place for interacting proteins, such as nucleolin, a nucleolar protein (Bharti et al. 1996), and to determine a specific enzyme localization at the fibrillar centers of nucleoli (Christensen et al. 2002) (see Chap. 2). As Top1 has a lower mobility in the nucleolus than in the nucleoplasm, it has been proposed that this differential enzyme mobility may contribute to the preferential accumulation in nucleoli (Christensen et al. 2002).

Nucleolar Top1 accumulation can likely reflect the engagement in rDNA transcription, as ribosomal RNA genes are by far the most highly transcribed genes in the cell. Interestingly, camptothecin very early affects nuclear enzyme localization as the drug causes a relocation from the nucleoli to the nucleoplasm of Top1 (Muller et al. 1985). As this was also observed with RNA synthesis inhibitors, it is likely that the phenomenon may be related to reduced activity of rRNA transcription in the nucleolus. Upon addition of camptothecin, Top1 relocates within 30 s from the nucleoli to nucleoplasmic structures. At these sites, Top1 mobility becomes reduced in a manner dependent on camptothecin concentration, whereas the enzyme mobility is much less affected inside nucleoli (Christensen et al. 2002). In agreement with previous papers (Desai et al. 1997; Li and Liu 2001), a recent proteomic study of the cellular response to camptothecin at the level of individual cells has provided clear evidence that Top1 is among the very first proteins undergoing a reduction of its cellular content, within 1 h of drug addition (Muller et al. 1985; Cohen et al. 2008). Less expected, a large fraction of all the tested proteins undergoes a significant decrease in fluorescence intensity in response to the drug, on diverse time scales (Cohen et al. 2008), indicating that protein degradation may be a general and important response to camptothecin. For instance, degradation of cytoskeleton proteins may be responsible for the loss of cell motility after 8–10 h of camptothecin treatment (Cohen et al. 2008). Moreover, Top1 shows rapid alterations of intracellular localization. Interestingly, a specific set of nucleolar proteins also showed rapid localization changes after camptothecin treatments, with timing similar to that of the drug target. The authors pointed out that similar changes of nucleolar proteins were also detected with unrelated inhibitors of transcription (Cohen et al. 2008). Thus, the findings indicate that early alterations of protein content and localization are likely related to ribosomal RNA transcription, and that cells quickly respond to altered transcription processes caused by camptothecin (Cohen et al. 2008).

14.6 Alterations of Gene Expression Patterns by Camptothecin-Induced Top1cc

We derived similar conclusion from our work showing that camptothecin specifically affects global gene expression profiles in yeast (Lotito et al. 2009). In order to define the cellular responses to CPT, we determined the global transcriptional consequences of Top1 inhibition by using a relatively low drug concentration, that is, a camptothecin dose with low cytotoxic activity. Such drug concentrations can be more relevant for drug antitumor activity as blood levels of drugs in patients and animal models are much lower than highly cytotoxic doses commonly used in cultured cells (Houghton et al. 1998; Zamboni et al. 1998).

We reported 95 yeast genes with an altered expression upon camptothecin treatments of cells expressing the wild-type TOP1 gene (Lotito et al. 2009). No significant gene alteration was reported in cells expressing an inactive Top1 enzyme. Thus, a relatively low camptothecin dose can alter global expression profiles only if a catalytically active Top1 is present in the cell demonstrating that drug inhibition of Top1 is still the sole trigger of the transcriptional response. Interestingly, the number of downregulated genes (73) was higher than the upregulated genes (22), indicating that a large part of the response is constituted by a relative reduction of the transcription of specific gene sets. These are mainly related to Gene Ontology components such as vesicle-mediated transport, organelle and cell wall organization, protein modifications, RNA synthesis and processing, and ribosome functions (Lotito et al. 2009). The findings may be consistent with the proteomic study of camptothecin effects in human cells (Cohen et al. 2008) showing that cells immediately respond to camptothecin inhibition of transcription, and particularly of ribosomal RNA synthesis.

Moreover, CPT was able to slow down the growth rate of yeast cells at the low cytotoxic dose used in the study. The findings showed that upon CPT inhibition of cell cycle progression, the yeast cells have a specific transcriptional response. This response likely triggers a new balance of global transcript levels depending, at least for the upregulated genes, on the Mbp1/Swi4 gene regulatory network. As established with MBP1 and SWI4 gene deletion experiments, the new transcription balance may then set a proper progression of the cell cycle in the presence of camptothecin (Lotito et al. 2009).

Interestingly, a similar approach in a human colon cancer cell line provided evidence that reversible cell cycle arrest in G_2-M after low-dose CPT treatment was associated with delayed upregulation of mitosis-related genes, normally upregulated during G_2 (Zhou et al. 2002; Daoud et al. 2003). In contrast, treatment with high-dose CPT increased the expression of some p53-responsive genes, and caused an interruption of the mitosis-related gene expression and G_2 arrest of cells. Thus, a fundamental difference can exist between gene expression profiles associated with reversible G_2 delay, which follows mild DNA damage, and permanent G_2 arrest, which follows more extensive DNA damage (Zhou et al. 2002).

14.7 Early Camptothecin Effects on RNA Polymerase II

A broad and general inhibition of transcription elongation is an immediate effect of camptothecin in cultured cells (Wu and Liu 1997; Pommier 2006). This is likely due to the stalling of elongating RNA polymerases by Top1ccs (Wu and Liu 1997; Pommier 2006; Sordet et al. 2008, 2009, 2010) and/or by persistent transcription-generated DNA supercoils (Darzacq et al. 2007). A kinetic analysis of RNA polymerase II (PolII) transcription at a gene-array locus showed that transcription can be inefficient and that Pol II often pauses during elongation (Darzacq et al. 2007). Interestingly, while leaving active the entire population of Pol IIs, camptothecin increased the efficiency of intragenic pausing but not the pause time, resulting in a reduction of the elongation rate to a ¼ of the normal rate (Darzacq et al. 2007). In contrast to other transcription inhibitors such as DRB, camptothecin is not able to fully block transcription at the studied gene array, thus documenting that some levels of nuclear RNA synthesis can occur in the presence of Top1 poisons (Darzacq et al. 2007).

Several groups described other unexpected effects of camptothecin at the transcriptional levels, such as the activation of the transcription initiation step (Ljungman and Hanawalt 1996) and the expression of specific genes in human cells (Collins et al. 2001). Strikingly, camptothecin-induced Top1ccs have immediate and specific effects on RNA polymerase II (Pol II). The poison triggers a high phosphorylation degree of the largest subunit (Rpb1) of Pol II (Desai et al. 2003; Khobta et al. 2006; Sordet et al. 2008), showing an effect on a critical step of transcription regulation. Apparently, hyperphosphorylation occurs selectively on Ser-5 residues of the conserved heptapeptide repeats of the carboxy-terminal domain (CTD) possibly mediated by Cdk7, component of TFIIH (Sordet et al. 2008). Interestingly, a recent report showed that camptothecin can disrupt the large inactive P-TEFb complex, thus releasing a free active P-TEFb complex (containing the Cdk9 subunit), which may then contribute to camptothecin-increased phosphorylation of Pol II (Amente et al. 2009). A second immediate effect of camptothecin on Pol II has been reported by us previously, and can be correlated to the hyperphosphorylation of Rpb1. Short cell treatments with camptothecin induce a redistribution of chromatin-bound Pol II along transcribed genes in human cancer cells, apparently by enhancing the escape of Pol II from promoter-proximal pausing sites (Khobta et al. 2006). Remarkably, this early specific camptothecin effect is independent from replication and replicative DNA damage.

Mainly based on *in vitro* findings, previous reports proposed that an elongating Pol II can collide with a Top1 trapped on the DNA template (Li and Liu 2001; Desai et al. 2003). It has also been shown that removal of Top1 cleavage complexes and DNA break processing are transcription-dependent, and coupled to ubiquitination and degradation of Top1 and Pol II through the 26S proteasome pathway (Desai et al. 2003) (see Chap. 17). Interestingly, transcription-dependent ubiquitination of the Pol II large subunit may also be triggered by RNA polymerase arrest following α-amanitin treatment or at sites of DNA damage caused by UV-irradiation or cisplatin. Nevertheless, in these studies drug concentrations were higher and time periods longer that those used by us (Khobta et al. 2006). We therefore propose that degradation of Top1 and Pol II is a later event than alterations of protein distribution at active chromatin regions. Interestingly, within the 1 h time frame of the study, camptothecin did not affect the morphology and intensity of nuclear Pol II foci, whereas replication factories were destroyed by the drug (Khobta et al. 2006). Unaffected nuclear transcriptional foci could therefore indicate that major destructive collisions do not often occur *in vivo*. This conclusion is also consistent with the observations that chromatin-bound Top1 levels are not increased at specific regions, but rather reduced, by camptothecin in ChIP experiments (Khobta et al. 2006), indicating that enzyme trapping is highly reversible in nuclear chromatin. Thus, given the highly reversible state of Top1–camptothecin–DNA complexes, an encounter between a trapped Top1 and an elongating Pol II could rather be a transient event in the chromatin fibers of living cells. Such an encounter could then transiently block polymerase movement without leading to irreversible strand cut and to RNA polymerase disassembly from the template. Nondestructive collisions are likely undetectable in *in vitro* investigations, even though, at high drug concentrations, they may become frequent enough to be detected leading to irreversible single-strand cuts in living cells.

14.8 Camptothecin Interference with Regulation of Transcriptional Pausing

To establish whether camptothecin-induced alterations of the distribution of Pol II along transcribed genes (Khobta et al. 2006) were due to an enhanced RNA polymerase escape from pause sites, we have determined nascent RNA levels downstream to the promoter-proximal pausing sites of the human HIF-1α and c-MYC genes in colon cancer cells (Baranello et al. 2010). Nascent RNA levels were determined with the

RIP method (RNA chromatin immunoprecipitation) following 1 h exposures of cells to 10 μM camptothecin. The data provide clear evidence that camptothecin increases transcription downstream to the studied promoter pausing sites while leaving unchanged transcription levels in other gene regions (Baranello et al. 2010). Because camptothecin induces Rpb1 hyperphosphorylation through Cdk7 and/or Cdk9 activity (Desai et al. 2003; Khobta et al. 2006; Sordet et al. 2008; Amente et al. 2009), we propose that Top1cc can increase the activity of Cdks, which can then phosphorylate Rpb1. This would promote transcription elongation at promoter-proximal pausing sites (Baranello et al. 2010).

Even though camptothecin is commonly considered an efficient inhibitor of transcription elongation, the molecular mechanism has not been fully established. Commonly, it is considered that transcription inhibition is due to the stalling of Pol II by Top1ccs (Wu and Liu 1997; Pommier 2006) and/or by persistent transcription-generated DNA supercoils (Darzacq et al. 2007). Nevertheless, transcription inhibition by camptothecin may be caused by other, not necessarily alternative, mechanisms. As Pol II pausing at promoters has been shown to favor the recruitment of further Pol II at promoters (Gilchrist et al. 2008), an attractive hypothesis is that camptothecin-stabilized Top1cc can interfere with a regulation mechanism at the initiation step of transcription by promoting Pol II escape from pausing sites. This may result in a reduction of Pol II density at promoters, in agreement with experimental data (Khobta et al. 2006; Baranello et al. 2010), contributing to decreased gene transcription. Such interference with initiation regulatory mechanisms is likely specific for Top1 and camptothecin, as VM-26 (a Top2 poison) and cisplatin (which promotes the formation of DNA strand crosslinks) caused a decrease in Pol II density both at promoters and along the transcribed genes (Baranello et al. 2010).

Moreover, a recent report showed that UV-induced DNA damage can alter alternative splicing at several genes in human cells by increasing the phosphorylation status of Rpb1 of Pol II. This is likely mediated by P-TEFb (Munoz et al. 2009), which has been shown to play an important role in coupling transcription elongation and alternative splicing (Barboric et al. 2009). Interestingly, UV-induced hyperphosphorylation of Pol II may cause a lower elongation rate of Pol II (Munoz et al. 2009), which may then affect alternative splicing by a kinetic coupling mechanism (Kornblihtt 2007). We have recently reported that camptothecin-induced Top1ccs can affect alternative splicing of the HIF-1α mRNA co-transcriptionally (Baranello et al. 2010). Moreover, Amente and coworkers showed that the active P-TEFb complex is markedly affected by camptothecin (Amente et al. 2009). Also, a recent study showed that camptothecin induces the rapid and selective splicing of genes involved in splicing regulation and that this effect was linked with Pol II hyperphosphorylation (Solier et al. 2010). Thus, based on these findings, an attractive hypothesis is that Top1ccs may reduce the elongation rate of Pol II by inducing the hyperphosphorylation of Pol II, similar to UV-induced DNA damage (Munoz et al. 2009). Clearly, the functional role of the camptothecin-induced hyperphosphorylation of Pol II must be established by definitive data to fully understand the mode of transcription inhibition by Top1 poisoning.

Intriguingly, some data have raised the possibility that Top1 may play a role during transcript maturation, particularly in splicing of messenger RNAs (Rossi et al. 1996; Pilch et al. 2001). A striking finding of our recent report is the demonstration that CPT-induced Top1ccs can affect alternative splicing of HIF-1α mRNA co-transcriptionally (Baranello et al. 2010). How an enzyme that regulates DNA topology may affect RNA processing remains undefined. However, other reports have shown evidence that Top1 activity may be critical for proper RNA maturation. Proteomic analyses of Top1-containing protein complexes aimed at identifying human Top1 partners has been performed by co-immunoprecipitation and affinity-chromatography combined with mass spectrometry (Czubaty et al. 2005). The N-terminal domain and the cap region of Top1 are the main regions that can interact with protein partners. Interestingly, 10 of the 36 proteins identified as interacting with Top1 are involved in RNA splicing. One of these splicing factors, PSF, has been shown to stimulate DNA relaxation activity of Top1 (Straub et al. 2000), in contrast to ASF/SF2 splicing factor that seems to inhibit enzyme activity (Andersen et al. 2002). Top1 activity and function can then be coupled to that of splicing factors. In a recent paper, Tuduri and coworkers showed that the subnuclear organization of ASF/SF2 speckles is profoundly altered in Top1-deficient cells (Tuduri et al. 2009). Moreover, depletion of ASF/SF2 induces fork arrest and chromosome breaks to a similar extent as in Top1-deficient cells. Because no additive effect of ASF/SF2 depletion and Top1 depletion was detected, the findings indicate that both proteins function in the same pathway. The authors proposed that Top1 could prevent R-loop formation both by relaxing DNA supercoiling and by promoting the ASF/SF2-dependent assembly of mRNPs. However, the precise functions of Top1 in RNA splicing remain to be completely established. Recently, Sordet et al. (2009, 2010) proposed that camptothecin-trapped Top1cc induces the formation of R-loops that induce the formation of transcription-dependent DNA double-strand breaks and Pol II arrest.

14.9 A Specific Transcriptional Stress Induced by Camptothecin

Intriguingly, the transcriptional consequences of Top1cc stabilized by camptothecin at relatively low concentrations are wider than those discussed above. 2–10 μM camptothecin can increase antisense transcript levels at the human *HIF-1α* gene locus, and levels of histone modifications marks of open chromatin conformations (Baranello et al. 2010). The events require Top1 and are independent from replication and replicative DNA damage. Remarkably, by using DRB, we showed that inhibition of Cdk9 and Cdk7 activity can suppress the camptothecin-induced activation of antisense transcription, and increased chromatin accessibility (Baranello et al. 2010). As increased Pol II escape and reduced elongation rate are earlier camptothecin effects, both of which are likely dependent on Cdk activation and Rpb1 hyperphosphorylation, we proposed that a sustained camptothecin interference with Pol II regulation may eventually lead to a more general transcriptional stress. Such a stress involves a more accessible chromatin conformation, de-repression of antisense transcription and reduced synthesis of mRNAs (Baranello et al. 2010).

Camptothecin-promoted Pol II escape, Cdk activation, and transcriptional stress can constitute a response to drug-promoted DNA strand cleavage or altered torsional tension of the DNA template. As discussed above, recent studies have shown that, when camptothecin freezes a Top1cc, the enzyme catalytic cycle is slowed down, in particular, when the enzyme removes positive supercoils (Koster et al. 2007). Consistently, the drug action results in the inhibition of enzyme catalytic activity leading to a marked torsional stress of the DNA template in living cells (Duann et al. 1999; Koster et al. 2007). Local DNA torsional stress can significantly regulate gene expression in mammalian cells as demonstrated in the case of the regulation of the human c-MYC gene (Kouzine et al. 2008), and of the divergent transcription at protein-coding gene promoters that has been proposed to be determined by negative supercoils generated by mRNA transcription (Seila et al. 2008). In particular, Kouzine and coworkers (Kouzine et al. 2008) showed that dynamic negative supercoiling upstream of c-MYC promoter can induce the formation of non-B-DNA structures in the susceptible FUSE (far upstream element) sequence, thus favoring the recruitment of transcription factors. Camptothecin inhibition of Top1 may then cause a supercoiling imbalance locally at promoters, and this may interfere with Pol II regulation as discussed above. Nevertheless, the precise mechanism is unknown, and in particular it remains to be established whether the drug-stabilized Top1cc or the altered torsional tension is the trigger of the reported drug effects.

In addition to the well-known effects on DNA replication and DNA damage checkpoints, camptothecin may interfere with transcription regulation leading to a specific transcriptional stress. This may result in alterations of gene expression patterns that can be relevant for cancer therapy, particularly at low drug concentrations. In future studies, one needs to further define the contribution of transcription-dependent effects on the antitumor activity of camptothecin and other Top1 inhibitors. We have reported that 2–10 μM camptothecin can impair the balance of cellular antisense and sense transcripts that may affect the cancer-related HIF-1 pathway (Baranello et al. 2010). HIF-1 is a transcription factor and a master regulator of the cell response to oxygen deprivation (Iyer et al. 1998; Semenza 2003), and a target of antiangiogenesis and anticancer agents (Melillo 2006). HIF-1 is a heterodimer constituted by HIF-1α or HIF-2α subunits, and a constitutively-expressed HIF-1β subunit. The HIF-1α subunits are degraded at high oxygen tensions by an oxygen-mediated hydroxylation of conserved prolyl and aspraginyl residues, to which the von Hippel-Lindau protein (pVHL) E3 ligase binds targeting HIF-1α to proteasomal degradation (Semenza 2003; Melillo 2006). Our recent findings show that the human HIF-1α gene locus is complex as at least two noncoding RNAs are present in the antisense orientation relative to the mRNA. We proposed that these RNAs may have a role in novel mechanisms of transcriptional and/or posttranscriptional regulation of HIF-1α activity (Lapidot and Pilpel 2006; Kapranov et al. 2007). Interestingly, previous reports demonstrated that camptothecin can markedly reduce HIF-1α protein accumulation in hypoxic cells in a manner independent from the

VHL pathway and from replicative DNA damage (Rapisarda et al. 2002, 2004a, b). Even though camptothecin has been shown to have antiangiogenesis activity independent from the cell killing activity, the mechanism of camptothecin interference with HIF-1α protein accumulation was not elucidated. Thus, one hypothesis is that de-repression or activation of antisense RNAs by camptothecin might regulate the activity of HIF-1α under certain conditions. The new mechanism may contribute to the control of tumor progression by Top1 poisons in animal models and human patients, and may constitute a different rational basis for the development of novel therapeutic approaches in patients.

Acknowledgments The authors thank Associazione Italiana per la Ricerca sul Cancro (Milan, Italy) for funding [IG 4494 to G.C.].

References

Amente, S., B. Gargano, et al. (2009). "Camptothecin releases P-TEFb from the inactive 7SK snRNP complex." *Cell Cycle* **8**(8): 1249–55.

Andersen, F. F., T. O. Tange, et al. (2002). "The RNA splicing factor ASF/SF2 inhibits human topoisomerase I mediated DNA relaxation." *J Mol Biol* **322**(4): 677–86.

Anderson, V. E. and N. Osheroff (2001). "Type II topoisomerases as targets for quinolone antibacterials: turning Dr. Jekyll into Mr. Hyde." *Curr Pharm Des* **7**(5): 337–53.

Baranello, L., D. Bertozzi, et al. (2010). "DNA topoisomerase I inhibition by camptothecin induces escape of RNA polymerase II from promoter-proximal pause site, antisense transcription and histone acetylation at the human HIF-1alpha gene locus." *Nucleic Acids Res* **38**(1): 159–71.

Barboric, M., T. Lenasi, et al. (2009). "7SK snRNP/P-TEFb couples transcription elongation with alternative splicing and is essential for vertebrate development." *Proc Natl Acad Sci USA* **106**(19): 7798–803.

Bermejo, R., T. Capra, et al. (2009). "Genome-organizing factors Top2 and Hmo1 prevent chromosome fragility at sites of S phase transcription." *Cell* **138**(5): 870–84.

Bharti, A. K., M. O. Olson, et al. (1996). "Identification of a nucleolin binding site in human topoisomerase I." *J Biol Chem* **271**(4): 1993–7.

Brill, S. J. and R. Sternglanz (1988). "Transcription-dependent DNA supercoiling in yeast DNA topoisomerase mutants." *Cell* **54**(3): 403–11.

Capranico, G., M. Binaschi, et al. (1997). "A protein-mediated mechanism for the DNA sequence-specific action of topoisomerase II poisons." *Trends Pharmacol Sci* **18**(9): 323–9.

Champoux, J. J. (2001). "DNA topoisomerases: structure, function, and mechanism." *Annu Rev Biochem* **70**: 369–413.

Choder, M. (1991). "A general topoisomerase I-dependent transcriptional repression in the stationary phase in yeast." *Genes Dev* **5**(12A): 2315–26.

Christensen, M. O., H. U. Barthelmes, et al. (2002). "Changes in mobility account for camptothecin-induced subnuclear relocation of topoisomerase I." *J Biol Chem* **277**(18): 15661–5.

Christman, M. F., F. S. Dietrich, et al. (1988). "Mitotic recombination in the rDNA of S. cerevisiae is suppressed by the combined action of DNA topoisomerases I and II." *Cell* **55**(3): 413–25.

Cohen, A. A., N. Geva-Zatorsky, et al. (2008). "Dynamic proteomics of individual cancer cells in response to a drug." *Science* **322**(5907): 1511–6.

Collins, I., A. Weber, et al. (2001). "Transcriptional consequences of topoisomerase inhibition." *Mol Cell Biol* **21**(24): 8437–51.

Covey, J. M., C. Jaxel, et al. (1989). "Protein-linked DNA strand breaks induced in mammalian cells by camptothecin, an inhibitor of topoisomerase I." *Cancer Res* **49**(18): 5016–22.

Czubaty, A., A. Girstun, et al. (2005). "Proteomic analysis of complexes formed by human topoisomerase I." *Biochim Biophys Acta* **1749**(1): 133–41.

Danks, M. K., K. E. Garrett, et al. (1996). "Subcellular redistribution of DNA topoisomerase I in anaplastic astrocytoma cells treated with topotecan." *Cancer Res* **56**(7): 1664–73.

Daoud, S. S., P. J. Munson, et al. (2003). "Impact of p53 knockout and topotecan treatment on gene expression profiles in human colon carcinoma cells: a pharmacogenomic study." *Cancer Res* **63**(11): 2782–93.

Darzacq, X., Y. Shav-Tal, et al. (2007). "In vivo dynamics of RNA polymerase II transcription." *Nat Struct Mol Biol* **14**(9): 796–806.

Desai, S. D., L. F. Liu, et al. (1997). "Ubiquitin-dependent destruction of topoisomerase I is stimulated by the antitumor drug camptothecin." *J Biol Chem* **272**(39): 24159–64.

Desai, S. D., H. Zhang, et al. (2003). "Transcription-dependent degradation of topoisomerase I-DNA covalent complexes." *Mol Cell Biol* **23**(7): 2341–50.

Drolet, M. (2006). "Growth inhibition mediated by excess negative supercoiling: the interplay between transcription elongation, R-loop formation and DNA topology." *Mol Microbiol* **59**(3): 723–30.

Duann, P., M. Sun, et al. (1999). "Plasmid linking number change induced by topoisomerase I-mediated DNA damage." *Nucleic Acids Res* **27**(14): 2905–11.

Felsenfeld, G., D. Clark, et al. (2000). "Transcription through nucleosomes." *Biophys Chem* **86**(2–3): 231–7.

French, S. L., M. L. Sikes, et al. (2011). "Distinguishing the roles of Topoisomerases I and II in relief of transcription-induced torsional stress in yeast rRNA genes." *Mol Cell Biol* **31**(3): 482–94.

Gilchrist, D. A., S. Nechaev, et al. (2008). "NELF-mediated stalling of Pol II can enhance gene expression by blocking promoter-proximal nucleosome assembly." *Genes Dev* **22**(14): 1921–33.

Grainge, I. and M. Jayaram (1999). "The integrase family of recombinase: organization and function of the active site." *Mol Microbiol* **33**(3): 449–56.

Houghton, P. J., C. F. Stewart, et al. (1998). "Extending principles learned in model systems to clinical trials design." *Oncology (Williston Park)* **12**(8 Suppl 6): 84–93.

Iyer, N. V., S. W. Leung, et al. (1998). "The human hypoxia-inducible factor 1alpha gene: HIF1A structure and evolutionary conservation." *Genomics* **52**(2): 159–65.

Kapranov, P., J. Cheng, et al. (2007). "RNA maps reveal new RNA classes and a possible function for pervasive transcription." *Science* **316**(5830): 1484–8.

Khobta, A., F. Ferri, et al. (2006). "Early effects of topoisomerase I inhibition on RNA polymerase II along transcribed genes in human cells." *J Mol Biol* **357**(1): 127–38.

Kornblihtt, A. R. (2007). "Coupling transcription and alternative splicing." *Adv Exp Med Biol* **623**: 175–89.

Koster, D. A., K. Palle, et al. (2007). "Antitumour drugs impede DNA uncoiling by topoisomerase I." *Nature* **448**(7150): 213–7.

Kouzine, F., S. Sanford, et al. (2008). "The functional response of upstream DNA to dynamic supercoiling in vivo." *Nat Struct Mol Biol* **15**(2): 146–54.

Kretzschmar, M., M. Meisterernst, et al. (1993). "Identification of human DNA topoisomerase I as a cofactor for activator-dependent transcription by RNA polymerase II." *Proc Natl Acad Sci USA* **90**(24): 11508–12.

Lapidot, M. and Y. Pilpel (2006). "Genome-wide natural antisense transcription: coupling its regulation to its different regulatory mechanisms." *EMBO Rep* **7**(12): 1216–22.

Lavelle, C. (2007). "Transcription elongation through a chromatin template." *Biochimie* **89**(4): 516–27.

Lee, M. S. and W. T. Garrard (1991). "Positive DNA supercoiling generates a chromatin conformation characteristic of highly active genes." *Proc Natl Acad Sci USA* **88**(21): 9675–9.

Li, T. K. and L. F. Liu (2001). "Tumor cell death induced by topoisomerase-targeting drugs." *Annu Rev Pharmacol Toxicol* **41**: 53–77.

Lisby, M., J. R. Olesen, et al. (2001). "Residues within the N-terminal domain of human topoisomerase I play a direct role in relaxation." *J Biol Chem* **276**(23): 20220–7.
Liu, L. F. and J. C. Wang (1987). "Supercoiling of the DNA template during transcription." *Proc Natl Acad Sci USA* **84**(20): 7024–7.
Ljungman, M. and P. C. Hanawalt (1996). "The anti-cancer drug camptothecin inhibits elongation but stimulates initiation of RNA polymerase II transcription." *Carcinogenesis* **17**(1): 31–5.
Lotito, L., A. Russo, et al. (2009). "A specific transcriptional response of yeast cells to camptothecin dependent on the Swi4 and Mbp1 factors." *Eur J Pharmacol* **603**(1–3): 29–36.
Lotito, L., A. Russo, et al. (2008). "Global transcription regulation by DNA topoisomerase I in exponentially growing Saccharomyces cerevisiae cells: activation of telomere-proximal genes by TOP1 deletion." *J Mol Biol* **377**(2): 311–22.
Melillo, G. (2006). "Inhibiting hypoxia-inducible factor 1 for cancer therapy." *Mol Cancer Res* **4**(9): 601–5.
Merino, A., K. R. Madden, et al. (1993). "DNA topoisomerase I is involved in both repression and activation of transcription." *Nature* **365**(6443): 227–32.
Mondal, N. and J. D. Parvin (2001). "DNA topoisomerase IIalpha is required for RNA polymerase II transcription on chromatin templates." *Nature* **413**(6854): 435–8.
Mondal, N., Y. Zhang, et al. (2003). "Elongation by RNA polymerase II on chromatin templates requires topoisomerase activity." *Nucleic Acids Res* **31**(17): 5016–24.
Muller, M. T., W. P. Pfund, et al. (1985). "Eukaryotic type I topoisomerase is enriched in the nucleolus and catalytically active on ribosomal DNA." *EMBO J* **4**(5): 1237–43.
Munoz, M. J., M. S. Perez Santangelo, et al. (2009). "DNA damage regulates alternative splicing through inhibition of RNA polymerase II elongation." *Cell* **137**(4): 708–20.
Pilch, B., E. Allemand, et al. (2001). "Specific inhibition of serine- and arginine-rich splicing factors phosphorylation, spliceosome assembly, and splicing by the antitumor drug NB-506." *Cancer Res* **61**(18): 6876–84.
Pommier, Y. (2006). "Topoisomerase I inhibitors: camptothecins and beyond." *Nat Rev Cancer* **6**(10): 789–802.
Pommier, Y., E. Leo, et al. (2010). "DNA topoisomerases and their poisoning by anticancer and antibacterial drugs." *Chem Biol* **17**(5): 421–33.
Pommier, Y., P. Pourquier, et al. (1998). "Mechanism of action of eukaryotic DNA topoisomerase I and drugs targeted to the enzyme." *Biochim Biophys Acta* **1400**(1–3): 83–105.
Rapisarda, A., B. Uranchimeg, et al. (2002). "Identification of small molecule inhibitors of hypoxia-inducible factor 1 transcriptional activation pathway." *Cancer Res* **62**(15): 4316–24.
Rapisarda, A., B. Uranchimeg, et al. (2004). "Topoisomerase I-mediated inhibition of hypoxia-inducible factor 1: mechanism and therapeutic implications." *Cancer Res* **64**(4): 1475–82.
Rapisarda, A., J. Zalek, et al. (2004). "Schedule-dependent inhibition of hypoxia-inducible factor-1alpha protein accumulation, angiogenesis, and tumor growth by topotecan in U251-HRE glioblastoma xenografts." *Cancer Res* **64**(19): 6845–8.
Rossi, F., E. Labourier, et al. (1996). "Specific phosphorylation of SR proteins by mammalian DNA topoisomerase I." *Nature* **381**(6577): 80–2.
Salceda, J., X. Fernandez, et al. (2006). "Topoisomerase II, not topoisomerase I, is the proficient relaxase of nucleosomal DNA." *EMBO J* **25**(11): 2575–83.
Sari, L. and I. Andricioaei (2005). "Rotation of DNA around intact strand in human topoisomerase I implies distinct mechanisms for positive and negative supercoil relaxation." *Nucleic Acids Res* **33**(20): 6621–34.
Seila, A. C., J. M. Calabrese, et al. (2008). "Divergent transcription from active promoters." *Science* **322**(5909): 1849–51.
Semenza, G. L. (2003). "Targeting HIF-1 for cancer therapy." *Nat Rev Cancer* **3**(10): 721–32.
Shuman, S. and B. Moss (1987). "Identification of a vaccinia virus gene encoding a type I DNA topoisomerase." *Proc Natl Acad Sci USA* **84**(21): 7478–82.
Shykind, B. M., J. Kim, et al. (1997). "Topoisomerase I enhances TFIID-TFIIA complex assembly during activation of transcription." *Genes Dev* **11**(3): 397–407.

Sims, R. J., 3 rd, R. Belotserkovskaya, et al. (2004). "Elongation by RNA polymerase II: the short and long of it." *Genes Dev* **18**(20): 2437–68.

Solier, S., J. Barb, et al. (2010). "Genome-wide analysis of novel splice variants induced by topoisomerase I poisoning shows preferential occurrence in genes encoding splicing factors." *Cancer Res* **70**(20): 8055–65.

Sordet, O., S. Larochelle, et al. (2008). "Hyperphosphorylation of RNA polymerase II in response to topoisomerase I cleavage complexes and its association with transcription- and BRCA1-dependent degradation of topoisomerase I." *J Mol Biol* **381**(3): 540–9.

Sordet, O., A. J. Nakamura, et al. (2010). "DNA double-strand breaks and ATM activation by transcription-blocking DNA lesions." *Cell Cycle* **9**(2): 274–8.

Sordet, O., C. E. Redon, et al. (2009). "Ataxia telangiectasia mutated activation by transcription- and topoisomerase I-induced DNA double-strand breaks." *EMBO Rep* **10**(8): 887–93.

Staker, B. L., K. Hjerrild, et al. (2002). "The mechanism of topoisomerase I poisoning by a camptothecin analog." *Proc Natl Acad Sci USA* **99**(24): 15387–92.

Straub, T., B. R. Knudsen, et al. (2000). "PSF/p54(nrb) stimulates "jumping" of DNA topoisomerase I between separate DNA helices." *Biochemistry* **39**(25): 7552–8.

Strumberg, D., A. A. Pilon, et al. (2000). "Conversion of topoisomerase I cleavage complexes on the leading strand of ribosomal DNA into 5′-phosphorylated DNA double-strand breaks by replication runoff." *Mol Cell Biol* **20**(11): 3977–87.

Tanizawa, A., A. Fujimori, et al. (1994). "Comparison of topoisomerase I inhibition, DNA damage, and cytotoxicity of camptothecin derivatives presently in clinical trials." *J Natl Cancer Inst* **86**(11): 836–42.

Tuduri, S., L. Crabbe, et al. (2009). "Topoisomerase I suppresses genomic instability by preventing interference between replication and transcription." *Nat Cell Biol* **11**(11): 1315–24.

Uemura, T. and M. Yanagida (1984). "Isolation of type I and II DNA topoisomerase mutants from fission yeast: single and double mutants show different phenotypes in cell growth and chromatin organization." *EMBO J* **3**(8): 1737–44.

Wang, J. C. (1996). "DNA topoisomerases." *Annu Rev Biochem* **65**: 635–92.

Wang, J. C. (2002). "Cellular roles of DNA topoisomerases: a molecular perspective." *Nat Rev Mol Cell Biol* **3**(6): 430–40.

Wang, J. C. and G. N. Giaever (1988). "Action at a distance along a DNA." *Science* **240**(4850): 300–4.

Wu, H. Y., S. H. Shyy, et al. (1988). "Transcription generates positively and negatively supercoiled domains in the template." *Cell* **53**(3): 433–40.

Wu, J. and L. F. Liu (1997). "Processing of topoisomerase I cleavable complexes into DNA damage by transcription." *Nucleic Acids Res* **25**(21): 4181–6.

Zamboni, W. C., C. F. Stewart, et al. (1998). "Relationship between topotecan systemic exposure and tumor response in human neuroblastoma xenografts." *J Natl Cancer Inst* **90**(7): 505–11.

Zhou, Y., F. G. Gwadry, et al. (2002). "Transcriptional regulation of mitotic genes by camptothecin-induced DNA damage: microarray analysis of dose- and time-dependent effects." *Cancer Res* **62**(6): 1688–95.

Chapter 15
Mechanisms Regulating Cellular Responses to DNA Topoisomerase I-Targeted Agents

Piero Benedetti and Mary-Ann Bjornsti

15.1 DNA Topoisomerase I-Targeted Therapeutics

Eukaryotic DNA topoisomerase I (Top1) is a monomeric enzyme that plays important roles in cellular processes involving DNA, such as DNA replication, transcription, and recombination and chromosome condensation (Bjornsti 2002; Wang 2002; Corbett and Berger 2004; Pommier 2009). For example, the enzyme provides a swivel to relieve the overwinding of DNA produced by advancing replication forks and the local DNA supercoiling produced by RNA polymerases during transcription. The nuclear enzyme, a type IB topoisomerase encoded by the *TOP1* gene, is highly conserved in terms of reaction mechanism, structure, and sensitivity to the camptothecin (CPT) class of chemotherapeutics (Corbett and Berger 2004; Pommier 2009). Top1 catalyzes the relaxation of supercoiled DNA through the transient breakage and rejoining of a single DNA strand in duplex DNA (see Chap. 2). As shown in Fig. 15.1, the monomeric enzyme first binds duplex DNA as a protein clamp. The nucleophilic attack of the active site tyrosine on a DNA phosphodiester bond subsequently generates a phosphotyrosyl bond between Top1 and the 3′ end of the cleaved DNA strand. The noncovalently bound 5′ DNA end is free to rotate about the intact, nonscissile strand to effect changes in the linkage of DNA strands. The 3′ phosphotyrosyl intermediate of this reaction mechanism distinguishes type IB enzymes from other topoisomerases (such as type IA and type II enzymes), whose active site tyrosines become transiently linked to a 5′ phosphoryl DNA end. Regardless of the DNA end bound, the phosphotyrosyl intermediate conserves the energy of phosphodiester bond, such that religation of the nicked DNA by a second transesterification reaction does not require ATP. Top1 is also the cellular target of several novel classes of antitumor agents (Li and Liu 2001; Thomas et al. 2004; Pommier et al. 2010) (see Chap. 10). As exemplified

M.-A. Bjornsti (✉)
Department of Pharmacology and Toxicology, University of Alabama at Birmingham, VH 140, 1530 3rd Ave S, Birmingham, AL 35294-0019, USA
e-mail: Bjornsti@uab.edu

Y. Pommier (ed.), *DNA Topoisomerases and Cancer*, Cancer Drug Discovery and Development, DOI 10.1007/978-1-4614-0323-4_15,

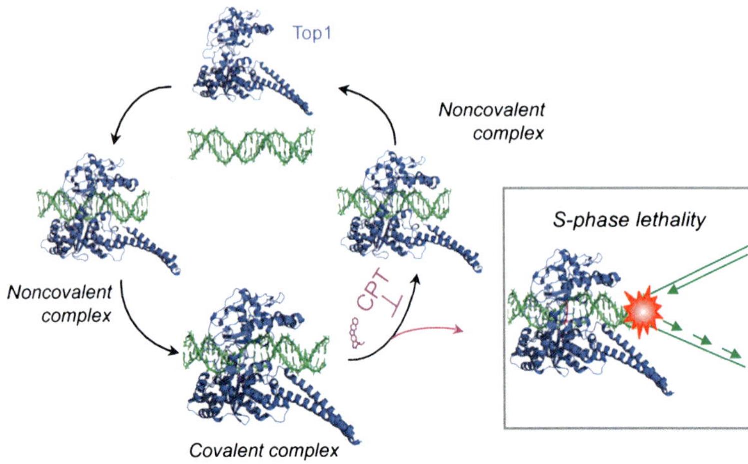

Fig. 15.1 The camptothecin (CPT) class of chemotherapeutucs interferes with Top1 by reversibly inhibiting the religation of cleaved DNA within the covalent Top1-DNA complex. Top1 (shown is the crystal structure of C-terminal 70 kDa fragment of human Top1 in *blue*) binds duplex DNA as a protein clamp. Cleavage of a single DNA strand by the active site tyrosine (*purple*) produces a transient phosphotyrosyl bond between Top1 and the 3′ end of the cleaved DNA. Changes in topology are accomplished by the rotation of the free 5′ DNA end about the nonscissile DNA strand. CPT (*magenta*) reversibly binds and stabilizes the covalent Top1-DNA complex. However, conversion of the ternary CPT-Top1-DNA complexes into the irreversible DNA lesions that induce cell death requires ongoing DNA replication. The ribbon diagrams of Top1 and DNA structures were generated using MacPyMol from PDB files 1K4T and 1A36

by CPT, these drugs poison Top1 by reversibly stabilizing the covalent enzyme-DNA intermediate. During S-phase, the collision of the advancing replication forks with CPT-stabilized complexes produces the DNA lesions that induce cell death.

CPT is a plant alkaloid with broad spectrum antitumor activity (Pommier et al. 2010; Venditto and Simanek 2010). Although early clinical trials with CPT were disappointing, the identification of Top1 as its cellular target renewed interest in the clinical potential of CPT (Hsiang and Liu 1988; Hertzberg et al. 1989). CPT analogs Topotecan (TPT) and CPT-11 have significant activity against adult and pediatric solid tumors and FDA approval for specific indications (Rodriguez-Galindo et al. 2000, Venditto and Simanek 2010; Pommier et al. 2010). Additional CPT analogs are in clinical trials, while structurally distinct Top1 poisons, such as triazachrysenes, indolocarbazoles, and ARC-111, are also being evaluated in preclinical models and clinical trials. A wealth of biochemical, structural and genetic data demonstrate the drug stabilization of covalent Top1-DNA complexes (Li and Liu 2001; Staker et al. 2002, 2005; Corbett and Berger 2004; Pommier 2009). Yet, we lack sufficient insight into the consequences of Top1 poisoning to explain the S-phase dependence of these chemotherapeutic drugs or even the basis for tumor selective toxicity. This chapter will focus on recent advances in our understanding of the cytotoxic mechanisms of Top1 targeted drugs and the pathways that dictate cellular responses to the DNA damage induced by these agents.

15.2 Model Systems and Approaches to Study Top1-Induced DNA Damage

15.2.1 The Yeast Saccharomyces cerevisiae

Critical components of the eukaryotic cell cycle machinery, DNA repair pathways, and DNA damage/replication checkpoints are well conserved in the budding yeast *S. cerevisiae* (Ulrich 2007; Harper and Elledge 2007; Branzei and Foiani 2010). Coupled with the ease of targeted gene deletion in otherwise isogenic haploid yeast strain backgrounds, and the availability of a wide range of mitotically stable expression vectors, this genetically tractable model has proven useful in dissecting the cytotoxic mechanism of Top1-targeted agents (Bjornsti 2002). In contrast to other genetic models, such as *Drosophila* and mouse, the *TOP1* gene in yeast is nonessential. Genetic studies have established that other gene products, such as DNA topoisomerase II, can compensate for the loss of Top1 function. Yet, yeast cells deleted for the *TOP1* gene (*top1*Δ strains) are resistant to CPT, while reintroducing *TOP1* on a plasmid restores drug sensitivity (Eng et al. 1988; Nitiss and Wang 1988; Bjornsti et al. 1989). As Top1 is not required to maintain yeast cell viability, these data indicate that CPT cytotoxicity is a consequence of stabilizing the covalent Top1-DNA complex, rather than the inhibition of Top1 activity. Consistent with this model of drug action, elevated levels of *TOP1* expression in isogenic yeast strains or human cells increases CPT sensitivity, while downregulation of Top1 protein levels confers resistance to CPT (Madden and Champoux 1992; Knab et al. 1993; Hann et al. 1998). This cytotoxic mechanism is further supported by the strong correlation of CPT analog potency with the production of Top1-DNA complexes and the toxicity of Top1 mutant protein that exhibit increased stabilization of covalent complexes in the absence of CPT (Megonigal et al. 1997; Fertala et al. 2000; Thomas et al. 2004; Colley et al. 2004; Pommier et al. 2010). However, in genetically diverse backgrounds, such as human tumor cells or yeast strains deleted for select DNA repair or checkpoint pathways, Top1 protein levels per se do not predict drug response.

Genetic and cell biology studies demonstrate that the mechanism of drug-induced cell killing is conserved in yeast and human cells, inducing similar effects on cell cycle progression, checkpoint activation, and DNA recombination (Fiorani and Bjornsti 2000; Bjornsti 2002; Pommier 2009). For instance, drug treatment of yeast or mammalian cells induces sister chromatid exchange and cell cycle arrest in G2. Experiments in yeast strains defective in double-strand break repair (due to deletion of *RAD52 or RAD51* genes) and mammalian cells exhibiting defects in homologous recombination implicate homologous recombination pathway function in the repair of drug-induced DNA lesions in S-phase. In yeast and mammalian cells, CPT sensitivity is abolished in the presence of the DNA synthesis inhibitor aphidicolin. So even though Top1 and drug stabilized Top1-DNA complexes remain constant throughout the cell cycle, CPT-induced cytotoxicity is highly S-phase dependent.

A key feature of the cell cycle is a series of conserved, dependent processes to ensure DNA replication occurs once per cell cycle (Bell and Dutta 2002; Blow and

Dutta 2005). The cell cycle machinery is further subject to the inhibitory activity of DNA damage and S-phase checkpoints (Harper and Elledge 2007; Branzei and Foiani 2010). Activation of the DNA damage checkpoint in response to DNA breaks or the S-phase checkpoint in response to replication fork damage/stalling results in the inhibition of origin firing, a slowing of fork progression and the maintenance of fork stability. Checkpoint components required for sensing the damage, amplifying the signal and inducing cellular responses through a kinase cascade are highly conserved and often involve components of the replication machinery. DNA damage and replication checkpoint proteins, such as yeast Mec1, Tel1, Mrc1, and Rad53 and mammalian orthologs ATM, ATR, MRC1, and CHK2, have been shown to modulate cell sensitivity to Top1 poisons (Bennett et al. 2001; Xiao et al. 2003; Furuta et al. 2003; Fiorani et al. 2004; Flatten et al. 2005; O'Connell et al. 2010). An increase in phosphorylated histone H_2AX (γH_2AX) in response to CPT treatment has also been reported in mammalian and yeast cells, consistent with the induction of Top1-induced DNA breaks (Furuta et al. 2003; Redon et al. 2005). Tyrosyl DNA phosphodiesterase I (Tdp1) is another conserved protein that cleaves the 3′ phosphotyrosyl linkage between Top1 and DNA (Pouliot et al. 1999). However, Tdp1 also resolves topoisomerase II-DNA complexes and 3′ phosphoglycolates (Interthal et al. 2005; Nitiss et al. 2006; He et al. 2007), and Tdp1 levels do not correlate with cell sensitivity to CPT. In yeast, additional genetic alterations, such as deletion of the Rad9 DNA damage checkpoint, are necessary to sensitize *tdp1Δ* cells to CPT (Liu et al. 2002; Fiorani et al. 2004).

More direct evidence for alterations in DNA replication affecting CPT cytotoxicity is the enhanced drug sensitivity of yeast strains mutated for *SGS1*, *MUS81*, *CTD1*, *CDC45*, or *DPB11* (Reid et al. 1999; Bennett et al. 2001; Vance and Wilson 2002; Bastin-Shanower et al. 2003; Fiorani et al. 2004). In the absence of the Sgs1 or Mus81 helicases, defects in replication fork stability may prevent repair of Top1-DNA lesions. In a yeast genetic screen for mutants with enhanced sensitivity to low levels of a self-poisoning Top1T_{722}A mutant enzyme, we identified conditional mutations in nine genes that function to protect cells from CPT, including gene products involved in replication (Cdt1, Cdc45, and Dbp11), ubiquitin degradation (Doa4), and SUMO conjugation (Ubc9) (Reid et al. 1999; Fiorani et al. 2004; Jacquiau et al. 2005). Cdt1 functions in G1-phase to license origins of replication, such that an origin will fire only once per cell cycle (Bell and Dutta 2002). The coordinated assembly of Cdc45 and Dpb11 is required for origin firing and for effective DNA polymerization (Blow and Dutta 2005). The human orthologs of these genes are human CDT1, CDC45L, and Top1BP1, respectively. As diagrammed in Fig. 15.2, Cdc45 functions in the recruitment of replicative polymerases and is a processivity factor for the Mcm2-7 replicative helicase. Dpb11 is associated with the replicative DNA polymerases Polε and δ, and plays a role in the S-phase checkpoint. Our studies further demonstrated genetic interactions between Cdc45, Dpb11, and the Rad9 DNA damage checkpoint (Reid et al. 1999). These data are consistent with a model of impaired replication fork stability in the temperature sensitive *cdc45* and *dpb11* mutants, which would enhance cell sensitivity to CPT. A similar function for human CDC45L in protecting cells from the cytotoxic activity of the

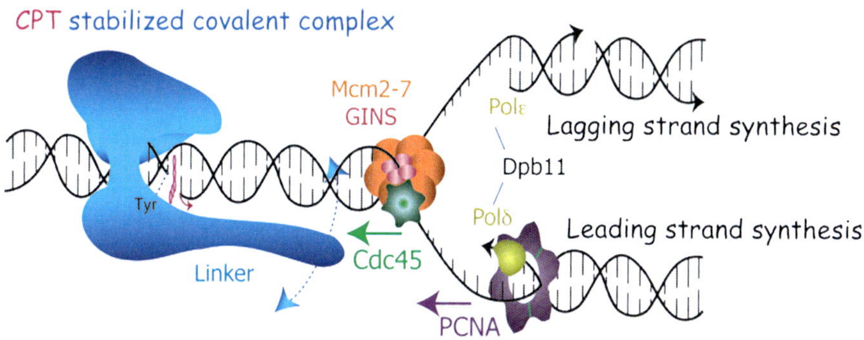

Fig. 15.2 CPT poisoning of Top1 and replication fork progression. Conditional temperture sensitive mutants of yeast *CDC45* and *DBP11* enhance cell sensitivity to Top1-induced DNA damage. Cdc45 acts as a processivity factor for the replicative Mcm2-7 helicase. Dpb11 associates with the replicative Polδ/ε polymerases. The flexibility of the Top1 linker domain had been correlated with CPT resistance

CPT analog Topotecan is also supported by preliminary studies using siRNA (Coric and Bjornsti, unpublished data). In a recent work describing high throughput plasmid transfer, Reid et al. (2010) introduced the same self-poisoning Top1T$_{722}$A enzyme into the yeast gene disruption library. In addition to previously identified gene products that regulate cell sensitivity to CPT, they also determined that gene disruptions of the Rpd3 histone deacetylase complex, the kinectochore and vesicular trafficking enhanced cell sensitivity to Top1-induced DNA damage.

The regulated expression of plasmid-borne yeast or human *TOP1* alleles in *top1Δ* strains has also been used to assess the effects of mutations and architecture on Top1 function and CPT sensitivity in the absence of the endogenous enzyme (Fiorani et al. 2003; Colley et al. 2004; Lossaso et al. 2007; van der Merwe and Bjornsti 2008). This approach has defined a number of amino acid substitutions in catalytically active enzymes that confer Top1 resistance to CPT, that alter the DNA cleavage/religation equilibrium in self-poisoning enzymes to mimic the action of CPT, or that enhance the intrinsic CPT sensitivity of Top1. Crystallographic and biochemical data reveal an unusual architecture for Top1 (Staker et al. 2002, 2005) (see Figs. 15.1 and 15.2), where an extended pair of alpha helices (linker domain) extend from a conserved protein core, which forms a clamp around duplex DNA. The linker connects the core with the C-terminal domain such that the active site tyrosine is positioned within the catalytic pocket of the Top1 protein clamp. Several studies implicate Top1 linker function as a determinant of CPT sensitivity. Increased linker flexibility, either as a consequence of mutation within the linker domain or combining a 58 kDa Top1 clamp with a 12 kDa linker/C-terminus to reconstitute an active enzyme, decreases Top1 sensitivity to CPT (Stewart et al. 1999; Fiorani et al. 2003). Our recent characterization of Top1 mutants involving substitutions of a conserved Gly that lies at the junction between the linker and the C-terminal domain, demonstrated an increase in Top1 enzyme sensitivity to CPT (van der Merwe and Bjornsti 2008). These data led up to posit that this conserved Gly provides the flexible hinge that enables linker movement and that restricting linker mobility enhances Top1 sensitivity to CPT in cells. In the context of the model shown in Fig. 15.2, it is tempting to speculate that the interaction of the flexible linker with the advancing replication machinery and/or processive Mcm2-7 complex may trigger the resolution of covalent Top1-DNA complexes to prevent the generation of potentially lethal DNA lesions.

In yeast experiments, the conserved serine-threonine TOR kinase (for **T**arget **o**f **R**apamycin) has also been shown to protect cells from genotoxic stress in S-phase, including that induced by CPT (Shen et al. 2007). The TOR signaling pathway has emerged as a central regulator of cellular responses to wide ranging environmental stresses, including amino acid deprivation, growth factor deprivation, hypoxia, and DNA damage through the action of two conserved protein complexes, TORC1 and TORC2 (Bjornsti and Houghton 2004; Wullschleger et al. 2005). TORC1 signaling is inhibited by the macrocyclic antibiotic rapamycin and several rapalogs have demonstrated antitumor activity in a variety of malignancies. When synchronized cultures of yeast cells were exposed to rapamycin and CPT, the inhibition of TORC1 dramatically enhanced the cytotoxic activity of CPT (Shen et al. 2007). The protective function of TORC1 against genotoxic stresses required the activation of replication/DNA damage checkpoints. Recent studies demonstrate that TORC1 signaling plays a similar protective role in mammalian cells (Cam et al. 2010), while the combination of rapamycin with CPT analogs has demonstrated remarkable additive or greater than additive antitumor activity in a panel of human pediatric tumor xenografts (Bjornsti and Houghton, unpublished data).

15.2.2 RNAi

The use of the genetically tractable yeast model obviates many of the complexities inherent in studies of transformed human cell lines. However, in human cells, RNAi technology allows for the targeted downregulation of gene expression, while avoiding the selection of other genetic changes that typically accompany plasmid integration or the clonal selection of drug resistant cell lines. A directed approach using specific siRNAs to target the human orthologs of genes identified in several yeast screens has confirmed the conservation of several pathways shown to protect cells from Top1-induced DNA damage, including CDC45L and the SUMO pathways as described above. However, recent studies highlight the utility of unbiased RNAi screens to define novel pathways that modulate cellular responses to CPT.

In independent studies, O'Connell et al. (2010) performed a human genome wide short hairpin (shRNA) screen for genes that altered HeLa cell responses to CPT, while O'Donnell et al. (2010) performed an siRNA screen for increased 53BP1 accumulation. In both cases, the investigators determined that a novel MMS22L-NFKBIL2 complex function in the recovery from replicative stress, such as that induced by CPT, and that depletion of components of this complex impairs Rad51-mediated homologous recombination. The same complex was also identified in an independent biochemical approach (Duro et al. 2010). Mammalian MMS22L is loosely related to yeast Mms22, depletion of which also impairs homologous recombinational repair of damage induced at replication forks (Duro et al. 2008). In the context of the model diagrammed in Fig. 15.2, it is interesting to note that NFKBIL2 (TONSL) also serves a scaffold for the histone chaperone ASF1 and MCM proteins.

15.2.3 Single Molecule Studies

The application of single molecule technologies to the study of enzyme and DNA dynamics has begun to provide unique perspectives on DNA topoisomerase catalysis and drug action (Koster et al. 2010; Neuman 2010). In the case of typeIB enzymes, magnetic tweezers have been used to query the dynamics of DNA unwinding in the context of individual Top1-DNA covalent complexes, both in the presence and absence of CPT (Koster et al. 2005; Koster et al. 2007; Taneja et al. 2007). These studies confirmed the increased half-life of the covalent Top1-DNA complex in the presence of CPT (Koster et al. 2007); The surprise finding was the decreased velocity with which Top1 removed positive supercoils in the presence of drug (by a factor of 20 relative to Top1-DNA complexes alone). Moreover, this drug-induced decrease was much more pronounced with positive supercoil removal than with negative supercoils.

To determine if CPT induced the same asymmetry in supercoil removal in eukaryotic cells, plasmid DNA topology was assessed in yeast cells expressing human Top1 in the presence or absence of CPT (Koster et al. 2007). Consistent with the single molecule studies, the presence of CPT induced the accumulation of positively supercoiled DNA, independent of cell cycle. However, this effect was dependent on the expression of a catalytically active, CPT sensitive Top1 enzyme. Since positive supercoils would preferentially accumulate in advance of an advancing replication fork, there data suggest that CPT-induced positive supercoils might contribute to the drug's cytotoxic activity.

15.3 Future Challenges

The application of wide-ranging approaches and technologies to the study of CPT-induced cytotoxicity continues to reveal the complexity of alterations in Top1 catalysis and the signaling and repair pathways that dictate cellular responses to Top1 poisons. Nevertheless, the picture emerging from these studies is that a critical determinant of cell survival in the face of Top1-mediated replicative stress is the effective sensing and repair of DNA at the replication fork. The current challenge is to translate these findings into predictive biomarkers and effective drug combinations for human tumor response in a clinical setting. For example, the apparent conservation of human CDC45L and TopBP1 in protecting cells from CPT-induced replicative stress provides the rationale for a systematic survey of CDC45L or TopBP11 protein levels in human tumor samples to assess whether this inversely correlates with therapeutic response. Similar arguments may relate to checkpoint proteins, such as BRCA1, Chk1, and ATR, or to components of the MMS22L-NFKBIL2 complex. In terms of drug combinations, the function of MMS22L-NFKBIL2 in the resolution of Top1-replicative lesions may help explain the activity of the alkylating agent Temozolomide with CPT analogs in the treatment of human gliomas (Venditto and Simanek 2010). The function of the TORC1 complexes in suppressing the cytotoxic activity of CPT (Shen et al. 2007) support the combination of rapamycin or TOR kinase inhibitors with CPT analogs in human cancer clinical trials. Indeed, this prediction of additive activity has been borne out in preclinical models of a range of human pediatric tumor xenografts (Bjornsti and Houghton, unpublished data). These finding refute the expectation of antagonistic activity that might have been predicted given the ability of rapamycin analogs to induce a transient arrest in G1 phase of the cell cycle and the strict S-phase dependence of CPT-induced toxicity and highlight the clinical benefits that may be gained from further mechanistic studies of Top1 poisons.

Acknowledgments We wish to thank past and present members of the Benedetti and Bjornsti labs for their many contributions. This work was supported in part by funds from PRIN Cofin MIUR (to P.B.) and NIH grants CA70406 and CA58755 (to M-A.B).

References

Bastin-Shanower SA et al (2003) The mechanism of Mus81-Mms4 cleavage site selection distinguishes it from the homologous endonuclease Rad1-Rad10. Mol Cell Biol 23:3487–3496

Bell SP and Dutta A (2002) DNA replication in eukaryotic cells. Annu Rev Biochem 71: 333–374

Bennett CB et al (2001) Genes required for ionizing radiation resistance in yeast. Nat Genet 29:426–434

Bjornsti M-A et al (1989) Expression of human DNA topoisomerase I in yeast cells lacking yeast DNA topoisomerase I: restoration of sensitivity of the cells to the antitumor drug camptothecin. Cancer Res 49:6318–6323

Bjornsti M-A (2002) Cancer therapeutics in yeast. Cancer Cell 2:267–273

Bjornsti M-A and Houghton PJ (2004) The TOR pathway: a target for cancer therapy. Nat Rev Cancer 4:335–348

Blow JJ and Dutta A (2005) Preventing re-replication of chromosomal DNA. Nat Rev Mol Cell Biol 6:476–486

Branzei D and Foiani M (2010) Maintaining genome stability at the replication fork. Nat Rev Mol Cell Biol 11:208–219

Cam H et al (2010) mTORC1 signaling under hypoxic conditions is controlled by ATM-dependent phosphorylation of HIF-1a. Mol Cell 40:509–520

Colley WC et al (2004) Substitution of conserved residues within the active site alters the cleavage-religation equilibrium of DNA topoisomerase I. J Biol Chem 279:54069–54078

Corbett KD and Berger JM (2004) Structure, molecular mechanisms, and evolutionary relationships in DNA topoisomerases. Annu Rev Biophys Biomol Struct 33:95–118

Duro E et al (2008) Budding yeast Mms22 and Mms1 regulate homologous recombination induced by replisome blockage. DNA repair (Amst) 7:811–818

Duro E et al (2010) Identification of the MMS22L-TONSL complex that promotes homologous recombination. Mol Cell 40:632–644

Eng W-K et al (1988) Evidence that DNA topoisomerase I is necessary for the cytotoxic effects of camptothecin. Mol Pharmacol 34:755–760

Fertala J et al (2000) Substitutions of Asn-726 in the active site of yeast DNA topoisomerase I define novel mechanisms of stabilizing the covalent enzyme-DNA intermediate. J Biol Chem 275:15246–15253

Fiorani P and Bjornsti M-A (2000) Mechanisms of DNA topoisomerase I-induced cell killing in the yeast Saccharomyces cerevisiae. Ann N Y Acad Sci 922:65–75

Fiorani P et al (2003) Single mutation in the linker domain confers protein flexibility and camptothecin resistance to human topoisomerase I. J Biol Chem 278:43268–43275

Fiorani P et al (2004) The deubiquitinating enzyme Doa4p protects cells from DNA topoisomerase I poisons. J Biol Chem 279:21271–21281

Flatten K et al (2005) The role of checkpoint kinase 1 in sensitivity to topoisomerase I poisons. J Biol Chem 280:14349–14355

Furuta T et al (2003) Phosphorylation of histone H2AX and activation of Mre11, Rad50, and Nbs1 in response to replication-dependent DNA double-strand breaks induced by mammalian DNA topoisomerase I cleavage complexes. J Biol Chem 278:20303–20312

Hann C et al (1998) Increased camptothecin toxicity in mammalian cells expressing *Saccharomyces cerevisiae* DNA topoisomerase I. J Biol Chem 273:8425–8433

Harper JW and Elledge SJ (2007) The DNA damage response: ten years after. Mol Cell 28:739–745

He X et al (2007) Mutation of a conserved active site residue converts tyrosyl-DNA phosphodiesterase I into a DMA topoisomerase I-dependent poison. J Mol Biol 372:1070–1081

Hertzberg RP, Caranfa MJ and Hecht SM (1989) On the mechanism of topoisomerase I inhibitions by camptothecin: evidence for binding to an enzyme-DNA complex. Biochem 28:4629–4638

Hsiang Y-H and Liu LF (1988) Identification of mammalian DNA topoisomerase I as an intracellular target of the anticancer drug camptothecin. Cancer Res 48:1722–1726

Interthal H, Chen HJ and Champoux JJ (2005) Human Tdp1 cleaves a broad spectrum of substrates, including phosphoamide linkages. J Biol Chem 280:36518–36528

Jacquiau HR et al (2005) Defects in SUMO (small ubiquitin-related modifier) conjugation and deconjugation alter cell sensitivity to DNA topoisomerase I-induced DNA damage. J Biol Chem 280:23566–23575

Knab AM, Fertala J and Bjornsti M-A (1993) Mechanisms of camptothecin resistance in yeast DNA topoisomerase I mutants. J Biol Chem 268:22322–22330

Koster DA et al (2005) Friction and torgue govern the relaxation of DNA supercoils by eukaryotic topoisomerase IB. Nature 434:671–674

Koster DA et al (2007) Antitumour drugs impede DNA uncoiling by topoisomerase I. Nature 448:213–217

Koster DA et al (2010) Cellular strategies for regulating DNA supercoiling: A single-molecule prespective. Cell 142:519–530

Li TK and Liu LF (2001) Tumor cell death induced by topoisomerase-targeting drugs. Annu Rev Pharmacol Toxicol 41:53–77

Liu C, Pouliot JJ and Nash HA (2002) Repair of topoisomerase I covalent complexes in the absence of the tyrosyl-DNA phosphodiesterase Tdp1. Proc Natl Acad Sci USA 99:14970–14975

Losasso CE et al (2007) Alterations in linker flexibility suppress DNA topoisomerase I mutant-induced cell lethality. J Biol Chem 282:9855–9864

Madden KR and Champoux JJ (1992) Overexpression of human topoisomerase I in baby hamster kidney cells: hypersensitivity of clonal isolates to camptothecin. Cancer Res 52:525–532

Megonigal MD, Fertala J and Bjornsti M-A (1997) Cell cycle arrest and lethality produced by alterations in the catalytic activity of yeast DNA topoisomerase I mutants. J Biol Chem 272:12801–12808

Neuman KC (2010) Single-molecule measurements of DNA topology and topoisomerases. J Biol Chem 285:18967–18971

Nitiss J and Wang JC (1988) DNA topoisomerase-targeting antitumor drugs can be studied in yeast. Proc Natl Acad Sci USA 85:7501–7505

Nitiss KC et al (2006) Tyrosyl-DNA phosphodiesterase (Tdp1) participates in the repair of Top2-mediated DNA damage. Proc Natl Acad Sci USA 103:8953–8958

O'Connell BC et al (2010) A genome-wide camptothecin sensitivity screen identifies a mammalian MMS22L-NFKBIL2 complex required for genomic stability. Mol Cell 40:645–657

O'Donnell L et al (2010) The MMS22L-TONSL complex mediates recovery from replication stress and homologous recombination. Mol Cell 40:619–631

Pommier Y (2009) DNA topoisomerase I inhibitors: chemistry, biology, and interfacial inhibition. Chem Rev 109:2894–2902

Pommier Y et al (2010) DNA topoisomerases and their poisoning by anticancer and antibacterial drugs. Chem Biol 17:421–433

Pouliot JJ et al (1999) Yeast gene for a Tyr-DNA phosphodiesterase that repairs topoisomerase I complexes. Science 286:552–555

Redon C, Pilch DR and Bonner WM (2005) Genetic analysis of Saccharomyces cerevisiae H2A serine 129 mutant suggests a functional relationship between H2A and the sister chromatid cohesion partners Csm3-Tof1 for the repair of Topoisomerase I-induced DNA damage. Genetics

Reid RJ et al (1999) CDC45 and DPB11 are required for processive DNA replication and resistance to DNA topoisomerase I-mediated DNA damage. Proc Natl Acad Sci USA 96:11440–11445

Reid RJD et al (2010) Selective ploidy abaltion, a high throughput plasmid transfer protocol, identifies new genes affecting repair of topoisomerase I-induced DNA damage. Genome Res (in press)

Rodriguez-Galindo C et al (2000) Clinical use of topoisomerase I inhibitors in anticancer treatment. Med Pediatr Oncol 35:385–402

Shen et al (2007) TOR signaling in a determinant of cell survival in response to DNA damage. Mol Cell Biol 27:7007–7017

Staker BL et al (2002) The mechanism of topoisomerase I poisoning by a camptothecin analog. Proc Natl Acad Sci USA 99:15387–15392

Staker BL et al (2005) Structures of three classes of anticancer agents bound to the human topoisomerase I-DNA covalent complex. J Med Chem 48:2336–2345

Stewart L, Ireton GC and Champoux JJ (1999) A functional linker in human topoisomerase I is required for maximum sensitivity to camptothecin in a DNA relaxation assay. J Biol Chem 274:32950–32960

Taneja B et al (2007) Topoisomerase V relaxes supercoiled DNA by a constrained swiveling mechanism. Proc Natl Acad Sci USA 104:14670–14675

Thomas CJ, Rahier NJ and Hecht SM (2004) Camptothecin: current perspectives. Bioorg Med Chem 12:1585–1604

Ulrich HD (2007) Conservation of DNA damage tolerance pathways from yeast to humans. Biochem Soc Trans 35:1334–1337

van der Merwe M and Bjornsti M-A (2008) Mutation of Gly721 alters DNA topoisomerase I active site architecture and sensitivity to camptothecin. J Biol Chem 283:3305–3315

Vance JR and Wilson TE (2002) Yeast Tdp1 and Rad1-Rad10 function as redundant pathways for repairing Top1 replicative damage. Proc Natl Acad Sci USA 99:13669–13774

Venditto VJ and Simanek EE (2010) Cancer therapies utilizing the camptothecins: A review of the in vivo literature. Mol Pharm 7:307–349

Wullschleger et al (2005) Molecular organization of target of rapamycin complex 2. J Biol Chem 280:30697–30704

Wang JC (2002) Cellular roles of DNA topoisomerases: a molecular perspective. Nat Rev Mol Cell Biol 3: 430–440

Xiao Z et al (2003) Chk1 mediates S and G2 arrests through Cdc25A degradation in response to DNA-damaging agents. J Biol Chem 278:21767–21773

Chapter 16
Tyrosyl-DNA-Phosphodiesterase

Thomas S. Dexheimer, Shar-yin N. Huang, Benu Brata Das, and Yves Pommier

16.1 Discovery of an Enzyme with 3′-Tyrosyl-Phosphodiesterase Activity

In all living organisms, there is a steady formation of DNA lesions that challenge the inherent stability of their genomes. To counteract this threat, cells have developed a diverse set of DNA repair systems that cope with a host of different types of DNA damage (Sancar et al. 2004). The most common form of DNA damage that arises in cells are single-strand breaks (SSBs) that can occur at a frequency of tens of thousands per cell per day (Lindahl 1993). However, these SSBs frequently are not proper substrates for DNA ligase, that is, a 3′-hydroxyl and 5′-phosphate. Instead, some DNA termini harbor blocking lesions or "dirty" ends that are not suitable for repair (Caldecott 2007). One such blocking lesion can emerge from the abortive activity of DNA topoisomerase I (Top1), resulting in a DNA strand break that is encumbered with a 3′-protein adduct. If not repaired, such breaks can result in the development of more dangerous double-strand breaks (DSBs) that can lead to chromosome loss, translocations, or truncations (see previous Chaps. 6–7). Thus, the initial "cleaning" or removal of this lesion is paramount to the repair of Top1-associated DNA strand breaks.

In 1996, Nash and colleagues (Yang et al. 1996) identified a phosphodiesterase activity in *Saccharomyces cerevisiae* that specifically hydrolyzed the phosphodiester bond between a single tyrosine residue and a terminal 3′-phosphate of DNA.

T.S. Dexheimer (✉)
National Chemical Genomic Center, National Institutes of Health, Rockville, MD, USA
e-mail: dexheimt@mail.nih.gov

Y. Pommier (ed.), *DNA Topoisomerases and Cancer*, Cancer Drug Discovery and Development, DOI 10.1007/978-1-4614-0323-4_16,

Given that the artificial substrate employed in vitro recapitulated the chemistry of the covalent linkage between Top1 and DNA, they hypothesized that the observed activity may be involved in the repair of abortive Top1-DNA cleavage complexes in vivo. This activity was named tyrosyl-DNA phosphodiesterase 1 (Tdp1). In addition to a single 3′-tyrosine residue, Nash and colleagues also demonstrated that an intact bacteriophage λ integrase protein-DNA complex, which also contains a 3′-phosphotyrosyl linkage, is cleaved by yeast Tdp1, albeit less efficiently (Yang et al. 1996). Moreover, in certain genetically altered backgrounds, Tdp1-defective yeast mutants showed increased sensitivity to conditions that produce high levels of Top1-DNA cleavage complexes (Pouliot et al. 1999, 2001). These results, in conjunction with the biochemical observations, confirmed the hypothesis that Tdp1 was explicitly involved in the repair of Top1-associated DNA damage.

Tdp1 has been found in all eukaryotes examined to date in which a Top1-3′-phosphodiester bond is formed, a finding compatible with the described activity of the enzyme (Pouliot et al. 1999). Most recently, Tdp1 orthologs have been documented in the kinetoplastid parasite *Leishmania donovani* (Banerjee et al. 2010) and in plants [i.e., *Medicago truncatula* (Macovei et al. 2010) and *Arabidopsis thaliana* (Lee et al. 2010)]. The human Tdp1 protein is encoded as a single copy gene (on chromosome 14q32.11) consisting of two 5′ noncoding exons and 15 coding exons. It is ubiquitously expressed in human tissues and has been shown to possess an analogous 3′-phosphotyrosyl processing activity to its yeast counterpart (Interthal et al. 2001), while having only minimal sequence identity (~15%) (Cheng et al. 2002). The majority of the sequence variance exists in the N-terminal domain, which is poorly conserved or absent in lower eukaryotes. The N-terminus (1–148) of human Tdp1 has been shown to be expendable for enzymatic activity, yet it appears to have evolved specific regulatory functions (see below) (Interthal et al. 2001).

The most conserved regions among the Tdp1 orthologs correspond to amino acids 262–289 and 492–522 of the human protein. Sequence alignments of these conserved regions revealed that Tdp1 is a member of the phospholipase D (PLD) superfamily (Interthal et al. 2001), which comprises a heterogeneous group of enzymes that catalyze phosphoryl transfer reactions. The defining feature of PLD enzymes is a highly conserved sequence [$HXK(X)_4D(X)_6GSXN$], known as the HKD motif. All PLDs contain two copies of this signature HKD motif, both of which are required for catalytic activity (Koonin 1996; Ponting and Kerr 1996). Human Tdp1 contains two such motifs that are spatially separated in the primary sequence (Fig. 16.1a). PLD enzymes encompass a broad range of substrate specificities (Liscovitch et al. 2000). However, whether the substrate is a phospholipid, a nucleic acid, or in the case of Tdp1, a polypeptide-DNA complex, the common feature of all PLD enzymes is their inherent ability to recognize, bind, and catalyze phosphodiester bond cleavage via a select number of critical active site residues.

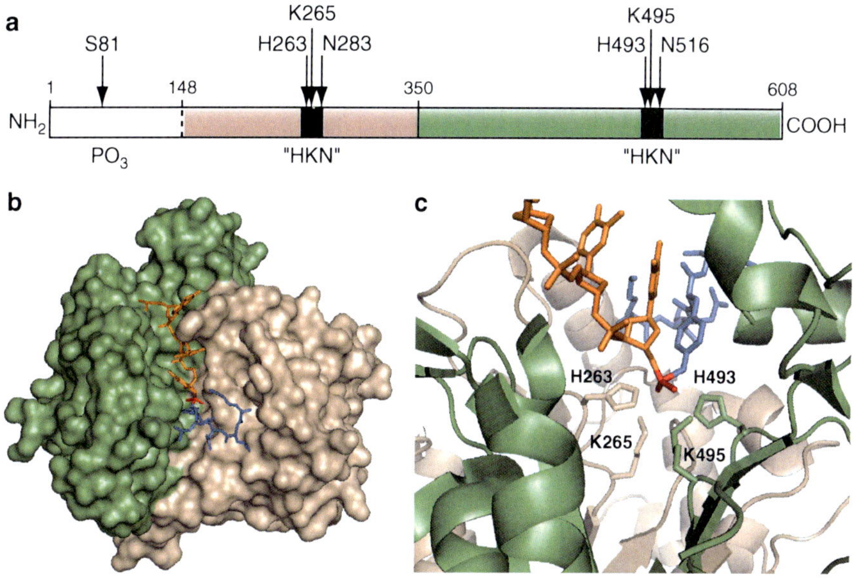

Fig. 16.1 (**a**) Schematic of the domain structure of human Tdp1. The N-terminal and C-terminal domains correspond to residues 1–350 and 351–608, respectively. Positions of the "HKN" motifs are shown in *black*. *Arrows* identify the active site residues and phosphorylation site at serine 81. Position of the physiological SCAN1 mutation (H493) is shown in *italics*. (**b**) Crystal structure of the quaternary complex consisting of truncated Tdp1 (Δ1-148), vanadate, a Top1 peptide, and single-strand DNA (PDB:1NOP). Shown as surface models, the N-terminal and C-terminal domains of Tdp1 are in *light brown* and *green*, respectively [*see* (**a**)]. Shown in stick structures are the substrate transition-state mimic consisting of single-strand DNA in *orange*, vanadate in *red*, and the peptide in *blue*. (**c**) The active site residues of Tdp1 are shown in stick structures with the rest of the protein shown in ribbon diagram; the domain colors correspond to those shown in (**a**) and (**b**). The substrate transition-state mimic structures are in the same colors as in (**b**), seen here from the bottom of the binding cleft projecting outward. For clarity, two loops in the N-terminal domain have been removed from the view (modified and updated from Dexheimer et al. (2008))

16.2 Structure and Catalytic Mechanism of Tdp1

Similar to other members of the PLD superfamily, mutagenic studies have demonstrated that the pair of HKD motifs in Tdp1 is responsible for its catalytic activity (Gottlin et al. 1998; Iwasaki et al. 1999; Rudolph et al. 1999; Sung et al. 1997). In human Tdp1, substituting H263 with alanine in the first HKD motif renders the enzyme inactive, while substituting H493 with arginine, alanine, or asparagine in the second HKD motif reduces the activity by 25-, 3,000- or 15,000-fold, respectively (Interthal et al. 2001, 2005b; Raymond et al. 2004). Likewise, mutation of lysine to serine (K265S) in the first HKD motif results in complete loss of Tdp1 activity, whereas an analogous mutation (K495S) in the second HKD motif leads to a 125-fold decrease in activity (Interthal et al. 2001; Raymond et al. 2004). Sequence alignments have revealed that Tdp1 lacks the invariant aspartic acid residues in its HKD motifs that otherwise appear to be important in protein folding and/or stabilization of certain PLD superfamily members (Interthal et al. 2001; Leiros et al. 2000; Stuckey and Dixon1999). Instead, Tdp1 orthologs have two highly conserved asparagine residues that cluster near the active site (N283 and N516, *see* Fig. 16.1a and c) and look to be important for substrate binding and stabilization of transition states (Davies et al. 2002a, 2004). Consequently, Tdp1 and its orthologs have been assigned to a distinct subclass within PLD superfamily based on these unique "HKN" motifs (Interthal et al. 2001).

Combined evidences from mutagenic and structural studies of Tdp1 (Davies et al. 2002a, 2003, 2004) have proposed that the hydrolysis of 3′-phosphotyrosyl bonds by Tdp1 proceeds via a two-step reaction similar to other PLD superfamily members (Gottlin et al. 1998; Rudolph et al. 1999; Stuckey and Dixon 1999; Waite 1999) (Fig. 16.2). The first step involves nucleophilic attack by H263 of the first HKN motif on the phosphate group linking the DNA and the tyrosyl-containing peptide, resulting in the formation of a phosphoenzyme intermediate. Indeed, a covalent Tdp1-DNA intermediate has been identified both structurally (Davies et al. 2003) and biochemically (Interthal et al. 2001, 2005b). The peptide then dissociates from the active site following protonation by the H493 of the second HKN motif acting as the general acid. Accordingly, the Tdp1 H493A mutant can only process substrates whose leaving group does not require protonation (Raymond et al. 2004). In the second step of the reaction, H493 acts as a general base and deprotonates a water molecule, which in turn attacks the phosphorous atom of the covalent intermediate. This results in hydrolysis of the phosphoamide bond between Tdp1 and the 3′-phosphate of the DNA.

The structures obtained from co-crystallizing human Tdp1 with the DNA-peptide substrate mimic also offer a detailed look into the active site geometry and substrate recognition of Tdp1 (Fig. 16.1b). For example, the structures demonstrate that Tdp1 consists of two similar domains related to each other through a pseudo-2-fold axis (Davies et al. 2002b). Each domain contributes a conserved HKN motif at the domain-domain interface, where the histidines and lysines of both HKN motifs juxtapose to form a single active site (Davies et al. 2002b, 2003) (Fig. 16.1c). The substrate mimic that was assembled from vanadate, single-strand DNA, and a Top1-derived peptide, binds in a cleft perpendicular to the interface of the two domains (Fig. 16.1b). In the co-crystal, vanadate is covalently bound to H263 at the catalytic site, which is situated at the center of the cleft. In addition, the vanadate, a phosphate transition state analog, assumes a trigonal bipyramidal configuration with the H263 of Tdp1 at one apical position and the tyrosine of the peptide at the other apical position. The structure is consistent with the transition state of an S_N2 attack, where the H263 of Tdp1 is the putative nucleophile and the tyrosine-containing peptide is the leaving group.

The single-strand DNA binds to the vanadate through its 3′-hydroxyl group at one of the three equatorial positions, while the rest of the oligonucleotide extends in one direction from the active site (Davies et al. 2003). The DNA-binding portion of

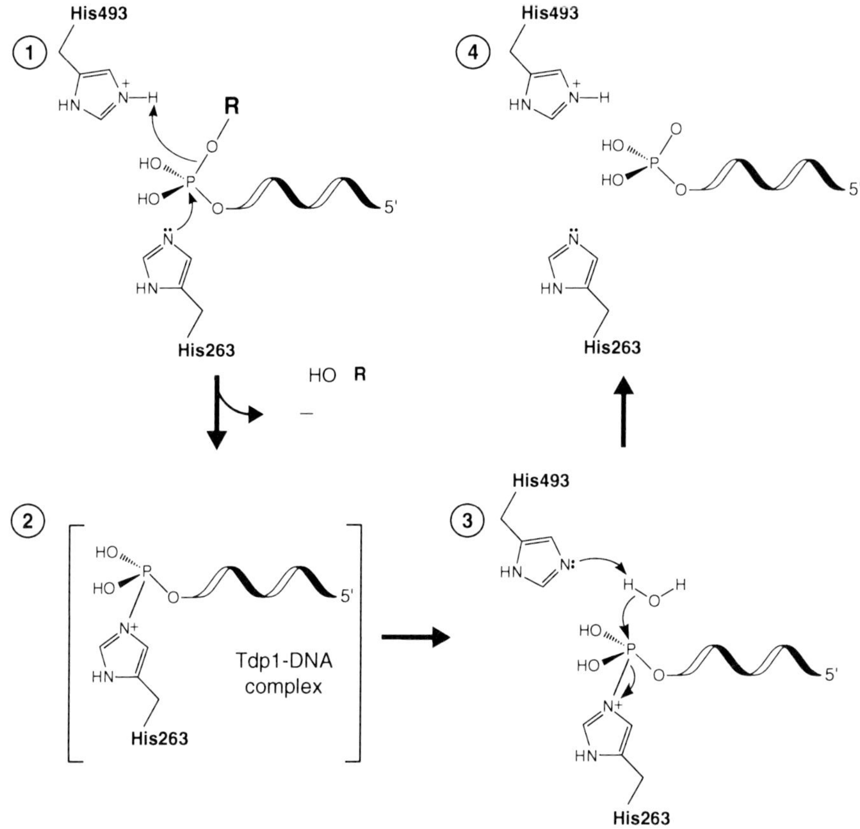

Fig. 16.2 Proposed two-step catalytic mechanism of human Tdp1. (1) In the first step of the reaction, His263 acts as a nucleophile, carrying out attack on the phosphorus atom in the phosphodiester bond between the 3′-lesion and the DNA 3′-oxygen. His493 donates a proton to the leaving group (HO-R). (2) After the first step of the catalytic reaction, a Tdp1-DNA intermediate remains wherein His263 is covalently bound to the 3′-end of the DNA via a phosphoamide bond. (3) In the second step of the reaction, the phosphohistidine intermediate is hydrolyzed via a second nucleophilic attack by a water molecule activated by His493, (4) resulting in the regeneration of the Tdp1 active site and the release of 3′-phosphate DNA end

the cleft is long and narrow in shape (20 × 10 × 15 Å^3) (Davies et al. 2002a, b, 2003) and is only able to accommodate single-strand DNA, although, an alternative model has been proposed for double-strand DNA (Raymond et al. 2005). A comparison of the Tdp1 crystal structures in complex with oligonucleotides of different sequences reveals very limited protein–DNA interactions, consistent with the fact that Tdp1 can act on broad range of substrates (Davies et al. 2004). Nevertheless, the DNA binding cleft is predominately positively charged and possesses three phosphate-binding sites in addition to the active site (Davies et al. 2003, 2004). The peptide moiety occupies only a small portion of the peptide-binding cleft, while additional residues on either end of the peptide could easily be accommodated given the arrangement of the peptide backbone (Davies et al. 2002b, 2003). Although the exact nature of Tdp1 substrate in vivo remains unknown, peptides or peptide analogs ranging from one to eight residues have successfully formed complexes with Tdp1 (Davies et al. 2004) and shown to be processed by the enzyme (Debethune et al. 2002). Surprisingly, the tyrosine residue only indirectly interacts with Tdp1 through the vanadate (phosphate mimic) atom in the active site (Davies et al. 2003). The only other interaction between Tdp1 and the peptide portion of an artificial substrate is the lysine residue of the sequence **K**LNYLDPR. Based on the characteristics of the DNA- and peptide-binding sites, the structural studies strongly suggest that Tdp1 likely can catalyze a broad spectrum of substrates with 3′-phosphodiester linkages Davies et al. (2003, 2004).

16.3 Recognized Substrates of Tdp1

16.3.1 Physiological 3′-Ends (Fig. 16.3a)

3′-phosphotyrosine/phosphotyrosyl peptide. Tdp1 can remove the 3′-tyrosine moiety from a variety of oligonucleotide constructs, including double-strand DNA with 3′-tyrosine at a nick or a gap, as well as a 3′-tyrosine at blunt, frayed, or tailed ends (Raymond et al. 2005; Yang et al. 1996). Single-strand DNA molecules of various lengths with 3′-peptidyl portions ranging from one to more than ten residues can also be processed by Tdp1 with varying efficiencies (Debethune et al. 2002; Interthal et al. 2005a). While Tdp1 cannot efficiently remove full-length Top1 enzyme linked to DNA molecules, prior denaturation or proteolytic digestion of Top1-DNA cleavage complex results in a much better substrate for Tdp1 (Debethune et al. 2002; Interthal et al. 2005a; Yang et al. 1996). Structural studies suggest that steric hindrance of the phosphodiester bond in native Top1-DNA cleavage complex likely accounts for its low processing efficiency (Davies et al. 2002a; Redinbo et al. 1998). In addition to 3′-phosphotyrosyl linkages, the yeast Tdp1 homolog has been reported to process 5′-phosphotyrosyl linkages (Nitiss et al. 2006). A human enzyme denoted Tdp2 has recently been shown to have robust 5′-tyrosyl-DNA phosphodiesterase activity (Cortes Ledesma et al. 2009; Zeng et al. 2010). Thus, the complementary catalytic activities of Tdp1 and Tdp2 provide a mechanism to mitigate DNA damage caused by trapped topoisomerase-DNA cleavage complexes on either DNA terminus.

3′-phosphoglycolate. Tdp1 has been shown to be a key enzyme for processing 3′-phosphoglycolate termini, which are commonly produced by oxidative DNA damage (Inamdar et al. 2002; Zhou et al. 2005, 2009). Although biochemical studies show that phosphoglycolate is a less efficient substrate than the phosphotyrosine substrate, further studies are needed to determine the relative importance of Tdp1 in the repair of oxidative DNA damage in cells (Inamdar et al. 2002). One reason the relative substrate processing efficiency may not correlate to relative repair frequency in vivo is that the substrates employed in these studies may not correspond exactly to the native Tdp1 substrates.

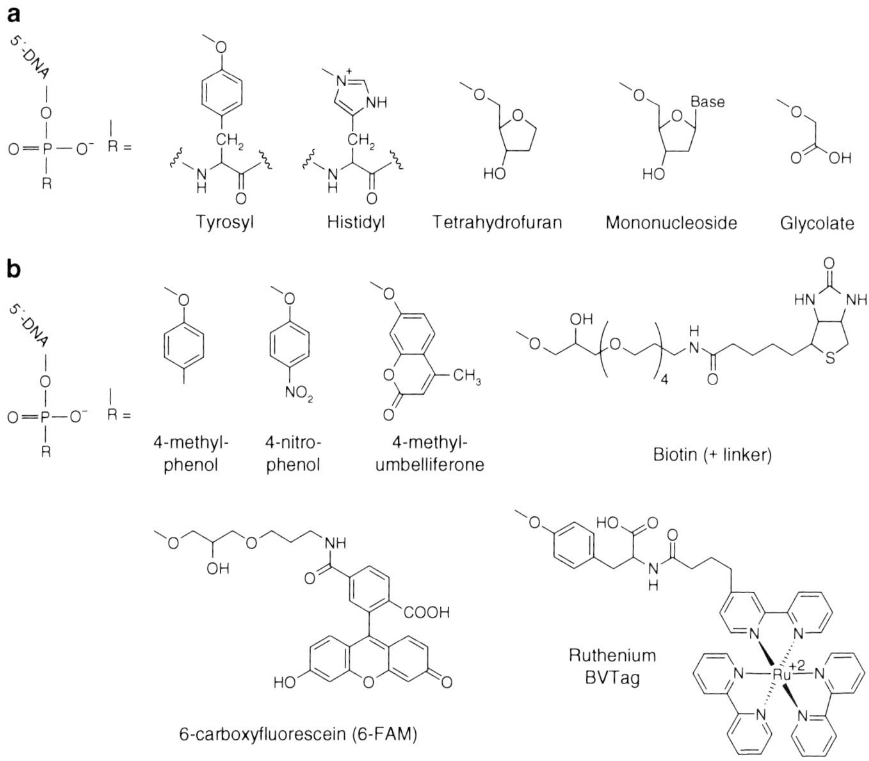

Fig. 16.3 (**a**) Physiological and (**b**) non-physiological Tdp1 substrates (modified and updated from Dexheimer et al. (2008))

3′-nucleoside/tetrahydrofuran. Tdp1 can also remove a single nucleoside from the 3′-end of DNA or RNA molecules, producing a polymer that is one nucleotide shorter and bears a 3′-phosphate group (Interthal et al. 2005a). Furthermore, a tetrahydrofuran moiety, the abasic mimic, can be removed by Tdp1 (Interthal et al. 2005a). While Tdp1 lacks intrinsic 3′-phosphatase activity, concerted actions by Tdp1 and the 3′-phosphatase activity of polynucleotide kinase 3′-phosphatase (PNKP) could conceivably serve as a 3′-exonuclease (Pommier et al. 2006).

16.3.2 Non-physiological 3′-Ends (Fig. 16.3b)

In addition to the endogenous substrates, Tdp1 can process a variety of synthetic DNA adducts on the 3′-end with varying efficiencies. The substrates identified to date include oligonucleotides with biotin and a variety of fluorophores attached to the 3′-phosphate (Antony et al. 2007; Dexheimer et al. 2010; Interthal et al. 2005a; Raymond et al. 2004; Rideout et al. 2004). These synthetic substrates are particularly useful in detailed mechanistic studies (Dexheimer et al. 2010) and screening for Tdp1 inhibitors (Antony et al. 2007; Marchand et al. 2009). In any case, the broad specificity of Tdp1 is indicative of the multiple roles that Tdp1 likely plays in a wide range of DNA repair pathways.

16.4 Physiological Consequences of Tdp1 Mutation: SCAN1

The association of human neurodegenerative disorders with inherited or acquired defects in DNA repair mechanisms has been well established (El-Khamisy 2011; McKinnon 2009; Rass et al. 2007). In 2002, a mutation in the human *Tdp1* gene was found to cause the rare heredity neurodegenerative disease spinocerebellar ataxia with axonal neuropathy (SCAN1). SCAN1 is inherited in an autosomal recessive manner (Takashima et al. 2002). To date, this disease has been identified only in nine patients from a single Saudi Arabian family, three of which have been clinically evaluated in detail. The affected individuals suffer from early onset ataxia (~15 years), cerebellum atrophy, and peripheral neuropathy, and eventually become wheelchair-bound but retain normal cognitive function (Takashima et al. 2002; Walton et al. 2010). In addition, SCAN1 patients present mild hypercholesterolemia and hypoalbuminemia (Takashima et al. 2002). In contrast to patients with other DNA repair-related disorders with neurological dysfunction, such as Ataxia telangiectasia (Lavin 2008) or xeroderma pigmentosum (Friedberg 2001), SCAN1 patients lack extra-neurological symptoms, most notably genomic instability and cancer predisposition (Takashima et al. 2002).

Genetic diagnosis of SCAN1 patients identified a homozygous transition mutation in exon 14 (A1478G) of the *Tdp1* gene, resulting in the substitution of histidine by arginine (H493R) within the second HKD motif of the Tdp1 active site (Takashima et al. 2002) (*see* Fig. 16.1a). This is currently the only mutation known to be associated with SCAN1. As previously mentioned, mutation of H493 results in a significant decrease in Tdp1 activity (Interthal et al. 2001), which strongly suggested that the SCAN1 phenotype results from a loss-of-function mutation. Indeed, a 25-fold decrease in Tdp1 activity has been demonstrated for the recombinant SCAN1 mutant H493R (Interthal et al. 2005b). However, three independently developed *Tdp1* knockout mouse models revealed no obvious behavioral phenotypes related to human SCAN1 patients (e.g., ataxia) (Hawkins et al. 2009; Hirano et al. 2007; Katyal et al. 2007). Nevertheless, in one of these mouse models, loss of Tdp1 resulted in gradual age-related cerebellar atrophy as well as hypoalbuminemia, which are neurological and extraneurological characteristics of SCAN1 individuals, respectively (Katyal et al. 2007). In addition, similar to human SCAN1 lymphoblasts, neural cells from *Tdp1*$^{-/-}$ mice exhibit a marked decrease in the repair of SSBs induced by camptothecin (CPT) and oxidative DNA damage (El-Khamisy et al. 2005; Hirano et al. 2007; Katyal et al. 2007; Miao et al. 2006). Another feature described for the SCAN1 mutant is the accumulation of the Tdp1-DNA intermediate

(Fig. 16.2), which has been observed using recombinant Tdp1 mutant H493R, extracts from SCAN1 cells (Interthal et al. 2005b), as well as *Tdp1*$^{-/-}$ extracts supplemented with Tdp1-H493R (Dexheimer et al. 2009; Hawkins et al. 2009). In addition, the trapping of Tdp1 on genomic DNA has also been demonstrated in SCAN1 cells treated with CPT (Hirano et al. 2007) and cells from SCAN1 patients are markedly defective in the repair of Top1-DNA complexes and hypersensitive to CPT (El-Khamisy et al. 2005; Miao et al. 2006).

16.5 Stepwise Repair of Top1-DNA Lesions by the Tdp1-Dependent Pathway

Progress has been remarkable in recent years regarding the elucidation of the repair pathways involved in the removal of Top1 cleavage complexes. The versatile base excision repair (BER) has been identified as one of the pathways responsible for repairing Top1-mediated DNA damage (Caldecott 2008; El-Khamisy et al. 2005; Plo et al. 2003; Pommier et al. 2006). To repair Top1 cleavage complexes as well as other 3′-DNA lesions, BER requires several other enzymes beside Tdp1, including PARP-1, PNKP, DNA polymerase β, ligase IIIα and the scaffolding protein XRCC1 (Caldecott 2008; El-Khamisy et al. 2005; Plo et al. 2003) (Fig. 16.4). Poly(ADP-ribose)polymerase 1(PARP-1) is involved in early detection of Top1-mediated DNA breaks (Chatterjee et al. 1989; Pommier et al. 2006; Schreiber et al. 2006). XRCC1 interacts with, stimulates, and/or stabilizes multiple enzymatic components of the repair pathway. Tdp1 is responsible for catalyzing the hydrolysis of the phosphodiester bond between the tyrosine moiety and a terminal 3′-phosphate of DNA (Miao et al. 2006). Next, PNKP hydrolyzes the resulting 3′-phosphate end and catalyzes the phosphorylation of the 5′-end of the DNA (Yang et al. 1996). Lastly, TDNA polymerase β fills in the missing TDNA segment and DNA ligase IIIα reseals the nicks in TDNA backbones.

Several studies have shown that PNKP functions in a concerted manner with Tdp1 to repair 3′-lesions. Consistent with the role of PNKP in the Tdp1-mediated BER pathway, it has been reported that PNKP-defective human cells and SCAN1 cells accrue similar levels of CPT-induced strand breaks (El-Khamisy et al. 2005). Furthermore, PNKP is known to interact with the XRCC1, polymerase β, ligase IIIα, and PARP-1 to form a multiprotein DNA repair complex in the BER pathway (Whitehouse et al. 2001). XRCC1-deficient cells have been shown to be defective in Tdp1 and PNKP activity, providing further evidence for involvement of XRCC1, Tdp1, and PNKP in the repair of Top1-mediated damage (Plo et al. 2003). Tdp1 has been shown to interact directly with ligase IIIα, which binds directly to XRCC1 and thus suggests all three proteins are in the same repair complex (El-Khamisy et al. 2005; Plo et al. 2003).

The primary transducers of the DNA damage response are the nuclear serine-threonine kinases, including ataxia-telangiectasia mutated (ATM) protein kinase (Lee and Paull 2007; Shiloh 2006), DNA-dependent protein kinase (DNA-PK), and ataxia-telangiectasia and Rad3-related (ATR) protein kinase (Cimprich and Cortez 2008). ATM is rapidly activated in response to DSBs (Bakkenist and Kastan 2003;

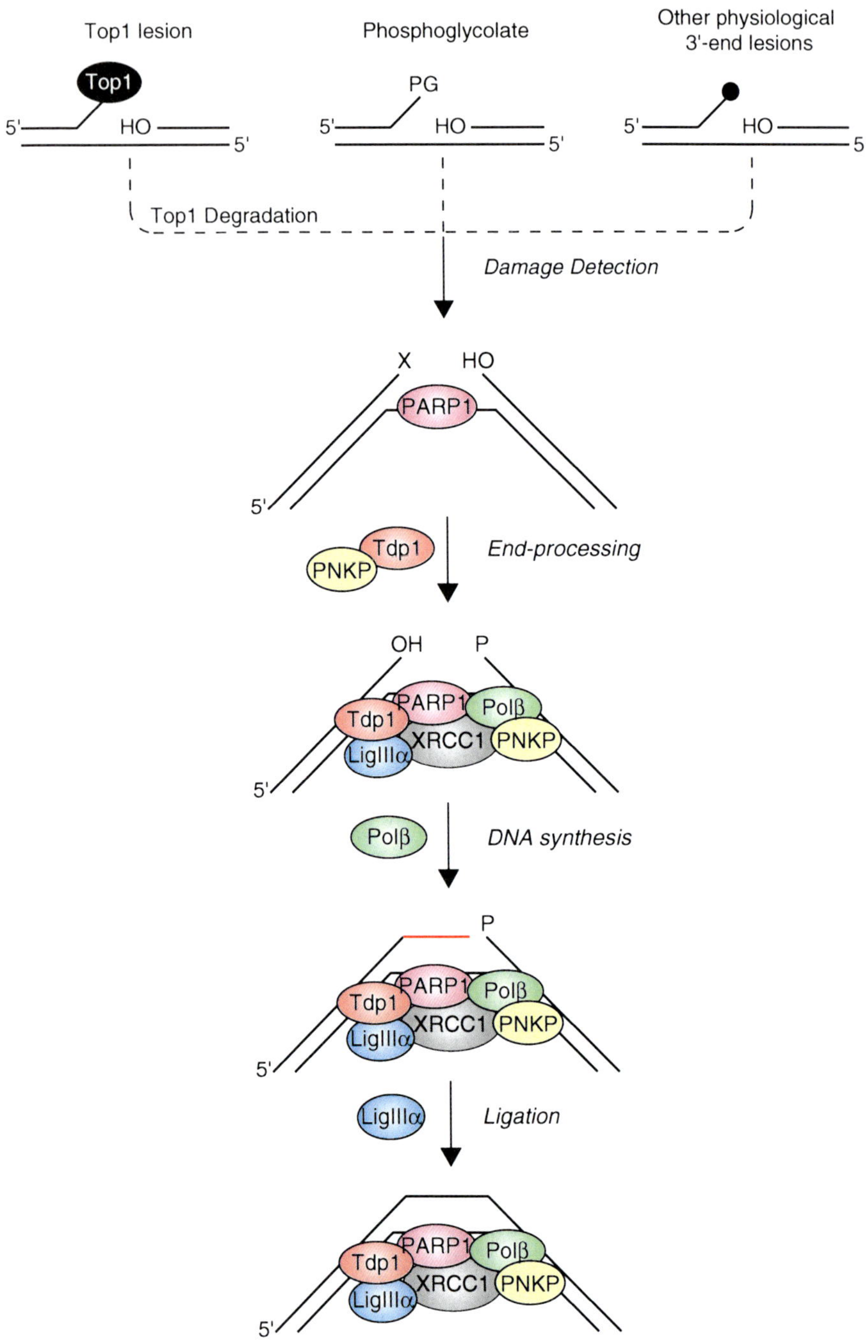

Fig. 16.4 Tdp1-dependent repair pathway of 3′-DNA lesions. The DNA damage/break is initially detected by PARP1. The 3′- and 5′-termini are then processed sequentially by TDP1 and PNKP, resulting in a 3′-hydroxyl and 5′-phosphate. The gap filling and ligation is conducted by DNA polymerase β and DNA ligase IIIα, respectively (modified from Caldecott (2008) and (Pommier et al. (2006))

Lee and Paull 2007) and phosphorylates a plethora of key players in the DNA damage response pathways (Matsuoka et al. 2007; Shiloh 2006), while DNA-PK is involved in the nonhomologous end-joining (NHEJ) of DSBs (Weterings and Chen 2007). In a recent study, both ATM and/or DNA-PK have been shown to regulate Tdp1 through phosphorylation of serine 81 (S81, *see* Fig. 16.1a) in response to DSBs associated with the Top1 cleavage complexes or with ionizing radiation (Das et al. 2009). The state of phosphorylation at Tdp1-S81 affects the stability and subcellular distribution of Tdp1 rather than directly affecting its catalytic activity (Chiang et al. 2010; Das et al. 2009). Phosphorylation at Tdp1-S81 promotes its interactions with XRCC1 and ligase IIIα, which potentially serves to prevent Tdp1 from degradation (Chiang et al. 2010; Das et al. 2009).

Although XRCC1 has been mainly implicated in SSB rejoining in the BER pathway (Caldecott 2008), it has been proposed that XRCC1 is also involved in DSB repair in an alternative end-joining pathway (Audebert et al. 2004; Rosidi et al. 2008). XRCC1-deficient cells display a significant defect in rejoining radiation-induced DSB (Nocentini 1999), and XRCC1 depletion sensitizes cells to the DSB-inducing agent bleomycin (Rosell et al. 2007). Accordingly, XRCC1- and/or PARP-1-deficient cells are hypersensitive to CPT (D'Onofrio et al. 2010; Horton et al. 2008; Plo et al. 2003; Pommier et al. 2006). Two recent reports describe a potential link between the ATM-Chk2 pathway and XRCC1 by phosphorylation of XRCC1 (Chou et al. 2008). Furthermore, DNA-PK has been shown to interact with XRCC1 and to phosphorylate XRCC1 at Serine 371 (Levy et al. 2006; Toulany et al. 2008). CPT-induced XRCC1 foci co-localize with the γH2AX and the pS81-TDP1 foci formed at DSBs (Das et al. 2009). These sites most likely correspond to the small fraction of the Top1 cleavage complexes that are converted into irreversible Top1-DNA lesions by replication (Furuta et al. 2003; Seiler et al. 2007; Strumberg et al. 2000) and transcription (Sordet et al. 2009). Thus, it is plausible that XRCC1 may have a specific role in the repair of lesions associated with Top1-linked DSBs. Phosphorylated Tdp1-S81 protects cells against CPT and IR-induced DNA damage, but it is still unclear whether this phosphorylation impacts SSB as well as DSB repair, since the phosphorylation appears to be driven by DSB formation (Chiang et al. 2010; Das et al. 2009).

Recently, Tdp1 has been identified in human mitochondria and the repair of oxidative DNA damage in mitochondrial DNA has been shown to be deficient in Tdp1 knockout cells (Das et al. 2010). The presence of Tdp1 in mitochondria is consistent with the presence of a specific mitochondrial type IB topoisomerase, Top1mt (see Chap. 3).

16.6 Redundancy of the Repair of Top1-DNA Lesions by Tdp1-Independent Repair Pathways

Each DNA repair pathway is directed to specific types of damage (for instance nucleotide excision repair for base alkylation and UV-induced DNA lesions) (Friedberg 2001). However, in the case of topoisomerase-mediated DNA damage, multiple pathways are involved (see Chap. 15). The choice of pathway is at least in part determined by the nature of the DNA lesion. For example, human cells have at least nine distinct DNA glycosylases, which are highly specific for a particular type of damaged base (Lindahl and Wood 1999). However, some degree of redundancy also occurs with respect to substrate specificities given that mice deficient in a specific DNA glycosylase lack evident phenotypic abnormalities (Nilsen et al. 2000; Parsons and Elder 2003; Takao et al. 2002). Both the 3′-lesion and the structure of the DNA containing the lesion contribute to the processing efficiency of Tdp1. For instance, Tdp1-mediated repair requires that the DNA-linked Top1 be proteolyzed or denatured to allow Tdp1 access to tyrosyl-DNA bond (Debethune et al. 2002; Interthal et al. 2005a; Yang et al. 1996) (see Chap. 17). Furthermore, Tdp1 has a preference for single-strand and blunt-end duplex substrates over nicked and tailed duplex substrate (Pouliot et al. 2001; Raymond et al. 2005). Thus, it is not surprising that alternative pathways exist for the removal of Top1 cleavage complexes, based on unique substrates that are preferential for Tdp1 action.

The initial understanding of the redundancy in the repair of Top1-mediated DNA damage emerged from studies using genetically altered yeast strains. Indeed, a plethora of genetic alterations in yeast confer hypersensitivity to Top1-mediated damage (Deng et al. 2005; Parsons et al. 2004; Pommier et al. 2006; Reid et al. 2011) (see Chap. 15). The budding yeast *Tdp1* knockout is viable and relatively insensitive to CPT (Pouliot et al. 1999). It is only sensitive to Top1 cleavage complexes when additional mutations in other DNA repair or checkpoint genes are also present. For example, CPT sensitivity in *Tdp1*-defective yeast was conditional to deficiencies in the checkpoint gene Rad9 (Pouliot et al. 1999, 2001). In addition, significant sensitization to CPT occurs when both Tdp1 and specific specialized endonucleases are inactivated, suggesting alternative or redundant pathways to excise Top1-mediated DNA damage. One such endonuclease is Rad1/Rad10 (Vance and Wilson 2002), an ortholog of the human XPF/ERCC1 that is involved in the nucleotide excision repair pathway (NER). XPF forms a heterodimer with its non-catalytic partner ERCC1 to generate a structure-specific endonuclease, which cleaves flap or branched DNA structures 5′ to the boundary of the 3′-single strand/duplex transition (de Laat et al. 1998; Sijbers et al. 1996) (Fig. 16.5). It is possible that Top1 cleavage complexes could assume a similar distorted 3′-boundary structure. In addition, XPF/ERCC1 has been suggested to be involved in the removal of 3′-blocking lesions induced by reactive oxygen species (Guzder et al. 2004). The XPF-related nuclease, Mus81, has also been suggested to be involved in the repair of Top1 lesions based on genetic evidence in yeast (Liu et al. 2002; Vance and Wilson 2002). Like XPF/ERCC1, Mus81 functions as a heterodimer by pairing with Eme1 in humans or Mms4 in budding yeast (Ciccia et al. 2008). The Mus81/Eme1 heterdimer cleaves similar flap or branched DNA intermediates, but typically cleaves 3–6 base pairs 5′ of the 3′single strand/duplex transition and requires the presence of a 5′-end of DNA at the flap junction (Bastin-Shanower et al. 2003). Based on genetic analysis, Tdp1 and XPF/ERCC1 appear to function in parallel and redundant pathways, while Mus81/Eme1 serves as an alternative pathway to Tdp1. Lastly, the MRN complex (Mre11/Rad50/Nbs1) has also been suggested as supplementary

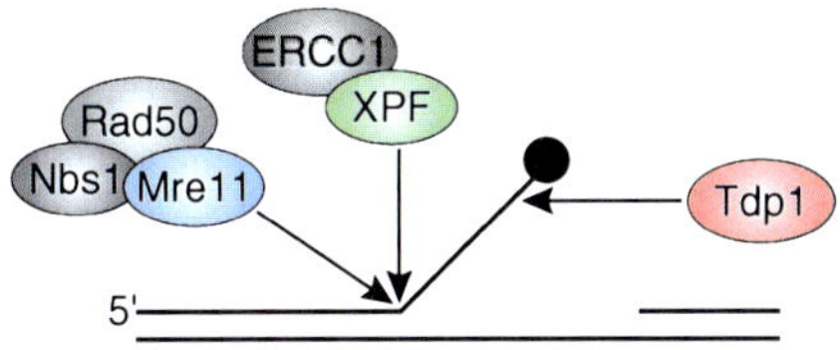

Fig. 16.5 Redundant enzymes involved in the removal of Top1-mediated DNA damage in mammalian cells. *Arrows* indicate the location of cleavage sites for different enzymes

pathway for the repair of Top1-mediated DNA damage (Deng et al. 2005; Liu et al. 2002). The MRN complex has been shown to be involved in the processing of both Top1 from 3′-DNA ends as well as Top2 from 5′-ends (Hamilton and Maizels 2010; Hartsuiker et al. 2009). With regard to Top1 lesions, Mre11, the nuclease of the MRN complex, preferentially cleaves 3′-single stranded branch structures. Like XPF/ERCC1, Mre11 requires a single-strand gap between the 3′-end to be processed and the 5′-end of the DNA (D'Amours and Jackson 2002) (Fig. 16.5). However, the MRN complex also possesses checkpoint functions that may contribute to the response to CPT.

Overall, the excision of Top1-DNA lesion can be accomplished by multiple different enzymes, which include Tdp1 and several 3′-flap endonuclease complexes (*see* Fig. 16.5). The activity of these enzymes is highly dependent on the structure of the Top1-DNA lesion. While Tdp1 is contingent upon the degradation of the Top1 prior to its action, the endonucleases have the propensity to remove a non-proteolyzed or intact Top1 from the 3′-end of the DNA. In addition, the presence of specific checkpoint genes (i.e., Rad9) (Pouliot et al. 1999, 2001) upstream in the DNA repair response cascade may also regulate excision enzyme selection (Pommier et al. 2003).

16.7 Tdp1 as a Target for Cancer Therapy

As emphasized above, eukaryotes have evolved a network of complex DNA repair mechanisms, consisting of redundant and partially overlapping pathways that function to maintain genomic integrity (Matsuoka et al. 2007). Underlying the importance of these pathways is the fact that their dysregulation can contribute to the initiation and progression of cancer. On the other hand, DNA repair can confer resistance to frontline cancer treatments (i.e., chemotherapy and radiation), which rely on the generation of DNA damage. For example, an apparent relationship exists between DNA repair activity and resistance to platinum-based therapies (Martin et al. 2008). Accordingly, the pharmacological inhibition of DNA damage repair pathways is currently being explored as a useful strategy to both prevent resistance and enhance the cytotoxic effects of conventional DNA-damage-based anticancer therapies (Helleday et al. 2008). DNA repair inhibitors could also be used as single agents to selectively kill cancer cells. This notion stems from the findings that cancer cells are often defective in particular DNA repair pathway(s), resulting in hyper-dependency on compensatory pathway(s). The concept of synthetic lethality can be used to identify these compensating pathways and to design novel treatment strategies that exploit these common weaknesses of tumor cells (Helleday et al. 2008; Kennedy and D'Andrea 2006). The success of this approach has been exemplified through the discovery of the PARP inhibitors, which have demonstrated significant therapeutic potential in BRCA-deficient tumors (Farmer et al. 2005).

Despite the clinical successes of Top1 inhibitors, inherent resistance has been reported. Since Top1 inhibitors induce cytotoxic DNA lesions, the repair of this damage is an important determinant in the cellular response to Top1 inhibition (Pommier 2009). Consequently, inhibitors of the DNA repair enzymes involved in the removal of Top1-mediated DNA damage, such as Tdp1, have been foreseen as an adjunct therapy to the clinically used Top1 inhibitors (Beretta et al. 2010; Dexheimer et al. 2008). CPT sensitivity has been established in human cells treated with Tdp1 siRNA (Das et al. 2009) as well as those harboring the physiologically relevant SCAN1 Tdp1 mutant (El-Khamisy et al. 2005; Interthal et al. 2005b; Miao et al. 2006). Moreover, overexpression of Tdp1 in human cells causes significant reduction in CPT-induced DNA damage (Barthelmes et al. 2004; Nivens et al. 2004). The marked hypersensitivity of Tdp1 knockout mice to the effects of both CPT (Hirano et al. 2007) and its water-soluble derivative topotecan (Katyal et al. 2007) provides further proof of principle for such combination therapy strategies. To date, several chemical families have already been reported as leads for discovery of Tdp1 inhibitors (Antony et al. 2007; Dexheimer et al. 2009; Marchand et al. 2009). The viability and mild phenotype of Tdp1 knockout mice suggests that Tdp1 inhibitors likely will have limited side effects (Hawkins et al. 2009; Hirano et al. 2007; Katyal et al. 2007). Taken together, these studies suggest that, in mammalian cells, a single defect in Tdp1 activity is sufficient for Top1 inhibitor hypersensitivity, which is in contrast to the conditional mutations required in Tdp1-deficient yeast cells.

References

Antony S, Marchand C, Stephen AG, Thibaut L, Agama KK, Fisher RJ, Pommier Y (2007) Novel high-throughput electrochemiluminescent assay for identification of human tyrosyl-DNA phosphodiesterase (Tdp1) inhibitors and characterization of furamidine (NSC 305831) as an inhibitor of Tdp1. *Nucleic Acids Res* **35**(13): 4474–4484

Audebert M, Salles B, Calsou P (2004) Involvement of poly(ADP-ribose) polymerase-1 and XRCC1/DNA ligase III in an alternative route for DNA double-strand breaks rejoining. *J Biol Chem* **279**(53): 55117–55126

Bakkenist CJ, Kastan MB (2003) DNA damage activates ATM through intermolecular autophosphorylation and dimer dissociation. *Nature* **421**(6922): 499–506

Banerjee B, Roy A, Sen N, Majumder HK (2010) A Tyrosyl DNA phosphodiesterase 1 from kinetoplastid parasite Leishmania donovani (LdTdp1) capable of removing Topo I-DNA covalent complexes. *Mol Microbiol*

Barthelmes HU, Habermeyer M, Christensen MO, Mielke C, Interthal H, Pouliot JJ, Boege F, Marko D (2004) TDP1 overexpression in human cells counteracts DNA damage mediated by topoisomerases I and II. *J Biol Chem* **279**(53): 55618–55625

Bastin-Shanower SA, Fricke WM, Mullen JR, Brill SJ (2003) The mechanism of Mus81-Mms4 cleavage site selection distinguishes it from the homologous endonuclease Rad1-Rad10. *Mol Cell Biol* **23**(10): 3487–3496

Beretta GL, Cossa G, Gatti L, Zunino F, Perego P (2010) Tyrosyl-DNA phosphodiesterase 1 targeting for modulation of camptothecin-based treatment. *Curr Med Chem* **17**(15): 1500–1508

Caldecott KW (2007) Mammalian single-strand break repair: mechanisms and links with chromatin. *DNA Repair (Amst)* **6**(4): 443–453

Caldecott KW (2008) Single-strand break repair and genetic disease. *Nat Rev Genet* **9**(8): 619–631

Chatterjee S, Cheng MF, Trivedi D, Petzold SJ, Berger NA (1989) Camptothecin hypersensitivity in poly(adenosine diphosphate-ribose) polymerase-deficient cell lines. *Cancer Commun* **1**(6): 389–394

Cheng TJ, Rey PG, Poon T, Kan CC (2002) Kinetic studies of human tyrosyl-DNA phosphodiesterase, an enzyme in the topoisomerase I DNA repair pathway. *Eur J Biochem* **269**(15): 3697–3704

Chiang SC, Carroll J, El-Khamisy SF (2010) TDP1 serine 81 promotes interaction with DNA ligase IIIalpha and facilitates cell survival following DNA damage. *Cell Cycle* **9**(3): 588–595

Chou WC, Wang HC, Wong FH, Ding SL, Wu PE, Shieh SY, Shen CY (2008) Chk2-dependent phosphorylation of XRCC1 in the DNA damage response promotes base excision repair. *EMBO J* **27**(23): 3140–3150

Ciccia A, McDonald N, West SC (2008) Structural and functional relationships of the XPF/MUS81 family of proteins. *Annu Rev Biochem* **77**: 259–287

Cimprich KA, Cortez D (2008) ATR: an essential regulator of genome integrity. *Nat Rev Mol Cell Biol* **9**(8): 616–627

Cortes Ledesma F, El Khamisy SF, Zuma MC, Osborn K, Caldecott KW (2009) A human 5'-tyrosyl DNA phosphodiesterase that repairs topoisomerase-mediated DNA damage. *Nature* **461**(7264): 674–678

D'Amours D, Jackson SP (2002) The Mre11 complex: at the crossroads of dna repair and checkpoint signalling. *Nat Rev Mol Cell Biol* **3**(5): 317–327

D'Onofrio G, Tramontano F, Dorio AS, Muzi A, Maselli V, Fulgione D, Graziani G, Malanga M, Quesada P (2010) Poly(Adp-ribose) polymerase signaling of topoisomerase 1-dependent DNA damage in carcinoma cells. *Biochem Pharmacol*

Das BB, Antony S, Gupta S, Dexheimer TS, Redon CE, Garfield S, Shiloh Y, Pommier Y (2009) Optimal function of the DNA repair enzyme TDP1 requires its phosphorylation by ATM and/or DNA-PK. *EMBO J* **28**(23): 3667–3680

Das BB, Dexheimer TS, Maddali K, Pommier Y (2010) Role of tyrosyl-DNA phosphodiesterase (TDP1) in mitochondria. *Proc Natl Acad Sci USA* **107**(46): 19790–19795

Davies DR, Interthal H, Champoux JJ, Hol WG (2002a) Insights into substrate binding and catalytic mechanism of human tyrosyl-DNA phosphodiesterase (Tdp1) from vanadate and tungstate-inhibited structures. *J Mol Biol* **324**(5): 917–932

Davies DR, Interthal H, Champoux JJ, Hol WG (2002b) The crystal structure of human tyrosyl-DNA phosphodiesterase, Tdp1. *Structure* **10**(2): 237–248

Davies DR, Interthal H, Champoux JJ, Hol WGJ (2003) Crystal structure of a transition state mimic for Tdp1 assembled from vanadate, DNA, and a topoisomerase I-derived peptide. *Chem Biol* **10**(2): 139–147

Davies DR, Interthal H, Champoux JJ, Hol WG (2004) Explorations of peptide and oligonucleotide binding sites of tyrosyl-DNA phosphodiesterase using vanadate complexes. *J Med Chem* **47**(4): 829–837

de Laat WL, Appeldoorn E, Jaspers NG, Hoeijmakers JH (1998) DNA structural elements required for ERCC1-XPF endonuclease activity. *J Biol Chem* **273**(14): 7835–7842

Debethune L, Kohlhagen G, Grandas A, Pommier Y (2002) Processing of nucleopeptides mimicking the topoisomerase I-DNA covalent complex by tyrosyl-DNA phosphodiesterase. *Nucleic Acids Res* **30**(5): 1198–1204

Deng C, Brown JA, You D, Brown JM (2005) Multiple endonucleases function to repair covalent topoisomerase I complexes in Saccharomyces cerevisiae. *Genetics* **170**(2): 591–600

Dexheimer TS, Antony S, Marchand C, Pommier Y (2008) Tyrosyl-DNA phosphodiesterase as a target for anticancer therapy. *Anticancer Agents Med Chem* **8**(4): 381–389

Dexheimer TS, Gediya LK, Stephen AG, Weidlich I, Antony S, Marchand C, Interthal H, Nicklaus M, Fisher RJ, Njar VC, Pommier Y (2009) 4-Pregnen-21-ol-3,20-dione-21-(4-bromobenzenesulfonate) (NSC 88915) and related novel steroid derivatives as tyrosyl-DNA phosphodiesterase (Tdp1) inhibitors. *J Med Chem* **52**(22): 7122–7131

Dexheimer TS, Stephen AG, Fivash MJ, Fisher RJ, Pommier Y (2010) The DNA binding and 3'-end preferential activity of human tyrosyl-DNA phosphodiesterase. *Nucleic Acids Res* **38**(7): 2444–2452

El-Khamisy SF (2011) To live or to die: a matter of processing damaged DNA termini in neurons. *Embo Mol Med* **3**(2): 78–88

El-Khamisy SF, Saifi GM, Weinfeld M, Johansson F, Helleday T, Lupski JR, Caldecott KW (2005) Defective DNA single-strand break repair in spinocerebellar ataxia with axonal neuropathy-1. *Nature* **434**(7029): 108–113

Farmer H, McCabe N, Lord CJ, Tutt AN, Johnson DA, Richardson TB, Santarosa M, Dillon KJ, Hickson I, Knights C, Martin NM, Jackson SP, Smith GC, Ashworth A (2005) Targeting the DNA repair defect in BRCA mutant cells as a therapeutic strategy. *Nature* **434**(7035): 917–921

Friedberg EC (2001) How nucleotide excision repair protects against cancer. *Nat Rev Cancer* **1**(1): 22–33

Furuta T, Takemura H, Liao ZY, Aune GJ, Redon C, Sedelnikova OA, Pilch DR, Rogakou EP, Celeste A, Chen HT, Nussenzweig A, Aladjem MI, Bonner WM, Pommier Y (2003) Phosphorylation of histone H2AX and activation of Mre11, Rad50, and Nbs1 in response to replication-dependent DNA double-strand breaks induced by mammalian DNA topoisomerase I cleavage complexes. *J Biol Chem* **278**(22): 20303–20312

Gottlin EB, Rudolph AE, Zhao Y, Matthews HR, Dixon JE (1998) Catalytic mechanism of the phospholipase D superfamily proceeds via a covalent phosphohistidine intermediate. *Proc Natl Acad Sci USA* **95**(16): 9202–9207

Guzder SN, Torres-Ramos C, Johnson RE, Haracska L, Prakash L, Prakash S (2004) Requirement of yeast Rad1-Rad10 nuclease for the removal of 3'-blocked termini from DNA strand breaks induced by reactive oxygen species. *Genes Dev* **18**(18): 2283–2291

Hamilton NK, Maizels N (2010) MRE11 Function in Response to Topoisomerase Poisons Is Independent of its Function in Double-Strand Break Repair in Saccharomyces cerevisiae. *PLoS One* **5**(10): e15387

Hartsuiker E, Neale MJ, Carr AM (2009) Distinct requirements for the Rad32(Mre11) nuclease and Ctp1(CtIP) in the removal of covalently bound topoisomerase I and II from DNA. *Mol Cell* **33**(1): 117–123

Hawkins AJ, Subler MA, Akopiants K, Wiley JL, Taylor SM, Rice AC, Windle JJ, Valerie K, Povirk LF (2009) In vitro complementation of Tdp1 deficiency indicates a stabilized enzyme-DNA adduct from tyrosyl but not glycolate lesions as a consequence of the SCAN1 mutation. *DNA Repair (Amst)* **8**(5): 654–663

Helleday T, Petermann E, Lundin C, Hodgson B, Sharma RA (2008) DNA repair pathways as targets for cancer therapy. *Nat Rev Cancer* **8**(3): 193–204

Hirano R, Interthal H, Huang C, Nakamura T, Deguchi K, Choi K, Bhattacharjee MB, Arimura K, Umehara F, Izumo S, Northrop JL, Salih MA, Inoue K, Armstrong DL, Champoux JJ, Takashima H, Boerkoel CF (2007) Spinocerebellar ataxia with axonal neuropathy: consequence of a Tdp1 recessive neomorphic mutation? *EMBO J* **26**(22): 4732–4743

Horton JK, Watson M, Stefanick DF, Shaughnessy DT, Taylor JA, Wilson SH (2008) XRCC1 and DNA polymerase beta in cellular protection against cytotoxic DNA single-strand breaks. *Cell Res* **18**(1): 48–63

Inamdar KV, Pouliot JJ, Zhou T, Lees-Miller SP, Rasouli-Nia A, Povirk LF (2002) Conversion of phosphoglycolate to phosphate termini on 3' overhangs of DNA double strand breaks by the human tyrosyl-DNA phosphodiesterase hTdp1. *J Biol Chem* **277**(30): 27162–27168

Interthal H, Chen HJ, Champoux JJ (2005a) Human Tdp1 cleaves a broad spectrum of substrates, including phosphoamide linkages. *J Biol Chem* **280**(43): 36518–36528

Interthal H, Chen HJ, Kehl-Fie TE, Zotzmann J, Leppard JB, Champoux JJ (2005b) SCAN1 mutant Tdp1 accumulates the enzyme--DNA intermediate and causes camptothecin hypersensitivity. *EMBO J* **24**(12): 2224–2233

Interthal H, Pouliot JJ, Champoux JJ (2001) The tyrosyl-DNA phosphodiesterase Tdp1 is a member of the phospholipase D superfamily. *Proc Natl Acad Sci USA* **98**(21): 12009–12014

Iwasaki Y, Horiike S, Matsushima K, Yamane T (1999) Location of the catalytic nucleophile of phospholipase D of Streptomyces antibioticus in the C-terminal half domain. *Eur J Biochem* **264**(2): 577–581

Katyal S, el-Khamisy SF, Russell HR, Li Y, Ju L, Caldecott KW, McKinnon PJ (2007) TDP1 facilitates chromosomal single-strand break repair in neurons and is neuroprotective in vivo. *EMBO J* **26**(22): 4720–4731

Kennedy RD, D'Andrea AD (2006) DNA repair pathways in clinical practice: lessons from pediatric cancer susceptibility syndromes. *J Clin Oncol* **24**(23): 3799–3808

Koonin EV (1996) A duplicated catalytic motif in a new superfamily of phosphohydrolases and phospholipid synthases that includes poxvirus envelope proteins. *Trends Biochem Sci* **21**(7): 242–243

Lavin MF (2008) Ataxia-telangiectasia: from a rare disorder to a paradigm for cell signalling and cancer. *Nat Rev Mol Cell Biol* **9**(10): 759–769

Lee JH, Paull TT (2007) Activation and regulation of ATM kinase activity in response to DNA double-strand breaks. *Oncogene* **26**(56): 7741–7748

Lee SY, Kim H, Hwang HJ, Jeong YM, Na SH, Woo JC, Kim SG (2010) Identification of tyrosyl-DNA phosphodiesterase as a novel DNA damage repair enzyme in Arabidopsis. *Plant Physiol* **154**(3): 1460–1469

Leiros I, Secundo F, Zambonelli C, Servi S, Hough E (2000) The first crystal structure of a phospholipase D. *Structure* **8**(6): 655–667

Levy N, Martz A, Bresson A, Spenlehauer C, de Murcia G, Menissier-de Murcia J (2006) XRCC1 is phosphorylated by DNA-dependent protein kinase in response to DNA damage. *Nucleic Acids Res* **34**(1): 32–41

Lindahl T (1993) Instability and decay of the primary structure of DNA. *Nature* **362**(6422): 709–715

Lindahl T, Wood RD (1999) Quality control by DNA repair. *Science* **286**(5446): 1897–1905

Liscovitch M, Czarny M, Fiucci G, Tang X (2000) Phospholipase D: molecular and cell biology of a novel gene family. *Biochem J* **345 Pt 3**: 401–415

Liu C, Pouliot JJ, Nash HA (2002) Repair of topoisomerase I covalent complexes in the absence of the tyrosyl-DNA phosphodiesterase Tdp1. *Proc Natl Acad Sci USA* **99**(23): 14970–14975

Macovei A, Balestrazzi A, Confalonieri M, Carbonera D (2010) The tyrosyl-DNA phosphodiesterase gene family in Medicago truncatula Gaertn.: bioinformatic investigation and expression profiles in response to copper- and PEG-mediated stress. *Planta* **232**(2): 393–407

Marchand C, Lea WA, Jadhav A, Dexheimer TS, Austin CP, Inglese J, Pommier Y, Simeonov A (2009) Identification of phosphotyrosine mimetic inhibitors of human tyrosyl-DNA phosphodiesterase I by a novel AlphaScreen high-throughput assay. *Mol Cancer Ther* **8**(1): 240–248

Martin LP, Hamilton TC, Schilder RJ (2008) Platinum resistance: the role of DNA repair pathways. *Clin Cancer Res* **14**(5): 1291–1295

Matsuoka S, Ballif BA, Smogorzewska A, McDonald ER, 3rd, Hurov KE, Luo J, Bakalarski CE, Zhao Z, Solimini N, Lerenthal Y, Shiloh Y, Gygi SP, Elledge SJ (2007) ATM and ATR substrate analysis reveals extensive protein networks responsive to DNA damage. *Science* **316**(5828): 1160–1166

McKinnon PJ (2009) DNA repair deficiency and neurological disease. *Nat Rev Neurosci* **10**(2): 100–112

Miao ZH, Agama K, Sordet O, Povirk L, Kohn KW, Pommier Y (2006) Hereditary ataxia SCAN1 cells are defective for the repair of transcription-dependent topoisomerase I cleavage complexes. *DNA Repair (Amst)* **5**(12): 1489–1494

Nilsen H, Rosewell I, Robins P, Skjelbred CF, Andersen S, Slupphaug G, Daly G, Krokan HE, Lindahl T, Barnes DE (2000) Uracil-DNA glycosylase (UNG)-deficient mice reveal a primary role of the enzyme during DNA replication. *Mol Cell* **5**(6): 1059–1065

Nitiss KC, Malik M, He X, White SW, Nitiss JL (2006) Tyrosyl-DNA phosphodiesterase (Tdp1) participates in the repair of Top2-mediated DNA damage. *Proc Natl Acad Sci USA* **103**(24): 8953–8958

Nivens MC, Felder T, Galloway AH, Pena MM, Pouliot JJ, Spencer HT (2004) Engineered resistance to camptothecin and antifolates by retroviral coexpression of tyrosyl DNA phosphodiesterase-I and thymidylate synthase. *Cancer Chemother Pharmacol* **53**(2): 107–115

Nocentini S (1999) Rejoining kinetics of DNA single- and double-strand breaks in normal and DNA ligase-deficient cells after exposure to ultraviolet C and gamma radiation: an evaluation of ligating activities involved in different DNA repair processes. *Radiat Res* **151**(4): 423–432

Parsons AB, Brost RL, Ding H, Li Z, Zhang C, Sheikh B, Brown GW, Kane PM, Hughes TR, Boone C (2004) Integration of chemical-genetic and genetic interaction data links bioactive compounds to cellular target pathways. *Nat Biotechnol* **22**(1): 62–69

Parsons JL, Elder RH (2003) DNA N-glycosylase deficient mice: a tale of redundancy. *Mutat Res* **531**(1–2): 165–175

Plo I, Liao ZY, Barcelo JM, Kohlhagen G, Caldecott KW, Weinfeld M, Pommier Y (2003) Association of XRCC1 and tyrosyl DNA phosphodiesterase (Tdp1) for the repair of topoisomerase I-mediated DNA lesions. *DNA Repair (Amst)* **2**(10): 1087–1100

Pommier Y (2009) DNA topoisomerase I inhibitors: chemistry, biology, and interfacial inhibition. *Chem Rev* **109**(7): 2894–2902

Pommier Y, Barcelo JM, Rao VA, Sordet O, Jobson AG, Thibaut L, Miao ZH, Seiler JA, Zhang H, Marchand C, Agama K, Nitiss JL, Redon C (2006) Repair of topoisomerase I-mediated DNA damage. *Prog Nucleic Acid Res Mol Biol* **81**: 179–229

Pommier Y, Redon C, Rao VA, Seiler JA, Sordet O, Takemura H, Antony S, Meng L, Liao Z, Kohlhagen G, Zhang H, Kohn KW (2003) Repair of and checkpoint response to topoisomerase I-mediated DNA damage. *Mutat Res* **532**(1–2): 173–203

Ponting CP, Kerr ID (1996) A novel family of phospholipase D homologues that includes phospholipid synthases and putative endonucleases: identification of duplicated repeats and potential active site residues. *Protein Sci* **5**(5): 914–922

Pouliot JJ, Robertson CA, Nash HA (2001) Pathways for repair of topoisomerase I covalent complexes in Saccharomyces cerevisiae. *Genes Cells* **6**(8): 677–687

Pouliot JJ, Yao KC, Robertson CA, Nash HA (1999) Yeast gene for a Tyr-DNA phosphodiesterase that repairs topoisomerase I complexes. *Science* **286**(5439): 552–555

Rass U, Ahel I, West SC (2007) Defective DNA repair and neurodegenerative disease. *Cell* **130**(6): 991–1004

Raymond AC, Rideout MC, Staker B, Hjerrild K, Burgin AB, Jr. (2004) Analysis of human tyrosyl-DNA phosphodiesterase I catalytic residues. *J Mol Biol* **338**(5): 895–906

Raymond AC, Staker BL, Burgin AB, Jr. (2005) Substrate specificity of tyrosyl-DNA phosphodiesterase I (Tdp1). *J Biol Chem* **280**(23): 22029–22035

Redinbo MR, Stewart L, Kuhn P, Champoux JJ, Hol WG (1998) Crystal structures of human topoisomerase I in covalent and noncovalent complexes with DNA. *Science* **279**(5356): 1504–1513

Reid RJ, Gonzalez-Barrera S, Sunjevaric I, Alvaro D, Ciccone S, Wagner M, Rothstein R (2011) Selective ploidy ablation, a high-throughput plasmid transfer protocol, identifies new genes affecting topoisomerase I-induced DNA damage. *Genome Res* **21**(3): 477–486

Rideout MC, Raymond AC, Burgin AB, Jr. (2004) Design and synthesis of fluorescent substrates for human tyrosyl-DNA phosphodiesterase I. *Nucleic Acids Res* **32**(15): 4657–4664

Rosell R, Skrzypski M, Jassem E, Taron M, Bartolucci R, Sanchez JJ, Mendez P, Chaib I, Perez-Roca L, Szymanowska A, Rzyman W, Puma F, Kobierska-Gulida G, Farabi R, Jassem J (2007) BRCA1: a novel prognostic factor in resected non-small-cell lung cancer. *PLoS ONE* **2**(11): e1129

Rosidi B, Wang M, Wu W, Sharma A, Wang H, Iliakis G (2008) Histone H1 functions as a stimulatory factor in backup pathways of NHEJ. *Nucleic Acids Res* **36**(5): 1610–1623

Rudolph AE, Stuckey JA, Zhao Y, Matthews HR, Patton WA, Moss J, Dixon JE (1999) Expression, characterization, and mutagenesis of the Yersinia pestis murine toxin, a phospholipase D superfamily member. *J Biol Chem* **274**(17): 11824–11831

Sancar A, Lindsey-Boltz LA, Unsal-Kacmaz K, Linn S (2004) Molecular mechanisms of mammalian DNA repair and the DNA damage checkpoints. *Annu Rev Biochem* **73:** 39–85

Schreiber V, Dantzer F, Ame JC, de Murcia G (2006) Poly(ADP-ribose): novel functions for an old molecule. *Nat Rev Mol Cell Biol* **7**(7): 517–528

Seiler JA, Conti C, Syed A, Aladjem MI, Pommier Y (2007) The intra-S-phase checkpoint affects both DNA replication initiation and elongation: single-cell and -DNA fiber analyses. *Mol Cell Biol* **27**(16): 5806–5818

Shiloh Y (2006) The ATM-mediated DNA-damage response: taking shape. *Trends Biochem Sci* **31**(7): 402–410

Sijbers AM, de Laat WL, Ariza RR, Biggerstaff M, Wei YF, Moggs JG, Carter KC, Shell BK, Evans E, de Jong MC, Rademakers S, de Rooij J, Jaspers NG, Hoeijmakers JH, Wood RD (1996) Xeroderma pigmentosum group F caused by a defect in a structure-specific DNA repair endonuclease. *Cell* **86**(5): 811–822

Sordet O, Redon CE, Guirouilh-Barbat J, Smith S, Solier S, Douarre C, Conti C, Nakamura AJ, Das BB, Nicolas E, Kohn KW, Bonner WM, Pommier Y (2009) Ataxia telangiectasia mutated activation by transcription- and topoisomerase I-induced DNA double-strand breaks. *EMBO Rep* **10**(8): 887–893

Strumberg D, Pilon AA, Smith M, Hickey R, Malkas L, Pommier Y (2000) Conversion of topoisomerase I cleavage complexes on the leading strand of ribosomal DNA into 5'-phosphorylated DNA double-strand breaks by replication runoff. *Mol Cell Biol* **20**(11): 3977–3987

Stuckey JA, Dixon JE (1999) Crystal structure of a phospholipase D family member. *Nat Struct Biol* **6**(3): 278–284

Sung TC, Roper RL, Zhang Y, Rudge SA, Temel R, Hammond SM, Morris AJ, Moss B, Engebrecht J, Frohman MA (1997) Mutagenesis of phospholipase D defines a superfamily including a trans-Golgi viral protein required for poxvirus pathogenicity. *EMBO J* **16**(15): 4519–4530

Takao M, Kanno S, Shiromoto T, Hasegawa R, Ide H, Ikeda S, Sarker AH, Seki S, Xing JZ, Le XC, Weinfeld M, Kobayashi K, Miyazaki J, Muijtjens M, Hoeijmakers JH, van der Horst G, Yasui A (2002) Novel nuclear and mitochondrial glycosylases revealed by disruption of the mouse Nth1 gene encoding an endonuclease III homolog for repair of thymine glycols. *EMBO J* **21**(13): 3486–3493

Takashima H, Boerkoel CF, John J, Saifi GM, Salih MA, Armstrong D, Mao Y, Quiocho FA, Roa BB, Nakagawa M, Stockton DW, Lupski JR (2002) Mutation of TDP1, encoding a topoisomerase I-dependent DNA damage repair enzyme, in spinocerebellar ataxia with axonal neuropathy. *Nat Genet* **32**(2): 267–272

Toulany M, Dittmann K, Fehrenbacher B, Schaller M, Baumann M, Rodemann HP (2008) PI3K-Akt signaling regulates basal, but MAP-kinase signaling regulates radiation-induced XRCC1 expression in human tumor cells in vitro. *DNA Repair (Amst)* **7**(10): 1746–1756

Vance JR, Wilson TE (2002) Yeast Tdp1 and Rad1-Rad10 function as redundant pathways for repairing Top1 replicative damage. *Proc Natl Acad Sci USA* **99**(21): 13669–13674

Waite M (1999) The PLD superfamily: insights into catalysis. *Biochim Biophys Acta* **1439**(2): 187–197

Walton C, Interthal H, Hirano R, Salih MA, Takashima H, Boerkoel CF (2010) Spinocerebellar ataxia with axonal neuropathy. *Adv Exp Med Biol* **685:** 75–83

Weterings E, Chen DJ (2007) DNA-dependent protein kinase in nonhomologous end joining: a lock with multiple keys? *J Cell Biol* **179**(2): 183–186

Whitehouse CJ, Taylor RM, Thistlethwaite A, Zhang H, Karimi-Busheri F, Lasko DD, Weinfeld M, Caldecott KW (2001) XRCC1 stimulates human polynucleotide kinase activity at damaged DNA termini and accelerates DNA single-strand break repair. *Cell* **104**(1): 107–117

Yang SW, Burgin AB, Jr., Huizenga BN, Robertson CA, Yao KC, Nash HA (1996) A eukaryotic enzyme that can disjoin dead-end covalent complexes between DNA and type I topoisomerases. *Proc Natl Acad Sci USA* **93**(21): 11534–11539

Zeng Z, Cortes-Ledesma F, El-Khamisy SF, Caldecott KW (2010) TDP2/TTRAP is the major 5'-tyrosyl DNA phosphodiesterase activity in vertebrate cells and is critical for cellular resistance to topoisomerase II-induced DNA damage. *J Biol Chembrsbrs*

Zhou T, Akopiants K, Mohapatra S, Lin PS, Valerie K, Ramsden DA, Lees-Miller SP, Povirk LF (2009) Tyrosyl-DNA phosphodiesterase and the repair of 3'-phosphoglycolate-terminated DNA double-strand breaks. *DNA Repair (Amst)* **8**(8): 901–911

Zhou T, Lee JW, Tatavarthi H, Lupski JR, Valerie K, Povirk LF (2005) Deficiency in 3'-phosphoglycolate processing in human cells with a hereditary mutation in tyrosyl-DNA phosphodiesterase (TDP1). *Nucleic Acids Res* **33**(1): 289–297

Chapter 17
Ubiquitin and Ubiquitin-Like Proteins in Repair of Topoisomerase-Mediated DNA Damage

Shyamal D. Desai

17.1 Human Topoisomerases and Their Functions

Topoisomerases are enzymes involved in various cellular DNA transactions (Chen and Liu 1994; Li and Liu 2001; Pommier 1996; Wang 2002) (see Chaps. 1–5). The main function of all topoisomerases is to dissipate the torsional stress (supercoiling of the DNA) generated during DNA transactions such as transcription, replication, chromosome condensation, and segregation (Castano et al. 1996; Champoux 2001; Leppard and Champoux 2005; Zhang et al. 1988, 2000). To date, four type I DNA topoisomerases have been identified and characterized in human cells: nuclear Top1 (Top1) (Liu 1983; Wang 2002), mitochondrial topoisomerase (Top1mt) (Zhang et al. 2001), Top3α (Li and Wang 1998), and Top3β (Wilson et al. 2000) (see Chap. 1). Two type II human topoisomerases have been identified: Top2α and Top2β (Nitiss 2009a). Human topoisomerase I (Top1) is a type IB topoisomerase (forms 3′-phosphotyrosyl linkage with DNA) that functions as a swivel in DNA replication, RNA transcription, and chromosome condensation and segregation (Champoux 2001; Liu 1983). Human Top3α (Top3α) is a type IA (forms 5′-DNA tyrosyl linkages) topoisomerase and is essential for early embryogenesis, as evidenced by mouse knockout studies (Li and Wang 1998). Human Top3β is also a type 1A topoisomerase; although the Top3β knockout mouse develops to maturity, its mean lifespan is reduced (Kwan and Wang 2001). Thus, it appears that Top3α and β do not complement each other despite of their very similar enzymatic characteristics.

S.D. Desai (✉)
Department of Biochemistry and Molecular Biology, LSU Health Sciences Center-School of Medicine, 1901 Perdido Street, New Orleans, LA 70112, USA
e-mail: sdesai@lsuhsc.edu

Y. Pommier (ed.), *DNA Topoisomerases and Cancer*, Cancer Drug Discovery and Development, DOI 10.1007/978-1-4614-0323-4_17,

Human topoisomerase IIα (Top2α) catalyzes ATP-dependent strand-passing reactions and functions in DNA replication, chromosome condensation, and segregation (Nitiss 2009a). The function of Top2β is unclear; however, recent studies have suggested that Top2β may play a role in transcription in early developing neurons (Yang et al. 2000).

All topoisomerases relax supercoiled DNA by performing controlled breakage and resealing reactions of DNA (Champoux 2001; Liu 1983; Nitiss 2009a). Type I topoisomerases nick one strand of the DNA and pass the intact DNA strand through the enzyme-linked strand break prior to resealing of the DNA ends to effectuate supercoil relaxation (Champoux 2001; Liu 1983; Nitiss 2009a). Type II topoisomerases cleave both strands of duplex DNA and the enzyme-linked duplex cleavage acts as a transient gate for the passage of a second duplex DNA molecule. This mechanism relaxes DNA supercoils and catenates/decatenates DNA circles (Champoux 2001; Liu 1983; Nitiss 2009a).

The dual function of topoisomerases, with their intrinsic nuclease and ligase ("nicking-closing") activities (see Chap. 6), is essential for the proper execution of many DNA transactions during normal cell growth. However, these dual enzymatic activities also make the enzymes highly vulnerable to various physiological and non-physiological stresses (e.g., exposure to topoisomerase poisons, acidic pH, and oxidative stresses) (Li and Liu 2001; Li et al. 1999; Nitiss 2009b; Pommier 2009; Xiao et al. 2003a). These stresses can convert DNA topoisomerases into DNA-breaking nucleases that can cause genomic instability and cell death. Hence, these enzymes are often referred to as "double-edged swords" (Deweese and Osheroff 2009; Pommier et al. 2006).

17.2 Topoisomerase-Mediated DNA Damage

All the human topoisomerases, except for Top3α and Top3β, are important molecular targets for anticancer drugs (Liu 1989; Nitiss 2009b; Pommier 1998, 2006, 2009; Pommier et al. 2010) (see Chaps. 10–13). Most of the clinically used anticancer drugs target ("poison") type I and II topoisomerases by trapping the target topoisomerase in a reaction intermediate, a ternary enzyme-drug-DNA complex, termed "the cleavable (or cleavage) complex," in which the topoisomerase is covalently linked to the cleaved DNA (e.g., Type I eukaryotic topoisomerases are linked to DNA via a 3′-phosphotyrosyl bond, and the type II and type III eukaryotic topoisomerases are linked to DNA via a 5′- phosphotyrosyl bond) (Hsiang and Liu 1988; Hsiang et al. 1985; Nitiss 2002; Nitiss and Nitiss 2001). For example, the chemotherapeutic inhibitors of Top1, the camptothecins (CPT), Topotecan (Hycamtin), and Irinotecan (Camptosar) trap the Top1 cleavable complex (Hsiang et al. 1985; Liu et al. 1996; Pommier 2006; Pommier et al. 1994) (see Chaps. 10 and 12). Similarly, the chemotherapeutic inhibitors of Top2, etoposide (VP-16), doxorubicin (Doxil), and mitoxantrone (Novantrone) trap the Top2 cleavable complex (Nitiss 2009b; Nitiss and Wang 1996, 1988; Nitiss et al. 1992) (see Chaps. 11 and 13).

All Top1 and Top2 cancer chemotherapeutics interfere with the DNA religation function of their target topoisomerase and thus enhance the retention time of cleavable complexes on the DNA (Anderson et al. 1991; Hsiang et al. 1985; Liu et al. 1996; Nitiss 2009b; Nitiss and Wang 1996, 1988; Nitiss et al. 1992; Pommier et al. 1994, 2006; Svejstrup et al. 1991). The majority of the drug-trapped, cleavable complexes of Top1 and Top2 readily reverse upon drug removal (Hsiang and Liu 1988, 1989; Tanizawa et al. 1994). However, elongating replication and transcription machineries can process the reversible, drug-trapped Top1- and Top2-cleavable complexes into irreversible, topoisomerase-DNA strand breaks, as has been demonstrated in vitro (Bendixen et al. 1990; Tsao et al. 1993; Wu and Liu 1997). DNA helicase has also been shown to convert the reversible Top2 cleavable complex into irreversible, topoisomerase-DNA strand breaks in vitro (Shea and Hiasa 1999).

In vivo as well, studies indicate that enzymatic machineries acting on DNA convert the drug-stabilized cleavable complexes of Top1 and Top2 into irreversible topoisomerase-DNA breaks that account for the lethality (Bendixen et al. 1990; D'Arpa et al. 1990; Holm et al. 1989; Hsiang et al. 1989; Pourquier et al. 1999; Strumberg et al. 2000; Tsao et al. 1992). These irreversible protein-linked-DNA strand breaks have been demonstrated to arrest cultured cells in the G2 phase of the cell cycle (D'Arpa et al. 1990; Hsiang et al. 1989; Shao et al. 1997, 1999; Tsao et al. 1992), to activate signal transduction molecules such as p53, and to induce apoptosis [reviewed in (Li and Liu 2001)]. In the case of CPT, high concentration treatments caused apoptotic cell death, that is, a cell killing mechanism independent of DNA replication (Alexandre et al. 2000; Davis et al. 1998; Morris and Geller 1996). In contrast, lower doses of CPT, achievable in patients, selectively kill S-phase cells (Davis et al. 1998; Morris and Geller 1996; Shao et al. 1997, 1999), that is, elongating replication forks are an essential component of the lethality of clinically achievable doses of CPT.

In contrast to these earlier findings, a recent report has shown lower-dose CPT to kill non-S-phase breast cancer cells (Davis et al. 1998; Desai et al. 2001), hypothesized to be due to elongating RNA polymerase converting reversible Top1-cleavable complexes into irreversible Top1-DNA strand breaks (Desai et al. 2003). Higher concentrations of CPT can also interfere with RNA polymerase and induce the formation of DNA double-strand breaks (Sordet et al. 2008, 2009, 2010). Another study has suggested that the transcription machinery can also convert Top2 cleavable complexes, especially Top2β cleavable complexes, into lethal DNA lesions in vivo (Xiao et al. 2003b).

In summary, active DNA replication and RNA transcription are involved in converting the drug-trapped Top1 and Top2 cleavable complexes into irreversible topoisomerase-linked DNA strand breaks that are lethal to cells. Several repair pathways for this topoisomerase-mediated DNA damage have been studied including tyrosyl DNA phosphodiesterase (Nitiss et al. 2006; Pommier et al. 2006) (see Chaps. 15 and 16). This chapter focuses on the current knowledge of the role of ubiquitin and ubiquitin-like proteins (Ubls) in processing/repair of topoisomerase-mediated DNA/protein damage.

17.3 Ubiquitin/26S Proteasome and Ubl Pathways

Ubiquitin: Ubiquitin is a highly conserved 8 kDa (76 amino acids) protein whose main function is to modify cellular proteins by covalent conjugation (ubiquitylation) marking them for degradation by the 26S proteasome (Hochstrasser 1996; Pickart 2001b; Schwartz and Ciechanover 2009; Varshavsky 1997). The 26S proteasome is the major cellular proteolytic machinery, which is present both in cytosol and nucleus (Palmer et al. 1994; Rivett 1998). The joint action of ubiquitylation and the 26S proteasome machineries regulates many cellular functions including cell cycle progression, development, apoptosis, signal transduction, and antigen presentation (Haas 1997).

Ubiquitin is expressed as an inactive precursor with C-terminal extensions (Jentsch and Pyrowolakis 2000). Cleavage of the extensions by ubiquitin proteases generates the mature form that has a conserved C-terminal RGG sequence (Jentsch and Pyrowolakis 2000). The C-terminus of ubiquitin is conjugated to cellular proteins in a three step enzymatic process (Pickart 2001a). In the first step, the C terminal Gly residue of ubiquitin is activated in an ATP-dependent manner to form a thiol ester linkage with a cysteine residue of ubiquitin-activating enzyme E1. In the second step, the activated ubiquitin is transferred to its cognate carrier enzyme E2. In the third step, ubiquitin is transferred either directly from E2, or indirectly with the help of ubiquitin ligase E3, to the target proteins (Haas and Siepmann 1997; Pickart 2001a). The transfer of ubiquitin to the ε-NH2 group of Lys on target proteins generates an isopeptide bond (Pickart 2000). The transfer of ubiquitin to an ubiquitin already conjugated to the target protein results in the synthesis of a polyubiquitin chain. Ubiquitin can be transferred to Lys48, 6, 11, 27, 29, 33, or 63 of another ubiquitin molecule to synthesize ubiquitin chains with different linkages (Pickart 2000; Pickart and Fushman 2004). The Lys48-linked polyubiquitin chain serves as a recognition marker for the 26S proteasome (Pickart 2000), a major cellular proteolytic machinery composed of the 20S core catalytic complex flanked on both sides by the 19S regulatory complexes (Baumeister et al. 1998; Seeger et al. 1997). Ubiquitin chains composed of more than four ubiquitin (Thrower et al. 2000) on the target substrates are recognized and then disassembled by the ubiquitin-specific proteases (UBPs) (e.g., DoA4 and Isopeptidase T) (Chung and Baek 1999; Papa and Hochstrasser 1993) prior to degradation of the target substrates. Degradation of the protein substrates occurs in the 20S core cylinder comprised of all proteolytic activities (Hershko and Ciechanover 1992). With some known exceptions (e.g., ornithine decarboxylase which is proteolyzed following association with its inhibitor antizyme but without prior ubiquitylation (Hoyt et al. 2003)), the 26S proteasome specifically recognizes Lys48-linked ubiquitin-tagged proteins (Young et al. 1998). As for other regulatory posttranslational modifications such as phosphorylation, ubiquitylation is reversible by enzymes associated with and independent of the 26S proteasome (Wilkinson 2009).

Ubiquitin-like proteins: In addition to ubiquitin, a number of proteins related in sequence to ubiquitin but functioning differently than ubiquitin in a variety of processes such as protein trafficking, protein degradation, DNA repair, cell division, autophagy, and apoptosis, have been identified (Herrmann et al. 2007; Hochstrasser 2000a; Jentsch and Pyrowolakis 2000; Yeh et al. 2000). The ubiquitin-like proteins fall into two separate classes: (1) ubiquitin-associated domain proteins (UBAs) that bear domains related to ubiquitin, but are not conjugated to cellular proteins, and (2) ubiquitin-like modifiers (Ubls) that modify cellular proteins similar to ubiquitin. The UBAs include RAD23/HHR23A/B, DSK2, PLIC-1, PLIC-2/Chap1, NUB1, among others [reviewed in (Jentsch and Pyrowolakis 2000)]. Known Ubls include SUMO1/2/3 (Small Ubiquitin like MOdifiers, also known as PIC1, sentrin, GMP1), NEDD8 (NEuronal precursor cell-expressed Developmentally Downregulated protein 8), FAT10, APG12, URM1, and ISG15 (**I**nterferon-**S**timulatory **G**ene **15**), among others [reviewed in (Jentsch and Pyrowolakis 2000)]. The biological functions of Ubls are mediated by their covalent conjugation to a subset of cellular proteins, whereas UBAs (mentioned above) are responsible for the shuttling of ubiquitylated substrates to the proteasome (Ferrier 2002; Herrmann et al. 2007; Hochstrasser 2000a; Jentsch and Pyrowolakis 2000; Yeh et al. 2000).

Similar to ubiquitin, Ubls are expressed as inactive precursors with C-terminal extensions (Jentsch and Pyrowolakis 2000; Yeh et al. 2000). These extensions are cleaved posttranslationally by UBL-specific proteases to generate their mature forms which, like ubiquitin, have a conserved RGG sequence at their C-termini (Ha and Kim 2008). Ubls are conjugated to cellular proteins by a mechanism similar to that of ubiquitin but with distinct E1, E2, and E3 enzymes (Herrmann et al. 2007; Jentsch and Pyrowolakis 2000; Yeh et al. 2000). Enzymes responsible for deconjugation of Ubls have also been identified (Hochstrasser 2000b). UBL conjugations to proteins have diverse functions, and are less well defined for many Ubls, as compared to the clearly defined role of ubiquitin conjugation in protein degradation. For example, SUMOylation of proteins functions in protein trafficking (Ulrich 2009), transcription regulation (Hay 2006), and antagonism of ubiquitylation (Buschmann et al. 2000; Desterro et al. 1998). Similarly, ISG15 is known to antagonize ubiquitylation (Desai et al. 2006; Okumura et al. 2008). By contrast, NEDDylation has been shown to facilitate ubiquitylation and proteasome-mediated degradation (Wu et al. 2000).

17.4 Ubiquitin Pathway in the Repair of Top1 and Top2-Mediated DNA Damage

Degradation of Top1 (Top1 downregulation) in CPT-treated cells was first reported by Beidler and Chang in 1995 (Beidler and Cheng 1995). In 1997, we demonstrated downregulation of Top1 via ubiquitin/26S proteasome in mammalian cells treated with CPT and in animals administered topotecan (Desai et al. 1997, 2001, 2003). The cellular content of Top1 was reduced in less than 6 h of CPT treatment (Desai et al. 1997). However, Top1 levels were restored back to normal levels within 12 h after CPT removal (Fu et al. 1999). The reduction of Top1 cellular content was dependent on active E1[ub] (ubiquitin-activating enzyme) (Desai et al. 1997), formation of Top1 cleavable complexes (Desai et al. 2003), and active 26S proteasome (Desai et al. 1997). In addition, CPT-induced Top1 degradation also required modification of Top1 with Lys48-linked polyubiquitin chains (Lin et al. 2009), a proteolysis signal that targets substrates to the 26S proteasome for degradation (Thrower et al. 2000). The CPT-induced degradation of Top1 was also blocked by the proteasome inhibitor and calpain inhibitor I, a Ca^{2+}-dependent cysteine protease inhibitor. By contrast, two other cysteine protease inhibitors, 1-*trans*-epoxysuccinyl-L-leucylamido-(4-guanidino) butane and IBU did not block degradation of Top1(Fu et al. 1999).

CPT-induced Top1 downregulation was found to be dependent on active transcription (Desai et al. 2003). Inhibitors of transcription [5,6-dichlorobenzimidazole riboside (DRB) and α-amanitin], but not replication (aphidicolin), blocked camptothecin-induced degradation of Top1 in CHO cells (Desai et al. 2003). In contrast, inhibitors of protein synthesis did not block CPT-induced degradation of Top1 (Desai et al. 2003). These data suggested a model wherein collision of transcription elongation complexes with reversible Top1 cleavable complexes converts them into long-lived Top1-DNA covalent complexes that are then multiubiquitylated and degraded by the 26S proteasome (Desai et al. 2003). The proteasomal degradation of Top1 cleavable complexes presumably makes accessible the otherwise Top1-concealed SSB to DNA repair enzymes such as TDP1 (see Chaps. 15 and 16) (Debethune et al. 2002; Interthal et al. 2005; Yang et al. 1996), ATM, and PARP1, thus facilitating DNA repair (Lin et al. 2009; Sordet et al. 2008, 2009, 2010). Evidence supporting these models include: (a) CPT treatment arrests transcription (Desai et al. 2003; Zhang et al. 1988); (b) the transcription inhibitor DRB blocks multiubiquitylation (Lin et al. 2008), PolII hyperphosphorylation (Sordet et al. 2008), and degradation of Top1 (Lin et al. 2008); (c) long-lived Top1-DNA cleavable complexes (irreversible strand breaks) are formed in vitro (Wu and Liu 1997); (d) Top1 and large subunit of RNA polymerase are multiubiquitylated and degraded via 26S proteasome in CPT-treated cells (Desai et al. 2003; Lin et al. 2008); and (e) the single- and double-strand DNA repair pathways are activated in CPT-treated cells (Lin et al. 2008; Sordet et al. 2009, 2010). Interestingly, Top1 is actively recruited onto genomic DNA following DNA damage by UV light without inducing ubiquitin-dependent degradation of Top1; thus it appears that downregulation of Top1 is specific for CPT-induced topoisomerase-mediated DNA damage (Subramanian et al. 1998).

Top1-ubiquitin conjugates are discernible after DNase treatment of cell lysates, suggesting that Top1 cleavable complexes are ubiquitylated on the DNA (Desai et al. 2003). However, it is not known whether ubiquitylated Top1 is degraded on DNA, and/or whether ubiquitylated Top1 is released from the DNA and then degraded in the nucleus by nuclear proteasomes, and/or ubiquitylated Top1 is transported to cytoplasm and degraded by cytoplasmic proteasomes. Increased cytoplasmic concentrations of Top1 protein (70 kDa fragment) was observed in cells treated with TPT (Danks et al. 1996). However, the purpose of the relocalization of this partially proteolyzed form of Top1 in the cytoplasm in this unique case is not known.

There are two plausible explanations for the downregulation of Top1 in response to CPT treatment: First, Top1 degradation may expose the Top1-concealed SSB to DNA repair enzymes to facilitate DNA repair as suggested in (Debethune et al. 2002; Dexheimer et al. 2008; Interthal et al. 2005; Lin et al. 2008; Yang et al. 1996) (see Chap. 16) and second, degradation may lower the total cellular pool of Top1 to reduce the level of Top1-mediated DNA damage as suggested in (Beidler and Cheng 1995). In agreement with the second notion, Top1 protein levels are commonly decreased in camptothecin-resistant cell lines selected for CPT resistance (Chang et al. 1992). It is possible that CPT-induced downregulation of Top1 is a mechanism of resistance for cells to avoid toxic levels of CPT-mediated accumulation of cleavable complexes. Indeed, ubiquitin/26S proteasome-mediated downregulation of Top1 was demonstrated to be correlated with CPT resistance in some tumor cells (Desai et al. 2001). Overexpression of cullin 3, a component of an SCF (Skip1-Cul-F-Box) E3 ligase, a putative E3^{ub} ligase for Top1, has been demonstrated to increase Top1 ubiquitylation and subsequent degradation resulting in CPT resistance (Zhang et al. 2004). In addition to cullin 3, the E3 ligase Brca1 has been involved in transcription-dependent Top1 degradation in response to CPT (Sordet et al. 2008) and Brca1 deficient cells are hypersensitive to CPT (Nakamura et al. 2010; Pommier et al. 2006). In line with this observation, it would be interesting to investigate whether the lack of Top1 degradation in cancers cells could be related to Brca1-inactivating mutations that occur frequently during tumorigenesis. Co-treatment of proteasome inhibitor MG132 inhibits Top1 downregulation and increases the sensitivity of tumor cells to the killing by CPT (Desai et al. 2001). The role of ubiquitin in determining CPT sensitivity/resistance in mammalian cells has also been corroborated by studies in yeast where two proteins related to the ubiquitylation pathway were discovered using genetic screens for mutants that alter CPT sensitivity. Overexpression of one of them, the ubiquitin-specific protease, Ubp11, conferred resistance to Top1-mediated DNA damage (Rasheed and Rubin 2003) and the loss of the other, DOA4, a 26S proteasome-associated C-terminal ubiquitin hydrolase, sensitized cells to Top1-mediated DNA damage (Fiorani et al. 2004).

We have demonstrated that CPT-induced Top1 downregulation is defective in many tumor cells (Desai et al. 2001). Tumor cells defective in CPT-induced degradation of Top1 are hypersensitive to CPT (Desai et al. 2001). In nontransformed cells, but not in many tumor cells, CPT treatment induces Top1 downregulation (Desai et al. 2001). Similarly, in a nude mouse model, topotecan treatment causes Top1 downregulation in many normal tissues (e.g., blood, brain, kidney, liver, and skin) but not in xenografted MDA-MB-435 breast cancer cells (Desai et al. 2003). Furthermore, patients with solid tumors receiving topotecan therapy exhibit reduced Top1 levels in normal peripheral blood cells (Rubin et al. 1995), which is not the case for leukemic cells obtained from patients with leukemia (Saleem et al. 2000). Thus, Top1 downregulation in normal tissues is associated with low sensitivity to the lethal effect of Top1-directed anticancer drugs. Most tumor cells are defective in CPT-induced Top1 downregulation, which could explain in part the increased sensitivity of tumor cells to CPTs (Desai et al. 2001). Together, these results suggest that the ubiquitin/proteasome pathway is an important determinant of CPT sensitivity/resistance.

Other compounds have been tested for their ability to trap the cleavable complex and induce degradation of topoisomerases in cultured cells (the indolocarbazole compound, NB-506 and VP-16, W1, and W2) (Fu et al. 1999). NB-506 and W1 did not induce Top1 degradation, although they trap the Top1 cleavable complex (Fu et al. 1999). Based on a crystal structure of CPT binding to Top1-DNA complexes (Staker et al. 2005) (see Chaps. 9 and 10), CPT and W1 may have different conformational effects on the Top1-DNA complex that may promote recognition by ubiquitin-conjugating enzymes (Fu et al. 1999). However, this possibility has not yet been tested.

Like Top1 poisons, the Top2 poison teniposide (VM-26) induces ubiquitylation and degradation of Top2 that is dependent upon the ubiquitin/26S proteasome pathway (Mao et al. 2001). Surprisingly, the Top2β isozyme is preferentially degraded over Top2α isozyme (Mao et al. 2001). Proteasome-mediated degradation of Top2β was demonstrated to be independent of replication or protein synthesis (Mao et al. 2001). By contrast, transcription inhibitors such as DRB and CPT blocked VM-26-induced Top2β degradation (Mao et al. 2001). Proteasome-mediated degradation of Top2β was found to be $E1^{ub}$-dependent and blocked by proteasome but not by caspase inhibitors (Mao et al. 2001). It is relatively unclear what the role of Top2β degradation is in response to Top2 poisons. However, by analogy with Top1, Top2β degradation could be an early step in the repair/excision of Top2 cleavable complexes (Mao et al. 2001) mediated by the recently discovered enzyme, tyrosyl-DNA-phosphodiesterase (TDP2/TTRAP) (Ledesma et al. 2009; Zeng et al. 2011).

Similar to VM-26, the Top2 catalytic inhibitors, ICRF-193 [4,4-(2,3-butanediyl)-bis(2,6-piperazinedione)], which trap Top2 into a circular clamp without inducing DNA damage, also arrested transcription and induced proteasomal degradation of Top2β (Xiao et al. 2003b). Hence, it was suggested that proteasomal degradation of Top2β induced by the Top2-DNA covalent complex or the Top2 circular clamp is due to transcriptional arrest, but not DNA damage (Xiao et al. 2003b). Interestingly, both VM-26 and ICRF-193 arrest elongation of RNA polymerase even though VM-26 induces Top2-mediated DNA breakage and ICRF-193 does not (Xiao et al. 2003b). But ICRF-193 did not induce degradation of the large subunit of RNA pol II via proteasome (Xiao et al. 2003b), as does VM-26 (Xiao et al. 2003b) and CPTs (Desai et al. 2003). Hence, the transcription arrest at the site of DNA damage together with the recruitment of DNA repair complexes might be responsible for the ubiquitin-mediated degradation of the large subunit of RNA pol II.

The role of Top2 downregulation in the sensitivity/resistance of normal/tumor cells to Top2 poisons has received somewhat less attention as compared to Top1. Ubiquitin-mediated downregulation of Top1 is deficient in most tumor cells (Desai et al. 2001). By contrast, the downregulation of Top2β following treatment with Top2 poisons has been found to be proficient in all tumor cells tested so far. The Top2β downregulation in response to both Top2 poisons and catalytic inhibitors suggests that Top2 downregulation may reflect the removal of protein that is linked to or clamped on DNA and is blocking the progression of the transcription machinery. The same idea may hold true for Top1 cleavable complexes.

The cleavable complexes of Top1 and Top2 and the Top2-circular clamp are reversible (Hsiang and Liu 1988, 1989). It is possible that reversible Top2 protein lesions are converted into irreversible forms upon collision with transcription machinery, as shown for Top1 in vitro (Wu and Liu 1997). Although, no such evidence for Top2β has been reported from in vitro studies, in vivo studies have shown that transcription inhibitors can block Top2β downregulation induced by VM-26 as well as ICRF 187, supporting the idea of such collisions (Mao et al. 2001; Xiao et al. 2003b). Although several lines of evidences suggest that ICRF derivatives inhibit Top2 catalytic activity without inducing cleavable complexes or binding to DNA (Roca et al. 1994), Snapka and colleagues have recently demonstrated that ICRF-193 can trap cleavable complex of Top2 (Huang et al. 2001). Hence, Top2β downregulation might also possibly be a repair response to some irreversible forms of Top2 cleavable complexes in response to Top2 catalytic inhibitors and poisons; however, such possibility needs further investigation.

17.5 UBL-SUMO Pathway in Top1 and Top2-Mediated DNA Damage

SUMO-1 was the first member of the SUMO family to be identified (Hay 2001). Two other SUMO paralogs, SUMO-2, SUMO-3 have only about 42–43% sequence identities to SUMO-1 but are about 96% identical to one another (Saitoh and Hinchey 2000). SUMO-1/2/3 are conjugated to cellular proteins in a way similar to ubiquitin but using distinct E1 /E2 /E3 enzymes (Ulrich 2009). By contrast, SUMO-4, another isoform of SUMO in mammalian cells does not conjugate to the cellular proteins in vivo (Ulrich 2009). As for ubiquitin, the activation of SUMO involves the formation of a thioester linkage with an E1 enzyme (SUMO-activating enzyme) (Ulrich 2009). SUMO is then transferred to the conjugating enzyme, Ubc9, an E2 enzyme for SUMO, in a transesterification reaction (Ulrich 2009). Ubc9 then transfers SUMO to a target protein, usually at ΨKX(E/D) (the sumoylation consensus sequence, where Ψ is a large hydrophobic amino acid, X is any amino acid, and the fourth amino acid is either E or D) (Ulrich 2009). Ubc9 can SUMOylate most target proteins in vitro; however, the majority of in vivo SUMOylation reactions require specific E3 enzymes to direct Ubc9 to specific protein targets (Hochstrasser 2001). SUMO-conjugation is reversible via enzymes that deconjugate SUMO from target proteins (Ulrich 2009). SUMO is involved in a variety of cellular functions such as antagonism of ubiquitin-dependent degradation, nuclear-cytoplasmic trafficking, regulation of transcription, mitochondrial fission, cell division, DNA damage and repair, and assembly of protein complexes reviewed in (Ulrich 2009).

Many SUMO targets have been identified. Among the earliest identified was Top1 (Mao et al. 2000b). The SUMO conjugates of Top1 were originally identified by Desai et al. as a ladder of bands above 100 kDa Top1 band on Western blots that immunoreacted with Top1 antibodies. This ladder of bands had 14–17 kDa spacing instead of the 8-kDa shifts known for ubiquitin conjugates (Desai et al. 1997). These bands disappeared upon prolonged treatment with CPT (4–6 h), and were absent in $E1^{ub}$ mutant cells ($E1^{ub}ts85$) at restrictive temperature (43°C) treated with CPT for 10 min (Desai et al. 1997). Later, following the discovery of SUMO-1 and the availability of SUMO-1-specific antibodies and HA-tagged SUMO-1 cDNA, the ladder of bands induced upon CPT treatment were shown to be Top1-SUMO-1 conjugates (Mao et al. 2000b). The disappearance of the Top1-SUMO-1 ladder from cells with increasing time of CPT treatment was later shown to be due to the degradation of cellular Top1, dependent on the ubiquitin/proteasome pathway (Mao et al. 2000b). However, the reason for the disappearance of Top1-SUMO-1 conjugates in $E1^{ub}ts85$ cells treated with CPT at restrictive temperature is still unclear. It may be due to heat-stress, which has been shown to abolish CPT-induced Top1-sumoylation (Mao et al. 2000a).

Within seconds of CPT treatment, Top1 is SUMOylated in normal and tumor cells (Mao et al. 2000b). The sites on human Top1 that are SUMOylated have been mapped to three N-terminal lysines, K103, K117, and K153, with K117 being the predominant site (Rallabhandi et al. 2002). The E3 ligase, Topors, a dual function E3 ligase shown to conjugate both ubiquitin and SUMO to p53 (Rajendra et al. 2004; Weger et al. 2005), has been demonstrated to polySUMOylate Top1 in vitro and in vivo (Hammer et al. 2007). Top1 of budding yeast is also SUMOylated in response to CPT (Jacquiau et al. 2005; Mao et al. 2000b). As with human Top1, budding yeast Top1 SUMOylation has been mapped to three N-terminal lysines (K65, K91, and K92) (Chen et al. 2007). The E3s acting in the SUMOylation of budding yeast Top1 were shown to be the PIAS family members Siz1 and Siz2 (Chen et al. 2007).

Supporting the possibility that the Top1-cleavable complex, rather than free Top1, is the substrate for SUMOylation are the observations that CPT-resistant cells defective in formation of the Top1 cleavable complex did not show SUMO-1-Top1 ladders (Desai et al. 2003), and DNase treatment is required to release SUMOylated Top1 from DNA in lysates of cells proficient in cleavable complex formation (Desai et al. 2003; Mao et al. 2000b). The SUMOylation of Top1 does not require ongoing DNA replication or transcription, as inhibitors of these cellular processes did not block Top1-SUMOylation (Mao et al. 2000b).

Various consequences of Top1 SUMOylation have been proposed by different groups. Initially, a budding yeast UBC9 mutant expressing human Top1 was shown to be hypersensitive to CPT, hence it was suggested that UBC9/SUMO-1 may be involved in the repair of Top1-mediated DNA damage (Mao et al. 2000b). Later, human Top1 SUMOylation site mutants were reported to be depleted from the nucleolus (Mo et al. 2002; Rallabhandi et al. 2002). However, other studies did not support a role for SUMOylation in Top1 nucleolar delocalization (Christensen et al. 2004). In yet another study, SUMO-1 conjugation to intact Top1 amplified cleavable complex formation induced by CPT in vivo, suggesting the role of SUMOylation in formation of cleavable complex (Horie et al. 2002). This conclusion was based on two observations: (1) substitutions of Lys117 and Lys153, identified as Top1 SUMOylation sites, reduced the CPT-induced cleavable complexes without influencing in vitro catalytic activity and (2) Top1 SUMOylation occurred independently of CPT when Top1 was inactivated by mutation of the active site tyrosine (Tyr723). Based on these observations, it was suggested that Top1 inactivation by CPT treatment can trigger Top1 SUMOylation, leading to enhanced cleavable complex formation. Similar to human Top1, catalytically inactive yeast Top 1, bearing mutations at the active site tyrosine, is extensively SUMO modified even in the absence of Top1 poisons (Chen et al. 2007). Thus it appears that Top1 SUMOylation is a consequence of the aberrant Top1 conformation.

Very recent studies have shown that CPT-induced Top1 cleavable complexes are heavily modified by ubiquitin and SUMO-2/3, but not by SUMO-1 in vivo (Kanagasabai et al. 2009). By contrast, previous studies by Liu and colleagues have demonstrated that Top1 is conjugated to SUMO-1 in cultured cells treated with CPT (Mao et al. 2000b). Several in vitro and in vivo studies from other groups are in agreement with this report that SUMO-1 is conjugated to both mammalian as well as yeast Top1 (Hammer et al. 2007; Jacquiau et al. 2005; Mao et al. 2000b; Rallabhandi et al. 2002; Yang et al. 2006). However, the reason for the failure to detect SUMO-1 peptides on purified Top1 cleavable complexes in earlier study is not clear. The recent studies have shown that SUMO-2/3 polychains serves as a signal for ubiquitin-mediated proteolysis on the target substrate (Weisshaar et al. 2008). The finding that Top1 is conjugated to both SUMO-2/3 and ubiquitin (Kanagasabai et al. 2009), and that poly-SUMO-2/3 chains serve as a signal for polyubiquitylation (mediated by RNF4) (Tatham et al. 2008) suggest that CPT-induced SUMO-2/3 conjugation to Top1 may signal ubiquitin-mediated degradation of Top1 cleavable complexes.

SUMOylation sites on Top1 have been mapped to three lysines in the unstructured N-terminus of Top1 after CPT treatment of both yeast (Chen et al. 2007) and human (Rallabhandi et al. 2002) cells. Mutations of a single SUMOylation site changes the pattern of the SUMOylated Top1 ladder in a way that suggests that a single SUMO (mono-SUMO-1) may be is conjugated to SUMOylation sites of Top1 (Rallabhandi et al. 2002). SUMO-1 does not form SUMO chains in vivo, whereas, SUMO-2/3 and Smt3 can form such chains because they possess internal consensus SUMO modification sites (Geoffroy and Hay 2009). Additionally, mono-SUMO is a poor substrate for polyubiquitination (Tatham et al. 2008). Together, these results suggest that Top1-SUMO-1 conjugation is unlikely to be for the purpose of degradation. On the other hand, CPT-induced rapid SUMOylation might possibly function to prevent Top1 reversible cleavable complexes from being converted into irreversible Top1-cleavable complexes (causing irreversible Top1-linked DNA strand breaks), which is dependent upon active replication, and associated with the lethality of Top1 poisons. Mono SUMOylation of multiple sites on reversible Top1 cleavable complexes may function to protect surface-exposed lysines. However, it is possible that after collision with replication/transcription machinery, these reversible cleavable complexes are converted into long-lived irreversible and lethal cleavable complexes. These in turn are conjugated to SUMO-2/3, to signal ubiquitylation (probably to RNF4 or RNF4-like E3-ligase) for the purpose of degradation via 26S proteasome (see Fig. 17.1 for

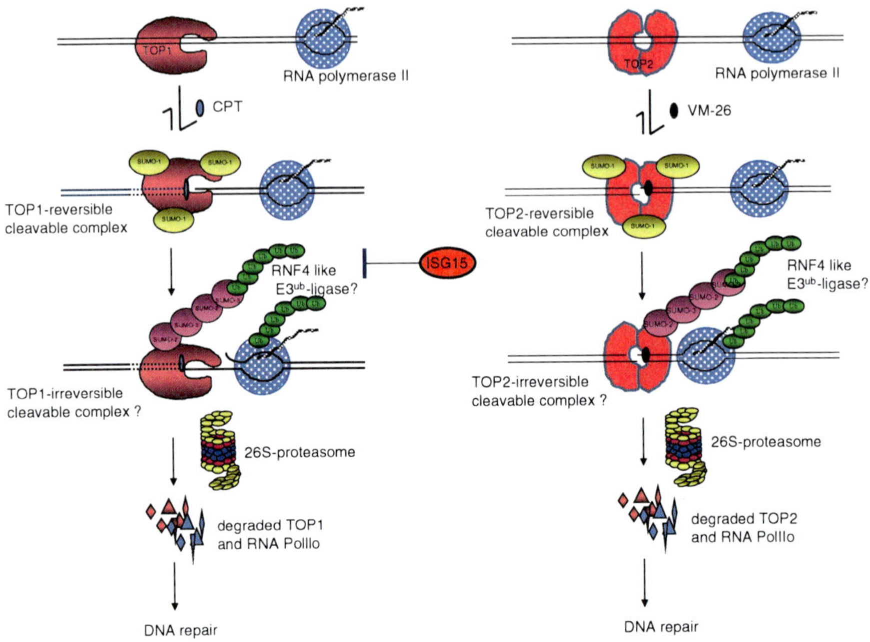

Fig. 17.1 The role(s) of the ubiquitin and ubiquitin-like proteins in the repair of topoisomerase-mediated DNA damage

schematic representation). It is possible that purified Top1 cleavable complexes isolated by Snapka's group used in their mass spectrophotometry study are irreversible Top1 cleavable complexes, and hence were devoid of SUMO-1, but contained SUMO-2/3 and ubiquitin. Of note, cells treated for 30 min with 10 μm CPT were used in this study to isolate purified cleavable complexes (Kanagasabai et al. 2009) and long-lived irreversible complexes are detected after 30 min of CPT treatment in tumor cells defective in degradation of Top1 (Desai and Liu, unpublished results). However, this interesting possibility needs further investigation.

In addition to Top1, the large subunit of RNA polymerase II is also ubiquitylated and degraded via 26S proteasome upon CPT treatment (Desai et al. 2003). Interestingly, the large subunit of RNA pol II is also SUMOylated in response to DNA damage (Chen et al. 2009). However, if this SUMOylation is for the purpose of ubiquitylation and large subunit of RNA pol II is SUMOylated in response to CPT is not known.

Like Top1, Top2 cleavable complexes are also SUMOylated in response to Top2 poisons (VM-26, VP16) and inhibitors (ICRF derivatives). ICRF-193, which does not induce topoisomerase II-mediated DNA damage, but traps topoisomerase II into a circular clamp conformation, was also shown to induce SUMO-1 conjugation to topoisomerase II isozymes, as does VM-26 (Isik et al. 2003; Mao et al. 2000a), which is known to induce DNA damage. It is not clear if SUMO-1 conjugation to topoisomerases is an indirect result of a DNA damage response or a direct result of protein conformational changes.

Various consequences of the SUMOylation of Top2 have been demonstrated by different groups. For example, the SUMO modification pathway was found to be essential for the ICRF-193-induced degradation of Top2β (Isik et al. 2003). Of note, Top2β was modified by multiple modifiers, SUMO-2/3, SUMO-1, and polyubiquitin in cells treated with ICRF-193 (Isik et al. 2003). One possibility is that SUMO-1 might be conjugated to drug-induced Top2 "reversible nonlethal" cleavable complexes (within seconds), to protect them from conversion to "irreversible lethal" Top2 cleavable complexes, as suggested for Top1. However, after collision with replication/transcription machinery, these Top2 reversible complexes are probably converted into long-lived irreversible and lethal complexes, which in turn are conjugated to SUMO-2/3, to signal ubiquitylation (probably by RNF4 or RNF4-like E3-ligase) for the purpose of degradation via 26S proteasome (see Fig. 17.1 for schematic representation). Additional genetic studies in yeast have shown that SUMO conjugation mutants show increased resistance to the Top2 poison doxorubicin (Huang et al. 2007) (see Chap. 18). However, specifically abolishing SUMOylation on Top2 by itself had no effect on doxorubicin toxicity (Huang et al. 2007).

In addition to the role of SUMOylation in proteolysis, SUMOylation has also been shown to occur as a normal aspect of Top2 regulation in mitosis in mitotic *Xenopus* egg extracts (Azuma et al. 2003, 2005) as well as in mitotic extracts from human and murine mitotic cells (Agostinho et al. 2008; Dawlaty et al. 2008). Top2α was found to be conjugated to SUMO-2/3 during interphase and mitosis in response to Top 2 inhibitors and poisons (ICRF-187, etoposide, and doxorubicin) (Agostinho et al. 2008). Formation of Top2α-SUMO-2/3 conjugates within mitotic chromosomes was strongly correlated with incomplete chromatid decatenation and decreased progressively as cells approach the metaphase-anaphase transition. In this case, whether SUMO-2/3 conjugated Top2α is targeted to destruction is not known. However, these studies indicate that SUMOylation of Top2 is essential for mitotic functions.

17.6 UBL-ISG15 in Top1 and Top2-Mediated DNA Damage

ISG15 is a 15 kDa protein that is induced by Type I interferons (IFN-α and IFN-β) (Haas et al. 1987) and is a member of the UBL (ubiquitin-like protein) superfamily of proteins (Andersen and Hassel 2006; Jentsch and Pyrowolakis 2000; Ritchie and Zhang 2004). It was the first ubiquitin-like protein to be identified (Haas et al. 1987; Loeb and Haas 1992). It was first discovered as a Ubiquitin Cross-Reactive Protein (UCRP) using antibodies specific to ubiquitin (Haas et al. 1987; Loeb and Haas 1992). Indeed, ISG15 is composed of two ubiquitin-like domains connected by a small linker region (Narasimhan et al. 2005). Each domain is roughly 30–40% homologous to ubiquitin (Narasimhan et al. 2005). These results explain its cross-reactivity to ubiquitin antisera. The carboxyl terminus of ISG15 retains the canonical LRLRGG ubiquitin sequence required for its conjugation to intracellular targets (Haas et al. 1987). ISG15 is conjugated to cellular proteins by a mechanism similar to that of ubiquitin but with distinct enzymes (Loeb and Haas 1992; Narasimhan et al. 1996). UBE1L, an E1-like protein, has been identified as the activating enzyme for ISG15 (Yuan and Krug 2001). UbcH8, a ubiquitin E2 enzyme, forms an obligate ISG15 thioester catalyzed by UBE1L, and has been identified as a major conjugating enzyme (E2) for ISG15 (Kim et al. 2004; Zhao et al. 2004). Although several E3s have been identified as possible ISG15 E3s, the major E3 for ISG15 appears to be HERC5 (Zou and Zhang 2006). Interestingly, many ISG15 E2 and E3s are thought to be dual function E2 and E3s that can conjugate both ubiquitin as well as ISG15 to their target substrates (Arimoto et al. 2008; Kim et al. 2004; Takeuchi et al. 2005; Zhao et al. 2004). UBP43 has been identified as an enzyme responsible for deconjugation of ISG15 from target substrates (Malakhov et al. 2002). It should be noted that all of the major enzymes in the ISG15 conjugation cascade are induced upon type I interferon treatment (Yuan and Krug 2001; Zhao et al. 2004; Zou and Zhang 2006).

The biological function of ISG15 is poorly understood. Initial studies suggested that extracellular ISG15 is an immunomodulatory cytokine (D'Cunha et al. 1996). However, the role of ISG15 in immunomodulation is not well understood. ISG15 is elevated after viral infections and has antiviral properties suggesting that it contributes to interferon's well-established immunological effects (Harty et al. 2009). ISG15 expression is also elevated in many human malignancies (Andersen and Hassel 2006; Desai et al. 2006; Harty et al. 2009), during pregnancy (Johnson et al. 1998) and in *Ataxia Telangiectasia* (A-T) (Siddoo-Atwal et al. 1996; Wood et al. 2011). However, the biological consequence(s) of elevated ISG15 upon viral infections, during pregnancy, in cancer and in *Ataxia Telangiectasia* are not known. Recent studies have suggested that ISG15, like ubiquitin, is involved in proteasomal degradation of PML/RARalpha (Pitha-Rowe et al. 2004). But, ISG15 conjugation to Serpin 2a, JAK, or STAT1 does not increase their degradation rates (Hamerman et al. 2002; Malakhova et al. 2003). On the other hand, other studies have shown that the constitutively elevated ISG15 pathway negatively regulates protein polyubiquitylation and subsequent degradation via 26S proteasome in tumor and *Ataxia Telangiectasia* cells (Desai et al. 2006; Wood et al. 2011). The precise mechanism by which ISG15 inhibits polyubiquitylation is not known. It has been suggested that ISGylation, which is elevated in many tumors, interferes with ubiquitylation through substrate competition at the E2/E3 level (Desai et al. 2006). Indeed, ISGylation of Ubc13 (ubiquitin E2) is shown to disrupt its ability to form the thioester bond with ubiquitin (Takeuchi and Yokosawa 2005; Zou et al. 2005). Whether other ubiquitin E2 functions are similarly inhibited by ISG15 through E2 ISGylation is not known. Analogous to ubiquitin E2, ubiquitin E1 has also been shown to be conjugated to ISG15 (supplementary data in (Giannakopoulos et al. 2005)). However, it is unclear whether ISGylation of ubiquitin E1 disrupts its ability to form the thioester bond with ubiquitin. It has also been reported that the ISG15 pathway converges with the ubiquitin pathway at E2/E3 (Arimoto et al. 2008; Kim et al. 2004; Zhao et al. 2004). Thus far, only one E2 (UbcH8) has been identified for ISG15 (Arimoto et al. 2008; Kim et al. 2004; Zhao et al. 2004). This ISG15 E2 is also a ubiquitin E2 (Arimoto et al. 2008; Dev et al. 2003). Consequently, it is possible that elevated expression of ISG15 may negatively interfere with the ubiquitin pathway by directly competing at a common site on this ISG15/ubiquitin E2 (UbcH8). However, although only one E2 has been identified for ISG15, there are many ubiquitin E2s (Haas and Siepmann 1997). It is not clear whether other ubiquitin E2s can also function as ISG15 E2s. It has been shown that ISG15/ubiquitin E2 (UbcH8) interacts with many ubiquitin E3s (e.g., Rsp5 E3 ligase and members of the HECT and single-subunit RING E3 families (Chin et al. 2002; Kumar et al. 1997)). It is also possible that these ISG15 E2-interacting ubiquitin E3s are dual function E3s, which could conjugate both ubiquitin and ISG15 to their respective substrates. Indeed, the ubiquitin E3 ligases (Rsp5, Efp), have been shown to be a dual function E3 ligases capable of conjugating ISG15 to a specific target (Zhao et al. 2004; Zou and Zhang 2006). Consequently, elevated expression of ISG15 in tumor cells may switch these ubiquitin E3s to ISG15 E3s, leading to decreased levels of polyubiquitylated proteins as demonstrated in (Desai et al. 2006; Wood et al. 2011).

CPT-induced Top1 degradation is proficient in normal cells (Desai et al. 2001). By contrast, many tumor cells are defective in degradation of Top1 (Desai et al. 2001). Tumor cells defective in Top1 degradation were found to be hypersensitive to CPT (Desai et al. 2001). However, the factors that determine CPT sensitivity/resistance are largely unknown. Recent studies by Desai et al. have demonstrated that ISG15 is an important determinant of CPT sensitivity/resistance, which might be due to ISG15 being an inhibitor of ubiquitin/proteasome-mediated repair of Top1-DNA covalent complexes. Two experimental evidences support this notion: (1) short hairpin RNA-mediated knockdown of either ISG15 or UbcH8 (major E2 for ISG15) in breast cancer ZR-75-1 cells reduce sensitivity to CPT, suggesting that ISG15 overexpression in tumors could be a factor affecting intrinsic CPT sensitivity in tumor cells (Desai et al. 2008), and (2) the level of ISG15 was found to be significantly reduced in several tumor cells selected for resistance to CPT, suggesting that altered ISG15 regulation could be a significant determinant for acquired CPT resistance (Desai et al. 2008). Parallel to reduced CPT sensitivity, short hairpin RNA-mediated knockdown of either ISG15 or UbcH8 in ZR-75-1 cells resulted in increased proteasomal degradation of CPT-induced Top1-DNA covalent complexes (Desai et al. 2008). Taken together, these results suggest that ISG15, by reducing general ubiquitylation, may interfere with ubiquitin/proteasome-mediated repair of Top1-DNA covalent complexes, and thereby confer CPT sensitivity to tumor cells (Desai et al. 2008). Indeed, interferon (IFN) has been shown to exhibit synergistic anticancer activity with CPT-11 against human colon cancer xenografts in nude mice (Kobayashi et al. 1996; Ohwada et al. 1996). Interferons are known to induce expression of more than 300 genes (Interferon-stimulated genes) including ISG15 (Kunzi and Pitha 2003). Hence, it is not known whether the synergistic anticancer activity observed with IFN and CPT administered to mice is due to an effect of a possible interaction between ISG15 and the ubiquitylation of Top1. Nevertheless, these results have significant implications in the clinic since both CPT analogs and interferons are used to manage cancers in clinic (Bracarda et al. 2009; Wall and Wani 1996), and ISG15 expression and CPT sensitivity are highly variable in variety of cancers (Desai et al. 2000, 2008). High expression of ISG15 and its conjugates in tumors may therefore be a useful predictor of tumor sensitivity to CPT.

The molecular mechanism of ISG15 interference with Top1 degradation is not clear. ISG15 could possibly interfere with Top1 degradation by competing with SUMO-2/3 (potential blocking of the degradation signal for ubiquitin) and/or ubiquitin for conjugation to the same lysine residue on Top1, or to putative lysines on SUMO-2/3 (potential proteolytic signal) for conjugation to ubiquitin. Alternatively, ISG15 may compete with ubiquitin to bind to Top1 $E2^{ub}/E3^{ub}$ ligases (Desai et al. 2006). ISGlyation of Top1 in response to CPT has not been reported, which suggests that it does not directly compete with ubiquitylation and SUMOylation for lysines on Top1. However, the constitutively elevated ISG15 pathway inhibits polyubiquitylation of cellular proteins in tumor and *Ataxia Telangiectasia* cells (Desai et al. 2006; Wood et al. 2011). This result supports the second possibility that ISG15 may interfere with polyubiquitylation of Top1 through competition at the E2/E3 level. Competition of ISG15 with the $E2^{ub}/E3^{ub}$ used for Top1 is expected to decrease polyubiquitylation and subsequent degradation of Top1. Indeed, subtle differences in CPT-induced polyubiquitylation of Top1 seen as smear above Top1 band have been observed in tumor cells that exhibit high expression of ISG15 (Desai et al. 2006). Interestingly, CPT was shown to induce free ISG15 and conjugates in a dose-dependent and time-dependent manner in cells (Liu et al. 2004). Whether there is concomitant decrease in polyubiquitylation under these experimental conditions is not known.

The role of ISGylation pathway in Top2 degradation has not been investigated to date. However, unlike the degradation of Top1, which is deficient in many tumor cells and suggested to be due in part to the elevated expression of ISG15, the defect in Top2 degradation has not been reported so far. It is possible that ISG15 specifically inhibits $E3^{ub}$ ligase responsible for ubiquitylating Top1 and does not inhibit $E3^{ub}$ ligase of Top2.

17.7 Other Ubiquitin-Like Proteins in the Repair of Topoisomerase-Mediated DNA Damage

Like ubiquitin, Nedd8 also facilitates substrate degradation via the 26S proteasome. However, unlike SUMO-1 and ubiquitin, NEDD8 conjugation to Top1 has not been reported in response to CPT treatment in mammalian cells. On the other hand, an intact NEDD8 pathway is required for Cullin-dependent ubiquitylation in mammalian cells (Zhang et al. 2004); Cullin 3 is a component of a SCF (Skip1-Cul-F-Box) E3 ligase used for ubiquitylation of Top1 in response to CPT treatment (Zhang et al. 2004). These results thus suggest a putative role of UBL Nedd8 in CPT-induced degradation of Top1.

17.8 Summary

The crosstalk between the ubiquitin and Ubl pathways in regulating various cellular processes (e.g., DNA repair) is evidenced by a rapidly emerging literature. This chapter covers the role(s) of the ubiquitin, SUMO, and ISG15 pathways in the repair of topoisomerase-mediated DNA damage. A hypothetical model for the role of ubiquitin and Ubls in the repair of topoisomerase-mediated DNA damage is shown in the schematic Fig. 17.1. Briefly, collision between elongating RNA polymerase and Top1 (Fig. 17.1, left panel) and/or Top2 (Fig. 17.1, right panel) trapped on DNA as cleavable complex (or closed circular clamp formed with Top2 inhibitors) activates both the SUMO and ubiquitin pathways. The ubiquitylation of Top1 and Top2 results in their degradation via the ubiquitin/26S proteasome pathway. The function of SUMOylation of both Top1 and Top2 is ambiguous. SUMO-1 and ubiquitin may compete for the same lysine residue on the target substrates, and/or SUMO-1 conjugation may protect and preserve initially formed, reversible, nonlethal, Top1 and Top2 cleavable complexes (and closed circular clamps of Top2), present during drug treatment, from being degraded via the ubiquitin-26S proteasome pathway. However, upon collision with elongating transcription machinery, reversible complexes are probably converted into lethal irreversible Top1 (Fig. 17.1, left panel)/ TOP2 (Fig. 17.1, right panel) cleavable complexes. The irreversible topoisomerase cleavable complexes linked to the broken ends of DNA have been shown conjugated to poly-SUMO-2/3. Polychains of SUMO-2/3 conjugated to the irreversible topoisomerase cleavable complexes may signal $E3^{ub}$ ligase to add ubiquitin chains to these lethal forms of Top1 (left panel) and Top2 (right panel), which is supported by the observation that SUMO-2/3 polychains can serve as a the signal for RNF4 $E3^{ub}$-ligase. The ubiquitylated forms of cleavable complexes can be recognized by the 26S proteasome and destroyed. Proteasomal degradation of cleavable complexes may be a necessary step to expose the DNA strand break for repair. ISG15 is shown to counteract ubiquitin-mediated degradation of Top1 and probably subsequent DNA repair. Most tumors that have the elevated ISG15 pathway are hypersensitive to Top1-targeting drugs, which may be due to reduced ubiquitylation-mediated repair of topoisomerase-linked DNA strand breaks.

References

Agostinho M, Santos V, Ferreira F, Costa R, Cardoso J, Pinheiro I, Rino J, Jaffray E, Hay RT, Ferreira J (2008) Conjugation of human topoisomerase 2 alpha with small ubiquitin-like modifiers 2/3 in response to topoisomerase inhibitors: cell cycle stage and chromosome domain specificity. *Cancer Res* **68**(7): 2409–2418

Alexandre S, Rast C, Nguyen-Ba G, Vasseur P (2000) Detection of apoptosis induced by topoisomerase inhibitors and serum deprivation in syrian hamster embryo cells. *Exp Cell Res* **255**(1): 30–39

Andersen JB, Hassel BA (2006) The interferon regulated ubiquitin-like protein, ISG15, in tumorigenesis: friend or foe? *Cytokine Growth Factor Rev* **17**(6): 411–421

Anderson AH, Sorensen BS, Christiansen K, Svejstrup JQ, Lund K, Westergaard O (1991) Studies of the topoisomerase II-mediated cleavage and religation reactions by use of a suicidal double-stranded DNA substrate. *J Biol Chem* **266**(14): 9203–9210

Arimoto K, Konishi H, Shimotohno K (2008) UbcH8 regulates ubiquitin and ISG15 conjugation to RIG-I. *Mol Immunol* **45**(4): 1078–1084

Azuma Y, Arnaoutov A, Anan T, Dasso M (2005) PIASy mediates SUMO-2 conjugation of Topoisomerase-II on mitotic chromosomes. *Embo J* **24**(12): 2172–2182

Azuma Y, Arnaoutov A, Dasso M (2003) SUMO-2/3 regulates topoisomerase II in mitosis. *J Cell Biol* **163**(3): 477–487

Baumeister W, Walz J, Zuhl F, Seemuller E (1998) The proteasome: paradigm of a self-compartmentalizing protease. *Cell* **92**(3): 367–380

Beidler DR, Cheng YC (1995) Camptothecin induction of a time- and concentration-dependent decrease of topoisomerase I and its implication in camptothecin activity. *Mol Pharmacol* **47**(5): 907–914

Bendixen C, Thomsen B, Alsner J, Westergaard O (1990) Camptothecin-stabilized topoisomerase I-DNA adducts cause premature termination of transcription. *Biochemistry* **29**(23): 5613–5619

Bracarda S, Eggermont AM, Samuelsson J (2009) Redefining the role of interferon in the treatment of malignant diseases. *Eur J Cancer*

Buschmann T, Fuchs SY, Lee CG, Pan ZQ, Ronai Z (2000) SUMO-1 modification of Mdm2 prevents its self-ubiquitination and increases Mdm2 ability to ubiquitinate p53. *Cell* **101**(7): 753–762

Castano IB, Brzoska PM, Sadoff BU, Chen H, Christman MF (1996) Mitotic chromosome condensation in the rDNA requires TRF4 and DNA topoisomerase I in Saccharomyces cerevisiae. *Genes Dev* **10**(20): 2564–2576

Champoux JJ (2001) DNA topoisomerases: structure, function, and mechanism. *Annu Rev Biochem* **70**: 369–413

Chang JY, Dethlefsen LA, Barley LR, Zhou BS, Cheng YC (1992) Characterization of camptothecin-resistant Chinese hamster lung cells. *Biochem Pharmacol* **43**(11): 2443–2452

Chen AY, Liu LF (1994) DNA topoisomerases: essential enzymes and lethal targets. *Annu RevPharmacolToxicol* **34**: 191–218

Chen X, Ding B, LeJeune D, Ruggiero C, Li S (2009) Rpb1 sumoylation in response to UV radiation or transcriptional impairment in yeast. *PLoS One* **4**(4): e5267

Chen XL, Silver HR, Xiong L, Belichenko I, Adegite C, Johnson ES (2007) Topoisomerase I-dependent viability loss in saccharomyces cerevisiae mutants defective in both SUMO conjugation and DNA repair. *Genetics* **177**(1): 17–30

Chin LS, Vavalle JP, Li L (2002) Staring, a novel E3 ubiquitin-protein ligase that targets syntaxin 1 for degradation. *J Biol Chem* **277**(38): 35071–35079

Christensen MO, Krokowski RM, Barthelmes HU, Hock R, Boege F, Mielke C (2004) Distinct effects of topoisomerase I and RNA polymerase I inhibitors suggest a dual mechanism of nucleolar/nucleoplasmic partitioning of topoisomerase I. *J Biol Chem* **279**(21): 21873–21882

Chung CH, Baek SH (1999) Deubiquitinating enzymes: their diversity and emerging roles. *Biochem Biophys Res Commun* **266**(3): 633–640

D'Arpa P, Beardmore C, Liu LF (1990) Involvement of nucleic acid synthesis in cell killing mechanisms of topoisomerase poisons. *Cancer Res* **50**(21): 6919–6924

D'Cunha J, Knight E, Jr., Haas AL, Truitt RL, Borden EC (1996) Immunoregulatory properties of ISG15, an interferon-induced cytokine. *Proc Natl Acad Sci USA* **93**(1): 211–215

Danks MK, Garrett KE, Marion RC, Whipple DO (1996) Subcellular redistribution of DNA topoisomerase I in anaplastic astrocytoma cells treated with topotecan. *Cancer Res* **56**(7): 1664–1673

Davis PL, Shaiu WL, Scott GL, Iglehart JD, Hsieh TS, Marks JR (1998) Complex response of breast epithelial cell lines to topoisomerase inhibitors. *Anticancer Res* **18**(4C): 2919–2932

Dawlaty MM, Malureanu L, Jeganathan KB, Kao E, Sustmann C, Tahk S, Shuai K, Grosschedl R, van Deursen JM (2008) Resolution of sister centromeres requires RanBP2-mediated SUMOylation of topoisomerase IIalpha. *Cell* **133**(1): 103–115

Debethune L, Kohlhagen G, Grandas A, Pommier Y (2002) Processing of nucleopeptides mimicking the topoisomerase I-DNA covalent complex by tyrosyl-DNA phosphodiesterase. *Nucleic Acids Res* **30**(5): 1198–1204

Desai SD, Haas AL, Wood LM, Tsai YC, Pestka S, Rubin EH, Saleem A, Nur EKA, Liu LF (2006) Elevated expression of ISG15 in tumor cells interferes with the ubiquitin/26S proteasome pathway. *Cancer Res* **66**(2): 921–928

Desai SD, Li TK, Rodriguez-Bauman A, Rubin EH, Liu LF (2001) Ubiquitin/26S proteasome-mediated degradation of topoisomerase I as a resistance mechanism to camptothecin in tumor cells. *Cancer Res* **61**(15): 5926–5932

Desai SD, Liu LF, Vazquez-Abad D, D'Arpa P (1997) Ubiquitin-dependent destruction of topoisomerase I is stimulated by the antitumor drug camptothecin. *J Biol Chem* **272**(39): 24159–24164

Desai SD, Mao Y, Sun M, Li TK, Wu J, Liu LF (2000) Ubiquitin, SUMO-1, and UCRP in camptothecin sensitivity and resistance. *Ann NY Acad Sci* **922**: 306–308

Desai SD, Wood LM, Tsai YC, Hsieh TS, Marks JR, Scott GL, Giovanella BC, Liu LF (2008) ISG15 as a novel tumor biomarker for drug sensitivity. *Mol Cancer Ther* **7**(6): 1430–1439

Desai SD, Zhang H, Rodriguez-Bauman A, Yang JM, Wu X, Gounder MK, Rubin EH, Liu LF (2003) Transcription-dependent degradation of topoisomerase I-DNA covalent complexes. *Mol Cell Biol* **23**(7): 2341–2350

Desterro JM, Rodriguez MS, Hay RT (1998) SUMO-1 modification of IkappaBalpha inhibits NF-kappaB activation. *Mol Cell* **2**(2): 233–239

Dev KK, van der Putten H, Sommer B, Rovelli G (2003) Part I: parkin-associated proteins and Parkinson's disease. *Neuropharmacology* **45**(1): 1–13

Deweese JE, Osheroff N (2009) The DNA cleavage reaction of topoisomerase II: wolf in sheep's clothing. *Nucleic Acids Res* **37**(3): 738–748

Dexheimer TS, Antony S, Marchand C, Pommier Y (2008) Tyrosyl-DNA phosphodiesterase as a target for anticancer therapy. *Anticancer Agents Med Chem* **8**(4): 381–389

Ferrier V (2002) Getting hit by SUMO. *NatCell Biol* **4**(3): E57

Fiorani P, Reid RJ, Schepis A, Jacquiau HR, Guo H, Thimmaiah P, Benedetti P, Bjornsti MA (2004) The deubiquitinating enzyme Doa4p protects cells from DNA topoisomerase I poisons. *J Biol Chem* **279**(20): 21271–21281

Fu Q, Kim SW, Chen HX, Grill S, Cheng YC (1999) Degradation of topoisomerase I induced by topoisomerase I inhibitors is dependent on inhibitor structure but independent of cell death. *Mol Pharmacol* **55**(4): 677–683

Geoffroy MC, Hay RT (2009) An additional role for SUMO in ubiquitin-mediated proteolysis. *Nat Rev Mol Cell Biol* **10**(8): 564–568

Giannakopoulos NV, Luo JK, Papov V, Zou W, Lenschow DJ, Jacobs BS, Borden EC, Li J, Virgin HW, Zhang DE (2005) Proteomic identification of proteins conjugated to ISG15 in mouse and human cells. *Biochem Biophys Res Commun*

Ha BH, Kim EE (2008) Structures of proteases for ubiqutin and ubiquitin-like modifiers. *BMB Rep* **41**(6): 435–443

Haas AL (1997) Introduction: evolving roles for ubiquitin in cellular regulation. *FASEB J* **11**(13): 1053–1054

Haas AL, Ahrens P, Bright PM, Ankel H (1987) Interferon induces a 15-kilodalton protein exhibiting marked homology to ubiquitin. *J Biol Chem* **262**(23): 11315–11323

Haas AL, Siepmann TJ (1997) Pathways of ubiquitin conjugation. *FASEB J* **11**(14): 1257–1268

Hamerman JA, Hayashi F, Schroeder LA, Gygi SP, Haas AL, Hampson L, Coughlin P, Aebersold R, Aderem A (2002) Serpin 2a is induced in activated macrophages and conjugates to a ubiquitin homolog. *J Immunol* **168**(5): 2415–2423

Hammer E, Heilbronn R, Weger S (2007) The E3 ligase Topors induces the accumulation of polysumoylated forms of DNA topoisomerase I in vitro and in vivo. *FEBS Lett* **581**(28): 5418–5424

Harty RN, Pitha PM, Okumura A (2009) Antiviral Activity of Innate Immune Protein ISG15. *J Innate Immun* **1**(5): 397–404

Hay RT (2001) Protein modification by SUMO. *Trends Biochem Sci* **26**(5): 332–333

Hay RT (2006) Role of ubiquitin-like proteins in transcriptional regulation. *Ernst Schering Res Found Workshop*(57): 173–192

Herrmann J, Lerman LO, Lerman A (2007) Ubiquitin and ubiquitin-like proteins in protein regulation. *Circ Res* **100**(9): 1276–1291

Hershko A, Ciechanover A (1992) The ubiquitin system for protein degradation. *Annu Rev Biochem* **61**: 761–807

Hochstrasser M (1996) Protein degradation or regulation: Ub the judge. *Cell* **84**(6): 813–815

Hochstrasser M (2000a) Biochemistry. All in the ubiquitin family. *Science* **289**(5479): 563–564

Hochstrasser M (2000b) Evolution and function of ubiquitin-like protein-conjugation systems. *Nat Cell Biol* **2**(8): E153-E157

Hochstrasser M (2001) SP-RING for SUMO: new functions bloom for a ubiquitin-like protein. *Cell* **107**(1): 5–8

Holm C, Covey JM, Kerrigan D, Pommier Y (1989) Differential requirement of DNA replication for the cytotoxicity of DNA topoisomerase I and II inhibitors in Chinese hamster DC3F cells. *Cancer Res* **49**: 6365–6368

Horie K, Tomida A, Sugimoto Y, Yasugi T, Yoshikawa H, Taketani Y, Tsuruo T (2002) SUMO-1 conjugation to intact DNA topoisomerase I amplifies cleavable complex formation induced by camptothecin. *Oncogene* **21**(52): 7913–7922

Hoyt MA, Zhang M, Coffino P (2003) Ubiquitin-independent mechanisms of mouse ornithine decarboxylase degradation are conserved between mammalian and fungal cells. *J Biol Chem* **278**(14): 12135–12143

Hsiang YH, Hertzberg R, Hecht S, Liu LF (1985) Camptothecin induces protein-linked DNA breaks via mammalian DNA topoisomerase I. *J Biol Chem* **260**(27): 14873–14878

Hsiang YH, Lihou MG, Liu LF (1989) Arrest of replication forks by drug-stabilized topoisomerase I-DNA cleavable complexes as a mechanism of cell killing by camptothecin. *Cancer Res* **49**(18): 5077–5082

Hsiang YH, Liu LF (1988) Identification of mammalian DNA topoisomerase I as an intracellular target of the anticancer drug camptothecin. *Cancer Res* **48**(7): 1722–1726

Hsiang YH, Liu LF (1989) Evidence for the reversibility of cellular DNA lesion induced by mammalian topoisomerase II poisons. *J Biol Chem* **264**(17): 9713–9715

Huang KC, Gao H, Yamasaki EF, Grabowski DR, Liu S, Shen LL, Chan KK, Ganapathi R, Snapka RM (2001) Topoisomerase II poisoning by ICRF-193. *J Biol Chem* **276**(48): 44488–44494

Huang RY, Kowalski D, Minderman H, Gandhi N, Johnson ES (2007) Small ubiquitin-related modifier pathway is a major determinant of doxorubicin cytotoxicity in Saccharomyces cerevisiae. *Cancer Res* **67**(2): 765–772

Interthal H, Chen HJ, Champoux JJ (2005) Human Tdp1 cleaves a broad spectrum of substrates including phosphoamide linkages. *J Biol Chem* **280**(Oct 28): 36518–36528

Isik S, Sano K, Tsutsui K, Seki M, Enomoto T, Saitoh H (2003) The SUMO pathway is required for selective degradation of DNA topoisomerase IIbeta induced by a catalytic inhibitor ICRF-193(1). *FEBS Lett* **546**(2–3): 374–378

Jacquiau HR, van Waardenburg RC, Reid RJ, Woo MH, Guo H, Johnson ES, Bjornsti MA (2005) Defects in SUMO (small ubiquitin-related modifier) conjugation and deconjugation alter cell sensitivity to DNA topoisomerase I-induced DNA damage. *J Biol Chem* **280**(25): 23566–23575

Jentsch S, Pyrowolakis G (2000) Ubiquitin and its kin: how close are the family ties? *Trends Cell Biol* **10**(8): 335–342

Johnson GA, Austin KJ, Van Kirk EA, Hansen TR (1998) Pregnancy and interferon-tau induce conjugation of bovine ubiquitin cross-reactive protein to cytosolic uterine proteins. *Biol Reprod* **58**(4): 898–904

Kanagasabai R, Liu S, Salama S, Yamasaki EF, Zhang L, Greenchurch KB, Snapka RM (2009) Ubiquitin-family modifications of topoisomerase I in camptothecin-treated human breast cancer cells. *Biochemistry* **48**(14): 3176–3185

Kim KI, Giannakopoulos NV, Virgin HW, Zhang DE (2004) Interferon-inducible ubiquitin E2, Ubc8, is a conjugating enzyme for protein ISGylation. *Mol Cell Biol* **24**(21): 9592–9600

Kobayashi I, Ohwada S, Maemura M (1996) Interferon-alpha potentiates the antiproliferative activity of CPT-11 against human colon cancer xenografts in nude mice. *Anticancer Res* **16**(5A): 2677–2680

Kumar S, Kao WH, Howley PM (1997) Physical interaction between specific E2 and Hect E3 enzymes determines functional cooperativity. *J Biol Chem* **272**(21): 13548–13554

Kunzi MS, Pitha PM (2003) Interferon targeted genes in host defense. *Autoimmunity* **36**(8): 457–461

Kwan KY, Wang JC (2001) Mice lacking DNA topoisomerase IIIbeta develop to maturity but show a reduced mean lifespan. *Proc Natl Acad Sci USA* **98**(10): 5717–5721

Ledesma FC, El Khamisy SF, Zuma MC, Osborn K, Caldecott KW (2009) A human 5′-tyrosyl DNA phosphodiesterase that repairs topoisomerase-mediated DNA damage. *Nature* **461**(7264): 674–678

Leppard JB, Champoux JJ (2005) Human DNA topoisomerase I: relaxation, roles, and damage control. *Chromosoma* **114**(2): 75–85

Li TK, Chen AY, Yu C, Mao Y, Wang H, Liu LF (1999) Activation of topoisomerase II-mediated excision of chromosomal DNA loops during oxidative stress. *Genes Dev* **13**(12): 1553–1560

Li TK, Liu LF (2001) Tumor cell death induced by topoisomerase-targeting drugs. *Annu Rev Pharmacol Toxicol* **41**: 53–77

Li W, Wang JC (1998) Mammalian DNA topoisomerase IIIalpha is essential in early embryogenesis. *Proc Natl Acad Sci USA* **95**(3): 1010–1013

Lin CP, Ban Y, Lyu YL, Desai SD, Liu LF (2008) A ubiquitin-proteasome pathway for the repair of topoisomerase I-DNA covalent complexes. *J Biol Chem* **283**(30): 21074–21083

Lin CP, Ban Y, Lyu YL, Liu LF (2009) Proteasome-dependent processing of topoisomerase I-DNA adducts into DNA double strand breaks at arrested replication forks. *J Biol Chem* **284**(41): 28084–28092

Liu LF (1983) DNA topoisomerases--enzymes that catalyse the breaking and rejoining of DNA. *CRC Crit Rev Biochem* **15**(1): 1–24

Liu LF (1989) DNA topoisomerase poisons as antitumor drugs. *Annu Rev Biochem* **58**: 351–375

Liu LF, Duann P, Lin CT, D'Arpa P, Wu J (1996) Mechanism of action of camptothecin. *Ann NY Acad Sci* **803**: 44–49

Liu M, Hummer BT, Li X, Hassel BA (2004) Camptothecin induces the ubiquitin-like protein, ISG15, and enhances ISG15 conjugation in response to interferon. *J Interferon Cytokine Res* **24**(11): 647–654

Loeb KR, Haas AL (1992) The interferon-inducible 15-kDa ubiquitin homolog conjugates to intracellular proteins. *J Biol Chem* **267**(11): 7806–7813

Malakhov MP, Malakhova OA, Kim KI, Ritchie KJ, Zhang DE (2002) UBP43 (USP18) specifically removes ISG15 from conjugated proteins. *J Biol Chem* **277**(12): 9976–9981

Malakhova OA, Yan M, Malakhov MP, Yuan Y, Ritchie KJ, Kim KI, Peterson LF, Shuai K, Zhang DE (2003) Protein ISGylation modulates the JAK-STAT signaling pathway. *Genes Dev* **17**(4): 455–460

Mao Y, Desai SD, Liu LF (2000a) SUMO-1 conjugation to human DNA topoisomerase II isozymes. *J Biol Chem* **275**(34): 26066–26073

Mao Y, Desai SD, Ting CY, Hwang J, Liu LF (2001) 26S proteasome-mediated degradation of topoisomerase II cleavable complexes. *J Biol Chem* **276**(44): 40652–40658

Mao Y, Sun M, Desai SD, Liu LF (2000b) SUMO-1 conjugation to topoisomerase I: A possible repair response to topoisomerase-mediated DNA damage. *Proc Natl Acad Sci USA* **97**(8): 4046–4051

Mo YY, Yu Y, Shen Z, Beck WT (2002) Nucleolar delocalization of human topoisomerase I in response to topotecan correlates with sumoylation of the protein. *J Biol Chem* **277**(4): 2958–2964

Morris EJ, Geller HM (1996) Induction of neuronal apoptosis by camptothecin, an inhibitor of DNA topoisomerase-I: evidence for cell cycle-independent toxicity. *J Cell Biol* **134**(3): 757–770

Nakamura K, Kogame T, Oshiumi H, Shinohara A, Sumitomo Y, Agama K, Pommier Y, Tsutsui KM, Tsutsui K, Hartsuiker E, Ogi T, Takeda S, Taniguchi Y (2010) Collaborative action of

Brca1 and CtIP in elimination of covalent modifications from double-strand breaks to facilitate subsequent break repair. *PLoS Genet* **6**(1): e1000828
Narasimhan J, Potter JL, Haas AL (1996) Conjugation of the 15-kDa interferon-induced ubiquitin homolog is distinct from that of ubiquitin. *J Biol Chem* **271**(1): 324–330
Narasimhan J, Wang M, Fu Z, Klein JM, Haas AL, Kim JJ (2005) Crystal structure of the interferon-induced ubiquitin-like protein ISG15. *J Biol Chem* **280**(29): 27356–27365
Nitiss J, Wang JC (1988) DNA topoisomerase-targeting antitumor drugs can be studied in yeast. *Proc Natl Acad Sci USA* **85**(20): 7501–7505
Nitiss JL (2002) DNA topoisomerases in cancer chemotherapy: using enzymes to generate selective DNA damage. *Curr Opin Investig Drugs* **3**(10): 1512–1516
Nitiss JL (2009a) DNA topoisomerase II and its growing repertoire of biological functions. *Nat Rev Cancer* **9**(5): 327–337
Nitiss JL (2009b) Targeting DNA topoisomerase II in cancer chemotherapy. *Nat Rev Cancer* **9**(5): 338–350
Nitiss JL, Liu YX, Harbury P, Jannatipour M, Wasserman R, Wang JC (1992) Amsacrine and etoposide hypersensitivity of yeast cells overexpressing DNA topoisomerase II. *Cancer Res* **52**(16): 4467–4472
Nitiss JL, Nitiss KC (2001) Yeast systems for demonstrating the targets of anti-topoisomerase II agents. *Methods Mol Biol* **95**: 315–327
Nitiss JL, Wang JC (1996) Mechanisms of cell killing by drugs that trap covalent complexes between DNA topoisomerases and DNA. *Mol Pharmacol* **50**(5): 1095–1102
Nitiss KC, Malik M, He X, White SW, Nitiss JL (2006) Tyrosyl-DNA phosphodiesterase (Tdp1) participates in the repair of Top2-mediated DNA damage. *Proc Natl Acad Sci USA* **103**(24): 8953–8958
Ohwada S, Kobayashi I, Maemura M, Satoh Y, Ogawa T, Iino Y, Morishita Y (1996) Interferon potentiates antiproliferative activity of CPT-11 against human colon cancer xenografts. *Cancer Lett* **110**(1–2): 149–154
Okumura A, Pitha PM, Harty RN (2008) ISG15 inhibits Ebola VP40 VLP budding in an L-domain-dependent manner by blocking Nedd4 ligase activity. *Proc Natl Acad Sci USA* **105**(10): 3974–3979
Palmer A, Mason GG, Paramio JM, Knecht E, Rivett AJ (1994) Changes in proteasome localization during the cell cycle. *Eur J Cell Biol* **64**(1): 163–175
Papa FR, Hochstrasser M (1993) The yeast DOA4 gene encodes a deubiquitinating enzyme related to a product of the human tre-2 oncogene. *Nature* **366**(6453): 313–319
Pickart CM (2000) Ubiquitin in chains. *Trends Biochem Sci* **25**(11): 544–548
Pickart CM (2001a) Mechanisms underlying ubiquitination. *Annu Rev Biochem* **70**: 503–533
Pickart CM (2001b) Ubiquitin enters the new millennium. *Mol Cell* **8**(3): 499–504
Pickart CM, Fushman D (2004) Polyubiquitin chains: polymeric protein signals. *Curr Opin Chem Biol* **8**(6): 610–616
Pitha-Rowe I, Hassel BA, Dmitrovsky E (2004) Involvement of UBE1L in ISG15 conjugation during retinoid-induced differentiation of acute promyelocytic leukemia. *J Biol Chem* **279**(18): 18178–18187
Pommier Y (1996) Eukaryotic DNA topoisomerase I: genome gatekeeper and its intruders, camptothecins. *Semin Oncol* **23**(1 Suppl 3): 3–10
Pommier Y (1998) Diversity of DNA topoisomerases I and inhibitors. *Biochimie* **80**(3): 255–270
Pommier Y (2006) Topoisomerase I inhibitors: camptothecins and beyond. *Nat Rev Cancer* **6**(10): 789–802
Pommier Y (2009) DNA topoisomerase I inhibitors: chemistry, biology, and interfacial inhibition. *Chem Rev* **109**(7): 2894–2902
Pommier Y, Barcelo JM, Rao VA, Sordet O, Jobson AG, Thibaut L, Miao ZH, Seiler JA, Zhang H, Marchand C, Agama K, Nitiss JL, Redon C (2006) Repair of topoisomerase I-mediated DNA damage. *Prog Nucleic Acid Res Mol Biol* **81**: 179–229
Pommier Y, Leo E, Zhang H, Marchand C (2010) DNA topoisomerases and their poisoning by anticancer and antibacterial drugs. *Chem Biol* **17**(5): 421–433

Pommier Y, Tanizawa A, Kohn KW (1994) Mechanisms of topoisomerase I inhibition by anticancer drugs. *Adv Pharmacol* **29B:** 73–92

Pourquier P, Jensen AD, Gong SS, Pommier Y, Rogler CE (1999) Human DNA topoisomerase I-mediated cleavage and recombination of duck hepatitis B virus DNA in vitro. *Nucleic Acids Res* **27**(8)**:** 1919–1925

Rajendra R, Malegaonkar D, Pungaliya P, Marshall H, Rasheed Z, Brownell J, Liu LF, Lutzker S, Saleem A, Rubin EH (2004) Topors functions as an E3 ubiquitin ligase with specific E2 enzymes and ubiquitinates p53. *J Biol Chem* **279**(35)**:** 36440–36444

Rallabhandi P, Hashimoto K, Mo YY, Beck WT, Moitra PK, D'Arpa P (2002) Sumoylation of topoisomerase I is involved in its partitioning between nucleoli and nucleoplasm and its clearing from nucleoli in response to camptothecin. *JBiolChem*

Rasheed ZA, Rubin EH (2003) Mechanisms of resistance to topoisomerase I-targeting drugs. *Oncogene* **22**(47)**:** 7296–7304

Ritchie KJ, Zhang DE (2004) ISG15: the immunological kin of ubiquitin. *Semin Cell Dev Biol* **15**(2)**:** 237–246

Rivett AJ (1998) Intracellular distribution of proteasomes. *Curr Opin Immunol* **10**(1)**:** 110–114

Roca J, Ishida R, Berger JM, Andoh T, Wang JC (1994) Antitumor bisdioxopiperazines inhibit yeast DNA topoisomerase II by trapping the enzyme in the form of a closed protein clamp. *Proc Natl Acad Sci USA* **91**(5)**:** 1781–1785

Rubin E, Wood V, Bharti A, Trites D, Lynch C, Hurwitz S, Bartel S, Levy S, Rosowsky A, Toppmeyer D, . (1995) A phase I and pharmacokinetic study of a new camptothecin derivative, 9- aminocamptothecin. *Clin Cancer Res* **1**(3)**:** 269–276

Saitoh H, Hinchey J (2000) Functional heterogeneity of small ubiquitin-related protein modifiers SUMO-1 versus SUMO-2/3. *J Biol Chem* **275**(9)**:** 6252–6258

Saleem A, Edwards TK, Rasheed Z, Rubin EH (2000) Mechanisms of resistance to camptothecins. *Ann NY Acad Sci* **922:** 46–55

Schwartz AL, Ciechanover A (2009) Targeting proteins for destruction by the ubiquitin system: implications for human pathobiology. *Annu Rev Pharmacol Toxicol* **49:** 73–96

Seeger M, Ferrell K, Dubiel W (1997) The 26S proteasome: a dynamic structure. *Mol Biol Rep* **24**(1–2)**:** 83–88

Shao R-G, Cao C-X, Shimizu T, O'Connor P, Kohn KW, Pommier Y (1997) Abrogation of an S-phase checkpoint and potentiation of camptothecin cytotoxicity by 7-hydroxystaurosporine (UCN-01) in human cancer cell lines, possibly influenced by p53. *Cancer Res* **57:** 4029–4035

Shao R-G, Cao C-X, Zhang H, Kohn KW, Wold MS, Pommier Y (1999) Replication-mediated DNA damage by camptothecin induces phosphorylation of RPA by DNA-dependent protein kinase and dissociates RPA:DNA-PK complexes. *EMBO J* **18:** 1397–1406

Shea ME, Hiasa H (1999) Interactions between DNA helicases and frozen topoisomerase IV- quinolone-DNA ternary complexes. *J Biol Chem* **274**(32)**:** 22747–22754

Siddoo-Atwal C, Haas AL, Rosin MP (1996) Elevation of interferon beta-inducible proteins in ataxia telangiectasia cells. *Cancer Res* **56**(3)**:** 443–447

Sordet O, Larochelle S, Nicolas E, Stevens EV, Zhang C, Shokat KM, Fisher RP, Pommier Y (2008) Hyperphosphorylation of RNA polymerase II in response to topoisomerase I cleavage complexes and its association with transcription- and BRCA1-dependent degradation of topoisomerase I. *J Mol Biol* **381**(3)**:** 540–549

Sordet O, Nakamura AJ, Redon CE, Pommier Y (2010) DNA double-strand breaks and ATM activation by transcription-blocking DNA lesions. *Cell Cycle* **9**(2)**:** 274–278

Sordet O, Redon CE, Guirouilh-Barbat J, Smith S, Solier S, Douarre C, Conti C, Nakamura AJ, Das BB, Nicolas E, Kohn KW, Bonner WM, Pommier Y (2009) Ataxia telangiectasia mutated activation by transcription- and topoisomerase I-induced DNA double-strand breaks. *EMBO Rep* **10**(8)**:** 887–893

Staker BL, Feese MD, Cushman M, Pommier Y, Zembower D, Stewart L, Burgin AB (2005) Structures of three classes of anticancer agents bound to the human topoisomerase I-DNA covalent complex. *J Med Chem* **48**(7)**:** 2336–2345

Strumberg D, Pilon AA, Smith M, Hickey R, Malkas L, Pommier Y (2000) Conversion of topoisomerase I cleavage complexes on the leading strand of ribosomal DNA into 5′-phosphorylated DNA double-strand breaks by replication runoff. *Mol Cell Biol* **20**(11)**:** 3977–3987

Subramanian D, Rosenstein BS, Muller MT (1998) Ultraviolet-induced DNA damage stimulates topoisomerase I-DNA complex formation in vivo: possible relationship with DNA repair. *Cancer Res* **58**(5)**:** 976–984

Svejstrup JQ, Christiansen K, Gromova, II, Andersen AH, Westergaard O (1991) New technique for uncoupling the cleavage and religation reactions of eukaryotic topoisomerase I. The mode of action of camptothecin at a specific recognition site. *J Mol Biol* **222**(3)**:** 669–678

Takeuchi T, Iwahara S, Saeki Y, Sasajima H, Yokosawa H (2005) Link between the Ubiquitin Conjugation System and the ISG15 Conjugation System: ISG15 Conjugation to the UbcH6 Ubiquitin E2 Enzyme. *J Biochem (Tokyo)* **138**(6)**:** 711–719

Takeuchi T, Yokosawa H (2005) ISG15 modification of Ubc13 suppresses its ubiquitin-conjugating activity. *Biochem Biophys Res Commun* **336**(1)**:** 9–13

Tanizawa A, Fujimori A, Fujimori Y, Pommier Y (1994) Comparison of topoisomerase I inhibition, DNA damage, and cytotoxicity of camptothecin derivatives presently in clinical trials. *J Natl Cancer Inst* **86:** 836–842

Tatham MH, Geoffroy MC, Shen L, Plechanovova A, Hattersley N, Jaffray EG, Palvimo JJ, Hay RT (2008) RNF4 is a poly-SUMO-specific E3 ubiquitin ligase required for arsenic-induced PML degradation. *Nat Cell Biol* **10**(5)**:** 538–546

Thrower JS, Hoffman L, Rechsteiner M, Pickart CM (2000) Recognition of the polyubiquitin proteolytic signal. *EMBO J* **19**(1)**:** 94–102

Tsao YP, D'Arpa P, Liu LF (1992) The involvement of active DNA synthesis in camptothecin-induced G2 arrest: altered regulation of p34cdc2/cyclin B. *Cancer Res* **52**(7)**:** 1823–1829

Tsao YP, Russo A, Nyamuswa G, Silber R, Liu LF (1993) Interaction between replication forks and topoisomerase I-DNA cleavable complexes: studies in a cell-free SV40 DNA replication system. *Cancer Res* **53**(24)**:** 5908–5914

Ulrich HD (2009) The SUMO system: an overview. *Methods Mol Biol* **497:** 3–16

Varshavsky A (1997) The ubiquitin system. *Trends Biochem Sci* **22**(10)**:** 383–387

Wall ME, Wani MC (1996) Camptothecin. Discovery to clinic. *Ann NY Acad Sci* **803:** 1–12

Wang JC (2002) Cellular roles of DNA topoisomerases: a molecular perspective. *Nat Rev Mol Cell Biol* **3**(6)**:** 430–440

Weger S, Hammer E, Heilbronn R (2005) Topors acts as a SUMO-1 E3 ligase for p53 in vitro and in vivo. *FEBS Lett* **579**(22)**:** 5007–5012

Weisshaar SR, Keusekotten K, Krause A, Horst C, Springer HM, Gottsche K, Dohmen RJ, Praefcke GJ (2008) Arsenic trioxide stimulates SUMO-2/3 modification leading to RNF4-dependent proteolytic targeting of PML. *FEBS Lett* **582**(21–22)**:** 3174–3178

Wilkinson KD (2009) DUBs at a glance. *J Cell Sci* **122**(Pt 14)**:** 2325–2329

Wilson TM, Chen AD, Hsieh T (2000) Cloning and characterization of Drosophila topoisomerase IIIbeta. Relaxation of hypernegatively supercoiled DNA. *J Biol Chem* **275**(3)**:** 1533–1540

Wood LM, Sankar S, Reed RE, Haas AL, Liu LF, McKinnon P, Desai SD (2011) A novel role for ATM in regulating proteasome-mediated protein degradation through suppression of the ISG15 conjugation pathway. *PLoS ONE* **6**:e16422

Wu J, Liu LF (1997) Processing of topoisomerase I cleavable complexes into DNA damage by transcription. *Nucleic Acids Res* **25**(21)**:** 4181–4186

Wu K, Chen A, Pan ZQ (2000) Conjugation of Nedd8 to CUL1 enhances the ability of the ROC1-CUL1 complex to promote ubiquitin polymerization. *J Biol Chem* **275**(41)**:** 32317–32324

Xiao H, Li TK, Yang JM, Liu LF (2003a) Acidic pH induces topoisomerase II-mediated DNA damage. *Proc Natl Acad Sci USA* **100**(9)**:** 5205–5210

Xiao H, Mao Y, Desai SD, Zhou N, Ting CY, Hwang J, Liu LF (2003b) The topoisomerase IIbeta circular clamp arrests transcription and signals a 26S proteasome pathway. *Proc Natl Acad Sci USA* **100**(6)**:** 3239–3244

Yang M, Hsu CT, Ting CY, Liu LF, Hwang J (2006) Assembly of a polymeric chain of SUMO1 on human topoisomerase I in vitro. *J Biol Chem* **281**(12)**:** 8264–8274

Yang S-W, Burgin AB, Huizenga BN, Robertson CA, Yao KC, Nash HA (1996) A eukaryotic enzyme that can disjoin dead-end covalent complexes between DNA and type I topoisomerases. *Proc Natl Acad Sci USA* **93:** 11534–11539

Yang X, Li W, Prescott ED, Burden SJ, Wang JC (2000) DNA topoisomerase IIbeta and neural development. *Science* **287**(5450)**:** 131–134

Yeh ET, Gong L, Kamitani T (2000) Ubiquitin-like proteins: new wines in new bottles. *Gene* **248**(1–2)**:** 1–14

Young P, Deveraux Q, Beal RE, Pickart CM, Rechsteiner M (1998) Characterization of two polyubiquitin binding sites in the 26S protease subunit 5a. *J Biol Chem* **273**(10)**:** 5461–5467

Yuan W, Krug RM (2001) Influenza B virus NS1 protein inhibits conjugation of the interferon (IFN)-induced ubiquitin-like ISG15 protein. *EMBO J* **20**(3)**:** 362–371

Zeng Z, Cortes-Ledesma F, El-Khamisy SF, Caldecott KW (2011) TDP2/TTRAP is the major 5′-tyrosyl DNA phosphodiesterase activity in vertebrate cells and is critical for cellular resistance to topoisomerase II-induced DNA damage. *J Biol Chem* **286:** 403–409

Zhang CX, Chen AD, Gettel NJ, Hsieh TS (2000) Essential functions of DNA topoisomerase I in Drosophila melanogaster. *Dev Biol* **222**(1)**:** 27–40

Zhang H, Barcelo JM, Lee B, Kohlhagen G, Zimonjic DB, Popescu NC, Pommier Y (2001) Human mitochondrial topoisomerase I. *Proc Natl Acad Sci USA* **98**(19)**:** 10608–10613

Zhang H, Wang JC, Liu LF (1988) Involvement of DNA topoisomerase I in transcription of human ribosomal RNA genes. *Proc Natl Acad Sci USA* **85**(4)**:** 1060–1064

Zhang HF, Tomida A, Koshimizu R, Ogiso Y, Lei S, Tsuruo T (2004) Cullin 3 promotes proteasomal degradation of the topoisomerase I-DNA covalent complex. *Cancer Res* **64**(3)**:** 1114–1121

Zhao C, Beaudenon SL, Kelley ML, Waddell MB, Yuan W, Schulman BA, Huibregtse JM, Krug RM (2004) The UbcH8 ubiquitin E2 enzyme is also the E2 enzyme for ISG15, an IFN-alpha/beta-induced ubiquitin-like protein. *Proc Natl Acad Sci USA* **101**(20)**:** 7578–7582

Zou W, Papov V, Malakhova O, Kim KI, Dao C, Li J, Zhang DE (2005) ISG15 modification of ubiquitin E2 Ubc13 disrupts its ability to form thioester bond with ubiquitin. *Biochem Biophys Res Commun* **336**(1)**:** 61–68

Zou W, Zhang DE (2006) The interferon-inducible ubiquitin-protein isopeptide ligase (E3) EFP also functions as an ISG15 E3 ligase. *J Biol Chem* **281**(7)**:** 3989–3994

Chapter 18
Repair of Topoisomerase II-Mediated DNA Damage: Fixing DNA Damage Arising from a Protein Covalently Trapped on DNA

John L. Nitiss, Eroica Soans, Jeffrey Berk, Aman Seth, Margarita Mishina, and Karin C. Nitiss

18.1 Introduction

Topoisomerase II (Top2) is an important anticancer drug target. Agents such as etoposide and doxorubicin are broadly used in a wide variety of malignancies (Baldwin and Osheroff 2005; Choi et al. 2008; Dombernowsky et al. 1996; Lieu et al. 2009; Verborg et al. 2008; Walker and Nitiss 2002). Most drugs that target Top2 generate DNA damage as a direct consequence of the catalytic activity of the enzyme. All topoisomerases cleave DNA by forming a covalent complex between the enzyme and DNA, and agents that perturb the catalytic cycle have the potential to trap the enzyme and introduce DNA damage. The DNA damage caused by interfering with a topoisomerase is unique because it includes both DNA strand breaks and protein covalently bound to DNA. Agents that lead to the trapping of topoisomerases on DNA have been termed topoisomerase poisons to highlight the importance of cellular damage induced by these agents. Because topoisomerase poisons lead to cell killing largely through enzyme-mediated damage, pathways that repair this damage are critical determinants of clinical response to these agents. A major goal of this chapter is to highlight our current understanding of how DNA repair pathways affect sensitivity to Top2 poisons. It is hoped that some of these concepts will lead to new approaches for the clinical application of Top2 targeting agents.

In addition to the clinical importance of Top2 targeting agents, these drugs have served as model compounds to study cellular responses to DNA damage. Unlike ionizing radiation or alkylating agents, many Top2 targeting drugs are highly specific,

J.L. Nitiss (✉)
Department of Biopharmaceutical Sciences, University of Illinois College of Pharmacy, 833 S. Wood Street, IL 60612-7231, Chicago
e-mail: jlnitiss@uic.edu

Y. Pommier (ed.), *DNA Topoisomerases and Cancer*, Cancer Drug Discovery and Development, DOI 10.1007/978-1-4614-0323-4_18,

and lead to a limited spectrum of DNA damage. This chapter will also highlight how Top2 targeting agents provide unique reagents for studying the repair and tolerance of DNA damage.

18.2 How Topoisomerase II Damages DNA

The topoisomerase II reaction cycle is addressed in detail in other chapters in this volume (see also (Schoeffler and Berger 2008; Wang 1998) for a detailed discussion of Top2 enzymology). The key points needed for the present discussion are that homodimeric Top2 cleaves both DNA strands (each monomer cleaving one strand) leading to a covalent intermediate with 5′ phosphotyrosyl linkages of both subunits to DNA. The generation of the phosphotyrosyl linkage preserves the energy of the phosphodiester bond, therefore resealing of the enzyme-induced break does not require a high-energy cofactor. Even though Top2 does not use ATP to reseal the enzyme-generated double-strand break, the complete catalytic cycle uses ATP hydrolysis to modulate the conformational changes required for the complete reaction cycle. The enzyme transiently opens a "gate" that allows for the passage of an intact DNA duplex. After this strand passage, the break is resealed by reversal of the phosphotyrosyl bonds reforming unbroken DNA.

Top2 poisons interfere with the breakage-reunion reactions of Top2. A major mechanism for interfering with the breakage-reunion reaction is inhibition of the enzyme-mediated religation (Robinson and Osheroff 1990). This mechanism operates for Top2 poisons such as mAMSA and etoposide. For other drugs such as ellipticines, there is no clear evidence for inhibition of religation, and it is thought that some drugs stimulate enzyme-mediated DNA cleavage (Froelich-Ammon et al. 1995; Robinson et al. 1991). It is important to remember that both mechanisms lead to a reversible enhancement of DNA cleavage (Tewey et al. 1984). If drug is removed, the enzyme carries out religation and the DNA returns to an undamaged state. If Top2 poisons are cytotoxic agents that introduce reversible DNA damage then there must be processes that convert the reversible DNA damage into irreversible damage. For Top2 targeting drugs, these processes include both replication and transcription, and may also involve other nuclear transactions such a chromosome condensation (Nitiss 2009).

While the Top2 reaction involves the generation of a transient double-strand break, the two subunits of Top2 can cleave DNA independently of each other (Andersen et al. 1989). For some Top2 targeting agents such as mAMSA, protein-linked single-strand breaks predominate over double breaks (Pommier et al. 1985). We recently showed that a Top2 molecule that could only generate single-strand breaks could nonetheless lead to cytotoxicity (Rogojina and Nitiss 2008). These results indicate that the spectrum of DNA damage induced by Top2 poisons includes covalent complexes with both single- and double-strand DNA cleavage. The generation of single-strand breaks by Top2 poisons is an important consideration for the repair of this damage, but it has not yet been carefully addressed.

18.3 The Biological Effects of Top2 Poisons

Top2 poisons fall into two categories: intercalating agents and agents that do not intercalate (and generally show weak to non-detectable DNA binding in the absence of Top2). Intercalating Top2 poisons have the potential to interfere with DNA metabolism by topoisomerase independent mechanisms. Both non-intercalating and intercalating Top2 poisons also have the potential to act on other cellular targets. This is especially the case for anthracyclines and anthracenediones, which can generate reactive oxygen species (ROS) (Injac and Strukej 2008). Therefore, assessment of drug action in vivo must allow for the possibility of drug effects (and DNA damage) that is not mediated by topoisomerases. Etoposide and other epipodophyllotoxins are non-intercalating, and in most studies these agents have been found to be very specific for Top2. This consideration does not mean that studies with intercalating agents are inherently suspect, since many intercalating Top2 poisons generate Top2-mediated damage at concentrations below those needed to produce significant Top2 independent effects. As described below, a strength of yeast model systems is the ability to rigorously demonstrate that the drug effects are specifically due to targeting Top2.

Top2 poisons generate DNA damage, but also inhibit Top2 catalytic activity. Several lines of evidence support the hypothesis that the DNA damage component of Top2 poisons is the major determinant for cell killing. In yeast, reduction of Top2 activity leads to resistance to etoposide and other Top2 targeting agents (Nitiss et al. 1992, 1993). In mammalian cells, drug resistant cell lines frequently have reduced Top2 activity (reviewed in (Nitiss and Beck 1996)). Taken together, these results indicate that Top2-mediated damage, rather than inhibition of enzyme activity, is most important for cell killing. Nonetheless, since it has been reported that cells have checkpoints that delay progression through mitosis when Top2 activity is limited (Downes et al. 1994), inhibition of enzyme activity may play a role in some of the drug-induced effects.

It is well established that cell killing by drugs targeting Top1 such as camptothecins kill cells predominantly during S phase (D'Arpa et al. 1990; Holm et al. 1989). These results have been explained by generation of double-strand breaks by collision of replication forks with trapped Top1 covalent complexes (Zhang et al. 1990). Consistent with this model, markers of double-strand breaks such as γH2AX phosphorylation do not occur in camptothecin-treated cells not undergoing DNA replication (Huang et al. 2003). By contrast, cell killing by Top2-targeting agents occurs at all points in the cell cycle. γH2AX phosphorylation can be detected in non-replicating cells (Huang et al. 2003). Nonetheless, replication plays an important role in cell killing by Top2-targeting agents. Early studies suggested that inhibiting replication reduced cell killing by Top2-targeting agents, and that progression through S phase enhanced cell killing by Top2-targeting agents (Holm et al. 1989; Markovits et al. 1987; Nitiss and Wang 1996).

The generation of DNA damage by Top2 poisons during S phase can arise by two related mechanisms. Models based on Top1 damage suggest that collision of a replication fork (or replication associated helicases (Howard et al. 1994)) lead to disruption of a Top2 covalent complex and the generation of a double-strand break. A second mechanism is that Top2 complexes block the progression of replication forks, and that collapse of a blocked fork generates double-strand breaks (Michel et al. 2004; Rothstein et al. 2000). An elaboration of both models is that the collision of a replication fork provokes processing of the Top2 covalent complex, and that the processing reactions are responsible for double-strand break formation. While it is not possible to directly distinguish between these possibilities at present, it is likely that a direct generation of double-strand breaks as well as replication fork collapse is partly responsible for generating Top2-mediated double-strand breaks. Double-strand breaks that arise entirely from collapsed replication forks would not lead to protein-linked double-strand breaks, and not confer a specific requirement for factors that remove protein covalently bound to DNA. As indicated in the sections below, there is now substantial evidence that removal of proteins covalently bound to DNA is an important element of repairing Top2-mediated damage. While there is no direct evidence of replication fork collapse due to Top2 targeting agent in eukaryotic cells, studies in *Escherichia coli* with fluoroquinolones suggest that trapped Top2 complexes can frequently block replication but not lead to disruption of the Top2 complex (Marians and Hiasa 1997).

Since Top2 poisons can kill non-replicating cells, other cellular processes, such as transcription, are also likely to be important in the generation of irreversible DNA damage. The detailed mechanism of how transcription could generate Top2-dependent DNA damage is unclear. The strongest evidence for a role for transcription in the generation of Top2 damage is the presence of proteolytic processing pathways of Top2 that are dependent on transcription (Fan et al. 2008; Zhang et al. 2006). An attractive hypothesis is based on the observation that RNA polymerase II stalling provokes substantial DNA repair responses (Hanawalt and Spivak 2008; Svejstrup 2003). One response is the targeted degradation of the large subunit of RNA polymerase II (Woudstra et al. 2002). The efficient recruitment of the proteasome may provoke proteolysis of proteins impeding the progression of the polymerase. Aspects of proteolytic processing of trapped Top2 are discussed in Sect. 18.5.

18.4 Nucleolytic Removal of Top2 from DNA

There are now two paradigms for removal of topoisomerases covalently bound to DNA. The first paradigm, endonucleolytic cleavage, is the mechanism used by the MRN(X) complex and Sae2/CtIP for removal of Spo11 as discussed below. The second mechanism, hydrolysis of the phosphotyrosyl linkage, was first described in the removal of 3′ phosphotyrosyl-linked peptides (i.e., peptides derived from trapped Top1) by Tdp1 (Yang et al. 1996). Both paradigms have been shown to be important for removal of Top2 covalent complexes although their relative importance in different contexts remains to be determined. Figure 18.1 summarizes the structures of the nucleolytic proteins.

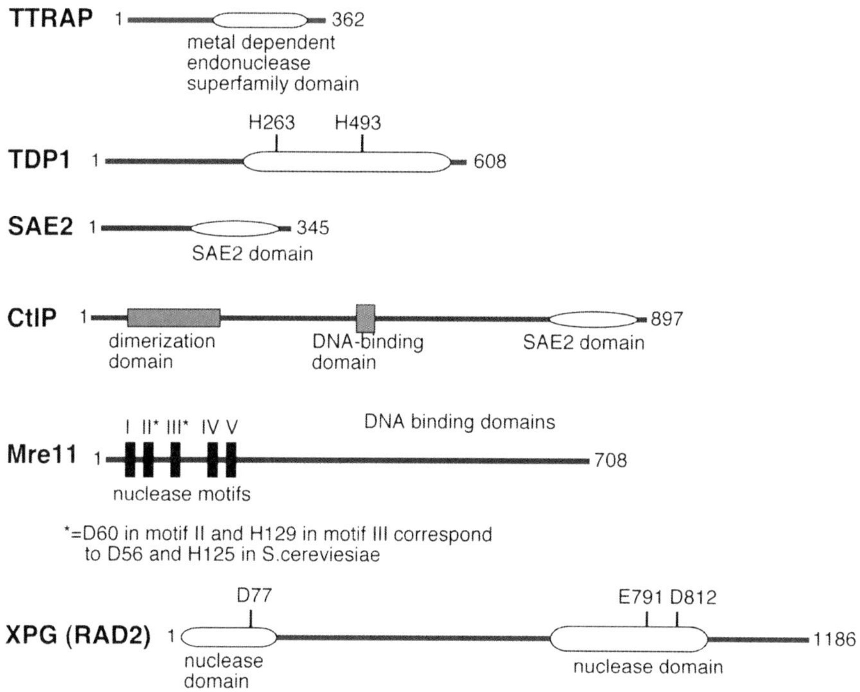

Fig. 18.1 Nucleolytic proteins that may play a role in removing Top2 covalently bound to DNA. The domains of nucleolytic proteins that can process Top2 are illustrated. As described in the text, TTRAP, Tdp1, Sae2/CtIP, and Mre11 have all been shown to contribute to Top2 processing. Genetic evidence in yeast suggests that Rad2 may also have a role in processing although there is no direct biochemical evidence at present

18.4.1 What We Learned from Spo11

An influential model for the repair of Top2-mediated DNA damage is the processing of double-strand breaks induced during meiotic recombination. Meiotic recombination is initiated by double-strand breaks that are induced by complexes that include the Spo11 protein. Spo11 is homologous to an archaebacterial type II topoisomerase (Bergerat et al. 1997) (termed TopVI). Genetic and biochemical studies, initially in yeast, showed that Spo11 is covalently bound to DNA by a 5′ phosphotyrosyl linkage (Keeney et al. 1997; Liu et al. 1995). Since Spo11 is linked to DNA in the same fashion as Top2, it has been widely thought that the processing of Top2 covalent complexes trapped by Top2 poisons could occur by pathways analogous to Spo11 processing pathways.

Induction of meiotic recombination requires a set of proteins required for chromosome pairing (Keeney and Neale 2006). The proteins required for initiating meiotic recombination include the **M**re11/**R**ad50/**N**bs1 complex (in yeast the Nbs1 homolog is termed Xrs2), although the details of the roles of MRN(X) complex may differ between yeasts and higher eukaryotes (Borde 2007). The MRN(X) complex orchestrates a wide range of responses to DNA double-strand breaks (Williams and Tainer 2007). The MRN(X) complex includes Rad50 a large coiled coil protein that has ATPase (Hopfner and Tainer 2003) and adenylate kinase activities (Bhaskara et al. 2007); Mre11, which carries 3′→5′ exonuclease and endonuclease activities, and Nbs1, thought to be a regulatory subunit. In the absence of the MRN(X) complex in yeast, Spo11-mediated cleavage does not occur and meiotic recombination fails to initiate. However, there are mutants of the MRN(X) complex that are competent for Spo11 cleavage, but which are unable to remove the covalently bound Spo11 protein. These include alleles of Rad50 (termed *rad50-S*, (Cao et al. 1990)) and nuclease-deficient alleles of Mre11 (Ajimura et al. 1993; Moreau et al. 1999). Interestingly, the same phenotype is seen in null alleles of *Sae2* (Keeney and Kleckner 1995; Prinz et al. 1997). Sae2 is homologous to the *Schizosaccharomyces pombe* Ctp1 and mammalian CtIP (Sartori et al. 2007; You and Bailis 2010), and is a single-strand specific endonuclease (Lengsfeld et al. 2007). These results suggested that a protein covalently bound by a 5′ phosphotyrosyl linkage could be removed by endonucleolytic cleavage, and that multiple nucleases might be required.

A strong confirmation of this model was obtained by analyzing the fate of the Spo11/oligonucleotide complex following excision from DNA. Keeney and colleagues immunoprecipitated Spo11 from meiotic cells and analyzed whether nucleotides are bound to release Spo11, and the nature of the bound oligonucleotide (Neale et al. 2005). They detected Spo11 protein covalently bound to a short oligonucleotide. Two different oligonucleotide lengths were observed, 12 nt and 21–37 nt, in equimolar ratios. The identification of Spo11 bound to an oligonucleotide demonstrated that removal of Spo11 occurred by an endonucleolytic cleavage, rather than hydrolysis of the phosphotyrosyl bond (as occurs with the Tdp1 and TTRAP/Tdp2 reactions discussed below). Importantly recovery of the Spo11 protein/oligonucleotide conjugate required both the MRN(X) complex and Sae2. Similar results were subsequently observed in *S. pombe*, although the differing oligonucleotide sizes were not seen (Milman et al. 2009). These results showed that there is a nucleolytic pathway for removing covalently bound Top2-like proteins from DNA. Since the Keeney assay relied on immune precipitation of Spo11, proteolytic degradation is not absolutely required for nucleolytic processing (although proteolytic processing of a subset of bound protein prior to nucleolytic excision obviously could not be excluded). A limitation of this model system is that it is unlikely to shed light on how trapped Top2 complexes are recognized. Since Spo11 is a meiosis-specific protein whose only function is generating double-strand breaks, there is no apparent need to limit its excision once it is covalently bound to DNA. Another current limitation of biochemical analysis of Spo11 removal has been the inability thus far to reconstitute Spo11 cleavage in vitro. Therefore, it has not been possible to examine the excision reaction using purified components.

18.4.2 Ctip and MRN(X) in Repair of Top2 Damage

The results described above for removal of Spo11 during meiosis provided an appealing model for the repair of trapped Top2. Until recently, there has been little direct evidence that either Ctip or MRN(X) is directly involved in nucleolytic Top2 removal. Hartsuiker and colleagues used *S. pombe* to analyze the importance of these nucleases in the repair of both Top1- and Top2-mediated DNA damage (Hartsuiker et al. 2009). Their central finding indicated that *rad50-S*, nuclease-deficient alleles of *mre11* (termed *rad32* in *S. pombe*, the specific allele used was D65N), and null alleles of CtIP (termed *ctp1* in *S. pombe*) increased sensitivity to the epipodophyllotoxin TOP-53, but not to either MMS or ionizing radiation. Importantly, all of the mutations also increased the level of Top2-DNA covalent complexes compared to isogenic wild-type strains. These results, taken together, show that an important pathway for removing covalently bound Top2 requires both the MRN(X) complex and CtIP.

A surprising result was seen by Hartsuiker and colleagues in the response of *ctp1*$^-$ cells to camptothecin (Hartsuiker et al. 2009). While *ctp1*$^-$ cells are hypersensitive to camptothecin, they are more proficient at removing Top1 covalent complexes than wild-type cells. Hartsuiker and colleagues suggested that Ctp1 might play a role in protecting 3′ ends from resection. Further studies will be needed to understand the orchestration of the two nuclease activities in the context of removing proteins from both the 5′ and 3′ ends of DNA.

Similar results have recently been reported at the genetic level in *Saccharomyces cerevisiae*. Hamilton and Maizels identified mutants in Mre11 that are hypersensitive to ionizing radiation and to hydroxyurea, but which had wild-type sensitivity to camptothecin and etoposide. By contrast, a nuclease-deficient allele (H125N) was hypersensitive to camptothecin and etoposide but not to ionizing radiation (Hamilton and Maizels 2010). Interestingly, they did not observe camptothecin or etoposide sensitivity in a *sae2* deletion (the *S. cerevisiae* CtIP homolog). This result needs to be interpreted with caution because we previously reported that *sae2* deletions were quite hypersensitive to etoposide (Stepanov et al. 2008). Neale and colleagues applied their immune precipitation assay to test whether they could detect an excised Top2 with bound oligonucleotide (Neale et al. 2005). While an oligonucleotide product was seen, it was not dependent on Rad50, Sae2, or other possible nucleases. This result leaves open the possibility that the Top2 oligonucleotide conjugate was not due to a repair event. Nonetheless, the results in yeast indicate that MRN(X) along with Sae2/CtIP constitute one important pathway for repairing trapped Top2.

Analysis of the role of MRN(X) and CtIP in mammalian cells is complicated by the fact that all of the MRN components (as well as CtIP) are essential for viability in higher eukaryotes (Nakamura et al. 2010; Yamaguchi-Iwai et al. 1999). Nakamura and colleagues analyzed the importance of CtIP for tolerance of topoisomerase-mediated damage in DT40 cells carrying a conditional knockout of CtIP. They found a large increase in sensitivity to both etoposide and camptothecin in DT40 cells hypomorphic for CtIP. By contrast, CtIP hypomorphic cells were not hypersensitive to MMS, again suggesting a specific defect in repairing topoisomerase-mediated damage. These results are consistent with studies in yeasts indicating that MRN(X) and CtIP are important for repairing topoisomerase-mediated damage beyond the roles of these proteins in double-strand break repair.

A critical question that remains to be answered is how MRN(X) and CtIP distinguish Top2 (and Top1) that are trapped versus the enzymes undergoing their normal reaction cycle. While recent results suggest that Sae2 processing of Spo11 is regulated by cyclin-dependent kinases (Manfrini et al. 2010), there must be some other marking of trapped covalent complexes beyond activation of Sae2. This issue is important not just for MRN(X) and CtIP, but also for any other processing pathway.

18.4.3 Tdp1: Is It Only for Top1?

Nash and colleagues identified a protein from yeast, Tdp1p (tyrosyl DNA phosphodiesterase), that could remove proteins such as topoisomerase I covalently bound to DNA, leaving a DNA molecule with a 3′ phosphate (Pouliot et al. 1999; Yang et al. 1996). Figure 18.2 summarizes the biochemical distinction between processing by tyrosyl DNA phosphodiesterases and conventional nuclease activity.

This protein was originally described as being inactive against oligonucleotides with a 3' phosphotyrosyl linkage. Mutants defective in this gene conferred slight sensitivity to camptothecin and when the *tdp1*⁻ mutation was combined with other DNA repair mutations, appreciable sensitivity to camptothecin was observed (Pouliot et al. 1999). For example, Vance and Wilson showed that combination of a *tdp1*⁻ mutation with mutations in the excision repair genes *RAD1* or *RAD10* also exhibited strong sensitivity to camptothecin (Vance and Wilson 2002).

In a screen of yeast mutants for sensitivity to Top2-targeting agents, we were surprised to find that *tdp1*⁻ mutants were hypersensitive to Top2-targeting agents (Nitiss et al. 2006). Despite the original failure to observe processing of a 5′phosphotyrosine linked to an oligonucleotide with the yeast enzyme (Yang et al. 1996), we tested the ability of yeast Tdp1p to remove peptides linked to DNA by a 5′phosphotyrosyl linkage. For these experiments, we used a peptidyl oligonucleotide substrate derived from Top2 cleavage of an oligonucleotide. Bacterially expressed yeast Tdp1 efficiently removed the covalently bound peptide, leaving a 5′ phosphate (Nitiss et al. 2006). The 5′ tyrosyl DNA phosphodiesterase was robust, with activity only slightly less than the enzyme's activity against 3′ substrates (K.C. Nitiss and J.L. Nitiss, unpublished results). Since tdp1-deficient mutants are hypersensitive to Top2 poisons, and since the yeast enzyme can efficiently remove proteins covalently bound by a 5′ phosphotyrosyl linkage, Tdp1 is clearly part of a yeast pathway that participates in repair of Top2 damage.

Does Tdp1 function in repairing Top2-mediated damage in higher eukaryotes? Most currently available evidence does not support a functional role for Tdp1 in affecting sensitivity to Top2-targeting drugs. Interthal and colleagues reported that they did not observe etoposide hypersensitivity in an RNAi knockdown of Tdp1

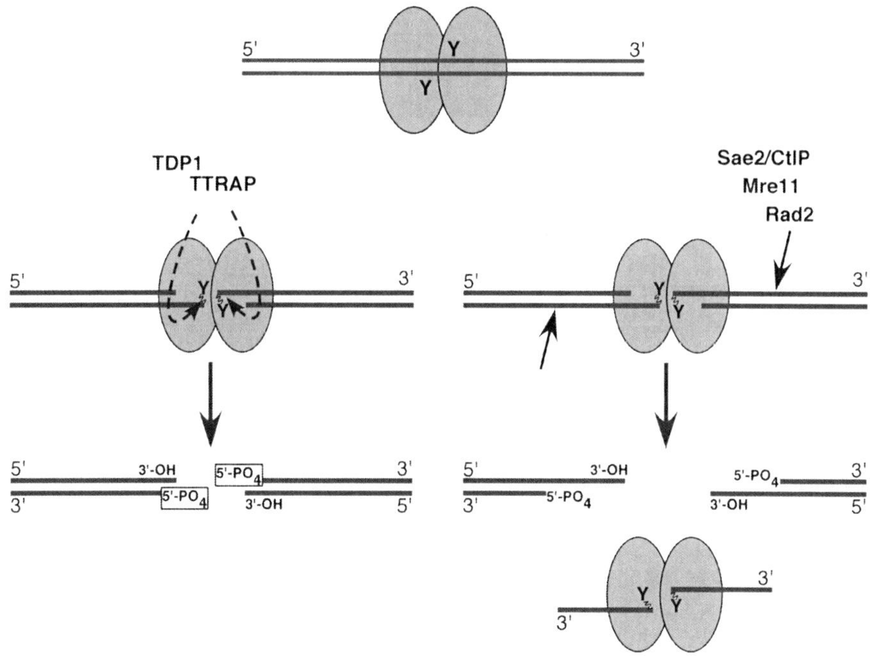

Fig. 18.2 Nucleolytic processing mechanisms for Top2 covalent complexes. Two classes of enzymes have been described that disjoin Top2 that is covalently bound to DNA. The first mechanism, exemplified by TTRAP/Tdp2 and Tdp1 is the direct nucleolytic reversal of the phosphotyrosyl bond. The resulting products are a DNA end with a 5′ PO_4, and nucleotide-free Top2. Repair nucleases that remove adducts from DNA use a mechanism related to that shown in the right pathway. A nuclease cuts 3′ of the trapped Top2, liberating Top2 still covalently bound to a short oligonucleotide. Both nucleolytic pathways generate DNA strand break(s) that are presumably repaired by single- or double-strand break repair pathways

(Interthal et al. 2005). More recently, Dexheimer and colleagues failed to observe processing of a 5′ fluorescein-labeled oligonucleotide by Tdp1 (Dexheimer et al. 2010). However, Boege and colleagues observed that Tdp1 overexpression could confer resistance to etoposide as well as camptothecin (Barthelmes et al. 2004). We have noted that 5′ fluorescein-labeled oligonucleotides are particularly poor substrates for the yeast Tdp1 reactions and are currently assessing the activity of human Tdp1 using 5′ peptidyl substrates (K.C. Nitiss and J.L. Nitiss, unpublished observations). Experiments with 5′ substrates that are efficiently used by yeast Tdp1 will address whether there are fundamental differences between yeast and mammalian Tdp1.

Another critical question for mammalian Tdp1 is whether the lack of sensitivity of Tdp1-deficient cells to Top2 poisons arises from multiple processing pathways that may occur in mammalian cells. As noted above, *S. cerevisiae* strains lacking Tdp1 are relatively insensitive to camptothecin unless they carry additional repair defects. As our understanding of functions needed to survive and repair Top2-mediated damage increases, it will be of considerable interest to test loss-of-function of Tdp1 alleles with other repair deficient alleles for sensitivity to Top2 poisons.

18.4.4 TTRAP/Tdp2

Since it is plausible that there are a number of nucleases that can remove topoisomerases that are covalently bound to DNA, it is a reasonable hypothesis that not all such enzymes have been discovered. Cortes Ledesma and colleagues followed this line of reasoning, and screened for additional proteins that could process Top1 covalent complexes (Cortes Ledesma et al. 2009). As noted above, while *tdp1* single mutants are not hypersensitive to camptothecin, *rad1 tdp1* double mutants are very hypersensitive compared to either single mutant. One protein new to the topoisomerase world was identified in this screen; a protein termed TTRAP. This protein had been previously identified as a CD40-binding protein (namely, **T**RAF and **T**NF **r**eceptor-**a**ssociated **p**rotein (Pype et al. 2000)). Purified TTRAP protein can remove a 3′phosphotyrosine from an oligonucleotide, although the reaction is relatively inefficient. Interestingly, TTRAP is very active with 5′ phosphotyrosyl modified oligonucleotides as a substrate. TTRAP is a metal ion-dependent phosphodiesterase related to apurinic/apyrimidinic (AP) endonuclease-1 (APE-1). The reaction products starting with either 3′ or 5′ phosphotyrosyl modified oligonucleotides are the same as for the (yeast) Tdp1 reaction, namely, oligonucleotides with either a 5′ phosphate or a 3′ phosphate.

Several genetic results supported a role for TTRAP in repairing Top2-mediated damage. Ectopic expression of TTRAP in yeast conferred resistance to etoposide, and the resistance required TTRAP catalytic activity. siRNA knockdown of TTRAP resulted in sensitivity to etoposide, but not to the Top1 targeting agent camptothecin. This result suggested that 5′ processing activity might be the most relevant biological activity of TTRAP. Given the biological similarities between Tdp1 and TTRAP, Cortes Ledesma and colleagues proposed the name Tdp2 for this protein (Cortes Ledesma et al. 2009).

Recent results support the hypothesis that Tdp2 plays important roles in processing Top2 complexes in higher eukaryotes. DT40 cells knocked out for Tdp2 are hypersensitive to etoposide but not to camptothecin or simple alkylating agents (Zeng et al. 2010). It has not yet been demonstrated whether Tdp2-deficient cells have elevated levels of Top2 covalent complexes following treatment with Top2 poisons.

18.4.5 Other Nucleases

In addition to the proteins described above, there are several other nucleases that have been indirectly implicated in processing Top2 complexes. In our studies with Tdp1 in yeast, we observed that *rad2 tdp1* double mutants showed enhanced sensitivity to etoposide but not to camptothecin. Yeast Rad2 is homologous to mammalian XPG. XPG, like yeast Rad2, participates in nucleotide excision repair and is the nuclease activity that incises the 3′ side of bulky adducts such as pyrimidine dimers (Prakash and Prakash 2000). The enzyme also possesses 5′→3′ exonuclease activity

(Habraken et al. 1994). The polarity of the Rad2 endonuclease activity would be consistent with processing Top2 covalent complexes. At present there is no biochemical evidence that Rad2 or XPG has activity against trapped Top2 complexes, and XPG mutant cells have not been reported to be etoposide hypersensitive.

A second nuclease that may have a role in processing Top2 covalent complexes is the structure-specific nuclease Slx1/Slx4. This nuclease was discovered by Brill and coworkers in a genetic screen in yeast for proteins that were required for viability when the recQ helicase Sgs1 was absent (Fricke and Brill 2003). Subsequent work has suggested that Slx1/Slx4 may function as a Holliday junction resolvase (Fekairi et al. 2009; Svendsen et al. 2009). Slx4 appears to act as a scaffold that interacts with several other nucleases and allows for the assembly of complexes that may be specific for aberrant DNA structures (Munoz et al. 2009). Slx1/Slx4 deficient mutant are camptothecin hypersensitive (Deng et al. 2005), and are also hypersensitive to Top2-targeting drugs (see Table 18.1 and the discussion in Sect. 18.7). Interestingly, the nuclease activity resides in the Slx1 subunit, and while Slx4 mutants are hypersensitive to other DNA damaging agents such as MMS, Slx1 mutants are not otherwise hypersensitive to DNA damage. Hence, Slx1 mutants show the same pattern of sensitivity that occurs in nuclease deficient alleles of Mre11.

Why are there so many nucleases that apparently process Top2 covalent complexes? Perhaps this result should not be surprising, since DNA damage processing at the ends of DNA is important for almost every repair pathway. In addition to the small molecules that have found use as anticancer and antibacterial therapeutics, many natural processes such as DNA damage also are able to trap topoisomerases (Kingma and Osheroff 1997; Nitiss et al. 2001; Pommier et al. 2000). A more interesting question will be to identify the regulators of the nucleases that can process Top2 covalent complexes and determine whether specific nucleases are associated with specific processes such as transcription and replication.

18.5 Repair Pathways: Proteolytic Degradation of Top2

Because Top2 covalent complexes include a large protein component, a plausible aspect of processing this damage is proteolytic degradation. Liu and colleagues found that Top2β, one of the two isozymes of human Top2 was rapidly degraded following treatment of HeLa cells with the epipodophyllotoxin teniposide (Mao et al. 2001). Degradation of Top2β depended on ubiquitination, and could be inhibited by the proteasome inhibitor MG132. Degradation was also blocked when cells were treated with either camptothecin or 5,6-dichlorobenzimidazole riboside (DRB), suggesting that transcription was critical for degradation. They found little degradation of Top2α under the same experimental conditions. Since Top2β is thought to play roles in transcription, while Top2α is more important for replication and chromosome disjunction (Nitiss 2009), these results suggested that the proteolytic pathway was particularly important when RNA polymerase collides with a trapped Top2 complex.

While Liu and colleagues failed to observe substantial degradation of Top2α, the protease pathway may also target trapped Top2α complexes (Fan et al. 2008). Top2α degradation was also blocked by either proteasome or transcription inhibitor. Inhibitors of DNA replication, such as the polymerase inhibitor aphidicolin did not block Top2α degradation.

An interesting aspect of the proteolytic processing pathway is that blocking proteasome-mediated degradation significantly reduces the induction of DNA damage responses. This attenuation of DNA damage signaling is especially apparent in postmitotic cells when Top2α is absent. This suggests that the proteolytic pathway may represent the major recognition pathway for Top2 covalent complexes in response to inhibition of transcription. Another consideration of the proteolytic pathway is that proteolysis is unable to completely remove all of the protein covalently bound to DNA. After proteolytic processing, a nucleolytic step is needed to generate a DNA end free of protein. Identification of the nucleases involved will be particularly challenging, since it is difficult to distinguish between a free DNA end and a DNA end bearing an attached phosphotyrosine residue.

18.6 Repair Pathways: Break Repair

Removal of Top2 by either nucleolytic pathways or proteolysis result in DNA strand breaks. When Top2 has cleaved both DNA strands, removal of the Top2 results in a double-strand break. Therefore, an important part of understanding the repair of Top2 damage includes understanding the double-strand break repair pathways that are used. In yeast, a deficiency in homologous recombination leads to very high levels of sensitivity to Top2-targeting agents, (Table 18.1, see also (Nitiss and Wang 1988; Nitiss et al. 1992)). While this result is in accord with repair of double-strand break repair in yeast from other DNA damaging agents such as ionizing radiation, it is interesting that yeast cells that are defective in nonhomologous end-joining (NHEJ) are also sensitive to Top2 poisons. Yeast NHEJ mutants have limited sensitivity to most DNA-damaging agents. Sensitivity is primarily seen when NHEJ mutants are combined with other mutants, especially mutants defective in homologous recombination (Critchlow and Jackson 1998; Lewis et al. 1998; Lewis and Resnick 2000). Since yeast NHEJ mutants are sensitive to Top2 poisons, some of the double-strand breaks generated by these agents are apparently not readily repairable by homologous recombination. By contrast, yeast NHEJ mutants show no increase in sensitivity to camptothecin.

In mammalian cells, NHEJ is the major pathway for repairing DNA damage due to ionizing radiation (Lieber 2010). Mammalian cells lacking NHEJ are clearly hypersensitive to Top2-targeting agents such as etoposide (Adachi et al. 2003; Jin et al. 1998). Not all NHEJ functions are required for repairing etoposide-mediated damage, for example, Artemis appears to play a limited role in repairing damage from etoposide (Adachi et al. 2004; Kurosawa et al. 2008).

Table 18.1 Yeast genes important for surviving exposure to topoisomerase II targeting drugs

Gene	Relative mAMSA Sens.	Doxo. Sens.	Cpt Sens.	Human homolog/paralog	Gene function
Double-strand break repair					
mre11	+++	NF	+	MRE11	MRN(X) complex
rad50	+++	S	+	RAD50	MRN(X) complex
rad51	++	S	+	RAD51	Recombination
rad52	+++	S	+	RAD52	Recombination
rad54	++	S	+	RAD54L	Recombination
rad55	++	S	+	RAD51 paralog	Recombination
rad57	++	S	+	RAD51 paralog	Recombination
rad59	+	S	+/−	RAD52	Rad52 homolog
rad61	+	NF	−	***	Mutation confers X-ray sensitivity
rdh54	+	NF	+/−	***	DNA-dependent ATPase, rad54 homolog
sae2	+	NF	+	CtIP	DNA end resection
xrs2	+	NF	+	NBS1	MRN(X) complex
yku70	+	NF	−	KU70	NHEJ
yku80	+	NF	−	KU80	NHEJ
dnl4	+	NF	−	DNL4	NHEJ
nej1	+	NF	−	XLF	NHEJ
Other repair functions					
asf1	++	S	+	ASF1A	Histone chaperone
ctf4	+++	S	+	HCTF4/WDHD1	DNA Polα-binding protein
ctf8	+	NF	+	HCTF8	Alternate RFC complex
ctf18	+++	NF	+	HCTF18	Alternate RFC complex
dcc1	+	NF	+	HDDC1	Alternate RFC complex

(continued)

Table 18.1 (continued)

Gene	Relative mAMSA Sens.	Doxo. Sens.	Cpt Sens.	Human homolog/paralog	Gene function
ddc1	+	NF	+	***	Checkpoint, interacts with Rad17 and Mec3
hnt3	+	NF	+	APTX	DNA 5′ AMP hydrolase
hpr5	++	NF	+	***	DNA helicase
mms1	++	S	+	***	DNA repair during S phase
mms4	+	S	+	EME1	Subunit of structure specific endonuclease
mms22	++	S	+	MMS22L	DNA repair during S phase
mus81	+	NF	+	MUS81	Subunit of structure specific endonuclease
pol32	+	NF	+	***	DNA polymerase δ complex subuint
rad5	+	NF	–	SHPRH	Post-replication repair
rad6	+	NF	–	HHR6A/HHR6B	Post-replication repair
rad17	+	NF	+	RAD1	Checkpoint
rad23	+	NF	+	RAD23B	Subunit of Nef2
rad24	+	NF	+	RAD17	Checkpoint protein
rtt101	+	NF	+	***	Cullin subunit of an E3 ubiquitin ligase, interacts with Mms22
rtt107	+	NF	+	***	Repair of S phase damage
rtt109/ rem50	++	S	+	***	Histone acetyl transferase
slx1	+	NF	+	SLX1	Subunit of structure-specific nuclease

slx4	+	NF	+	BTB12/SLX4	Subunit of structure-specific nuclease
slx5/hex3	+	S	+	***	Forms a complex with Slx8
slx8	+	S	+	***	RING finger protein forms a complex with Slx5
top3	++	S	+	TOP3A	Type 1A topoisomerase, resolution of crossovers
tdp1	+	NF	+/–	TDP1	Tyrosyl DNA phosphodiesterase 1
Other nuclear functions					
arp8	+	NF	+	ACTR8	Nuclear actin-related protein involved in chromatin remodeling
asm4	++	NF	+	***	Nuclear pore complex
ccr4	+	S	+	CNOT6/CNOT6L	CCR4-NOT Complex Transcription
kre28	+	NF	+	***	Subunit of a kinetochore-microtubule-binding complex
not4	+	NF	+	CNOT4	CCR4-NOT Complex Transcription
rsc7/npl6	+	NF	+	***	RSC chromatin-remodeling complex
nup84	+	NF	+	NUP107	Nuclear pore complex
rsc2	+	NF	–	PBRM1	RSC chromatin-remodeling complex

(continued)

Table 18.1 (continued)

Gene	Relative mAMSA Sens.	Doxo. Sens.	Cpt Sens.	Human homolog/paralog	Gene function
swd1	+	NF	–	RBBP5	Subunit of COMPASS (histone H3 methylation complex)
vid21/ eaf1	+	NF	+	***	NuA4 histone acetyltransferase
Transcription					
ada2	+	NF	+	TADA2A	Component of the ADA and SAGA complexes
bur2	+	NF	+	***	Transcription
gcn5	+	NF	–	GCN5L2	Histone acetyltransferase, catalytic subunit of the ADA and SAGA complexes
rtf1	++	NF	–	RTF1	PAF transcription complex
spt10	++	NF	+	***	Putative histone acetyl transferase
spt20	++	S	+	***	Subunit of the SAGA transcriptional complex
srb5	+	NF	+	***	Subunit of RNA polymerase II holoenzyme/mediator complex
swi6	++	S	+	***	Transcription factor component involved in G1/S transition

taf14	++	S	+	***	Transcription complex subunit
ydl041 (sir2)	+	S	+	SIRT1 (Sir2 ortholog)	Small open reading frame whose disruption partly ablates Sir2 function
Ubiquitin, SUMO, and protein degradation					
doc1	+	S	+	APC10	Ubiquitination of APC
shp1	+	S	+	NSFL1C	UBX domain containing protein
ubp6	+	NF	+	USP14	Ubiquitin-specific protease
Other cellular functions					
aat2	++	NF	+	GOT1	Aspartate aminotransferase
akr1	+	S	+	ZDHHC17	Palmitoyltransferase activity
ard1	+	NF	+	ARD1B/ARD2	Protein acetylation
atp4	+	NF	+	ATP5F1	Subunit b of the mitochondrial F1F0 ATP synthase
bck1	++	S	+	***	MAP kinase kinase kinase
gon7	++	S	+	***	KEOPS complex; telomere maintenance
ilm1	++	NF	+	***	Unknown, mitochondrial DNA?
lsm6	+	NF	+	***	RNA processing, mRNA decay

(continued)

Table 18.1 (continued)

Gene	Relative mAMSA Sens.	Doxo. Sens.	Cpt Sens.	Human homolog/paralog	Gene function
pep12	+	NF	+	STX7	t-SNARE protein
plc1	+	S	+	PLCD1/PLCD3 PLCD4	Phospholipase C
rpl12B	++	NF	+	RPL12	60S Ribosome subunit
rpl22A	++	NF	+	RPL22/RPL22L	60S Ribosome subunit
rpl34B	+	NF	+	RPL34	60S Ribosome subunit
rsa1	+	S	–	***	Ribosome assembly
rvs161	++	NF	+	AMPH	Amphiphysin-like
she1	+	NF	–	***	Mitotic spindle protein
tif4631	+	NF	–	***	Translation initiation factor eIF4G
tom37	+	NF	+	***	Outer mitochondrial membrane translocase
tpk1	++	NF	+	PRKACA	cAMP-dependent protein kinase
ume6	+	NF	+	***	Transcriptional regulator of meiosis

Sensitivity to either mAMSA or doxorubicin was determined as described in the text. The doxorubicin results are from (Westmoreland et al. 2009). The genes listed in this table do not comprise the complete set of mAMSA or doxorubicin hypersensitive genes. For mAMSA hypersensitivity, +++ indicates mutants that result in a reduction in cell survival to below 1% after a 24 h drug exposure, ++ indicates mutants that result in a reduction in cell survival to below 1% after a 24 h drug exposure, and + indicates mutants that result in a reduction in cell survival to below 1% after a 24 h drug exposure. The doxorubicin sensitivity is listed as either *S*, indicating sensitive, or *NF* (not found) indicating the mutant was not identified in the screen. The failure to find the mutant in the screen should not be interpreted as the mutant is not sensitive. Camptothecin sensitivity was determined by Berk and Nitiss (unpublished results) and the overall level of sensitivity is not indicated except a small number of mutants that showed equivocal sensitivity (denoted +/–). The human homologs or paralogs were mainly identified using the Princeton Protein Orthology Database (http://ppod.princeton.edu). Homologs/orthologs marked *** did not yield convincing orthologs. Gene functions were annotated in part using the descriptions found at the yeast genome database (http://www.yeastgenome.org/). Homologs/orthologs marked did not yield convincing orthologs

The NHEJ pathway may be of particular importance in the use of Top2-targeting agents because etoposide and other Top2-targeting agents can cause secondary malignancies (Felix et al. 2006; Mistry et al. 2005). While it has not been clearly demonstrated whether NHEJ functions mediate translocations arising from Top2-targeting agents, it is clear that nonhomologous recombination is a pathway that may limit the usefulness of Top2-targeting agents (Kantidze and Razin 2007).

The importance of homologous recombination in repairing Top2 damage in mammalian cells is less clear. Recent results indicate that mutants that show defects in homologous recombination are hypersensitive to etoposide (Powell and Kachnic 2008; Schonn et al. 2010; Treszezamsky et al. 2007). The sensitive mutants include rad51, Brca1, and Brca2 cells; therefore, it may be possible to specifically exploit repair deficiencies in human tumors that are defective in homologous recombination (Powell and Kachnic 2008).

18.7 Identification of Other Genes Required for Surviving Top2-Mediated DNA Damage

Our understanding of cellular pathways that are involved in repairing Top2-mediated DNA damage has been enhanced by several key model systems. Yeast has been particularly useful in understanding biological aspects of topoisomerases and topoisomerase poisons (Bjornsti 2002; Nitiss 1994; Nitiss et al. 1996), and recent advances in RNAi open up the possibility of using yeast-like genetic screens to identify human genes important for repairing Top2-mediated damage. This section emphasizes the potential for learning aspects of repair of Top2 damage, rather than mechanistic or biochemical details.

18.7.1 Yeast Repair Pathways

Yeast has served as a powerful model system for understanding DNA repair pathways in eukaryotic cells. Yeast has also been used extensively to study Top2 (and Top1)-targeting agents. Early work in yeast helped to establish the importance of enzyme-mediated DNA damage in the action of Top2-targeting drugs, the roles of various double-strand break repair pathways, and was instrumental in the identification of covalent complex processing factors such as Tdp1 and Sae2/CtIP. The results described in this section highlight the power of yeast to identify repair functions on a genomic scale.

The simplicity of the yeast genome and the ability to carry out gene replacement in yeast has led to the development of powerful tools to carry out systematic functional analysis on a genome wide scale. The yeast community collaborated to construct a set of strains that carry precise deletion of all of the nonessential open reading frames of the yeast genome (Winzeler et al. 1999). This deletion set has been used to identify yeast genes important for many processes, and has been an especially powerful resource for identifying genes that confer sensitivity to DNA-damaging agents (Bennett et al. 2001; Chang et al. 2002; Deng et al. 2005). Osheroff and colleagues carried out the first screen of the yeast deletion set for mutants that were hypersensitive to etoposide. The relative insensitivity of yeast cells to etoposide limited the number of genes identified in this screen. In addition to genes required for homologous recombination, this screen showed that deletion of *MMS22* conferred hypersensitivity to etoposide (Baldwin et al. 2005). Subsequent screens assessed sensitivity to doxorubicin, which led to the identification of a much greater number of yeast genes (Westmoreland et al. 2009). An interesting aspect of this screen was that many genes were identified that conferred hypersensitivity to doxorubicin in diploid but not haploid cells.

Doxorubicin is a potent cytotoxic agent against yeast cells, but it generates DNA damage by a variety of mechanisms including Top2 targeting and generation of reactive oxygen species. As an alternate approach, we used a mechanism-specific screen to identify yeast genes that were specifically sensitive to Top2-mediated damage. This screen used overexpression of Top2 and sensitivity to mAMSA, an intercalating Top2 poison (J. Berk and J.L. Nitiss, unpublished results). In addition, we also carried out a screen where the overexpressed allele of Top2 was mAMSA hypersensitive. The use of either of the Top2 overexpression vectors greatly enhanced the sensitivity of the screen. Since hypersensitivity was not seen (for most mutants) in the absence of Top2 overexpression, this screen specifically identified mutants that were hypersensitive to Top2 poisons.

The doxorubicin and mAMSA screens described above generated a large number of genes that are required for survival following Top2-mediated DNA damage. A subset of the genes identified in yeast is shown in Table 18.1. While it is beyond the scope of this chapter to discuss all of the genes in detail, there are several important conclusions from these screens. First, many of the genes that have been shown to be important for surviving Top2-mediated DNA damage are also important for surviving other types of DNA damage such as ionizing radiation or simple alkylating agents. Essentially, all of the genes known to be required for repairing double-strand breaks by homologous recombination or nonhomologous end-joining were identified in yeast screens, or by a direct examination of null mutants (Malik et al. 2006; Sabourin et al. 2003). As expected, several nucleases confer hypersensitivity to Top2-targeting agents. These include the components of the MRN(X) complex, the Sae2 nuclease, and the structure-specific nucleases Slx1/Slx4 and Mms4/Mus81.

Other repair functions identified in the doxorubicin and mAMSA screens include some components of the Rad6 pathway. The Rad5 and Rad6 genes are of particular interest because deletions of these genes do not confer sensitivity to camptothecin. Most of the yeast genes that confer sensitivity to Top2 drugs also confer sensitivity to camptothecin, but the components of the Rad6 pathway are an interesting exception. Another pathway that is important for Top2-targeting agents that is not important for camptothecin sensitivity is NHEJ. The importance of NHEJ likely reflects the induction of Top2-mediated double-strand breaks when a sister chromatid is unavailable as a template for repair, as discussed above.

Finally, it is interesting to note some of the unexpected genes that were identified as conferring high levels of sensitivity to Top2 targeting agents.

18.8 Consequences of Topoisomerase II DNA Damage: Repair as a Determinant of Clinical Response

A major challenge in the clinical application of any anticancer drug is to identify the tumors that are most likely to respond to drug treatment. The discovery that Top2-targeting drugs acted by generation of enzyme-mediated DNA damage led to the prediction that Top2 levels might predict sensitivity to Top2-targeting drugs. While Top2 levels predicted sensitivity in some cases, it was clear that many tumors expressing relatively low Top2 protein levels were quite sensitive, while other tumors with much higher levels of Top2 were relatively resistant to Top2 poisons. The results summarized in this chapter indicate that there are a large number of genes that profoundly affect sensitivity to Top2targeting agents

One of the areas of great excitement in cancer chemotherapy is the concept of synthetic lethality. Cells have multiple pathways for survival and protection from genotoxic stress. As cancer cells evolve and obtain a proliferative advantage, they acquire mutations in repair pathways that render them more dependent on alternative pathways. One way to exploit this sensitivity is the direct inhibition of a second repair pathway as was found for PARP inhibitors that are highly active against BRCA deficient tumors (Banerjee et al. 2010; Rehman et al. 2010). An alternate application of the synthetic lethality concept that is relevant to Top2-targeting agents is the identification of repair genes in mutated tumors that are important for repairing Top2-mediated damage. A reason why Top2-targeting drugs are useful in many tumor types is the diversity of repair pathways that is required for repairing damage arising from trapping the enzyme.

18.9 Future Prospects

Our understanding of the repair of Top2-mediated damage has increased enormously in the last few years. The results with yeast-based screens as described in Sect. 18.7 suggest that there are many genes that play important roles whose biochemical functions in repair remain unclear. The elaboration of siRNA screens to identify genes conferring hypersensitivity to small molecules will allow investigators to do yeast-like screens in mammalian cells. These screens should lead to the identification of genetic markers that will predict the response of individual tumors to Top2-targeting drugs. As understanding of repair pathways for Top2 damage increase, it is plausible that the clinical utility of Top2 as an anticancer drug target will undergo a renaissance.

Acknowledgments Work from our laboratory described in this chapter was supported by grants from the NIH (CA82313 and CA52814, and core grant CA21765) and the American Lebanese Syrian Associated Charities (ALSAC).

References

Adachi, N., Iiizumi, S., So, S., and Koyama, H. (2004). Genetic evidence for involvement of two distinct nonhomologous end-joining pathways in repair of topoisomerase II-mediated DNA damage. Biochem Biophys Res Commun *318*, 856–861.

Adachi, N., Suzuki, H., Iiizumi, S., and Koyama, H. (2003). Hypersensitivity of nonhomologous DNA end-joining mutants to VP-16 and ICRF-193: implications for the repair of topoisomerase II-mediated DNA damage. J Biol Chem *278*, 35897–35902.

Ajimura, M., Leem, S.H., and Ogawa, H. (1993). Identification of new genes required for meiotic recombination in Saccharomyces cerevisiae. Genetics *133*, 51–66.

Andersen, A.H., Christiansen, K., Zechiedrich, E.L., Jensen, P.S., Osheroff, N., and Westergaard, O. (1989). Strand specificity of the topoisomerase II mediated double-stranded DNA cleavage reaction. Biochemistry *28*, 6237–6244.

Baldwin, E.L., Berger, A.C., Corbett, A.H., and Osheroff, N. (2005). Mms22p protects Saccharomyces cerevisiae from DNA damage induced by topoisomerase II. Nucleic Acids Res *33*, 1021–1030.

Baldwin, E.L., and Osheroff, N. (2005). Etoposide, topoisomerase II and cancer. Curr Med Chem Anticancer Agents *5*, 363–372.

Banerjee, S., Kaye, S.B., and Ashworth, A. (2010). Making the best of PARP inhibitors in ovarian cancer. Nat Rev Clin Oncol *7*, 508–519.

Barthelmes, H.U., Habermeyer, M., Christensen, M.O., Mielke, C., Interthal, H., Pouliot, J.J., Boege, F., and Marko, D. (2004). TDP1 overexpression in human cells counteracts DNA damage mediated by topoisomerases I and II. J Biol Chem *279*, 55618–55625.

Bennett, C.B., Lewis, L.K., Karthikeyan, G., Lobachev, K.S., Jin, Y.H., Sterling, J.F., Snipe, J.R., and Resnick, M.A. (2001). Genes required for ionizing radiation resistance in yeast. Nat Genet *29*, 426–434.

Bergerat, A., de Massy, B., Gadelle, D., Varoutas, P.C., Nicolas, A., and Forterre, P. (1997). An atypical topoisomerase II from Archaea with implications for meiotic recombination. Nature *386*, 414–417.

Bhaskara, V., Dupre, A., Lengsfeld, B., Hopkins, B.B., Chan, A., Lee, J.H., Zhang, X., Gautier, J., Zakian, V., and Paull, T.T. (2007). Rad50 adenylate kinase activity regulates DNA tethering by Mre11/Rad50 complexes. Mol Cell *25*, 647–661.

Bjornsti, M.A. (2002). Cancer therapeutics in yeast. Cancer Cell *2*, 267–273.

Borde, V. (2007). The multiple roles of the Mre11 complex for meiotic recombination. Chromosome Res *15*, 551–563.

Cao, L., Alani, E., and Kleckner, N. (1990). A pathway for generation and processing of double-strand breaks during meiotic recombination in S. cerevisiae. Cell *61*, 1089–1101.

Chang, M., Bellaoui, M., Boone, C., and Brown, G.W. (2002). A genome-wide screen for methyl methanesulfonate-sensitive mutants reveals genes required for S phase progression in the presence of DNA damage. Proc Natl Acad Sci USA *99*, 16934–16939.

Choi, H.J., Cho, B.C., Shin, S.J., Cheon, S.H., Jung, J.Y., Chang, J., Kim, S.K., Sohn, J.H., and Kim, J.H. (2008). Combination of topotecan and etoposide as a salvage treatment for patients with recurrent small cell lung cancer following irinotecan and platinum first-line chemotherapy. Cancer Chemotherapy and Pharmacology *61*, 309–313.

Cortes Ledesma, F., El Khamisy, S.F., Zuma, M.C., Osborn, K., and Caldecott, K.W. (2009). A human 5′-tyrosyl DNA phosphodiesterase that repairs topoisomerase-mediated DNA damage. Nature *461*, 674–678.

Critchlow, S.E., and Jackson, S.P. (1998). DNA end-joining: from yeast to man. Trends Biochem Sci *23*, 394–398.

D'Arpa, P., Beardmore, C., and Liu, L.F. (1990). Involvement of nucleic acid synthesis in cell killing mechanisms of topoisomerase poisons. Cancer Res *50*, 6919–6924.

Deng, C., Brown, J.A., You, D., and Brown, J.M. (2005). Multiple endonucleases function to repair covalent topoisomerase I complexes in Saccharomyces cerevisiae. Genetics *170*, 591–600.

Dexheimer, T.S., Stephen, A.G., Fivash, M.J., Fisher, R.J., and Pommier, Y. (2010). The DNA binding and 3′-end preferential activity of human tyrosyl-DNA phosphodiesterase. Nucleic Acids Res *38*, 2444–2452.

Dombernowsky, P., Gehl, J., Boesgaard, M., Paaske, T., and Jensen, B.V. (1996). Doxorubicin and paclitaxel, a highly active combination in the treatment of metastatic breast cancer. Seminars in Oncology *23*, 23–27.

Downes, C.S., Clarke, D.J., Mullinger, A.M., Gimenez-Abian, J.F., Creighton, A.M., and Johnson, R.T. (1994). A topoisomerase II-dependent G2 cycle checkpoint in mammalian cells/ [published erratum appears in Nature 1994 Dec 15;372(6507):710]. Nature *372*, 467–470.

Fan, J.R., Peng, A.L., Chen, H.C., Lo, S.C., Huang, T.H., and Li, T.K. (2008). Cellular processing pathways contribute to the activation of etoposide-induced DNA damage responses. DNA Repair *7*, 452–463.

Fekairi, S., Scaglione, S., Chahwan, C., Taylor, E.R., Tissier, A., Coulon, S., Dong, M.Q., Ruse, C., Yates, J.R., 3rd, Russell, P., *et al.* (2009). Human SLX4 is a Holliday junction resolvase subunit that binds multiple DNA repair/recombination endonucleases. Cell *138*, 78–89.

Felix, C.A., Kolaris, C.P., and Osheroff, N. (2006). Topoisomerase II and the etiology of chromosomal translocations. DNA Repair (Amst) *5*, 1093–1108.

Fricke, W.M., and Brill, S.J. (2003). Slx1-Slx4 is a second structure-specific endonuclease functionally redundant with Sgs1-Top3. Genes Dev *17*, 1768–1778.

Froelich-Ammon, S.J., Patchan, M.W., Osheroff, N., and Thompson, R.B. (1995). Topoisomerase II binds to ellipticine in the absence or presence of DNA. Characterization of enzyme-drug interactions by fluorescence spectroscopy. J Biol Chem *270*, 14998–15004.

Habraken, Y., Sung, P., Prakash, L., and Prakash, S. (1994). A conserved 5′ to 3′ exonuclease activity in the yeast and human nucleotide excision repair proteins RAD2 and XPG. J Biol Chem *269*, 31342–31345.

Hamilton, N.K., and Maizels, N. (2010). MRE11 function in response to topoisomerase poisons is independent of its function in double-strand break repair in Saccharomyces cerevisiae. PLoS One *5*, e15387.

Hanawalt, P.C., and Spivak, G. (2008). Transcription-coupled DNA repair: two decades of progress and surprises. Nat Rev Mol Cell Biol *9*, 958–970.

Hartsuiker, E., Neale, M.J., and Carr, A.M. (2009). Distinct requirements for the Rad32(Mre11) nuclease and Ctp1(CtIP) in the removal of covalently bound topoisomerase I and II from DNA. Mol Cell *33*, 117–123.

Holm, C., Covey, J.M., Kerrigan, D., and Pommier, Y. (1989). Differential requirement of DNA replication for the cytotoxicity of DNA topoisomerase I and II inhibitors in Chinese hamster DC3F cells. Cancer Res *49*, 6365–6368.

Hopfner, K.P., and Tainer, J.A. (2003). Rad50/SMC proteins and ABC transporters: unifying concepts from high-resolution structures. Curr Opin Struct Biol *13*, 249–255.

Howard, M.T., Neece, S.H., Matson, S.W., and Kreuzer, K.N. (1994). Disruption of a topoisomerase-DNA cleavage complex by a DNA helicase. Proc Natl Acad Sci USA *91*, 12031–12035.

Huang, X., Traganos, F., and Darzynkiewicz, Z. (2003). DNA damage induced by DNA topoisomerase I- and topoisomerase II-inhibitors detected by histone H2AX phosphorylation in relation to the cell cycle phase and apoptosis. Cell Cycle *2*, 614–619.

Injac, R., and Strukej, B. (2008). Recent Advances in Protection Against Doxorubicin-induced Toxicity. Technology in Cancer Research & Treatment *7*, 497–516.

Interthal, H., Chen, H.J., Kehl-Fie, T.E., Zotzmann, J., Leppard, J.B., and Champoux, J.J. (2005). SCAN1 mutant Tdp1 accumulates the enzyme--DNA intermediate and causes camptothecin hypersensitivity. EMBO J *24*, 2224–2233.

Jin, S., Inoue, S., and Weaver, D.T. (1998). Differential etoposide sensitivity of cells deficient in the Ku and DNA-PKcs components of the DNA-dependent protein kinase. Carcinogenesis *19*, 965–971.

Kantidze, O.L., and Razin, S.V. (2007). Chemotherapy-related secondary leukemias: A role for DNA repair by error-prone non-homologous end joining in topoisomerase II - Induced chromosomal rearrangements. Gene *391*, 76–79.

Keeney, S., Giroux, C.N., and Kleckner, N. (1997). Meiosis-specific DNA double-strand breaks are catalyzed by Spo11, a member of a widely conserved protein family. Cell *88*, 375–384.

Keeney, S., and Kleckner, N. (1995). Covalent protein-DNA complexes at the 5′ strand termini of meiosis-specific double-strand breaks in yeast. Proc Natl Acad Sci USA *92*, 11274–11278.

Keeney, S., and Neale, M.J. (2006). Initiation of meiotic recombination by formation of DNA double-strand breaks: mechanism and regulation. Biochem Soc Trans *34*, 523–525.

Kingma, P.S., and Osheroff, N. (1997). Apurinic sites are position-specific topoisomerase II poisons. J Biol Chem *272*, 1148–1155.

Kurosawa, A., Koyama, H., Takayama, S., Miki, K., Ayusawa, D., Fujii, M., Iiizumi, S., and Adachi, N. (2008). The requirement of Artemis in double-strand break repair depends on the type of DNA damage. DNA Cell Biol *27*, 55–61.

Lengsfeld, B.M., Rattray, A.J., Bhaskara, V., Ghirlando, R., and Paull, T.T. (2007). Sae2 is an endonuclease that processes hairpin DNA cooperatively with the Mre11/Rad50/Xrs2 complex. Mol Cell *28*, 638–651.

Lewis, L.K., Kirchner, J.M., and Resnick, M.A. (1998). Requirement for end-joining and checkpoint functions, but not RAD52-mediated recombination, after EcoRI endonuclease cleavage of Saccharomyces cerevisiae DNA. Mol Cell Biol *18*, 1891–1902.

Lewis, L.K., and Resnick, M.A. (2000). Tying up loose ends: nonhomologous end-joining in Saccharomyces cerevisiae. Mutat Res *451*, 71–89.

Lieber, M. (2010). The mechanism of double-strand DNA break repair by the nonhomologous DNA end-joining pathway. Annu Rev Biochem *79*, 181–211.

Lieu, C., Chow, L., Pierson, A., Eckhardt, S., O'Bryant, C., Morrow, M., Tran, Z., Wright, J., and Gore, L. (2009). A phase I study of bortezomib, etoposide and carboplatin in patients with advanced solid tumors refractory to standard therapy. Investigational New Drugs *27*, 53–62.

Liu, J., Wu, T.C., and Lichten, M. (1995). The location and structure of double-strand DNA breaks induced during yeast meiosis: evidence for a covalently linked DNA-protein intermediate. EMBO J *14*, 4599–4608.

Malik, M., Nitiss, K.C., Enriquez-Rios, V., and Nitiss, J.L. (2006). Roles of nonhomologous end-joining pathways in surviving topoisomerase II-mediated DNA damage. Mol Cancer Ther *5*, 1405–1414.

Manfrini, N., Guerini, I., Citterio, A., Lucchini, G., and Longhese, M.P. (2010). Processing of meiotic DNA double strand breaks requires cyclin-dependent kinase and multiple nucleases. J Biol Chem *285*, 11628–11637.

Mao, Y., Desai, S.D., Ting, C.Y., Hwang, J., and Liu, L.F. (2001). 26S proteasome-mediated degradation of topoisomerase II cleavable complexes. J Biol Chem *276*, 40652–40658.

Marians, K.J., and Hiasa, H. (1997). Mechanism of quinolone action. A drug-induced structural perturbation of the DNA precedes strand cleavage by topoisomerase IV. J Biol Chem *272*, 9401–9409.

Markovits, J., Pommier, Y., Kerrigan, D., Covey, J.M., Tilchen, E.J., and Kohn, K.W. (1987). Topoisomerase II-mediated DNA breaks and cytotoxicity in relation to cell proliferation and the cell cycle in NIH 3T3 fibroblasts and L1210 leukemia cells. Cancer Res *47*, 2050–2055.

Michel, B., Grompone, G., Flores, M.J., and Bidnenko, V. (2004). Multiple pathways process stalled replication forks. Proc Natl Acad Sci USA *101*, 12783–12788.

Milman, N., Higuchi, E., and Smith, G.R. (2009). Meiotic DNA double-strand break repair requires two nucleases, MRN and Ctp1, to produce a single size class of Rec12 (Spo11)-oligonucleotide complexes. Mol Cell Biol *29*, 5998–6005.

Mistry, A.R., Felix, C.A., Whitmarsh, R.J., Mason, A., Reiter, A., Cassinat, B., Parry, A., Walz, C., Wiemels, J.L., Segal, M.R., *et al.* (2005). DNA topoisomerase II in therapy-related acute promyelocytic leukemia. N Engl J Med *352*, 1529–1538.

Moreau, S., Ferguson, J.R., and Symington, L.S. (1999). The nuclease activity of Mre11 is required for meiosis but not for mating type switching, end joining, or telomere maintenance. Mol Cell Biol *19*, 556–566.

Munoz, I.M., Hain, K., Declais, A.C., Gardiner, M., Toh, G.W., Sanchez-Pulido, L., Heuckmann, J.M., Toth, R., Macartney, T., Eppink, B., *et al.* (2009). Coordination of structure-specific nucleases by human SLX4/BTBD12 is required for DNA repair. Mol Cell *35*, 116–127.

Nakamura, K., Kogame, T., Oshiumi, H., Shinohara, A., Sumitomo, Y., Agama, K., Pommier, Y., Tsutsui, K.M., Tsutsui, K., Hartsuiker, E., *et al.* (2010). Collaborative action of Brca1 and CtIP in elimination of covalent modifications from double-strand breaks to facilitate subsequent break repair. PLoS Genet *6*, e1000828.

Neale, M.J., Pan, J., and Keeney, S. (2005). Endonucleolytic processing of covalent protein-linked DNA double-strand breaks. Nature *436*, 1053–1057.

Nitiss, J., and Wang, J.C. (1988). DNA topoisomerase-targeting antitumor drugs can be studied in yeast. Proc Natl Acad Sci USA *85*, 7501–7505.

Nitiss, J.L. (1994). Yeast as a genetic model system for studying topoisomerase inhibitors. Advances in Pharmacology *29B*, 201–226.

Nitiss, J.L. (2009). DNA topoisomerase II and its growing repertoire of biological functions. Nat Rev Cancer *9*, 327–337.

Nitiss, J.L., and Beck, W.T. (1996). Antitopoisomerase drug action and resistance. Eur J Cancer *32A*, 958–966.

Nitiss, J.L., Liu, Y.X., Harbury, P., Jannatipour, M., Wasserman, R., and Wang, J.C. (1992). Amsacrine and etoposide hypersensitivity of yeast cells overexpressing DNA topoisomerase II. Cancer Res *52*, 4467–4472.

Nitiss, J.L., Liu, Y.X., and Hsiung, Y. (1993). A temperature sensitive topoisomerase II allele confers temperature dependent drug resistance on amsacrine and etoposide: a genetic system for determining the targets of topoisomerase II inhibitors. Cancer Res *53*, 89–93.

Nitiss, J.L., Nitiss, K.C., Rose, A., and Waltman, J.L. (2001). Overexpression of type I topoisomerases sensitizes yeast cells to DNA damage. J Biol Chem *276*, 26708–26714.

Nitiss, J.L., Rose, A., Sykes, K.C., Harris, J., and Zhou, J. (1996). Using yeast to understand drugs that target topoisomerases. Ann NY Acad Sci *803*, 32–43.

Nitiss, J.L., and Wang, J.C. (1996). Mechanisms of cell killing by drugs that trap covalent complexes between DNA topoisomerases and DNA. Mol Pharmacol *50*, 1095–1102.

Nitiss, K.C., Malik, M., He, X., White, S.W., and Nitiss, J.L. (2006). Tyrosyl-DNA phosphodiesterase (Tdp1) participates in the repair of Top2-mediated DNA damage. Proc Natl Acad Sci USA *103*, 8953–8958.

Pommier, Y., Laco, G.S., Kohlhagen, G., Sayer, J.M., Kroth, H., and Jerina, D.M. (2000). Position-specific trapping of topoisomerase I-DNA cleavage complexes by intercalated benzo[a]- pyrene diol epoxide adducts at the 6-amino group of adenine. Proc Natl Acad Sci USA *97*, 10739–10744.

Pommier, Y., Minford, J.K., Schwartz, R.E., Zwelling, L.A., and Kohn, K.W. (1985). Effects of the DNA intercalators 4′-(9-acridinylamino)methanesulfon-m- anisidide and 2-methyl-9-hydroxyellipticinium on topoisomerase II mediated DNA strand cleavage and strand passage. Biochemistry *24*, 6410–6416.

Pouliot, J.J., Yao, K.C., Robertson, C.A., and Nash, H.A. (1999). Yeast gene for a Tyr-DNA phosphodiesterase that repairs topoisomerase I complexes. Science *286*, 552–555.

Powell, S.N., and Kachnic, L.A. (2008). Therapeutic exploitation of tumor cell defects in homologous recombination. Anticancer Agents Med Chem *8*, 448–460.

Prakash, S., and Prakash, L. (2000). Nucleotide excision repair in yeast. Mutat Res *451*, 13–24.

Prinz, S., Amon, A., and Klein, F. (1997). Isolation of COM1, a new gene required to complete meiotic double-strand break-induced recombination in Saccharomyces cerevisiae. Genetics *146*, 781–795.

Pype, S., Declercq, W., Ibrahimi, A., Michiels, C., Van Rietschoten, J.G., Dewulf, N., de Boer, M., Vandenabeele, P., Huylebroeck, D., and Remacle, J.E. (2000). TTRAP, a novel protein that associates with CD40, tumor necrosis factor (TNF) receptor-75 and TNF receptor-associated factors (TRAFs), and that inhibits nuclear factor-kappa B activation. J Biol Chem *275*, 18586–18593.

Rehman, F.L., Lord, C.J., and Ashworth, A. (2010). Synthetic lethal approaches to breast cancer therapy. Nat Rev Clin Oncol *7*, 718–724.

Robinson, M.J., Martin, B.A., Gootz, T.D., McGuirk, P.R., Moynihan, M., Sutcliffe, J.A., and Osheroff, N. (1991). Effects of quinolone derivatives on eukaryotic topoisomerase II. A novel mechanism for enhancement of enzyme-mediated DNA cleavage. J Biol Chem *266*, 14585–14592.

Robinson, M.J., and Osheroff, N. (1990). Stabilization of the topoisomerase II-DNA cleavage complex by antineoplastic drugs: inhibition of enzyme-mediated DNA religation by 4′-(9-acridinylamino)methanesulfon-m-anisidide. Biochemistry *29*, 2511–2515.

Rogojina, A.T., and Nitiss, J.L. (2008). Isolation and Characterization of mAMSA-hypersensitive Mutants CYTOTOXICITY OF Top2 COVALENT COMPLEXES CONTAINING DNA SINGLE STRAND BREAKS. Journal of Biological Chemistry *283*, 29239–29250.

Rothstein, R., Michel, B., and Gangloff, S. (2000). Replication fork pausing and recombination or "gimme a break". Genes Dev *14*, 1–10.

Sabourin, M., Nitiss, J.L., Nitiss, K.C., Tatebayashi, K., Ikeda, H., and Osheroff, N. (2003). Yeast recombination pathways triggered by topoisomerase II-mediated DNA breaks. Nucleic Acids Res *31*, 4373–4384.

Sartori, A.A., Lukas, C., Coates, J., Mistrik, M., Fu, S., Bartek, J., Baer, R., Lukas, J., and Jackson, S.P. (2007). Human CtIP promotes DNA end resection. Nature *450*, 509–514.

Schoeffler, A.J., and Berger, J.M. (2008). DNA topoisomerases: harnessing and constraining energy to govern chromosome topology. Q Rev Biophys *41*, 41–101.

Schonn, I., Hennesen, J., and Dartsch, D.C. (2010). Ku70 and Rad51 vary in their importance for the repair of doxorubicin- versus etoposide-induced DNA damage. Apoptosis.

Stepanov, A., Nitiss, K.C., Neale, G., and Nitiss, J.L. (2008). Enhancing drug accumulation in S. cerevisiae by repression of pleiotropic drug resistance genes with chimeric transcription repressors. Mol Pharmacol.

Svejstrup, J.Q. (2003). Rescue of arrested RNA polymerase II complexes. J Cell Sci *116*, 447–451.

Svendsen, J.M., Smogorzewska, A., Sowa, M.E., O'Connell, B.C., Gygi, S.P., Elledge, S.J., and Harper, J.W. (2009). Mammalian BTBD12/SLX4 assembles a Holliday junction resolvase and is required for DNA repair. Cell *138*, 63–77.

Tewey, K.M., Chen, G.L., Nelson, E.M., and Liu, L.F. (1984). Intercalative antitumor drugs interfere with the breakage-reunion reaction of mammalian DNA topoisomerase II. J Biol Chem *259*, 9182–9187.

Treszezamsky, A.D., Kachnic, L.A., Feng, Z., Zhang, J., Tokadjian, C., and Powell, S.N. (2007). BRCA1- and BRCA2-deficient cells are sensitive to etoposide-induced DNA double-strand breaks via topoisomerase II. Cancer Res *67*, 7078–7081.

Vance, J.R., and Wilson, T.E. (2002). Yeast Tdp1 and Rad1-Rad10 function as redundant pathways for repairing Top1 replicative damage. Proc Natl Acad Sci USA *99*, 13669–13674.

Verborg, W.A., Campbell, L.R., Highley, M.S., and Rankin, E.M. (2008). Weekly cisplatin with oral etoposide: a well-tolerated and highly effective regimen in relapsed ovarian cancer. International Journal of Gynecological Cancer *18*, 228–234.

Walker, J.V., and Nitiss, J.L. (2002). DNA topoisomerase II as a target for cancer chemotherapy. Cancer Invest *20*, 570–589.

Wang, J.C. (1998). Moving one DNA double helix through another by a type II DNA topoisomerase: the story of a simple molecular machine. Q Rev Biophys *31*, 107–144.

Westmoreland, T.J., Wickramasekara, S.M., Guo, A.Y., Selim, A.L., Winsor, T.S., Greenleaf, A.L., Blackwell, K.L., Olson, J.A., Jr., Marks, J.R., and Bennett, C.B. (2009). Comparative genome-wide screening identifies a conserved doxorubicin repair network that is diploid specific in Saccharomyces cerevisiae. PLoS One *4*, e5830.

Williams, R.S., and Tainer, J.A. (2007). Learning our ABCs: Rad50 directs MRN repair functions via adenylate kinase activity from the conserved ATP binding cassette. Mol Cell *25*, 789–791.

Winzeler, E.A., Shoemaker, D.D., Astromoff, A., Liang, H., Anderson, K., Andre, B., Bangham, R., Benito, R., Boeke, J.D., Bussey, H., *et al.* (1999). Functional characterization of the S. cerevisiae genome by gene deletion and parallel analysis. Science *285*, 901–906.

Woudstra, E.C., Gilbert, C., Fellows, J., Jansen, L., Brouwer, J., Erdjument Bromage, H., Tempst, P., and Svejstrup, J.Q. (2002). A Rad26-Def1 complex coordinates repair and RNA pol II proteolysis in response to DNA damage. Nature *415*, 929–933.

Yamaguchi-Iwai, Y., Sonoda, E., Sasaki, M.S., Morrison, C., Haraguchi, T., Hiraoka, Y., Yamashita, Y.M., Yagi, T., Takata, M., Price, C., *et al.* (1999). Mre11 is essential for the maintenance of chromosomal DNA in vertebrate cells. EMBO J *18*, 6619–6629.

Yang, S.W., Burgin, A.B., Jr., Huizenga, B.N., Robertson, C.A., Yao, K.C., and Nash, H.A. (1996). A eukaryotic enzyme that can disjoin dead-end covalent complexes between DNA and type I topoisomerases. Proc Natl Acad Sci USA *93*, 11534–11539.

You, Z., and Bailis, J.M. (2010). DNA damage and decisions: CtIP coordinates DNA repair and cell cycle checkpoints. Trends Cell Biol *20*, 402–409.

Zeng, Z., Cortes-Ledesma, F., El-Khamisy, S.F., and Caldecott, K.W. (2010). TDP2/TTRAP is the major 5′-tyrosyl DNA phosphodiesterase activity in vertebrate cells and is critical for cellular resistance to topoisomerase II-induced DNA damage. J Biol Chem.

Zhang, A.L., Lyu, Y.L., Lin, C.P., Zhou, N., Azarova, A.M., Wood, L.M., and Liu, L.F. (2006). A protease pathway for the repair of topoisomerase II-DNA covalent complexes. Journal of Biological Chemistry *281*, 35997–36003.

Zhang, H., D'Arpa, P., and Liu, L.F. (1990). A model for tumor cell killing by topoisomerase poisons. Cancer Cells *2*, 23–27.

Chapter 19
Topoisomerases and Apoptosis

Olivier Sordet and Stéphanie Solier

19.1 Introduction

Topoisomerases are ubiquitous enzymes that induce transient DNA breaks (Champoux 2001; Wang 2002; Pommier et al. 2010) (see Chaps. 1–5). Among them, topoisomerases I (Top1) and II (Top2) are particularly relevant to apoptosis owing to the discovery that they are targeted by a broad range of anticancer drugs (see Chaps. 10–13). Most clinical drugs that target Top1 or Top2 convert the topoisomerase-associated DNA breaks (known as topoisomerase cleavage complexes) into irreversible DNA damage that initiates the apoptotic program (Liu 1989; Pommier 2006; Nitiss 2009). These topoisomerase-targeted drugs, referred to as topoisomerase poisons, stabilize the topoisomerase cleavage complexes by preventing DNA religation (Pommier et al. 2010). Camptothecins are highly specific and selective Top1 inhibitors (Pommier 2006, 2009) and among the Top2 inhibitors, the most specific are etoposide and its derivative teniposide (Nitiss 2009). Besides their role in the initiation of apoptosis, recent studies showed that Top1 and Top2 participate directly in the execution of the apoptotic program (Sordet et al. 2004b, 2007; Samejima and Earnshaw 2005).

This chapter focuses on the role of topoisomerases in both the induction and the execution of apoptosis. We will first describe the apoptotic pathways activated by topoisomerase inhibitors-mediated DNA damage. Emphasis will be given to the transmission of the apoptotic signal from the nucleus (DNA lesions) to the cytoplasm

O. Sordet (✉)
Cancer Research Center of Toulouse, INSERM-Université de Toulouse UMR1037,
Institut Claudius Regaud, 20-24 rue du Pont-Saint-Pierre, 31052, Toulouse Cedex, France
e-mail: olivier.sordet@inserm.fr

S. Solier (✉)
Laboratory of Molecular Pharmacology, Center for Cancer Research,
National Cancer Institute, National Institutes of Health,
37 Convent Drive, Bethesda, MD 20892-4255, USA
e-mail: soliers@mail.nih.gov

Y. Pommier (ed.), *DNA Topoisomerases and Cancer*, Cancer Drug Discovery and Development, DOI 10.1007/978-1-4614-0323-4_19,

(mitochondrial permeabilization). Then, we will review the current knowledge on the role of topoisomerases in nuclear dismantling during the execution of apoptosis.

19.2 DNA Damage Induced by Topoisomerase Inhibitors

Top1 cleavage complexes (Top1cc) are readily reversible after camptothecin removal, and short exposures to camptothecin (for less than 1 h) are relatively non-cytotoxic (Covey et al. 1989; Tanizawa et al. 1994; Goldwasser et al. 1996). Persistent camptothecin exposure is required to induce apoptosis, as Top1cc are converted into irreversible DNA lesions by cellular metabolism (Holm et al. 1989; Hsiang, Lihou and Liu 1989) (Fig. 19.1). During replication, stalled Top1cc are

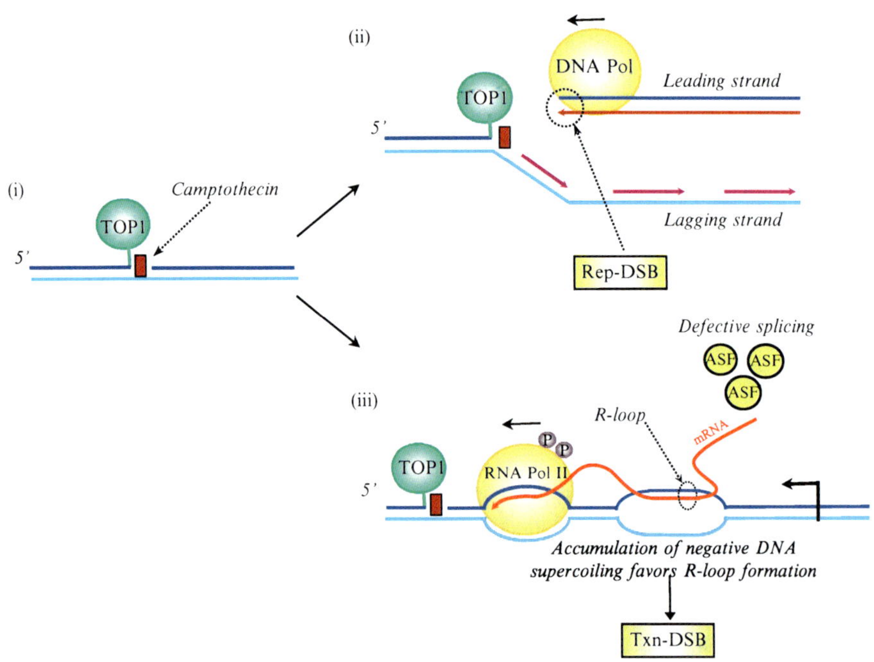

Fig. 19.1 Conversion of stabilized Top1cc into DSBs during replication and transcription. (i) Schematic representation of a Top1cc trapped by camptothecin. Top1 is covalently bound to the 3′-end of the broken DNA. (ii) When a trapped Top1cc is on the leading strand (*dark blue*) for DNA synthesis, DNA polymerase elongates the nascent leading strand (*red*) up to the last base flanking the Top1cc, thereby generating a replication double-strand break (Rep-DSB). (iii) When a trapped Top1cc is on the transcribed strand, RNA polymerase II arrests RNA elongation (*orange*) and becomes hyperphosphorylated. A hybrid RNA-DNA (R-loop) forms behind the arrested RNA polymerase II generating a transcription double-strand break (Txn-DSB). R-loops may form as negative supercoiling, which facilitates DNA strand opening, accumulates behind the transcription complexes arrested by Top1cc. Inhibition of Top1 SR-kinase activity by camptothecin may also promote R-loops by interfering with splicing because of ASF hypophosphorylation [for reviews, see (Pommier 2006; Sordet et al. 2010)]

converted to DNA double-strand breaks (DSBs) by "replication run-off" (Strumberg et al. 2000) as the leading strand is replicated up to the last nucleotide at the 5′ end of the Top1cc (Fig. 19.1). Transcription arrest by stalled Top1cc (Bendixen et al. 1990; Wu and Liu 1997; Capranico et al. 2007; Sordet et al. 2008b) also leads to DSBs by an R-loop-dependent mechanism (Sordet et al. 2009, 2010; French et al. 2011) (Fig. 19.1). R-loops are RNA-DNA hybrids known to induce DSBs and genomic instability (Huertas and Aguilera 2003; Li and Manley 2005). They result from the extended pairing of nascent mRNA with the corresponding unwound DNA template behind the elongating RNA polymerase II (Huertas and Aguilera 2003). The transcription-dependent DSBs associated with Top1cc have been detected in postmitotic primary neurons and lymphocytes (Sordet et al. 2009), as well as in the non-S phase population of dividing cells (Sordet et al. 2009; Sakasai et al., 2010).

Replication-mediated DSBs seem to be the primary cytotoxic mechanism of Top1 inhibitors in dividing cells. Indeed, cancer cells in culture tend to be resistant to camptothecin when they are outside of S-phase (Horwitz and Horwitz 1973; O'Connor et al. 1991) or when replication is arrested at the time of camptothecin treatment (Holm et al. 1989; Hsiang et al. 1989). It is only at high (>1 μM) concentrations that the cytotoxicity of camptothecin becomes independent of replication (Holm et al. 1989; O'Connor et al. 1991). Nevertheless, transcription-dependent DSBs associated with Top1cc (Sordet et al. 2009) can induce apoptosis in postmitotic cells such as neurons (Morris and Geller 1996) and lymphocytes (O. Sordet and Y. Pommier, unpublished observations).

Trapped Top2cc by Top2 inhibitors (e.g., etoposide) correspond to DSBs that are concealed with the Top2 heterodimeric complex and covalently linked to Top2 at their 5′-ends (Nelson et al. 1984; Tewey et al. 1984; Long et al. 1985; Kerrigan et al. 1987; Covey et al. 1988; Pommier et al. 2010) (see Chaps. 3 and 11). The DSBs associated with Top2cc do not require ongoing DNA replication (Holm et al. 1989) and have been detected in postmitotic neurons (Zhang et al. 2006).

19.3 Sensing DNA Damage Induced by Topoisomerase Inhibitors

After DNA damage occurs, the lesions activate the checkpoint proteins and the effector pathways for DNA repair, cell cycle arrest, and/or apoptosis (Kastan and Bartek 2004; Jackson and Bartek 2009). "DNA sensors" allow the detection of lesions. They bind to (or at the proximity of) DNA lesions and activate checkpoint and repair proteins. DNA sensors activated by topoisomerase-mediated DNA damage include the kinases ATM, ATR, and DNA-PK (Pommier 2006; Nitiss 2009). The DNA-PK (DNA-dependent Protein Kinase) complex consists of the Ku heterodimer (Ku70 and Ku80) and the large catalytic serine-threonine kinase subunit (DNA-PKcs) (Mimori et al. 1986; Meek et al. 2008). Ku initially binds to the two ends of a double-strand break, each of which then recruits DNA-PKcs. DNA-PK can regulate end access both positively and negatively, via distinct autophosphorylations with opposite effects on DNA end access. Some autophosphorylations of

DNA-PK can also impact on its kinase activity and complex dissociation. Moreover, the phosphorylation status of DNA-PK can affect repair pathway choice (NHEJ or HR) (Meek et al. 2008). ATM (Ataxia Telangiectasia Mutated) is recruited very rapidly to the damaged site, initially associating with DNA regions that flank the break, before associating with the MRN (Mre11-Rad50-Nbs1) complex, which facilitates the full activation of ATM and amplifies its localization to DNA breaks (Berkovich et al. 2007; Lavin 2008). ATR (Ataxia Telangiectasia and Rad 3-related) is associated with replication complexes and is activated by replication-associated DSBs and single-stranded DNA regions (Sordet et al. 2003; MacDougall et al. 2007; Kinner et al. 2008).

DNA-PK, ATM, and ATR mediate their proapoptotic effects by phosphorylating a large number of substrates, including p53 and Chk2, which can activate by themselves apoptosis.

19.4 Mitochondrial and Plasma Membrane Death Receptor Pathways Are Activated by Topoisomerase-Mediated DNA Damage

Topoisomerase inhibitors are among the most efficient inducers of apoptosis (Solary et al. 1994; Kaufmann 1998; Sordet et al. 2003). They mainly activate the intrinsic pathway, and in some cell types, the extrinsic pathway. The intrinsic pathway implicates the mitochondria and the formation of the apoptosome that contains cytochrome c, the apoptosis protease-activating factor-1 (Apaf-1) and caspase-9 (Green 2005). The extrinsic pathway or death receptor-dependent pathway implicates the formation of the death-inducing signaling complex (DISC) that contains the adaptor protein Fas-associated death domain (FADD) and caspase-8 (Johnstone et al. 2008; Taylor et al. 2008). Both pathways share the effector caspases (caspase-3, caspase-6, and caspase-7), which cleave intracellular substrates to elicit the biochemical and morphological apoptotic changes (Fig. 19.2).

We will first describe the main signaling pathway leading from topoisomerase-mediated DNA damage to apoptosis, which is the one that involves mitochondria; and in a second part we will introduce the pathway involving the death receptors.

19.4.1 The Mitochondrial Intrinsic Pathway

Most chemotherapeutic drugs, including Top1 and Top2 inhibitors, increase the permeability of the outer mitochondrial membrane (OMM) as they induce apoptosis (Solary et al. 2000, 2001; Sordet et al. 2001). This process is under the control of the Bcl-2 family that includes more than 30 anti-apoptotic and pro-apoptotic molecules

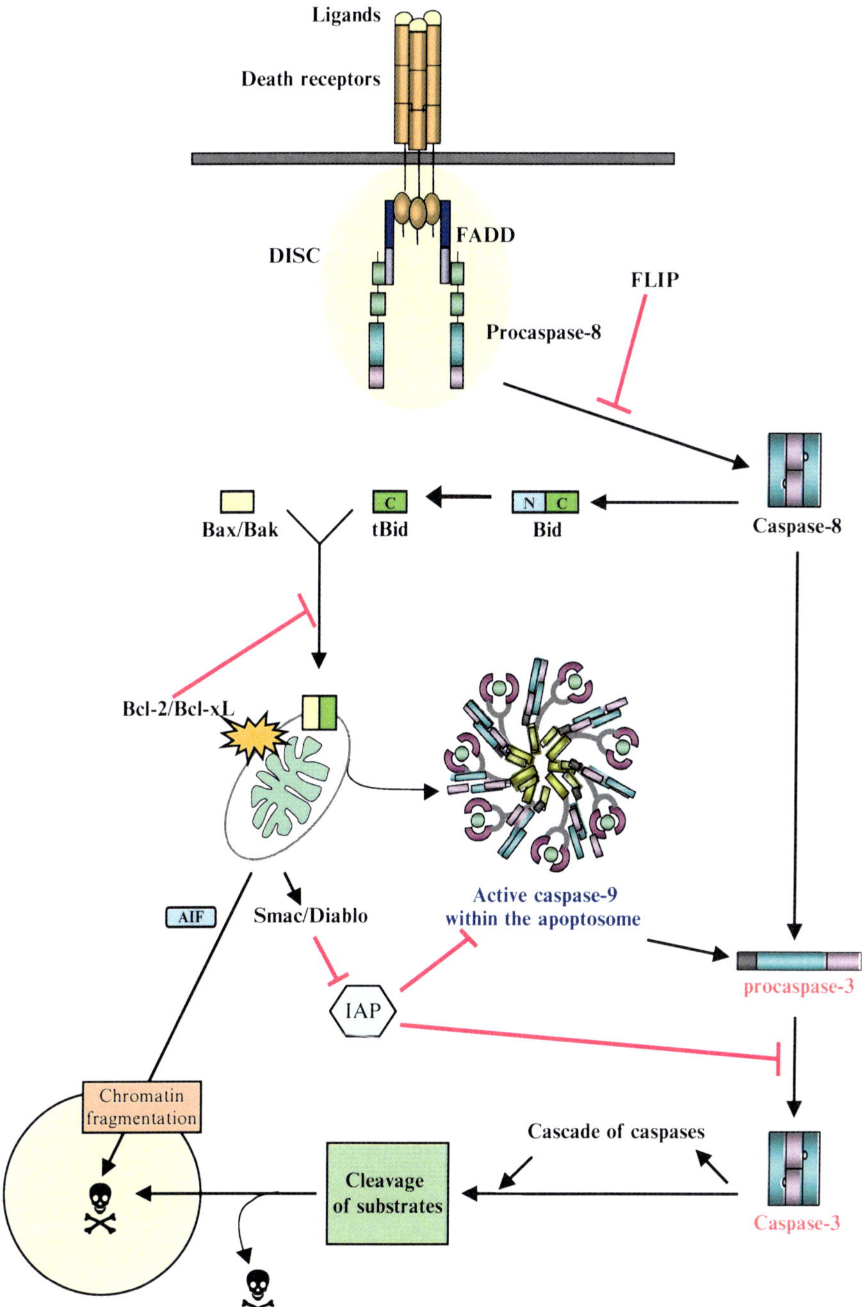

Fig. 19.2 Apoptotic pathways activated by topoisomerase-mediated DNA damage

characterized by the presence of one to four conserved Bcl-2 homology (BH) domains (BH1 to BH4) (Green and Kroemer 2004; Chipuk et al. 2010; Tait and Green 2010). The anti-apoptotic proteins (e.g., Bcl-2, Bcl-xL, Bcl-2A1, Bcl-w, Mcl-1) preserve the OMM integrity. The pro-apoptotic proteins are divided into the effectors "multidomains" proteins (e.g., Bax, Bak) and the BH3-only proteins (e.g., Bad, Noxa, Bid, Bim). Bad and Noxa interact with the anti-apoptotic Bcl-2 proteins whereas Bid and Bim can interact with both the anti-apoptotic Bcl-2 proteins and the pro-apoptotic Bax and Bak proteins. Bax (Bcl-2 associated X protein) and Bak (Bcl-2 antagonist or killer) are essential for mitochondrial outer membrane permeabilization (MOMP). Following activation, Bax and Bak undergo conformational changes that target Bax to mitochondria and promote homo-oligomerization of Bak and Bax (Hsu et al. 1997; Eskes et al. 2000; Wei et al. 2000; Tait and Green 2010). Ku70, in addition to its involvement in DNA repair, can suppress the apoptotic translocation of Bax to mitochondria (Sawada et al. 2003). Histone H1.2, released from the nucleus upon X-ray-induced DNA damage, can trigger MOMP in a Bak-dependent manner (Konishi et al. 2003; Green and Kroemer 2004). p53, in addition to be a transcriptional regulator of multiple apoptotic genes, exerts a direct mitochondrial pro-apoptotic role by engaging in protein–protein interactions with anti- and pro-apoptotic Bcl-2 family members (Moll et al. 2006). The transcription factor Nur77 becomes a potent killer when certain death stimuli induce its migration to mitochondria, where it binds to Bcl-2 and conformationally converts it to a killer that triggers cytochrome c release and apoptosis (Moll et al. 2006). After DNA damage, Rad9 can also traffic to mitochondria, interact with Bcl-2 and Bcl-xL, and induce apoptosis (Komatsu et al. 2000; Yoshida et al. 2002). It is noteworthy, that MOMP is under the control of the Bcl-2 proteins but equally involve mitochondrial lipids that regulate bioenergetic metabolite flux, and components of the permeability transition pore (Green and Kroemer 2004).

MOMP allows soluble molecules to diffuse from the mitochondrial intermembrane space into the cytosol. These molecules include AIF (apoptosis inducing factor) and endonuclease G, which after migration to the nucleus induce chromatin condensation and DNA fragmentation. Other mitochondrial proteins also cooperate in the cytosol to activate caspases (cytochrome c, Smac–Diablo and Htra2–Omi) (Tait and Green 2010). Cytochrome c engages Apaf-1 to oligomerize in the presence of ATP (Li et al. 1997). Apaf-1 oligomers recruit procaspase-9 in a complex termed the "apoptosome" where juxtaposition of procaspase-9 molecules results in autoactivation (Srinivasula et al. 1998; Saleh et al. 1999). Mature caspase-9 activates additional caspase-9 molecules as well as caspase-3 and caspase-7. In turn, caspase-3 activates downstream caspases in a proteolytic cascade (Slee et al. 1999). Smac–Diablo and Htra2–Omi, released simultaneously with cytochrome c, neutralize the inhibitors of apoptosis protein (IAPs) family. Some of these IAPs associate with procaspase-9, caspase-3, and caspase-7 to inhibit their proteolytic activity, at least in part by triggering their proteosomal degradation after ubiquitinylation (Vaux and Silke 2003). Mitochondrial caspases and some heat shock proteins (Hsp60 and Hsp10) are also released from mitochondria and facilitate the activation of caspase-3 (Samali et al. 1999). Caspase-2 plays a role upstream of MOMP (Kumar 2009).

19.4.2 The Extrinsic Plasma Membrane Receptor Pathway

In some cell types, apoptosis implicates the membrane death receptor Fas (also known as APO-1 and CD95). Fas is a member of the tumor necrosis factor (TNF) family. Cross-linking of Fas by its natural ligand (FasL) induces the clustering of Fas, which in turn recruits the adaptor protein FADD (Chinnaiyan et al. 1995) that links to procaspase-8 (Medema et al. 1997) to form the DISC. When oligomerized in the DISC, procaspase-8 auto-activates (Salvesen and Dixit 1999). DISC-activated caspase-8 engages apoptosis by two different pathways depending on the cell type (Scaffidi et al. 1998). In type I cells, DISC assembly is sufficient for caspase-8 to cleave and activate downstream effector caspases. In type II cells, DISC assembly activates smaller amounts of caspase-8 and requires amplification of the apoptotic signal through the mitochondrial apoptotic pathway. Activation of this mitochondrial amplification loop is achieved through cleavage of Bid, a proapoptotic member of the Bcl-2 family. Cleaved Bid binds to and activates Bax and Bak, which causes the release of apoptogenic factors such as cytochrome c from mitochondria. In turn, cytochrome c activates effector caspases via Apaf-1 and caspase 9 in the apoptosome (Li et al. 1998; Luo et al. 1998) (Fig. 19.2).

Top1 and Top2 inhibitors can activate the extrinsic pathway by enhancing the expression of Fas and FasL (Chatterjee et al. 2001; Shao et al. 2001; Ciusani et al. 2002; Menendez et al. 2006). At least in some cell types, this upregulation is transcription-dependent and implicates p53 (Muller et al. 1998). Binding of FasL to Fas at the cell surface defines an autocrine-paracrine pathway similar to that observed in activation-induced cell death in T lymphocytes. However, the role of FasL in drug-induced apoptosis is probably not essential because antagonist antibodies or molecules that prevent FasL interaction with Fas do not suppress apoptosis (Eischen et al. 1997; Shao et al. 2001). Anticancer drugs can induce Fas clustering at the cell surface of tumor cells in the absence of FasL (Micheau et al. 1997). This clustering could take place in lipid rafts at the plasma membrane (Lacour et al. 2004). However, apoptosis induced by topoisomerase inhibitors is not altered in embryonic fibroblasts from FADD and caspase-8 knockout mice indicating only a partial role for the death receptor pathway (Varfolomeev et al. 1998; Yeh et al. 1998).

In summary, topoisomerase inhibitors mainly induce apoptosis by the intrinsic (mitochondrial) pathway. This pathway can be amplified, at least in some cell types, by the transmembrane extrinsic pathway. The following section will provide examples of molecules that transmit apoptotic signals from the nucleus (DNA lesions) to the cytoplasm (mitochondria) (Fig. 19.3).

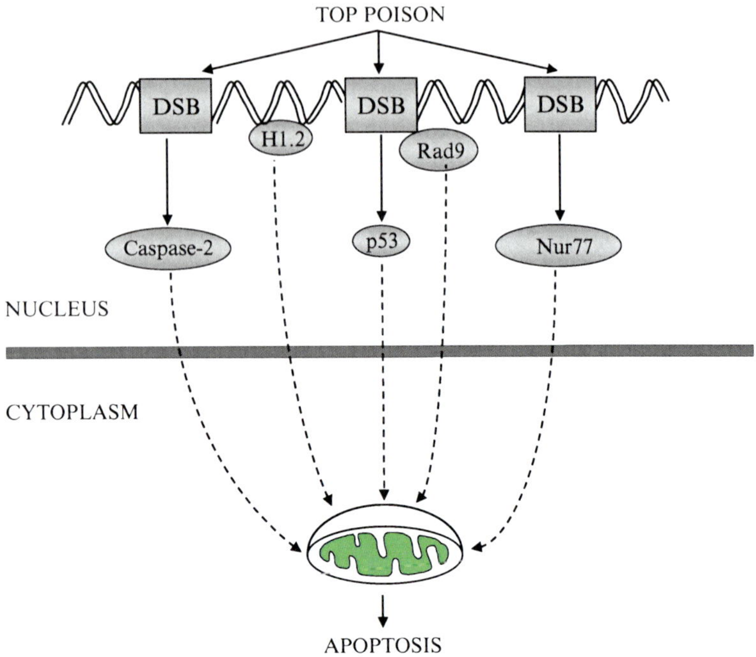

Fig. 19.3 Transmission of topoisomerase inhibitors-mediated DNA damage signals from the nucleus to mitochondria

19.5 From DNA Damage in the Nucleus to Apoptosis in the Cytoplasm

As discussed above, ATM (and also ATR and DNA-PK) responds preferentially to the DSBs produced by Top1 and Top2 cleavage complexes. At least four known substrates of ATM are implicated in apoptosis: p53, Chk2, E2F1, and c-Abl (http://discover.nci.nih.gov/mim/view.jsp?MIM=ATMChk2&selection=map) [see also (Sordet et al. 2003)]. ATM phosphorylates–activates directly p53 and E2F1 thereby enhancing their stability and transcriptional activity. ATM can also activate p53 and E2F1 indirectly by phosphorylating-–activating the checkpoint kinase Chk2. The third Chk2 substrate implicated in apoptosis is PML. ATM also phosphorylates–activates c-Abl. PML-, c-Abl-, and E2F1-mediated apoptosis can occur through both p53-dependent and p53-independent pathways. Thus, apoptosis induced by topoisomerase inhibitors can schematically be divided into a p53-dependent manner and–or p53-independent manner.

19.5.1 p53-Dependent Apoptosis

p53 is a transcription factor (Green and Kroemer 2009; Menendez et al. 2009) for a set of genes encoding the pro-apoptotic proteins from the Bcl-2 family (Bax, Bid, Noxa, and Puma). Puma also controls the sequestration of cytoplasmic p53 by the anti-apoptotic Bcl-xL protein, releasing p53 to activate Bax (Chipuk et al. 2005; Green and Kroemer 2009); consequently, without transcription, regulated by nuclear p53, endogenous cytoplasmic p53 may not function (Green and Kroemer 2009). p53 also induces the apoptosis-associated speck-like protein (ASC) that associates with Bax and promotes its translocation to mitochondria where it induces the release of cytochrome c (Ohtsuka et al. 2004). Several other mitochondria-targeting proteins are induced by p53. Some of these, such as ferrodoxin reductase (Yang et al. 2006), are involved in the production of reactive oxygen species (ROS), while others induce mitochondrial permeabilization. These proteins include p53-regulated apoptosis-inducing protein-1 (p53AIP1), chloride intracellular channel 4 (CLIC4), p53-induced protein with a death domain (PIDD; implicated in caspase-2 activation; see below). p53AIP1 plays a role in mediating p53-dependent apoptosis, and p53 phosphorylation at Ser-46 regulates the transcriptional activation of this apoptosis-inducing gene (Oda et al. 2000; Ekert and Vaux 2005). CLIC4 can be cytoplasmic or mitochondrial. Cytoplasmic CLIC4 translocates to the nucleus in response to DNA damage, and this translocation is associated with apoptosis (Suh et al. 2007). Mitochondrial CLIC4, which associates with the inner mitochondrial membrane is upregulated after DNA damage and also induces apoptosis (Fernandez-Salas et al. 2002). In addition, p53 can upregulate Fas, which in turn may play a role in the activation of Apaf-1 and caspase-9 (Shinoura et al. 2002). p53 induces scotin, a pro-apoptotic protein localized in the endoplasmic reticulum and the nuclear membrane (Bourdon et al. 2002). On the other hand, p53 represses the transcription of the anti-apoptotic proteins Bcl-2 (Miyashita et al. 1994) and survivin (an IAP that prevents caspase activity and regulates cell cycle) (Hoffman et al. 2002).

p53 also induces apoptosis in a transcription-independent manner by directly targeting mitochondria (Fig. 19.3). After DNA damage, a fraction of p53 is exported from the nucleus and binds to the OMM (Mihara et al. 2003). Mitochondrial p53 binds to Bcl-2 and Bcl-xL and neutralizes their inhibitory effect on Bak (and Bax), resulting in Bax oligomerization and subsequent mitochondrial permeabilization (Mihara et al. 2003). Bcl-2 and Bcl-xL interact with the DNA-binding region of p53, the same region that harbors the vast majority of "hot spots" mutations in human cancer cells. Thus, some p53 mutations that interfere with DNA binding also interfere with p53 binding to Bcl-2 and Bcl-xL. In addition, p53 itself can bind to DNA strand breaks and might be therefore involved in DNA damage detection and repair (Bakalkin et al. 1994).

A specific isoform of the linker histone, histone H1.2, has also been reported to localize to mitochondria following DSBs (Yan and Shi 2003) (Fig. 19.3). This process requires the stabilization of p53 by Chk2 but is independent of p53 transcriptional activity (Chen et al. 2005). Mitochondria H1.2 induces conformational activation and oligomerization of Bak. In mitochondria isolated from Bak-deficient cells, H1.2 fails to induce cytochrome c release (Konishi et al. 2003; Okamura et al. 2008). The mechanism for H1.2 to cause the conformational change of Bak and the subsequent cytochrome c release remains to be determined. H1.2 seems to play also a role downstream of the mitochondria by interacting with the apoptosome and promoting caspase-3 and −7 activation (Ruiz-Vela and Korsmeyer 2007). H1.2 appears to respond specifically to DSBs as downregulation of H1.2 by antisense RNA or small interfering RNA (siRNA) reduces apoptosis induced by X-rays or the Top2 inhibitor etoposide, but not by TNF-α or UV radiation (Konishi et al. 2003).

Procaspase-2 might also link DNA damage and mitochondria (Lassus et al. 2002) (Fig. 19.3). The "PIDDosome," a molecular complex containing PIDD, whose expression is induced by p53, and RAIDD–CRAIDD, an adaptor protein with a death domain, activate procaspase-2 in the nucleus (Tinel and Tschopp 2004; Baptiste-Okoh et al. 2008). Increased PIDD expression results in spontaneous activation of procaspase-2 and sensitization to apoptosis by genotoxic stress (Tinel and Tschopp 2004; Baptiste-Okoh et al. 2008). In the nucleus, juxtaposition of procaspase-2 molecules (dimerization) results in auto-cleavage–activation (Baliga et al. 2003), a similar mechanism of activation to the initiator procaspase-8 and procaspase-9. Release of mature caspase-2 can stimulate directly mitochondrial release of cytochrome c. This process requires the processing of procaspase-2 but not its enzymatic activity and is also independent of Bax, Bak, and Bcl-2 (Robertson et al. 2004). It is noteworthy that caspase-2 can induce apoptosis independently of p53 when Chk1 is suppressed (Kumar 2009). Moreover, besides its role in apoptosis, caspase-2 has also a role in promoting G2–M arrest and DNA repair by NHEJ in response to DSBs (Kumar 2009).

Nam et al. showed that the Top2 inhibitor, etoposide, induces G2–M arrest and apoptosis in neural progenitor cells via an ATM–p53-related pathway (Nam et al. 2010). p53-mediated cell cycle arrest response might in some cases antagonize the p53-mediated apoptotic response. Activation of p21, which was among the first isolated p53-dependent genes (El-Deiry et al. 1993), induces both cell cycle arrest in response to low doses of camptothecin and blocks DNA damage-induced apoptosis (Gupta et al. 1997; Han et al. 2002). p53 may selectively induce apoptosis in cells with elevated E2F1 activity, such as pRb-deficient cells. p53 binds to the cyclin A box of E2F1, and this complex induces apoptosis when cyclin A is low (Hsieh et al. 2002). E2F1, like p53, is negatively regulated by Mdm2, and both E2F1 and p53 are upregulated in response to DNA damage (Blattner et al. 1999). p53 may also specifically promote apoptosis when it is transcribed as an N-terminal truncated variant, designated p53–47. In contrast to p53, p53–47 lacks the Mdm2-binding domain. Thus Mdm2 expression increases the ratio p53–47 to p53. P53–47 has a different gene expression profile: upregulation of Bax and downregulation of p21 (Yin et al. 2002). It is therefore possible that specific modifications of p53 might selectively activate one set of genes or the other. The pleiotropic regulation of p53 (Kohn and Pommier 2005) could allow fine tuned adjustments of p53 levels and p53 phosphorylation (depending on the intensity of DNA damage), which could account for the selectivity of p53 for transactivating cell cycle arrest and/or apoptotic genes.

19.5.2 p53-Independent Apoptosis

In spite of the apparent pivotal role of p53 in apoptosis (Chipuk and Green 2006), the p53-null leukemia cells HL60 and U937 undergo apoptosis readily in response to topoisomerase inhibitors (Bertrand et al. 1991, 1993, 1994; Solary et al. 1993, 1994; Shimizu and Pommier 1997; Sordet et al. 1999, 2001). In these cells, the p53-related protein p73 does not compensate the lack of p53 since apoptosis is also transcription-independent. Moreover, more than 50% of human tumors contain mutated and defective p53. Although such tumors might be defective in their apoptotic response in vivo, experiments performed in cell cultures demonstrate that these tumors can readily undergo apoptosis in response to topoisomerase inhibitors (Solary et al. 1994; Nieves-Neira and Pommier 1999). p53-independent apoptosis involves the receptor Nur77 and the checkpoint kinase Rad9 that target directly mitochondria in response to DNA damage, and also the DNA repair protein Ku70 (see above). Other p53-independent pathways include Chk2, E2F1, PML, and c-Abl [for review see (Sordet et al. 2003; Pommier et al. 2006)].

The orphan receptor Nur77 (also known as TR3 or NGFI-B) is a transcription factor of the steroid–thyroid receptor superfamily. Nur77 is involved in promoting cell proliferation (Kolluri et al. 2003). It is also a critical inducer of apoptosis [for review see (Zhang 2007)]. *Nur77* gene is rapidly induced by different inducers of apoptosis, and overexpression of a dominant-negative Nur77 protein (Woronicz et al. 1994) or inhibition of Nur77 expression by antisense Nur77 mRNA (Liu et al. 1994) inhibits apoptosis. By contrast, constitutive expression of Nur77 induces apoptosis (Xue et al. 1997). Although the mitogenic effect of Nur77 occurs in the nucleus through target gene regulation, the pro-apoptotic effect of Nur77 occurs in the cytoplasm independently of its transactivating activity. In response to various apoptotic stimuli, including DSBs, Nur77 translocates from the nucleus to the cytoplasm (Liu et al. 2002) (Fig. 19.3). Phosphorylation of the N-terminal domain of Nur77 by JNK (Han et al. 2006) and at Ser-354 by ribosomal S6 kinase (RSK) (Wang et al. 2009), together with inhibition of Akt phosphorylation of Nur77 at Ser-105 (Han et al. 2006) contribute to Nur77 nuclear export. In the cytoplasm, Nur77 targets mitochondria where it induces the mitochondrial release of cytochrome c and apoptosis (Li et al. 2000). The binding of Nur77 to retinoic X receptor-α (RXRα) is required for Nur77 nuclear export and mitochondrial targeting in response to apoptotic stimuli (Cao et al. 2004). Despite lacking classical mitochondria-targeting sequences, Nur77 relocates to mitochondria by binding to anti-apoptotic members of the Bcl-2 family including Bcl-2 itself (Lin et al. 2004), Bcl-B and Bfl-1 (Luciano et al. 2007). At the mitochondria, the interaction of Nur77 to Bcl-2 causes a Bcl-2 conformational change that exposes its pro-apoptotic BH3 domain (Lin et al. 2004). Nur77 could therefore activate the apoptotic mitochondrial pathway by converting Bcl-2, and probably also Bcl-B and Bfl-1, from anti-apoptotic to pro-apoptotic members of the Bcl-2 family.

Another molecule that directly targets mitochondria is the cell cycle checkpoint Rad9 (Fig. 19.3). Rad9 is loaded as a complex with Hus1 and Rad1 (known as 9-1-1 complex) onto damaged chromatin by a clamp loader consisting of Rad17 and replication factor C (Roos-Mattjus et al. 2002). The 9-1-1 complex promotes the phosphorylation/activation of Chk1 by ATR, which in turn induces cell cycle arrest and survival. Following DNA damage, Rad9 can also migrate from the nucleus to mitochondria where the N-terminal BH3-like domain of Rad9 interacts with Bcl-2 and Bcl-xL, which induces apoptosis (Komatsu et al. 2000; Ishii et al. 2005). Dual phosphorylation of Rad9 by c-Abl (Yoshida et al. 2002) (which is itself activated by ATM) and PKCδ (Yoshida et al. 2003) are important for the binding of Rad9 to Bcl-2 and Bcl-xL. The cleavage of Rad-9 by caspase-3 has been involved in Rad9 nuclear export and apoptosis in response to DNA damage (Lee et al. 2003). Caspase-3-mediated cleavage of Rad-9 generates an N-terminal fragment that still possesses the BH3-like domain and binds to Bcl-xL (Lee et al. 2003). Because the N- and the C-terminal domains of Rad9 interact with Rad1 and Hus1, respectively (Burtelow et al. 2001), it is likely that caspase-mediated cleavage of Rad9 disrupts the 9-1-1 complex and therefore prevents cell cycle arrest and repair in cells undergoing apoptosis. Thus, Rad9 seems to have two opposite functions: 1/ cell survival by activation of Chk1 and cell cycle arrest, and 2/ cell death by activation of the proapoptotic Bcl-2 proteins. The predominant role of Rad9 is likely to promote cell survival after topoisomerase inhibitors-mediated DNA damage since *Rad9−/−* ES cells are hypersensitive to camptothecin and etoposide (Loegering et al. 2004).

Ku70 is a protein that acts as part of a heterodimer with Ku80 in the repair of DSBs by the nonhomologous end-joining (NHEJ) pathway (Lieber et al. 2003). In addition to its nuclear localization, Ku70 resides in the cytoplasm where it regulates Bax-mediated apoptosis, independently of Ku80 [for review, see (Nothwehr and Martinou 2003)]. Bax ubiquitylation negatively regulates its pro-apoptotic functions by targeting it for proteosomal degradation (Amsel et al. 2008). Under normal growth conditions, cytosolic Ku70 interacts with and de-ubiquitylates Bax preventing its degradation. Binding of Bax to Ku70 also prevents Bax mitochondrial localization and pro-apoptotic activity (Nothwehr and Martinou 2003; Sawada et al. 2003). In response to apoptotic stimuli, un-ubiquitinylated Bax is released from Ku70 (Sawada et al. 2003). Acetylation of Ku70 by the acetyl transferases 300–CBP and PCAF–GCN5 has been involved in this dissociation (Cohen et al. 2004). Nbs1, a component of the MRN (Mre11–Rad50–Nbs1) complex involved in ATM activation by DSBs (Lee and Paull 2005), also promotes the dissociation of Bax from Ku (Iijima et al. 2008). The release of Bax from Ku70 causes Bax to form a large complex, called the "baxosome," containing Bax itself, BH3-only proteins, cardiolipin, and probably other unidentified proteins. In the baxosome, Bax undergoes conformational changes, allowing its insertion into the OMM, where it promotes the release of cytochrome c and other proapoptotic molecules. Because Ku70 accumulates following DSBs, it is possible that Ku70 would prevent Bax from inducing premature apoptosis (if the cell can still repair). However, beyond a certain threshold of DNA damage, Ku70 might release Bax to induce apoptosis.

The relative importance of these pathways in p53-deficient cells is not known. Thus, it will be interesting to use genetically altered cells and /or selective pharmacological inhibitors to determine the relative contribution of each of these pathways.

19.6 Impact of Topoisomerases on the Splicing of Apoptotic Genes Can Regulate Apoptosis

Several studies have shown the implication of Top1 in splicing. First, Rossi et al. demonstrated that Top1 can phosphorylate the SR splicing proteins (Rossi et al. 1996; Tazi et al. 1997), and two domains of Top1 were implicated in this activity: one as an ATP-binding site in the carboxy-terminal region of Top1 and the other as a binding site for SF2–ASF and a protein kinase domain in the amino-terminal region of Top1 (Tazi et al. 1997). The induction of Top1cc by camptothecin has been shown to impact on RNA splicing (Solier et al. 2004, 2008, 2010; Shkreta et al. 2008; Eisenreich et al. 2009). Transcription could regulate alternative splicing by modulation of RNA polymerase II elongation rates (kinetic coupling) (de la Mata et al. 2003) and by the association of splicing factors to the transcribing polymerase (recruitment coupling) (de la Mata and Kornblihtt 2006; Solier et al. 2010). Camptothecin has been shown to impact on the splicing of apoptotic genes (Solier et al. 2004, 2008, 2010; Shkreta et al. 2008). For example, concerning caspase-2, camptothecin decreases the *CASP-2 L–CASP-2 S* ratio, therefore decreasing the pro-apoptotic isoform (Solier et al. 2004, 2008, 2010). The Top2 inhibitor etoposide can also impact on the splicing of caspase-2 (Solier et al. 2004, 2008), probably by the fact that during mitosis, Top2 is associated with the kinase SRPK1 (serine–arginine-rich protein-specific kinase-1) and some splicing factors (PRP8, hnRNP C) within the toposome (Borowiec 2004; Lee et al. 2004).

19.7 Role of Topoisomerases as Nuclear Effectors of Apoptosis

Besides the role of Top1 and Top2 in the initiation of apoptosis, recent studies have revealed their participation in the execution of the apoptotic program.

Stabilization of Top1-DNA covalent complexes has been observed in cells undergoing apoptosis. These cleavage complexes termed "apoptotic Top1cc" have been detected in different mammalian cells exposed to a wide range of apoptotic inducers, which by themselves do not act directly as Top1 inhibitors (Soe et al. 2004; Sordet et al. 2004a, c, 2006, 2008a; Ganguly et al. 2007; Rockstroh et al. 2007) [for reviews, see (Sordet et al. 2004b, 2007)]. Table 19.1 summarizes the various agents that have been identified as producing apoptotic Top1cc. The formation of apoptotic Top1cc is conserved in the parasite *Leshmania donovani* (Sen et al. 2007). Hence, stabilization of Top1cc appears as a general response of cells undergoing apoptosis.

The formation of apoptotic Top1cc is likely related to DNA alterations produced during apoptosis that interfere with Top1's nicking-closing activities. Indeed, oxidative DNA lesions, which are known to readily stabilize Top1cc (Pourquier et al. 1999; Pourquier and Pommier 2001; Daroui et al. 2004; Dexheimer et al. 2008) (see Chap. 6), are produced in apoptotic cells as a result of ROS accumulation, and modulation of ROS levels is directly correlated with the formation of apoptotic Top1cc (Sordet

Table 19.1 Agents known to induce apoptotic Top1cc

Agents	Cellular target(s)	References
Etoposide, Doxorubicin, m-AMSA	Stabilization of Top2cc	Sordet Goldman and Pommier. (2006)
Vinblatine, Taxol, Colcemid	Binding at the interface of the tubulin heterodimer	Sordet Goldman and Pommier. (2006); Rockstroh et al. (2007)
TRAIL	Binds to and activates the plasma membrane receptors DR4 and DR5	Rockstroh et al. (2007); Sordet et al. (2008a)
Fas ligand	Binds to and activates the plasma membrane receptors Fas	
TNF-α	Binds to and activates the plasma membrane receptors TNFR1	
Antimycin, BH3I-2′	BH3 mimetics that bind to and inhibit the antiapoptotic effect of Bcl-xL at the mitochondria	Sordet et al. (2008a)
Arsenic trioxide	Induces the intracellular accumulation of ROS	Sordet et al. (2004c)
Staurosporine	Inhibitor of protein kinases: Chk1, Chk2, PDK1, PKC	Sordet et al. (2004a); Ganguly et al. (2007); Sen et al. (2007)
UV radiation	Production of pyrimidine dimers, 4,6-photoproducts and oxidative DNA lesions	Soe et al. (2004)

TNF-α tumor necrosis factor α, *TRAIL* tumor necrosis factor-related apoptosis ligand, *DR4* death receptor 4, *DR5* death receptor 5, *TNFR1* tumor necrosis factor receptor 1, *BH3* Bcl-2 homology domain 3, *PDK1* phosphoinositide-dependent kinase 1, *PKC* protein kinase C, *Chk1* checkpoint kinase 1, *Chk2* checkpoint kinase 2

et al. 2004a, c, 2006, 2008a; Sen et al. 2007). It has been proposed that apoptosis-inducing agents induce the intracellular accumulation of ROS that damage DNA (oxidized bases, abasic sites), thereby stabilizing Top1cc in apoptotic cells (Fig. 19.4). Besides oxidized nucleobases, the DNA breaks produced by ROS and apoptotic nucleases (Samejima and Earnshaw 2005) may also contribute to the apoptotic Top1cc as Top1 can be directly trapped by DNA breaks (Pourquier et al. 1997).

Mitochondria are likely to participate in the production of the ROS and the Top1cc during apoptosis as Bcl-2 overexpression (Sordet et al. 2004c) or Bax deficiency (Sordet et al. 2008a) prevent their formation. By contrast, direct inhibition of Bcl-xL (a Bcl-2 homolog) by BH3-mimetics is sufficient to induce apoptotic Top1cc (Sordet et al. 2008a). Bcl-2 and Bcl-xL prevents MOMP, and therefore the release of cytochrome c and the downstream activation of caspases, whereas Bax exerts the opposite effect (see Sect. 19.4.1). Activated caspase-3 feeds back on permeabilized mitochondria, which further dissipates the mitochondrial membrane potential ($\Delta\Psi$m) and induces the further accumulation of intracellular ROS (Ricci et al. 2003, 2004). Caspase activation is involved in the production of apoptotic Top1cc as their inhibition prevents the production of ROS, oxidative DNA lesions, and Top1cc in response to various apoptotic stimuli (Sordet et al. 2004a, c, 2006, 2008a). Activation of caspases could therefore serve to generate the ROS that lead to apoptotic Top1cc (Fig. 19.4).

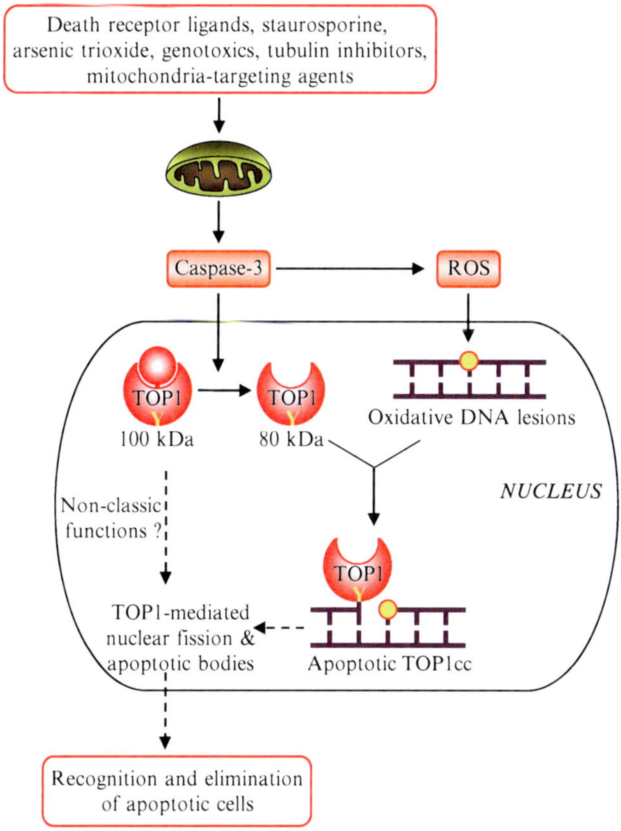

Fig. 19.4 Proposed molecular pathways for the formation of apoptotic Top1cc. Most apoptotic stimuli activate the apoptotic mitochondrial pathway, causing caspase-3 activation and accumulation of ROS. Activated caspase-3 cleaves Top1 and further generates ROS, which produce oxidative DNA lesions (8-oxoguanine, abasic sites, and strand breaks). Caspase-cleaved Top1 binds at the proximity of oxidative DNA lesions by forming apoptotic Top1cc. The tyrosine 723 of Top1 (Y) covalently bound to DNA is indicated in yellow. Those complexes may participate in apoptotic-related nuclear modifications including nuclear fission and the release of nuclear bodies in the extracellular space and may therefore contribute to the recognition and elimination of apoptotic cells. It is possible that these apoptotic events could depend in nonclassic functions of Top1, independently of its nicking closing activity

Besides their role in ROS production, caspases cleave Top1 during apoptosis. The 100-kDa native Top1 protein was among the first identified substrate of caspase-3 (Samejima et al. 1999). Caspase-3 cleaves Top1 after aspartate residue 146, and generates an 80-kDa C-terminal fragment that remains capable of forming Top1cc (Samejima et al. 1999; Pommier et al. 2000) and still possesses one functional nuclear localization signal (Mo et al. 2000). Apoptotic Top1cc consists preferentially in the 80-kDa C-terminal fragment of Top1 generated by caspase-3 (Sordet et al. 2008a) (Fig. 19.4), although it is not clear whether caspase-3-mediated cleavage of

Top1 contributes to or results from Top1cc formation. Together, these studies suggest a model for the formation of apoptotic Top1cc, in which activation of the apoptotic mitochondrial pathway causes caspase-3 activation and accumulation of ROS. Activated caspase-3 cleaves Top1 and induces the further accumulation of ROS, which produces oxidative DNA lesions. Caspase-3-cleaved Top1 binds at the proximity of oxidative DNA lesions by forming apoptotic Top1cc (Fig. 19.4).

Top1 downregulation experiments by small interfering RNA (siRNA) and small hairpins RNA (shRNA) suggest that the apoptotic Top1cc contribute to nuclear fission and the release of apoptotic nuclear bodies in the extracellular space. Indeed, the number of nuclei with sub-G1 DNA content is reduced in Top1 downregulated cells exposed to various apoptotic stimuli (Sordet et al. 2004a, c, 2008a). Typically, apoptotic cells are comprised in the sub-G1 fraction as they release apoptotic nuclear bodies. Analysis of apoptotic nuclei by electron microscopy revealed that Top1 deficiency is further associated with nuclear envelope distension (Sordet et al. 2008a). It is currently not known whether distension of the nuclear envelope is involved in preventing nuclear fission. In addition, it has been shown that siRNA-mediated Top1 downregulation prevents apoptosis-associated histone accumulation (Ganguly et al. 2007). Although histone release seems to precede apoptotic nuclear fission (Gabler et al. 2004), it is still unclear whether these two events are connected or separated in two independent processes. It is unlikely that apoptotic Top1cc participate in the direct breakdown of genomic DNA as apoptosis-related global and oligonucleosomal DNA fragmentation, as well as phosphorylation of histone H2AX at Ser-139 (γ-H2AX), a landmark marker for DSBs (Bonner et al. 2008; Solier et al. 2009), are unaffected by siRNA-induced Top1 downregulation in cells undergoing apoptosis (Sordet et al. 2008a). In agreement with these observations, the number of apoptotic Top1cc per genome scores relatively low as compared with the observed DSBs frequency produced by apoptotic endonucleases (Samejima and Earnshaw 2005) with an average of approximately one Top1cc–100 kpb and one Top1cc–10 kpb in early and late apoptotic cells, respectively (Rockstroh et al. 2007; Sordet et al. 2008a).

Although the Top1 siRNA and shRNA experiments are consistent with the involvement of Top1cc in nuclear fission and apoptotic body release, it is possible that these apoptotic events could depend in nonclassic functions of Top1, independently of its nicking-closing activity. Nonclassical functions of Top1 have been associated with transcription initiation (Merino et al. 1993; Shykind et al. 1997), phosphorylation of splicing factors (Rossi et al. 1996; Soret et al. 2003), DNA replication and genomic stability, nucleolar structure, and gene-specific transcription (Miao et al. 2007). Further experiments are required to determine which function(s) of Top1 is responsible for these nuclear events. They are however not straightforward because there is presently no known specific catalytic inhibitor of Top1, and the lethality of knocking out Top1 in eukaryotic cells (Morham et al. 1996) is a major obstacle for genetic approaches.

Top2 has been reported to participate in the excision of DNA-loops and in chromatin condensation during apoptosis (Li et al. 1999; Durrieu et al. 2000; Solovyan et al. 2002). In response to oxidative stress, Top2 itself produces reversible high molecular weight (HMW) DNA fragments of approximately 50–100 kb in size within minutes. This early step is followed by the production of irreversible HMW DNA fragments as cells undergo apoptosis (Li et al. 1999). Experiments in Top2β deficient cells suggest that Top2 can also participate in the irreversible HMW DNA cleavage during apoptosis (Solovyan et al. 2002). It is still unclear how Top2 is activated during apoptosis. Although Top2α interacts with the apoptotic nuclease CAD (also known as DFF40) (Durrieu et al. 2000), and stimulate CAD activity in vitro (Widlak et al. 2000), the significance of this interaction in the condensation and fragmentation of genomic DNA during apoptosis is not known. Unlike Top1 that is stabilized as cleavage complexes during apoptosis (see above), Top2cc (α or β) have not been detected in apoptotic cells (Sordet et al. 2004c, 2006, 2008a), which raises the possibility that the catalytic activity of Top2, rather than its stabilization as Top2cc, contributes to the excision of DNA-loops during apoptosis.

The role of Top1 and Top2 in promoting apoptotic nuclear events (nuclear fission and nuclear bodies release, chromatin condensation, HMW DNA fragments) suggest that topoisomerases may contribute to the full apoptotic program required for the proper recognition and elimination of apoptotic cells. At the organism level, the complete elimination of apoptotic cells is essential to prevent autoimmune disease (Napirei et al. 2000), as well as chronic inflammation that may lead to cancer (Coussens and Werb 2002).

19.8 Conclusion

Cellular responses to topoisomerase inhibitors include DNA repair, cell cycle arrest, and/or apoptosis, and thus determine cell survival or cell death. It is becoming increasingly clear that cell cycle checkpoint and DNA repair pathways such as the ATM–Chk2, Rad9 (9-1-1), and Ku70 pathways are also connected to the apoptotic pathways. Likewise, apoptotic proteins such as caspase-2 also play a role in cell cycle arrest and DNA repair. A more complete molecular interaction network connecting these pathways is warranted. One of the challenges is to understand how these pathways are integrated, and how in the presence of extensive DNA damage, the same DNA damage sensors and checkpoints that stop cell cycle progression and promote DNA repair, can activate apoptosis. Thus, a promising new area of research is the elucidation of the relationships between specific DNA lesions, sensor proteins, checkpoints, DNA repair and apoptosis. Integration of these pathways in comprehensive molecular interaction maps (Kohn 1998, 1999; Pommier et al. 2002, 2003, 2005, 2006; Reinhold et al. 2003; Sordet et al. 2003; Aladjem et al. 2004; Kohn and Pommier 2005; Kohn et al. 2004a, b, 2006a, b, 2008, 2009) (see also http://discover.nci.nih.gov/mim/) should reveal the interplays between the cellular determinants of cellular response to topoisomerase inhibitors and other types of DNA damage. They should also provide opportunities to develop novel therapeutic strategies and markers to better predict and follow tumor responses to therapeutic agents.

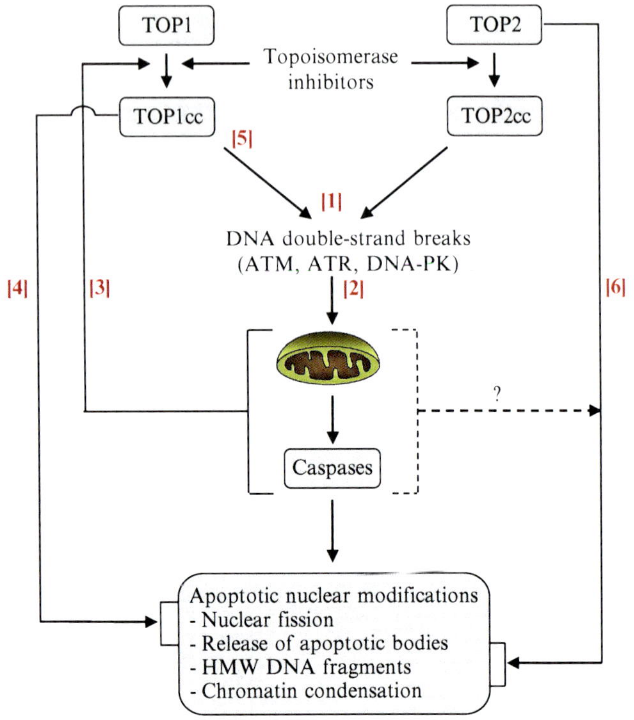

Fig. 19.5 Role of topoisomerases in both the induction and the execution of apoptosis. [1] Stabilization of Top1cc and Top2cc by topoisomerase inhibitors leads to the production of DSBs with activation of ATM, ATR, and DNA-PK (for details, see Sects. 19.2 and 19.3 and Fig. 19.1). [2] The signalization to these DSBs activates the apoptotic mitochondrial pathway and the subsequent activation of caspases, which contribute to the induction of apoptotic nuclear modifications (for details, see Sects. 19.4 and 19.5 and Figs. 19.2 and 19.3). [3] Activation of the apoptotic mitochondrial pathway further stabilizes Top1cc (for details, see Sect. 19.7 and Fig. 19.4). These cleavage complexes, termed "apoptotic Top1cc" contribute to apoptotic nuclear modifications by promoting nuclear fission and the release of apoptotic bodies [4], and by further engaging the apoptotic machinery in trans [5]. [6] Top2 also contributes to apoptotic nuclear modifications by promoting HMW DNA fragments and chromatin condensation. It is still not known how activation of the apoptotic machinery stimulates these Top2-dependent apoptotic nuclear modifications

In addition to their role in the initiation of apoptosis, a growing number of studies show that Top1 and Top2 also participate in the execution of apoptosis by contributing to the apoptotic-associated nuclear modifications including nuclear fission, apoptotic body release, DNA fragmentation, and chromatin condensation. A pending issue is whether stabilization of topoisomerases as cleavage complexes is required for these nuclear events. If this is the case, the stabilized apoptotic topoisomerase cleavage complexes may further engage the apoptotic process in trans to amplify the apoptotic response (Fig. 19.5).

Acknowledgments The authors wish to thank Y. Pommier for many years of supervision, inspiration, and encouragement, as well as for editing this chapter.

References

Aladjem MI, Pasa S, Parodi S et al (2004) Molecular interaction maps--a diagrammatic graphical language for bioregulatory networks. Science STKE 2004:pe8

Amsel AD, Rathaus M, Kronman N et al (2008) Regulation of the proapoptotic factor Bax by Ku70-dependent deubiquitylation. Proc Natl Acad Sci USA 105:5117–5122

Bakalkin G, Yakovleva T, Selivanova G et al (1994) p53 binds single-stranded DNA ends and catalyzes DNA renaturation and strand transfer. Proc Natl Acad Sci USA 91:413–417

Baliga BC, Colussi PA, Read SH et al (2003) Role of prodomain in importin-mediated nuclear localization and activation of caspase-2. J Biol Chem 278:4899–4905

Baptiste-Okoh N, Barsotti AM, Prives C (2008) A role for caspase 2 and PIDD in the process of p53-mediated apoptosis. Proc Natl Acad Sci USA 105:1937–1942

Bendixen C, Thomsen B, Alsner J et al (1990) Camptothecin-stabilized topoisomerase I-DNA adducts cause premature termination of transcription. Biochemistry 29:5613–5619

Berkovich E, Monnat RJ, Jr., Kastan MB (2007) Roles of ATM and NBS1 in chromatin structure modulation and DNA double-strand break repair. Nat Cell Biol 9:683–690

Bertrand R, Kerrigan D, Sarang M et al (1991) Cell death induced by topoisomerase inhibitors. Role of calcium in mammalian cells. Biochem Pharmacol 42:77–85

Bertrand R, Solary E, Jenkins J et al (1993) Apoptosis and its modulation in human promyelocytic HL-60 cells treated with DNA topoisomerase I and II inhibitors. Exp Cell Res 207:388–397

Bertrand R, Solary E, Kohn KW et al (1994) Induction of a common pathway to apoptosis by staurosporine. Exp Cell Res 211:314–321

Blattner C, Sparks A, Lane D (1999) Transcription factor E2F-1 is upregulated in response to DNA damage in a manner analogous to that of p53. Mol Cell Biol 19:3704–3713

Bonner WM, Redon CE, Dickey JS et al (2008) gammaH2AX and cancer. Nat Rev Cancer 8:957–967

Borowiec JA (2004) The toposome: a new twist on topoisomerase IIalpha. Cell Cycle 3:627–628

Bourdon JC, Renzing J, Robertson PL et al (2002) Scotin, a novel p53-inducible proapoptotic protein located in the ER and the nuclear membrane. J Cell Biol 158:235–246

Burtelow MA, Roos-Mattjus PM, Rauen M et al (2001) Reconstitution and molecular analysis of the hRad9-hHus1-hRad1 (9-1-1) DNA damage responsive checkpoint complex. J Biol Chem 276:25903–25909

Cao X, Liu W, Lin F et al (2004) Retinoid X receptor regulates Nur77/TR3-dependent apoptosis [corrected] by modulating its nuclear export and mitochondrial targeting. Mol Cell Biol 24:9705–9725

Capranico G, Ferri F, Fogli MV et al (2007) The effects of camptothecin on RNA polymerase II transcription: roles of DNA topoisomerase I. Biochimie 89:482–489

Champoux JJ (2001) DNA TOPOISOMERASES: Structure, Function, and Mechanism. Annu Rev Biochem 70:369–413

Chatterjee D, Schmitz I, Krueger A et al (2001) Induction of apoptosis in 9-nitrocamptothecin-treated DU145 human prostate carcinoma cells correlates with de novo synthesis of CD95 and CD95 ligand and down-regulation of c-FLIP(short). Cancer Res 61:7148–7154

Chen C, Shimizu S, Tsujimoto Y et al (2005) Chk2 regulates transcription-independent p53-mediated apoptosis in response to DNA damage. Biochem Biophys Res Commun 333:427–431

Chinnaiyan AM, O'Rourke K, Tewari M et al (1995) FADD, a novel death domain-containing protein, interacts with the death domain of Fas and initiates apoptosis. Cell 81:505–512

Chipuk JE, Bouchier-Hayes L, Kuwana T et al (2005) PUMA couples the nuclear and cytoplasmic proapoptotic function of p53. Science 309:1732–1735

Chipuk JE, Green DR (2006) Dissecting p53-dependent apoptosis. Cell Death Differ 13:994–1002

Chipuk JE, Moldoveanu T, Llambi F et al (2010) The BCL-2 family reunion. Mol Cell 37:299–310

Ciusani E, Perego P, Carenini N et al (2002) Fas/CD95-mediated apoptosis in human glioblastoma cells: a target for sensitisation to topoisomerase I inhibitors. Biochem Pharmacol 63:881–887

Cohen HY, Lavu S, Bitterman KJ et al (2004) Acetylation of the C terminus of Ku70 by CBP and PCAF controls Bax-mediated apoptosis. Mol Cell 13:627–638

Coussens LM, Werb Z (2002) Inflammation and cancer. Nature 420:860–867

Covey JM, Kohn KW, Kerrigan D et al (1988) Topoisomerase II-mediated DNA damage produced by 4′-(9-acridinylamino)methanesulfon-m-anisidide and related acridines in L1210 cells and isolated nuclei: relation to cytotoxicity. Cancer Res 48:860–865

Covey JM, Jaxel C, Kohn KW et al (1989) Protein-linked DNA strand breaks induced in mammalian cells by camptothecin, an inhibitor of topoisomerase I. Cancer Res 49:5016–5022

Daroui P, Desai SD, Li TK et al (2004) Hydrogen peroxide induces topoisomerase I-mediated DNA damage and cell death. J Biol Chem 279:14587–14594

de la Mata M, Alonso CR, Kadener S et al (2003) A slow RNA polymerase II affects alternative splicing in vivo. Mol Cell 12:525–532

de la Mata M, Kornblihtt AR (2006) RNA polymerase II C-terminal domain mediates regulation of alternative splicing by SRp20. Nat Struct Mol Biol 13:973–980

Dexheimer TS, Kozekova A, Rizzo CJ et al (2008) The modulation of topoisomerase I-mediated DNA cleavage and the induction of DNA-topoisomerase I crosslinks by crotonaldehyde-derived DNA adducts. Nucleic Acids Res 36:4128–4136

Durrieu F, Samejima K, Fortune JM et al (2000) DNA topoisomerase IIalpha interacts with CAD nuclease and is involved in chromatin condensation during apoptotic execution. Curr Biol 10:923–926

Eischen CM, Kottke TJ, Martins LM et al (1997) Comparison of apoptosis in wild-type and Fas-resistant cells: chemotherapy-induced apoptosis is not dependent on Fas/Fas ligand interactions. Blood 90:935–943

Eisenreich A, Bogdanov VY, Zakrzewicz A et al (2009) Cdc2-like kinases and DNA topoisomerase I regulate alternative splicing of tissue factor in human endothelial cells. Circ Res 104:589–599

Ekert PG, Vaux DL (2005) The mitochondrial death squad: hardened killers or innocent bystanders? Curr Opin Cell Biol 17:626–630

El-Deiry WS, Tokino T, Velculescu VE et al (1993) WAF1, a potential mediator of p53 tumor suppression. Cell 75:817–825

Eskes R, Desagher S, Antonsson B et al (2000) Bid induces the oligomerization and insertion of Bax into the outer mitochondrial membrane. Mol Cell Biol 20:929–935

Fernandez-Salas E, Suh KS, Speransky VV et al (2002) mtCLIC/CLIC4, an organellular chloride channel protein, is increased by DNA damage and participates in the apoptotic response to p53. Mol Cell Biol 22:3610–3620

French SL, Sikes ML, Hontz RD et al (2011) Distinguishing the roles of Topoisomerases I and II in relief of transcription-induced torsional stress in yeast rRNA genes. Mol Cell Biol 31:482–494

Gabler C, Blank N, Hieronymus T et al (2004) Extranuclear detection of histones and nucleosomes in activated human lymphoblasts as an early event in apoptosis. Ann Rheum Dis 63:1135–1144

Ganguly A, Das B, Roy A et al (2007) Betulinic acid, a catalytic inhibitor of topoisomerase I, inhibits reactive oxygen species-mediated apoptotic topoisomerase I-DNA cleavable complex formation in prostate cancer cells but does not affect the process of cell death. Cancer Res 67:11848–11858

Goldwasser F, Shimizu T, Jackman J et al (1996) Correlations between S- and G2-phase arrest and cytotoxicity of camptothecin in human colon carcinoma cells. Cancer Res 56:4430–4437

Green DR, Kroemer G (2004) The pathophysiology of mitochondrial cell death. Science 305:626–629
Green DR (2005) Apoptotic pathways: ten minutes to dead. Cell 121:671–674
Green DR, Kroemer G (2009) Cytoplasmic functions of the tumour suppressor p53. Nature 458:1127–1130
Gupta M, Fan S, Zhan Q et al (1997) Inactivation of p53 increases the cytotoxicity of camptothecin in human colon HCT116 and breast MCF-7 cancer cells. Clin Cancer Res 3:1653–1660
Han YH, Cao X, Lin B et al (2006) Regulation of Nur77 nuclear export by c-Jun N-terminal kinase and Akt. Oncogene 25:2974–2986
Han Z, Wei W, Dunaway S et al (2002) Role of p21 in apoptosis and senescence of human colon cancer cells treated with camptothecin. J Biol Chem 277:17154–17160
Hoffman WH, Biade S, Zilfou JT et al (2002) Transcriptional repression of the anti-apoptotic survivin gene by wild type p53. J Biol Chem 277:3247–3257
Holm C, Covey JM, Kerrigan D et al (1989) Differential requirement of DNA replication for the cytotoxicity of DNA topoisomerase I and II inhibitors in Chinese hamster DC3F cells. Cancer Res 49:6365–6368
Horwitz SB, Horwitz MS (1973) Effects of camptothecin on the breakage and repair of DNA during the cell cycle. Cancer Res 33:2834–2836
Hsiang YH, Lihou MG, Liu LF (1989) Arrest of replication forks by drug-stabilized topoisomerase I-DNA cleavable complexes as a mechanism of cell killing by camptothecin. Cancer Res 49:5077–5082
Hsieh JK, Yap D, O'Connor DJ et al (2002) Novel function of the cyclin A binding site of E2F in regulating p53-induced apoptosis in response to DNA damage. Mol Cell Biol 22:78–93
Hsu YT, Wolter KG, Youle RJ (1997) Cytosol-to-membrane redistribution of Bax and Bcl-X(L) during apoptosis. Proc Natl Acad Sci USA 94:3668–3672
Huertas P, Aguilera A (2003) Cotranscriptionally formed DNA:RNA hybrids mediate transcription elongation impairment and transcription-associated recombination. Mol Cell 12:711–721
Iijima K, Muranaka C, Kobayashi J et al (2008) NBS1 regulates a novel apoptotic pathway through Bax activation. DNA Repair (Amst) 7:1705–1716
Ishii H, Inageta T, Mimori K et al (2005) Frag1, a homolog of alternative replication factor C subunits, links replication stress surveillance with apoptosis. Proc Natl Acad Sci USA 102:9655–9660
Jackson SP, Bartek J (2009) The DNA-damage response in human biology and disease. Nature 461:1071–1078
Johnstone RW, Frew AJ, Smyth MJ (2008) The TRAIL apoptotic pathway in cancer onset, progression and therapy. Nat Rev Cancer 8:782–798
Kastan MB, Bartek J (2004) Cell-cycle checkpoints and cancer. Nature 432:316–323
Kaufmann SH (1998) Cell death induced by topoisomerase-targeted drugs: more questions than answers. Biochim Biophys Acta 1400:195–211
Kerrigan D, Pommier Y, Kohn KW (1987) Protein-linked DNA strand breaks produced by etoposide and teniposide in mouse L1210 and human VA-13 and HT-29 cell lines: relationship to cytotoxicity. NCI Monogr:117–121
Kinner A, Wu W, Staudt C et al (2008) Gamma-H2AX in recognition and signaling of DNA double-strand breaks in the context of chromatin. Nucleic Acids Res 36:5678–5694
Kohn KW (1998) Functional capabilities of molecular network components controlling the mammalian G1/S cell cycle phase transition. Oncogene 16:1065–1075
Kohn KW (1999) Molecular interaction map of the mammalian cell cycle control and DNA repair systems. Mol Biol Cell 10:2703–2734
Kohn KW, Aladjem MI, Pasa S et al (2004a) Cell cycle control: molecular interaction map. Nature Encyclopedia of the Human Genome 1:457–474
Kohn KW, Riss J, Aprelikova O et al (2004b) Properties of switch-like bioregulatory networks studied by simulation of the hypoxia response control system. Mol Biol Cell 15:3042–3052
Kohn KW, Pommier Y (2005) Molecular interaction map of the p53 and Mdm2 logic elements, which control the Off-On switch of p53 in response to DNA damage. Biochem Biophys Res Commun 331:816–827

Kohn KW, Aladjem MI, Kim S et al (2006a) Depicting combinatorial complexity with the molecular interaction map notation. Mol Syst Biol 2:51
Kohn KW, Aladjem MI, Weinstein JN et al (2006b) Molecular interaction maps of bioregulatory networks: a general rubric for systems biology. Mol Biol Cell 17:1–13
Kohn KW, Aladjem MI, Weinstein JN et al (2008) Chromatin challenges during DNA replication: a systems representation. Mol Biol Cell 19:1–7
Kohn KW, Aladjem MI, Weinstein JN et al (2009) Network architecture of signaling from uncoupled helicase-polymerase to cell cycle checkpoints and trans-lesion DNA synthesis. Cell Cycle 8:2281–2299
Kolluri SK, Bruey-Sedano N, Cao X et al (2003) Mitogenic effect of orphan receptor TR3 and its regulation by MEKK1 in lung cancer cells. Mol Cell Biol 23:8651–8667
Komatsu K, Miyashita T, Hang H et al (2000) Human homologue of S. pombe Rad9 interacts with BCL-2/BCL-xL and promotes apoptosis. Nat Cell Biol 2:1–6
Konishi A, Shimizu S, Hirota J et al (2003) Involvement of histone H1.2 in apoptosis induced by DNA double-strand breaks. Cell 114:673–688
Kumar S (2009) Caspase 2 in apoptosis, the DNA damage response and tumour suppression: enigma no more? Nat Rev Cancer 9:897–903
Lacour S, Hammann A, Grazide S et al (2004) Cisplatin-induced CD95 redistribution into membrane lipid rafts of HT29 human colon cancer cells. Cancer Res 64:3593–3598
Lassus P, Opitz-Araya X, Lazebnik Y (2002) Requirement for caspase-2 in stress-induced apoptosis before mitochondrial permeabilization. Science 297:1352–1354
Lavin MF (2008) Ataxia-telangiectasia: from a rare disorder to a paradigm for cell signalling and cancer. Nat Rev Mol Cell Biol 9:759–769
Lee CG, Hague LK, Li H et al (2004) Identification of toposome, a novel multisubunit complex containing topoisomerase IIalpha. Cell Cycle 3:638–647
Lee JH, Paull TT (2005) ATM activation by DNA double-strand breaks through the Mre11-Rad50-Nbs1 complex. Science 308:551–554
Lee MW, Hirai I, Wang HG (2003) Caspase-3-mediated cleavage of Rad9 during apoptosis. Oncogene 22:6340–6346
Li H, Zhu H, Xu CJ et al (1998) Cleavage of BID by caspase 8 mediates the mitochondrial damage in the Fas pathway of apoptosis. Cell 94:491–501
Li H, Kolluri SK, Gu J et al (2000) Cytochrome c release and apoptosis induced by mitochondrial targeting of nuclear orphan receptor TR3. Science 289:1159–1164
Li P, Nijhawan D, Budihardjo I et al (1997) Cytochrome c and dATP-dependent formation of Apaf-1/caspase-9 complex initiates an apoptotic protease cascade. Cell 91:479–489
Li TK, Chen AY, Yu C et al (1999) Activation of topoisomerase II-mediated excision of chromosomal DNA loops during oxidative stress. Genes Dev 13:1553–1560
Li X, Manley JL (2005) Inactivation of the SR protein splicing factor ASF/SF2 results in genomic instability. Cell 122:365–378
Lieber MR, Ma Y, Pannicke U et al (2003) Mechanism and regulation of human non-homologous DNA end-joining. Nat Rev Mol Cell Biol 4:712–720
Lin B, Kolluri SK, Lin F et al (2004) Conversion of Bcl-2 from protector to killer by interaction with nuclear orphan receptor Nur77/TR3. Cell 116:527–540
Liu LF (1989) DNA topoisomerase poisons as antitumor drugs. Annu Rev Biochem 58:351–375
Liu S, Wu Q, Ye XF et al (2002) Induction of apoptosis by TPA and VP-16 is through translocation of TR3. World J Gastroenterol 8:446–450
Liu ZG, Smith SW, McLaughlin KA et al (1994) Apoptotic signals delivered through the T-cell receptor of a T-cell hybrid require the immediate-early gene nur77. Nature 367:281–284
Loegering D, Arlander SJ, Hackbarth J et al (2004) Rad9 protects cells from topoisomerase poison-induced cell death. J Biol Chem 279:18641–18647
Long BH, Musial ST, Brattain MG (1985) Single- and double-strand DNA breakage and repair in human lung adenocarcinoma cells exposed to etoposide and teniposide. Cancer Res 45:3106–3112
Luciano F, Krajewska M, Ortiz-Rubio P et al (2007) Nur77 converts phenotype of Bcl-B, an anti-apoptotic protein expressed in plasma cells and myeloma. Blood 109:3849–3855

Luo X, Budihardjo I, Zou H et al (1998) Bid, a Bcl2 interacting protein, mediates cytochrome c release from mitochondria in response to activation of cell surface death receptors. Cell 94:481–490

MacDougall CA, Byun TS, Van C et al (2007) The structural determinants of checkpoint activation. Genes Dev 21:898–903

Medema JP, Scaffidi C, Kischkel FC et al (1997) FLICE is activated by association with the CD95 death-inducing signaling complex (DISC). Embo J 16:2794–2804

Meek K, Dang V, Lees-Miller SP (2008) DNA-PK: the means to justify the ends? Adv Immunol 99:33–58

Menendez D, Inga A, Resnick MA (2009) The expanding universe of p53 targets. Nat Rev Cancer 9:724–737

Menendez JA, Vellon L, Lupu R (2006) DNA topoisomerase IIalpha (TOP2A) inhibitors up-regulate fatty acid synthase gene expression in SK-Br3 breast cancer cells: in vitro evidence for a 'functional amplicon' involving FAS, Her-2/neu and TOP2A genes. Int J Mol Med 18:1081–1087

Merino A, Madden KR, Lane WS et al (1993) DNA topoisomerase I is involved in both repression and activation of transcription. Nature 365:227–232

Miao ZH, Player A, Shankavaram U et al (2007) Nonclassic functions of human topoisomerase I: genome-wide and pharmacologic analyses. Cancer Res 67:8752–8761

Micheau O, Solary E, Hammann A et al (1997) Sensitization of cancer cells treated with cytotoxic drugs to fas-mediated cytotoxicity. J Natl Cancer Inst 89:783–789

Mihara M, Erster S, Zaika A et al (2003) p53 has a direct apoptogenic role at the mitochondria. Mol Cell 11:577–590

Mimori T, Hardin JA, Steitz JA (1986) Characterization of the DNA-binding protein antigen Ku recognized by autoantibodies from patients with rheumatic disorders. J Biol Chem 261:2274–2278

Miyashita T, Harigai M, Hanada M et al (1994) Identification of a p53-dependent negative response element in the bcl-2 gene. Cancer Res 54:3131–3135

Mo YY, Wang C, Beck WT (2000) A novel nuclear localization signal in human DNA topoisomerase I. J Biol Chem 275:41107–41113

Moll UM, Marchenko N, Zhang XK (2006) p53 and Nur77/TR3 - transcription factors that directly target mitochondria for cell death induction. Oncogene 25:4725–4743

Morham SG, Kluckman KD, Voulomanos N et al (1996) Targeted disruption of the mouse topoisomerase I gene by camptothecin selection. Mol Cell Biol 16:6804–6809

Morris EJ, Geller HM (1996) Induction of neuronal apoptosis by camptothecin, an inhibitor of DNA topoisomerase-I: evidence for cell cycle-independent toxicity. J Cell Biol 134:757–770

Muller M, Wilder S, Bannasch D et al (1998) p53 activates the CD95 (APO-1/Fas) gene in response to DNA damage by anticancer drugs. J Exp Med 188:2033–2045

Nam C, Doi K, Nakayama H (2010) Etoposide induces G2/M arrest and apoptosis in neural progenitor cells via DNA damage and an ATM/p53-related pathway. Histol Histopathol 25:485–493

Napirei M, Karsunky H, Zevnik B et al (2000) Features of systemic lupus erythematosus in Dnase1-deficient mice. Nat Genet 25:177–181

Nelson EM, Tewey KM, Liu LF (1984) Mechanism of antitumor drug action: poisoning of mammalian DNA topoisomerase II on DNA by 4′-(9-acridinylamino)-methanesulfon-m-anisidide. Proc Natl Acad Sci USA 81:1361–1365

Nieves-Neira W, Pommier Y (1999) Apoptotic response to camptothecin and 7-hydroxystaurosporine (UCN-01) in the 8 human breast cancer cell lines of the NCI Anticancer Drug Screen: multifactorial relationships with topoisomerase I, protein kinase C, Bcl-2, p53, MDM-2 and caspase pathways. Int J Cancer 82:396–404

Nitiss JL (2009) Targeting DNA topoisomerase II in cancer chemotherapy. Nat Rev Cancer 9:338–350

Nothwehr SF, Martinou JC (2003) A retention factor keeps death at bay. Nat Cell Biol 5:281–283

O'Connor PM, Nieves-Neira W, Kerrigan D et al (1991) S-phase population analysis does not correlate with the cytotoxicity of camptothecin and 10,11-methylenedioxycamptothecin in human colon carcinoma HT-29 cells. Cancer Commun 3:233–240

Oda K, Arakawa H, Tanaka T et al (2000) p53AIP1, a potential mediator of p53-dependent apoptosis, and its regulation by Ser-46-phosphorylated p53. Cell 102:849–862
Ohtsuka T, Ryu H, Minamishima YA et al (2004) ASC is a Bax adaptor and regulates the p53-Bax mitochondrial apoptosis pathway. Nat Cell Biol 6:121–128
Okamura H, Yoshida K, Amorim BR et al (2008) Histone H1.2 is translocated to mitochondria and associates with Bak in bleomycin-induced apoptotic cells. J Cell Biochem 103:1488–1496
Pommier Y, Laco GS, Kohlhagen G et al (2000) Position-specific trapping of topoisomerase I-DNA cleavage complexes by intercalated benzo[a]- pyrene diol epoxide adducts at the 6-amino group of adenine. Proc Natl Acad Sci USA 97:10739–10744
Pommier Y, Yu Q, Kohn KW (2002) Novel targets in the cell cycle and cell cycle checkpoints. Anticancer Drug Development:13–30
Pommier Y, Redon C, Rao VA et al (2003) Repair of and checkpoint response to topoisomerase I-mediated DNA damage. Mutat Res 532:173–203
Pommier Y, Sordet O, Rao VA et al (2005) Targeting chk2 kinase: molecular interaction maps and therapeutic rationale. Curr Pharm Des 11:2855–2872
Pommier Y (2006) Topoisomerase I inhibitors: camptothecins and beyond. Nat Rev Cancer 6:789–802
Pommier Y, Weinstein JN, Aladjem MI et al (2006) Chk2 molecular interaction map and rationale for Chk2 inhibitors. Clin Cancer Res 12:2657–2661
Pommier Y (2009) DNA topoisomerase I inhibitors: chemistry, biology, and interfacial inhibition. Chem Rev 109:2894–2902
Pommier Y, Leo E, Zhang H et al (2010) DNA topoisomerases and their poisoning by anticancer and antibacterial drugs. Chem Biol 17:421–433
Pourquier P, Pilon AA, Kohlhagen G et al (1997) Trapping of mammalian topoisomerase I and recombinations induced by damaged DNA containing nicks or gaps. Importance of DNA end phosphorylation and camptothecin effects. J Biol Chem 272:26441–26447
Pourquier P, Ueng L-M, Fertala J et al (1999) Induction of reversible complexes between eukaryotic DNA topoisomerase I and DNA-containing oxidative base damages. J Biol Chem 274:8516–8523
Pourquier P, Pommier Y (2001) Topoisomerase I-mediated DNA damage. Adv Cancer Res 80:189–216
Reinhold WC, Kouros-Mehr H, Kohn KW et al (2003) Apoptotic Susceptibility of Cancer Cells Selected for Camptothecin Resistance: Gene Expression Profiling, Functional Analysis, and Molecular Interaction Mapping. Cancer Res 63:1000–1011
Ricci JE, Gottlieb RA, Green DR (2003) Caspase-mediated loss of mitochondrial function and generation of reactive oxygen species during apoptosis. J Cell Biol 160:65–75
Ricci JE, Munoz-Pinedo C, Fitzgerald P et al (2004) Disruption of Mitochondrial Function during Apoptosis Is Mediated by Caspase Cleavage of the p75 Subunit of Complex I of the Electron Transport Chain. Cell 117:773–786
Robertson JD, Gogvadze V, Kropotov A et al (2004) Processed caspase-2 can induce mitochondria-mediated apoptosis independently of its enzymatic activity. EMBO Rep 5:643–648
Rockstroh A, Kleinert A, Kramer M et al (2007) Cellular stress triggers the human topoisomerase I damage response independently of DNA damage in a p53 controlled manner. Oncogene 26:123–131
Roos-Mattjus P, Vroman BT, Burtelow MA et al (2002) Genotoxin-induced Rad9-Hus1-Rad1 (9-1-1) chromatin association is an early checkpoint signaling event. J Biol Chem 277:43809–43812
Rossi F, Labourier E, Forne T et al (1996) Specific phosphorylation of SR proteins by mammalian DNA topoisomerase I. Nature 381:80–82
Ruiz-Vela A, Korsmeyer SJ (2007) Proapoptotic histone H1.2 induces CASP-3 and –7 activation by forming a protein complex with CYT c, APAF-1 and CASP-9. FEBS Lett 581:3422–3428
Sakasai R, Teraoka H, Takagi M et al (2010) Transcription-dependent activation of ataxia telangiectasia mutated prevents DNA-dependent protein kinase-mediated cell death in response to topoisomerase I poison. J Biol Chem 285:15201–15208

Saleh A, Srinivasula SM, Acharya S et al (1999) Cytochrome c and dATP-mediated oligomerization of Apaf-1 is a prerequisite for procaspase-9 activation. J Biol Chem 274:17941–17945
Salvesen GS, Dixit VM (1999) Caspase activation: The induced-proximity model. Proc Natl Acad Sci USA 96:10964–10967
Samali A, Cai J, Zhivotovsky B et al (1999) Presence of a pre-apoptotic complex of pro-caspase-3, Hsp60 and Hsp10 in the mitochondrial fraction of jurkat cells. EMBO J 18:2040–2048
Samejima K, Svingen PA, Basi GS et al (1999) Caspase-mediated cleavage of DNA topoisomerase I at unconventional sites during apoptosis. J Biol Chem 274:4335–4340
Samejima K, Earnshaw WC (2005) Trashing the genome: the role of nucleases during apoptosis. Nat Rev Mol Cell Biol 6:677–688
Sawada M, Sun W, Hayes P et al (2003) Ku70 suppresses the apoptotic translocation of Bax to mitochondria. Nat Cell Biol 5:320–329
Scaffidi C, Fulda S, Srinivasan A et al (1998) Two CD95 (APO-1/Fas) signaling pathways. Embo J 17:1675–1687
Sen N, Banerjee B, Das BB et al (2007) Apoptosis is induced in leishmanial cells by a novel protein kinase inhibitor withaferin A and is facilitated by apoptotic topoisomerase I-DNA complex. Cell Death Differ 14:358–367
Shao RG, Cao CX, Nieves-Neira W et al (2001) Activation of the Fas pathway independently of Fas ligand during apoptosis induced by camptothecin in p53 mutant human colon carcinoma cells. Oncogene 20:1852–1859
Shimizu T, Pommier Y (1997) Camptothecin-induced apoptosis in p53-null human leukemia HL60 cells and their isolated nuclei: effects of the protease inhibitors Z-VAD-fmk and dichloroisocoumarin suggest an involvement of both caspases and serine proteases. Leukemia 11:1238–1244
Shinoura N, Sakurai S, Shibasaki F et al (2002) Co-transduction of Apaf-1 and caspase-9 highly enhances p53-mediated apoptosis in gliomas. Br J Cancer 86:587–595
Shkreta L, Froehlich U, Paquet ER et al (2008) Anticancer drugs affect the alternative splicing of Bcl-x and other human apoptotic genes. Mol Cancer Ther 7:1398–1409
Shykind BM, Kim J, Stewart L et al (1997) Topoisomerase I enhances TFIID-TFIIA complex assembly during activation of transcription. Genes Dev 11:397–407
Slee EA, Harte MT, Kluck RM et al (1999) Ordering the cytochrome c-initiated caspase cascade: hierarchical activation of caspases-2, -3, -6, -7, -8, and −10 in a caspase-9-dependent manner. J Cell Biol 144:281–292
Soe K, Rockstroh A, Schache P et al (2004) The human topoisomerase I damage response plays a role in apoptosis. DNA Repair (Amst) 3:387–393
Solary E, Bertrand R, Kohn KW et al (1993) Differential induction of apoptosis in undifferentiated and differentiated HL-60 cells by DNA topoisomerase I and II inhibitors. Blood 81:1359–1368
Solary E, Bertrand R, Pommier Y (1994) Apoptosis induced by DNA topoisomerase I and II inhibitors in human leukemic HL-60 cells. Leuk Lymphoma 15:21–32
Solary E, Droin N, Bettaieb A et al (2000) Positive and negative regulation of apoptotic pathways by cytotoxic agents in hematological malignancies. Leukemia 14:1833–1849
Solary E, Plenchette S, Sordet O et al (2001) Modulation of apoptotic pathways triggered by cytotoxic agents. Therapie 56:511–518
Solier S, Lansiaux A, Logette E et al (2004) Topoisomerase I and II inhibitors control caspase-2 pre-messenger RNA splicing in human cells. Mol Cancer Res 2:53–61
Solier S, De Cian MC, Bettaieb A et al (2008) PKC zeta controls DNA topoisomerase-dependent human caspase-2 pre-mRNA splicing. FEBS Lett 582:372–378
Solier S, Sordet O, Kohn KW et al (2009) Death receptor-induced activation of the Chk2- and histone H2AX-associated DNA damage response pathways. Mol Cell Biol 29:68–82
Solier S, Barb J, Zeeberg BR et al (2010) Genome-wide analysis of novel splice variants induced by topoisomerase I poisoning shows preferential occurrence in genes encoding splicing factors. Cancer Res 70:8055–8065
Solovyan VT, Bezvenyuk ZA, Salminen A et al (2002) The role of topoisomerase II in the excision of DNA loop domains during apoptosis. J Biol Chem 277:21458–21467

Sordet O, Bettaieb A, Bruey JM et al (1999) Selective inhibition of apoptosis by TPA-induced differentiation of U937 leukemic cells. Cell Death Differ 6:351–361

Sordet O, Rebe C, Leroy I et al (2001) Mitochondria-targeting drugs arsenic trioxide and lonidamine bypass the resistance of TPA-differentiated leukemic cells to apoptosis. Blood 97:3931–3940

Sordet O, Khan QA, Kohn KW et al (2003) Apoptosis induced by topoisomerase inhibitors. Curr Med Chem Anticancer Agents 3:271–290

Sordet O, Khan QA, Plo I et al (2004a) Apoptotic topoisomerase I-DNA complexes induced by staurosporine-mediated oxygen radicals. J Biol Chem 279:50499–50504

Sordet O, Khan QA, Pommier Y (2004b) Apoptotic topoisomerase I-DNA complexes induced by oxygen radicals and mitochondrial dysfunction. Cell Cycle 3:1095–1097

Sordet O, Liao Z, Liu H et al (2004c) Topoisomerase I-DNA complexes contribute to arsenic trioxide-induced apoptosis. J Biol Chem 279:33968–33975

Sordet O, Goldman A, Pommier Y (2006) Topoisomerase II and tubulin inhibitors both induce the formation of apoptotic topoisomerase I cleavage complexes. Mol Cancer Ther 5:3139–3144

Sordet O, Pommier Y, Solary E (2007) Topoisomerase I poisons and apoptotic Topoisomerase I cleavage complexes. In Gewirtz DA, Holt SE, and Grant S (eds) Apoptosis and Senescence and Cancer, Humana Press Inc., Totowa, NJ.

Sordet O, Goldman A, Redon C et al (2008a) Topoisomerase I requirement for death receptor-induced apoptotic nuclear fission. J Biol Chem 283:23200–23208

Sordet O, Larochelle S, Nicolas E et al (2008b) Hyperphosphorylation of RNA polymerase II in response to topoisomerase I cleavage complexes and its association with transcription- and BRCA1-dependent degradation of topoisomerase I. J Mol Biol 381:540–549

Sordet O, Redon CE, Guirouilh-Barbat J et al (2009) Ataxia telangiectasia mutated activation by transcription- and topoisomerase I-induced DNA double-strand breaks. EMBO Rep 10:887–893

Sordet O, Nakamura AJ, Redon CE et al (2010) DNA double-strand breaks and ATM activation by transcription-blocking DNA lesions. Cell Cycle 9:274–278

Soret J, Gabut M, Dupon C et al (2003) Altered serine/arginine-rich protein phosphorylation and exonic enhancer-dependent splicing in Mammalian cells lacking topoisomerase I. Cancer Res 63:8203–8211

Srinivasula SM, Ahmad M, Fernandes-Alnemri T et al (1998) Autoactivation of procaspase-9 by Apaf-1-mediated oligomerization. Mol Cell 1:949–957

Strumberg D, Pilon AA, Smith M et al (2000) Conversion of topoisomerase I cleavage complexes on the leading strand of ribosomal DNA into 5′-phosphorylated DNA double-strand breaks by replication runoff. Mol Cell Biol 20:3977–3987

Suh KS, Malik M, Shukla A et al (2007) CLIC4, skin homeostasis and cutaneous cancer: surprising connections. Mol Carcinog 46:599–604

Tait SW, Green DR (2010) Mitochondria and cell death: outer membrane permeabilization and beyond. Nat Rev Mol Cell Biol 11:621–632

Tanizawa A, Fujimori A, Fujimori Y et al (1994) Comparison of topoisomerase I inhibition, DNA damage, and cytotoxicity of camptothecin derivatives presently in clinical trials. J Natl Cancer Inst 86:836–842

Taylor RC, Cullen SP, Martin SJ (2008) Apoptosis: controlled demolition at the cellular level. Nat Rev Mol Cell Biol 9:231–241

Tazi J, Rossi F, Labourier E et al (1997) DNA topoisomerase I: customs officer at the border between DNA and RNA worlds? J Mol Med 75:786–800

Tewey KM, Chen GL, Nelson EM et al (1984) Intercalative antitumor drugs interfere with the breakage-reunion reaction of mammalian DNA topoisomerase II. J Biol Chem 259:9182–9187

Tinel A, Tschopp J (2004) The PIDDosome, a protein complex implicated in activation of caspase-2 in response to genotoxic stress. Science 304:843–846

Varfolomeev EE, Schuchmann M, Luria V et al (1998) Targeted disruption of the mouse Caspase 8 gene ablates cell death induction by the TNF receptors, Fas/Apo1, and DR3 and is lethal prenatally. Immunity 9:267–276

Vaux DL, Silke Jfrs (2003) Mammalian mitochondrial IAP binding proteins. Biochem Biophys Res Commun 304:499–504

Wang A, Rud J, Olson CM, Jr. et al (2009) Phosphorylation of Nur77 by the MEK-ERK-RSK cascade induces mitochondrial translocation and apoptosis in T cells. J Immunol 183:3268–3277

Wang JC (2002) Cellular roles of DNA topoisomerases: a molecular perspective. Nat Rev Mol Cell Biol 3:430–440

Wei MC, Lindsten T, Mootha VK et al (2000) tBID, a membrane-targeted death ligand, oligomerizes BAK to release cytochrome c. Genes Dev 14:2060–2071

Widlak P, Li P, Wang X et al (2000) Cleavage preferences of the apoptotic endonuclease DFF40 (caspase-activated DNase or nuclease) on naked DNA and chromatin substrates. J Biol Chem 275:8226–8232

Woronicz JD, Calnan B, Ngo V et al (1994) Requirement for the orphan steroid receptor Nur77 in apoptosis of T-cell hybridomas. Nature 367:277–281

Wu J, Liu LF (1997) Processing of topoisomerase I cleavable complexes into DNA damage by transcription. Nucleic Acids Res 25:4181–4186

Xue Y, Chomez P, Castanos-Velez E et al (1997) Positive and negative thymic selection in T cell receptor-transgenic mice correlate with Nur77 mRNA expression. Eur J Immunol 27:2048–2056

Yan N, Shi Y (2003) Histone H1.2 as a trigger for apoptosis. Nat Struct Biol 10:983–985

Yang G, Zhang G, Pittelkow MR et al (2006) Expression profiling of UVB response in melanocytes identifies a set of p53-target genes. J Invest Dermatol 126:2490–2506

Yeh WC, Pompa JL, McCurrach ME et al (1998) FADD: essential for embryo development and signaling from some, but not all, inducers of apoptosis. Science 279:1954–1958

Yin Y, Stephen CW, Luciani MG et al (2002) p53 Stability and activity is regulated by Mdm2-mediated induction of alternative p53 translation products. Nat Cell Biol 4:462–467

Yoshida K, Komatsu K, Wang HG et al (2002) c-Abl tyrosine kinase regulates the human Rad9 checkpoint protein in response to DNA damage. Mol Cell Biol 22:3292–3300

Yoshida K, Wang HG, Miki Y et al (2003) Protein kinase Cdelta is responsible for constitutive and DNA damage-induced phosphorylation of Rad9. Embo J 22:1431–1441

Zhang A, Lyu YL, Lin CP et al (2006) A protease pathway for the repair of topoisomerase II-DNA covalent complexes. J Biol Chem 281:35997–36003

Zhang XK (2007) Targeting Nur77 translocation. Expert Opin Ther Targets 11:69–79

Index

Y. Pommier (ed.), *DNA Topoisomerases and Cancer*, Cancer Drug Discovery and Development, DOI 10.1007/978-1-4614-0323-4,

Cancer Drug Discovery and Development

Series Editor

Beverly A. Teicher
Genyzme Corporation, Framingham, MA, USA

For further volumes:
http://www.springer.com/series/7625